Case-based Review in
Critical Care Medicine
A Comprehensive Preparatory Book for the Examinee

Case-based Review in Critical Care Medicine
A Comprehensive Preparatory Book for the Examinee

SECOND EDITION

Editors

Atul Prabhakar Kulkarni
MD (Anesthesiology) FISCCM PGDHHM FICCM
Professor and Head
Division of Critical Care Medicine
Department of Anesthesiology, Critical Care and Pain
Tata Memorial Hospital
Homi Bhabha National Institute
Mumbai, Maharashtra, India

Kapil Gangadhar Zirpe
MBBS MD (Chest) FICCM FCCM FSNCC
Head
Department of Neuro-Trauma Intensive Care Unit
Grant Medical Foundation
Ruby Hall Clinic
Pune, Maharashtra, India

Subhal Bhalchandra Dixit
MD (Medicine) FCCM FICCM FICP
Director
Department of Critical Care ICU
Sanjeevan and MJM Hospital
Pune, Maharashtra, India

Rahul Anil Pandit
MD FJFICM FCICM IFCCM EDIC DA
Chair
Department of Critical Care Medicine
Sir HN Reliance Foundation Hospital and all other
Reliance Foundation Healthcare Initiatives
Mumbai, Maharashtra, India

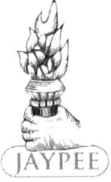

JAYPEE BROTHERS MEDICAL PUBLISHERS
The Health Sciences Publisher
New Delhi | London

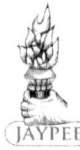

Jaypee Brothers Medical Publishers (P) Ltd.

Headquarters

Jaypee Brothers Medical Publishers (P) Ltd
EMCA House, 23/23-B
Ansari Road, Daryaganj
New Delhi 110 002, India
Landline: +91-11-23272143, +91-11-23272703
+91-11-23282021, +91-11-23245672
Email: jaypee@jaypeebrothers.com

Corporate Office

Jaypee Brothers Medical Publishers (P) Ltd
4838/24, Ansari Road, Daryaganj
New Delhi 110 002, India
Phone: +91-11-43574357
Fax: +91-11-43574314
Email: jaypee@jaypeebrothers.com

Overseas Office

JP Medical Ltd.
83, Victoria Street, London
SW1H 0HW (UK)
Phone: +44 20 3170 8910
Fax: +44 (0)20 3008 6180
Email: info@jpmedpub.com

Website: www.jaypeebrothers.com
Website: www.jaypeedigital.com

© 2024, Jaypee Brothers Medical Publishers

The views and opinions expressed in this book are solely those of the original contributor(s)/author(s) and do not necessarily represent those of editor(s) or publisher of the book.

All rights reserved. No part of this publication may be reproduced, stored or transmitted in any form or by any means, electronic, mechanical, photo copying, recording or otherwise, without the prior permission in writing of the publishers.

All brand names and product names used in this book are trade names, service marks, trademarks or registered trademarks of their respective owners. The publisher is not associated with any product or vendor mentioned in this book.

Medical knowledge and practice change constantly. This book is designed to provide accurate, authoritative information about the subject matter in question. However, readers are advised to check the most current information available on procedures included and check information from the manufacturer of each product to be administered, to verify the recommended dose, formula, method and duration of administration, adverse effects and contra indications. It is the responsibility of the practitioner to take all appropriate safety precautions. Neither the publisher nor the author(s)/editor(s) assume any liability for any injury and/or damage to persons or property arising from or related to use of material in this book.

This book is sold on the understanding that the publisher is not engaged in providing professional medical services. If such advice or services are required, the services of a competent medical professional should be sought.

Every effort has been made where necessary to contact holders of copyright to obtain permission to reproduce copyright material. If any have been inadvertently overlooked, the publisher will be pleased to make the necessary arrangements at the first opportunity.

Inquiries for bulk sales may be solicited at: jaypee@jaypeebrothers.com

Case-based Review in Critical Care Medicine: A Comprehensive Preparatory Book for the Examinee

First Edition: 2019

Second Edition: **2024**

ISBN: 978-93-5696-387-0

Dedicated to
*All the hardworking, caring and sincere residents
in the field of critical care medicine, with grounded feet and
stars in their eyes, who provide compassionate care to the critically ill.*

Contributors

Akshaya Ramaswami
MD (Emergency Medicine) DM 1st year Critical Care Medicine
Senior Registrar in Critical Care Medicine
Department of Anesthesia, Critical Care and Pain
Tata Memorial Hospital
Mumbai, Maharashtra, India

Amit Madhukar Narkhede MD DNB DM (Critical Care Medicine)
Specialist Senior Registrar
Division of Critical Care Medicine
Department of Anesthesiology, Critical Care and Pain
Tata Memorial Hospital, Homi Bhabha National Institute
Mumbai, Maharashtra, India

Anand M Tiwari
MBBS DA DNB (Anesthesiology) IDCCM FNB (Critical Care Medicine)
Chief Intensivist
Department of Critical Care
IMH, Pune, Maharashtra, India

Ashit Hegde MD MRCP
Consultant
Department of Medicine and Critical Care
PD Hinduja Hospital and Medical Research Centre
Mumbai, Maharashtra, India

Atul Prabhakar Kulkarni
MD (Anesthesiology) FISCCM PGDHHM FICCM
Professor and Head
Division of Critical Care Medicine
Department of Anesthesiology, Critical Care and Pain
Tata Memorial Hospital
Homi Bhabha National Institute
Mumbai, Maharashtra, India

Babu K Abraham
MD (General Medicine) MRCP (UK) FCCM (University of Toronto) FICCM
Senior Consultant
Department of Critical Care Medicine
Apollo Hospitals
Chennai, Tamil Nadu, India

Balkrishna D Nimavat
MD DNB (Anesthesiology) IDCCM FNB (Critical Care) EDIC EDAIC
Intensivist
Department of Critical Care
Apollo Hospitals
Navi Mumbai, Maharashtra, India

Bindu M MD IDCCM
Chief Intensivist
Department: Critical Care
Sir HN Reliance Foundation Hospital
Mumbai, Maharashtra, India

Binila Chacko MD DNB FCICM FICCM DM (Critical Care)
Professor and Head
Division of Critical Care
Medical Intensive Care Unit
Christian Medical College, Vellore
Medical ICU, CMC Hospital
Vellore, Tamil Nadu, India

Carol Shayne Dsilva
MD (Anesthesiology) FNB (Critical Care Medicine)
Assistant Professor
Department of Critical Care Medicine
St John's Medical College Hospital
Bengaluru, Karnataka, India

Deeksha Singh Tomar DA IDCCM IFCCM EDIC
Senior Consultant
Department of Critical Care Medicine
Narayana Superspeciality Hospital
Gurugram, Haryana, India

Deepak Govil MD EDIC FCCM
Vice Chairman
Department of Critical Care Medicine
Medanta—The Medicity
Gurugram, Haryana, India

Dilip R Karnad MD FACP FRCP (Glasgow)
Senior Consultant
Department of Critical Care Medicine
Jupiter Hospital
Thane, Maharashtra, India

Dinesh Ekambaram MD (Anesthesiology) IDCCM
Senior Consultant
Department of Anesthesia and Critical Care
Antrang Institute of Gastroenterology
Kolhapur, Maharashtra, India

Divya Pal MD IDCCM FNB
Consultant
Department of Critical Care Medicine
Medanta—The Medicity
Gurugram, Haryana, India

Contributors

Gautam Gondal MBBS MD (Pulmonary Medicine) DM
Critical Care Fellow
Department of Critical Care
Tata Memorial Hospital
Mumbai, Maharashtra, India

Harish Mallapura Maheshwarappa
MBBS MD DNB DM (Critical Care Medicine) IDCCM EDICM
Fellowship in Infectious Diseases MBA
Director
Institute of Critical Care Medicine
Department of Critical Care Medicine
Kauvery Hospitals
Bengaluru, Karnataka, India

Jacob George Pulinilkunnathil
MBBS MD DM DrNB IDCCM IFCCM EDIC FCCP
Medical Superintendent and Consultant
Department of Critical Care
Mar Sleeva Medicity Palai
Ettumanoor, Kerala, India

Jagdeep Sharma MBBS MD
Assistant Professor
Department of Anesthesia, Critical Care and Pain
Homi Bhabha Cancer Hospital and Research Centre
Chandigarh, India

Jigeeshu Vashisth Divatia MD FICCM FCCM
Professor and Head
Department of Anesthesiology, Critical Care and Pain
Tata Memorial Hospital
Mumbai, Maharashtra, India
Editor-in-Chief, Indian Journal of Anesthesia
Past President, Indian Society of Critical Care Medicine

Jitendra Choudhary MD (Anesthesia) IDCCM FNB (Critical Care) EDIC
Consultant
Department of Critical Care
Fortis Hospital
Mumbai, Maharashtra, India

JV Peter
MD DNB FRACP FJFICM FCICM FICCM FRCP (Edinburgh) FAMS MPhil
Professor
Department of Critical Care
Medical Intensive Care Unit
Christian Medical College
Vellore, Tamil Nadu, India

Kapil Gangadhar Zirpe MBBS MD (Chest) FICCM FCCM FSNCC
Head
Department of Neuro-Trauma Intensive Care Unit
Grant Medical Foundation
Ruby Hall Clinic
Pune, Maharashtra, India

Kapil Sharad Borawake MBBS DNB (Medicine) IDCCM
Director
Department of Medicine and ICU
Vishwaraj Hospital and Research Institute
Pune, Maharashtra, India

Keyur Shah MD (Medicine) DM (Critical Care Medicine)
Senior Resident
Department of Anesthesiology, Critical Care and Pain
Tata Memorial Hospital, Homi Bhabha National Institute
Mumbai, Maharashtra, India

Khalid Ismail Khatib MD (Medicine) FICCM FICP
Professor
Department of Medicine
SKN Medical College
Pune, Maharashtra, India

Kushal Rajeev Kalvit MD (Medicine) DM (Critical Care Medicine)
Assistant Professor
Department of Anesthesiology, Critical Care and Pain
Tata Memorial Hospital
Mumbai, Maharashtra, India

Lalita Gouri Mitra MBBS DA MD DNB FICCM
Professor and Officer In-charge
Department of Anesthesia, Critical Care and Pain
Homi Bhabha Cancer Hospital and Research Centre
Chandigarh, India

Meghena Mathew
DNB (Respiratory Medicine) IDCCM IFCCM EDIC EDRM
Consultant
Department of Critical Care and Pulmonology
Apollo First Med Hospitals
Chennai, Tamil Nadu, India

Natesh Prabu R
MD DNB (Anesthesiology) DM (Critical Care Medicine) EDIC
Assistant Professor
Department of Critical Care Medicine
St John's Medical College Hospital
Bengaluru, Karnataka, India

Naveen Salins MD PhD FRCP
Professor
Department of Palliative Medicine
Kasturba Medical College
Manipal Academy of Higher Education
Manipal, Karnataka, India

Niteen D Karnik MD FCPS
Professor and Head—Medical ICU
Department of General Medicine
LTM Medical College and General Hospital
Mumbai, Maharashtra, India

Pradnya Atul Kulkarni DPB
Blood Transfusion Officer
Department of Pathology
KJ Somaiya Medical College and Research Center
Mumbai, Maharashtra, India

Priyanshu D Shah MD
Assistant Professor
Department of General Medicine
Lokmanya Tilak Municipal Medical College and General Hospital
Mumbai, Maharashtra, India

Rahul Anil Pandit MD FJFICM FCICM IFCCM EDIC DA
Chair
Department of Critical Care Medicine
Sir HN Reliance Foundation Hospital and all other
Reliance Foundation Healthcare Initiatives
Mumbai, Maharashtra, India

Rakesh Mohanty
MD (Anesthesia) FAEM (CMC Vellore) MRCEM EDAIC EDIC
Senior Resident
Department of Anesthesia, Critical Care and Pain
Tata Memorial Hospital
Mumbai, Maharashtra, India

Raymond Dominic Savio MD DM EDIC FICCM
Lead Consultant
Critical Care Services
Apollo Proton Cancer Centre
Chennai, Tamil Nadu, India

Richa Narang MD (Anesthesia)
DrNB Resident
Department of Critical Care Medicine
Medanta—The Medicity
Gurugram, Haryana, India

Ruchira Wasudeo Khasne MBBS DA DNB IDCCM EDAIC EDIC
Consultant and Head
Department of Critical Care Medicine
SMBT Institute of Medical Sciences and Research Center
Nashik, Maharashtra, India

Rupak Banerjee MBBS CTCCM IDCCM EDIC
Clinical Associate
Department of Critical Care
Apollo Multispeciality Hospital
Kolkata, West Bengal, India

Sachin Gupta MD IDCCM IFCCM EDIC FCCM FICCM
Director
Department of Critical Care
Narayana Superspeciality Hospital
Gurugram, Haryana, India

Sheila Nainan Myatra MD FCCM FICCM
Professor
Department of Anesthesiology, Critical Care and Pain
Tata Memorial Hospital, Homi Bhabha National Institute
Mumbai, Maharashtra, India

Shilpushp Jagannath Bhosale
MD (Anesthesiology) DM (Critical Care Medicine)
Professor
Department of Anesthesiology, Critical Care and Pain
Tata Memorial Hospital, Homi Bhabha National Institute
Mumbai, Maharashtra, India

Srinivas Samavedam MD FRCP DNB FNB EDIC FICCM
Consultant Intensivist
Internal Medicine and Critical Care
TX Hospital
Hyderabad, Telangana, India

Subhal Bhalchandra Dixit MD (Medicine) FCCM FICCM FICP
Director
Department of Critical Care ICU
Sanjeevan and MJM Hospital
Pune, Maharashtra, India

Suhail Sarwar Siddiqui
MD Fellow (Critical Care) DM (Critical Care Medicine) EDIC
Associate Professor
Department of Critical Care Medicine
King George's Medical University
Lucknow, Uttar Pradesh, India

Suresh Ramasubban
AB (Internal Medicine, Pulmonary and Critical Care Medicine)
Director and Senior Consultant
Department of Critical Care
Apollo Multispeciality Hospitals
Kolkata, West Bengal, India

Syed Nabeel Muzaffar MD PDCC DM EDIC
Assistant Professor
Department of Critical Care Medicine
King George's Medical University
Lucknow, Uttar Pradesh, India

Vijaya Patil MBBS DA MD DHA
Professor and Head
Division of Anesthesiology
Department of Clinical Anesthesia, Critical Care and Pain
Tata Memorial Hospital, Homi Bhabha National Institute
Mumbai, Maharashtra, India

Preface to the Second Edition

न चौरहार्यं न च राजहार्यं न च भ्रातृभाज्यं न च भारकारि।
व्यये कृते वर्धत एव नित्यं विद्याधनं सर्वधनप्रधानम्।।3।।

It can neither be plundered by a thief, nor can be squeezed by the king, can be divided by brothers or not, and does not fall on consumption. The more the education is spent, the more it grows.

We are glad and feel highly privileged to present the second edition of the *Case-based Review in Critical Care Medicine: A Comprehensive Preparatory Book for the Examinee* to our strict, loving and the most discriminating critiques, the exam-going trainees. The first edition of the book was published in 2019, and almost immediately, we started getting enquiries, about the second edition.

The field of Medicine, and in particular Critical Care Medicine, is ever expanding, that too at a rapid pace. Yesterday's bright ideas become passé very quickly and new technologies are emerging. It is extremely hard to keep up with these fast-paced developments in a book. Therefore, this delay of almost 4 years. The first edition of this book seemed to fill an essential but glaringly vacant niche, in the plethora of books available in the specialty. We hope that it will continue to be popular with the students and this edition is liked as much as its predecessor was liked.

We have added a few more cases which we had missed and few suggested by the readers. We have tried to keep up with the latest evidence available at the time of writing. However, we are fully aware of that by the time this reaches you some more new studies will have been published. We hope that this book gives you a solid grounding in most the basics in clinical management and we know today's netizens are better than us at keeping abreast of the latest developments.

As we suggested in the last preface, please do not read only this book, except to brush up the cobwebs at the time of examination, otherwise continue reading your regular standard textbooks. We wish you all the very best for your examinations, and hope, in the future some of you will be contributing to the future editions of the book.

Atul Prabhakar Kulkarni
Kapil Gangadhar Zirpe
Subhal Bhalchandra Dixit
Rahul Anil Pandit

Preface to the First Edition

कामधेनुगुणा विद्या
ह्यकाले फलदायिनी।
प्रवासे मातृसदृशा
विद्या गुप्तं धनं स्मृतम्।।

(विद्या अर्जन करना यह एक कामधेनु के समान है जो हर मौसम में अमृत प्रदान करती है वह विदेश में माता के समान रक्षक एवं हितकारी होती है इसीलिए विद्या को एक गुप्त धन कहा जाता है)

There are two parents (as the nature dictates) to the idea of this book. The Department of Anesthesiology, Critical Care and Pain, Tata Memorial Hospital, Mumbai, Maharashtra, India, published a book, titled *Objective Anesthesia Review* for examinees in Anesthesiology, many years back (and newer editions are continuing). This book became hugely popular and became one of essential reading companion to all examinees. The second parent was a discussion amongst us; i.e., me, Rahul Anil Pandit, Subhal Bhalchandra Dixit, and Kapil Gangadhar Zirpe; regarding the lack of a concise book for the examinees in Critical Care Medicine.

There are many books in the field of Critical Care Medicine, some excellent, some very good and so on. None of them is specifically oriented towards helping the exam-going student, who is forced to read from multiple sources, just before the practical examination. This leads to haphazard study, making the stress levels increase even further. On top of all of this, they are expected to know the latest literature, which is ever changing and makes the life of the trainees more difficult. There are many review courses, but even there our boys and girls are made to work hard, to take down notes, and nowadays take snaps of the slides on their proud possession, the smartphone. This distracts them from understanding what is being discussed. Therefore this book! We have made an attempt to cover all the cases the examinee is likely to come across in most examinations, in the form of case vignettes. The book follows a question and answer format, as close to the real life as we can get, in the examination. The latest evidence is included in all answers throughout the book and the references quoted can be looked up for further information by examinees.

As a bonus, there are 100 OSCEs (The Objective Structured Clinical Examination) for practice in the book, which will be extremely helpful to all.

Does this mean the examinees should read only this book? Not at all, this book is a distilled essence of all that is there in the standard textbooks, which are a must read for all of us. There is added fragrance of updated knowledge and we can proudly say that these references are updated.

We wish that this book proves an enviable successor to its older brother, *Objective Anesthesia Review*, and helps you in your exit examinations. We wish you all the very best for your examinations, and hope, in future some of you will be contributing the book itself when we are writing the future editions of the book.

Atul Prabhakar Kulkarni
Kapil Gangadhar Zirpe
Subhal Bhalchandra Dixit
Rahul Anil Pandit

Acknowledgments

I wish to thank all my co-editors, in particular Dr Kapil Gangadhar Zirpe, and contributors from all over India, for their efforts in contributing the chapters to the first ever book published for the exam-going students in the field of critical care medicine. This book would not have been possible without their hard work, put in, in spite of their busy clinical schedule. I must acknowledge the fact that they have been amicable to me (and continue to be so) in spite of persistent, irritating pestering, throughout all the stages of the book being shaped.

We are lucky to have trainees in our department who in their quest of learning keep us on our toes. While doing this, we learn from them and also get to know what changes are needed in our books. Similar to the previous edition, when Jacob George Pulinilkunnathil, Ruchira Wasudeo Khasne, Suhail Sarwar Siddiqui, Harish Mallapura Maheshwarappa and others, for this edition, Kushal Rajeev Kalvit, Rakesh Mohanty, and others gave valuable inputs. Many students who read the previous editions also suggested changes and corrections. I hope this edition will be better because of them. Therefore, a request to all readers to be critical of the presentation and suggest changes for the next edition.

I would also like to extend our appreciation to Shri Jitendar P Vij (Group Chairman), Mr Ankit Vij (Managing Director), Mr MS Mani (Group President), Ms Chetna Malhotra (Senior Director—Professional Publishing, Marketing, and Business Development), Ms Pooja Bhandari (Director-Production), Ms Manpreet Kaur (Development Editor), and all the staff of M/s Jaypee Brothers Medical Publishers (P) Ltd, New Delhi, India, for their efforts and input enabling timely publication of the book.

Atul Prabhakar Kulkarni

Contents

1. **How to Examine an ICU Patient in the Examination?**..........1
   Rahul Anil Pandit, Atul Prabhakar Kulkarni

2. **Community-acquired Pneumonia**..........6
   Ruchira Wasudeo Khasne, Atul Prabhakar Kulkarni

3. **Liberation from Mechanical Ventilation, Ventilator-associated Pneumonia, and ICU-acquired Weakness**....25
   Jacob George Pulinilkunnathil, Vijaya Patil

4. **Acute Exacerbation of Chronic Obstructive Pulmonary Disease**..........41
   Gautam Gondal, Jacob George Pulinilkunnathil, Kapil Gangadhar Zirpe, Atul Prabhakar Kulkarni

5. **Acute Severe Asthma**..........60
   Babu K Abraham, Meghena Mathew

6. **Pulmonary Embolism**..........70
   Jacob George Pulinilkunnathil, Shilpushp Jagannath Bhosale, Atul Prabhakar Kulkarni

7. **Acute Respiratory Distress Syndrome**..........86
   Jigeeshu Vashisth Divatia, Kushal Rajeev Kalvit

8. **Approach to Tropical Infections in the ICU**..........109
   Ashit Hegde

9. **Sepsis and Septic Shock**..........117
   Divya Pal, Deepak Govil

10. **Acute Coronary Syndrome**..........141
    Kushal Rajeev Kalvit, Akshaya Ramaswami, Atul Prabhakar Kulkarni

11. **Eclampsia and Cerebral Venous Thrombosis**..........146
    Dilip R Karnad

12. **Subarachnoid Hemorrhage**..........156
    Suresh Ramasubban, Rupak Banerjee

13. **Acute Ischemic Stroke**..........174
    Keyur Shah, Kapil Gangadhar Zirpe, Atul Prabhakar Kulkarni

14. **Spontaneous Intracerebral Hemorrhage**..........189
    Keyur Shah, Atul Prabhakar Kulkarni

15. **Meningoencephalitis and Status Epilepticus**..........197
    Kushal Rajeev Kalvit, Atul Prabhakar Kulkarni

16. **Traumatic Brain Injury**..........204
    Rakesh Mohanty, Amit Madhukar Narkhede, Kapil Sharad Borawake, Kapil Gangadhar Zirpe

17. **Polytrauma**..........215
    Jacob George Pulinilkunnathil, Balkrishna D Nimavat, Pradnya Atul Kulkarni, Atul Prabhakar Kulkarni, Kapil Gangadhar Zirpe

18. **Snake and Scorpion Bites**..........234
    Niteen D Karnik, Priyanshu D Shah

19. **Infective Endocarditis** 243
    Sachin Gupta, Deeksha Singh Tomar

20. **Acute Aortic Emergencies** 252
    Khalid Ismail Khatib

21. **Hyponatremia** 255
    Harish Mallapura Maheshwarappa, Richa Narang

22. **Guillain–Barré Syndrome** 271
    Jitendra Choudhary, Rahul Anil Pandit

23. **Approach to a Patient with Unknown Poisoning** 277
    Bindu M, Rahul Anil Pandit

24. **Organophosphorus Poisoning** 282
    JV Peter, Binila Chacko

25. **Acute Kidney Injury** 289
    Srinivas Samavedam

26. **Upper Gastrointestinal Bleeding** 293
    Lalita Gouri Mitra, Jagdeep Sharma, Atul Prabhakar Kulkarni

27. **Oncologic Emergencies** 307
    Suhail Sarwar Siddiqui, Syed Nabeel Muzaffar, Atul Prabhakar Kulkarni

28. **Acute Heart Failure and Cardiogenic Shock** 330
    Kushal Rajeev Kalvit, Atul Prabhakar Kulkarni

29. **Severe Acute Pancreatitis** 334
    Subhal Bhalchandra Dixit, Khalid Ismail Khatib

30. **Acute Liver Failure** 339
    Dinesh Ekambaram, Raymond Dominic Savio

31. **Diabetic Ketoacidosis** 354
    Natesh Prabu R, Carol Shayne D Silva, Atul Prabhakar Kulkarni

32. **Out-of-Hospital Cardiac Arrest, Brain Death, and Organ Donation** 367
    Anand M Tiwari, Kapil Gangadhar Zirpe

33. **End-of-life Care in Intensive Care Unit** 374
    Sheila Nainan Myatra, Suhail Sarwar Siddiqui, Naveen Salins

34. **Tips and Tricks for the Table Viva Voce** 380
    Khalid Ismail Khatib, Subhal Bhalchandra Dixit, Rahul Anil Pandit, Atul Prabhakar Kulkarni

Index *383*

CHAPTER 1

How to Examine an ICU Patient in the Examination?

Rahul Anil Pandit, Atul Prabhakar Kulkarni

INTRODUCTION

Intensive care patients are very complex and sick. They also have a confusing array of monitoring and tubes attached that can change in a very short span of time.

The key to clinical examination of intensive care unit (ICU) patient lies in integrating the information available from the medical technology and correlate it with patient's clinical findings and arrive at diagnosis and treatment plan.

A large amount of information is available at bedside, in order to assimilate all this, it is important to have a structured approach toward examination of patient. Following approach would be one of the ways toward a structured examination.

SYSTEM-BASED APPROACH

- *Airway:* Tube type, size, and position (at which fixed)
- *Breathing:* Lungs, ventilation, and oxygen delivery systems
- *Circulation:* Heart, vascular devices, and cardiovascular drugs
- *Disability:* Central and peripheral neurological examination, pain, and sedation
- Exposure
- *Fluids:* Status, balance, and management
- *Gastrointestinal (GI):* Abdominal examination, nutritional examination, and renal examination
- Examination of the peripheries.

APPROACH TOWARD CLINICAL EXAMINATION OF THE PATIENT

When one approaches the patient, it is very important to adhere to infection control policies of that ICU. Handwashing practice is imperative, either with alcohol-based rub or soap and water. Some ICUs insist on gowns and gloves for all patients or for contact isolation only. If any respiratory infection precaution is to be taken then it must be strictly adhered to.

The initial urge to approach the patient straight away should be curbed. Take a step back and have a good look at the patient and the patient's surroundings in the cubical. There is a lot of information which one could gain just by been observant. It is most important to know that this information once missed is likely to stay missed and not picked up. This may result on one missing the broad focus of the examination. Sometimes a lead question may be asked as an introduction toward clinical examination. It is important to focus on this lead question when one is approaching clinical examination.

Look at the patient, his position in bed, and for any sign of pain, discomfort, and distress. Observe the tubes that are attached such as drains, urine, and color of drains. Look at the monitors, ventilator settings, and the infusion or syringe pumps. Ask relevant questions, if permitted, e.g., dilution of vasopressors, or type of nasogastric feed that is being administered.

Ensure patient privacy, by drawing up curtains. Lower the bed and bed railings to an appropriate height so that you are comfortable. Expose the patient completely for a thorough examination, taking care that private body parts are shielded with bed sheet or towels. Please introduce yourself and any other observers to the patient. Be polite and ask their permission to examine them if the patient is awake. "Hello Sir/Madam, I am Dr, I would like to examine you, are you OK with that? Warn them if you are going to use a stethoscope (often cold due to AC in the ICU), "Sir this might feel a bit cold". Alternatively, you can warm the diaphragm of the stethoscope by rubbing against the back of your hand (after handwashing of course). Similarly, also ask their permission if you are going to expose them, "Sir, I need to see your chest or abdomen, and I need to remove your clothes. May I do that?" Make sure a female nurse or doctor is present when you examine a female patient, particularly if you are going to expose her body. Always draw the curtains of the cubicle closed. A similar warning needs to be given if you are going to perform an ultrasonographic examination, please tell the patient that you are going to use cold and sticky jelly. Make sure you clean the probe with Clinisept® or other antiseptic solution (nonalcohol-based, so as to not damage the probe), and the patient's body part has to be wiped with tissue to clean the jelly after the ultrasonography (USG).

Ask them to perform some simple task like opening the mouth. This will immediately give you an idea about the patient's condition, especially the neurology, while observing the surroundings you would have definitely checked whether sedation is being administered. Inform them about your plan to examine.

Airway

After introduction, assess if the patient is capable of maintaining his airway or not. Examine the airway of the patient: Intubated or not intubated? Is the patient on noninvasive ventilation? A simple way to assess that is to check neurological status, pattern and rate of respiration, and clearance of secretions.

If patient has an endotracheal tube in place then, look at the size of tube, smaller size tubes often pose difficulty in suctioning and weaning process. Look at the position of endotracheal tube at angle of mouth and compare it with the insertion position recorded in the chart. Assess the cuff pressure; it should be <30 cmH$_2$O. Assess the ties of the tube; make sure they are not too tight or loose. Some patients may have a tracheostomy in place. Quite frequently, it is inserted for comfort and weaning. However, sometimes it may be inserted for anatomical or pathological reasons. In such case understand the reason for insertion of tracheostomy. Complete a cuff and tie check for tracheostomy as well. Look for the skin at the insertion site.

Breathing

Start the analysis of respiratory system with *observation:*
- Paradoxical breathing
- Unequal rise of hemithorax with inspiration
- Work of breathing
- Rate of breathing.

Respiratory distress may present with following signs:
- Sweating
- Tachycardia
- Agitation
- *Patient ventilator dyssynchrony:* Often obvious to people who possess the knowledge about it, however, the incidence is fairly common. Unfortunately the most common response to ventilatory dyssynchrony is often sedation, which in some cases may be an inappropriate response.

Look at any chest drains that may be present, observe any bubbling, swinging of column, and color of drain fluid.

Study the ventilator:
- Look at settings—note, if patient is breathing spontaneously, or on a controlled mode.
- Study the fraction of inspired oxygen (FiO$_2$), positive end-expiratory pressure (PEEP), mode and other settings on the ventilator.
- Look at the ventilator graphs, loops, and understand the resistance and compliance of the lung.
- A detailed look at the history of these graphics will give important information of the respiratory mechanics over time.
- Special tests such as compliance, plateau pressure, and intrinsic PEEP (iPEEP) may be estimated to have a better understanding of patient's current respiratory status.

Oxygenation
- Observe the saturation on monitor and try to correlate it with FiO$_2$ and PEEP settings.
- If available, now is the time to look at the arterial blood gas for pH, partial pressure of oxygen (PaO$_2$), partial pressure of carbon dioxide (PaCO$_2$), and bicarbonate.

Palpation and Percussion
- In critically ill ICU patients, both palpation and percussion may be unhelpful in providing you good clinical information.
- Specifically, if you are wearing gloves, percussion is often difficult to elicit.
- However, if the patient is not ventilated then it is an important tool to complete your respiratory system examination.
- Examine the trachea and determine if it is in center.
- Palpate both sides of the chest and see if the respiratory mechanics are equal.

Auscultation
- Auscultate both the lungs fields completely.
- Quite often this may be challenging, due to presence of dressings, positioning of patients, etc.
- Rolling patients on one side or in awake patients sitting them up will allow a complete auscultation on the back as well.
- Hear the breath sounds, compare if they are equal on both sides.
- Any rhonchi, crepitation, or abnormal breath sounds are important findings.

Secretions
- Look at the quantity, consistency, and color of secretions.
- Observe the chart to look at the secretions history.

- A trend is often helpful to determine a decision for extubation, decannulation, or development or progress of a new respiratory problem.

Other
- If patient is awake, then try and assess the patient's ability to cough. Look at the strength and force of cough.
- Ask patient to take a big breathe in and out to determine the forced vital capacity (FVC). Usually if a patient is able to generate >15 mL/kg of tidal volume on minimal ventilator settings then they should be able to breathe comfortably postextubation as well.
- If possible and available and if you know how and permitted by examiner you should try to do USG of the lungs. If you do not know how, keep your trap shut!

Circulation

Observation
- Start with a look at the monitor.
- Note the heart rate and blood pressure on the monitor.
- Is the rhythm paced, are there arrhythmias on the monitor?
- Look at the blood pressure, importantly the mean arterial pressure. It is more importantly physiologically.
- If any other indices such as central venous pressure (CVP) and stroke volume variation (SVV) are being monitored, then study them, note them down, and check the trend, if available.
- A very high or low CVP would be of significance. Similarly, SVV and cardiac index assessment will give details about the patient's volume and hemodynamic status.

Palpation
- Start with peripheral circulation.
- Temperature of the hands and legs, if cold, note up to what level the extremities are cold, ankle, knees, thighs, etc.
- Check that there is no difference in temperature of limbs on either side.
- Check the color of the periphery, note down capillary refill time.
- Check for peripheral pulses.
- Feel for and observe pulsations over the precordium and any other abnormal pulsations elsewhere.

Percussion
Limited utility in circulatory system examination in the critically ill patient.

Auscultation
- Carefully listen to the heart sounds.
- This may be challenging specifically due to distracting noises and sounds in ICU.

Other
- Other features of circulatory adequacy are mentation in absence of sedation, urine output, and the acid–base balance, importantly lactate level.
- If permitted, available, and if you know how, try to perform a transthoracic echocardiography. Otherwise keep your mouth shut about this too!

Interpretation
- All this needs to be interpreted in the context of several variables.
- Vasoactive drugs
- Inotropes
- Intra-aortic balloon pump
- Cardiac medications
- Fluid balance

Fluid Balance
- It is important to look at the fluid balance. Especially the cumulative fluid balance and daily weight of patient, if it is possible or the input and output chart.
- Skin turgor, peripheral edema, raised jugular venous pressure (JVP), or CVP are other coarse methods for assessing fluid status.

Devices
- Always look at the site of intravascular devices.
- Look for signs of infection, thrombosis or ischemia.

Neurological System

Important Considerations
- Level of sedation, pain relief with opioids or analogs, and use of muscle relaxants (sometimes).
- This needs to be considered before embarking on a neurological examination.

Examination
- Start with trying to elicit some response with verbal commands.
- If no response then a gradual graded painful stimulus starting from periphery to central would be necessary to give a good understanding of Glasgow Coma Scale (GCS). Calculate the GCS score for components and total score and note it down.
- If patient is responsive then ask them to perform simple tasks, assess their limb muscle tone and power.

- Spend some time eliciting deep tendon reflexes and plantar response.
- Pupillary examination, looking for size, response to light is important.
- Look at signs which suggest lateralizing signs. This will help in assessing the complete neurological system.
- Look at any neuromonitoring devices, such as intracranial pressure monitors or operative wounds incisions (fresh) and scars (old).
- Look at the chart and compare your neurological findings to those noted before, this will give an objective assessment of the further course.

Abdominal, Renal, and Nutrition

As opposed to the cardiovascular and respiratory system a continuous monitoring of GI and renal system is not possible. However, pathologies may be hidden and could be difficult to assess. Hence a careful examination of the abdomen is absolutely necessary.

Observation

- Observe the general shape and respiratory movements of the abdomen.
- Look for any distension, presence of surgical wounds, scars, drains, stoma, and their contents.
- Look for Foley's catheter and in male patients always look for any signs of phimosis.

Palpation

- Make the patient fully supine.
- Carefully palpate the abdomen, looking for any organomegaly.
- Watch for any signs of pain or distress during palpation.
- Note if patient is on pain medication or has received muscle relaxant.

Percussion

- Percussion in ICU patients may help determine the presence of ascites.
- Otherwise percussion is of limited clinical benefit.

Auscultation

Hear carefully for presence or absence of bowel sounds, note if they are abnormally high pitched and increased.

Sometimes the intra-abdominal pressure may be an important marker to measure. It is best measured using a three-way Foley, or special intra-abdominal measuring kits. Remember to note that an absolute value and trend both are important in decision making. Check if it is being measured, not the value and trend of available.

Nutrition

- Look if the patient is being fed by the nasogastric, nasojejunal, or by percutaneous gastrostomy or jejunostomy route. Ask and note if the feeds are given as continuous drip or by bolus method.
- Note the type of feeds, volume, and rate at which it is delivered.
- It is important to ask for gastric residual volumes which tell a lot about feed absorption.
- If patient is not being fed then look at nasogastric aspirates, study the trend and the aspirates.
- Ask for bowel movements, as diarrhea and constipation, both are common in ICU patients.
- Always look for any evidence of GI bleed in the form of altered blood in nasogastric tube or melena.

Exposure and Periphery

- Look for any rashes, eschar, ecchymosis, petechiae, blebs, etc., all over the body. If present, check for any anatomical distribution.
- Relevant history and bite marks are necessary to be ruled out.
- Note the type, feel, and location of rash.
- Some rashes are specific, e.g., malar rash is seen over the face.
- Observe for any ulcers or sore in the pressure areas.
- Specific spots, such as heels, sacrum, and back should be examined meticulously.
- Look for any peripheral signs which may be relevant in the clinical examination such as presence of clubbing, cyanosis, icterus, or presence of lymphadenopathy.
- Try and correlate these signs with your clinical examination to arrive at a conclusion.

Documentation

It is important to note down the relevant history points and document positive findings in your examination. *Do not rely on memory; write it down for later reference* during viva. Always look at the ICU monitoring chart, this gives a wealth of information on trends, medications, and how the patient has progressed.

Always review the blood investigations, it is important to review them in a tabular form if possible to understand the trends. Special investigations such as echocardiography, computed tomography (CT) scan or magnetic resonance imaging (MRI) should be reviewed and reports seen wherever relevant. Always review the X-ray of chest; airway, breathing, and circulation (ABG); and electrocardiograph (ECG) of patient.

Review the medication chart and look at specific medications, such as antibiotics, cardiac medicines, and their dosages. If trade names are written which are unfamiliar to you, ask for the actual name of the drug.

Housekeeping

Fast hug has become a standard for ICU practitioners. A number of variants have been developed and in other units you will hear some of them. Here is an example of what they cover:

F—feeding
Ensuring the patient is appropriately fed is an important care issue. We will deal with this in more detail in a subsequent module, but suffice to say that you should at least consider the need for feeding for each patient.

F is also sometimes used for feces management and fluids.

A—analgesia
Check if the patient is formally assessed for their level of pain and note their current analgesia regimen. Perhaps there are other agents you could consider, or even a regional pain solution such as an epidural might help.

S—sedation
Sedation is an important component of ICU care, because it enables patients to tolerate some of the more uncomfortable treatments they require (e.g., mechanical ventilation). In the past, clinicians have taken a "if little bit is good, more must be better" approach. Try to note the sedation and delirium score of the patient, if written. If not assess with the score you are familiar with and note the score.

However, it is also important to remember that most therapies also have complications, and so it is true for sedatives. Increasingly, we are becoming aware of the risks of over sedation, including prolongation of mechanical ventilation, and there is evidence that reducing it to the minimum level required results in better outcomes for patients.

T—thromboprophylaxis
All patients in the ICU should be considered high risk for the development of deep venous thrombosis (DVT). In fact, in a sentinel paper of mechanically ventilated patients in ICU, up to 2.7% *already had* significant proximal leg DVT on admission! The need for chemical and physical thromboprophylaxis should be considered on a daily basis, and the risks versus benefits carefully analyzed.

H—head up to 30°
It may sound a little strange, but such a simple maneuver (45% head up) can reduce the risk of hospital-acquired pneumonia, an important ICU complication. Unless there is a good reason not to, all ventilated patients should be nursed with their head and torso at 30° from the horizontal.

U—ulcer prophylaxis
There are a number of factors common in ICU patients that predispose them to developing gastric stress ulcers, with the consequent potential for GI bleeding. Consider the need for prophylaxis, something we will come back to in a later module.

G—glucose control
Hyperglycemia has been associated with a higher risk of complications for ICU patients. In fact, this has been associated with worse outcomes in many other patient groups too, such as acute myocardial infarction and stroke. For a while, very tight glycemic control was advocated in ICU patients. However, subsequent research has suggested that tight control is no better than standard range targets, and may even worsen outcome, possibly due to hypoglycemic episodes. You should check your unit's policy on this and ensure it is followed.

Check the patient's blood sugar level, if recorded, look at trend and see if the patient is on insulin infusion.

Final Thoughts

Always complete your examination by thanking the patient and leaving the bedside as neat and clean as possible. Postexamination handwashing is compulsory.

Try and formulate a problem list, separate the problems which are active and inactive. Formulate a treatment plan or investigation plan as per the priority of problem, e.g., if oxygenation or hypotension is the problem then it needs to be addressed with priority over other non-life-threatening problems.

Remember there are no trick questions in an examination. Usually the lead question is formulated by the examiner with intent to lead the candidate to a problem.

Enjoy your work in ICU so you are happy in your chosen life work; remember there are no shortcuts to success.

All the best for your examinations!!!

If your examination going soon, we *do not* wish to see you again next year as a delegate!!!

FURTHER READING

1. Cook DJ, Crowther M, Meade M, Rabbat C, Schiff D, Geerts W, et al. Deep venous thrombosis in medical-surgical ICU patients: prevalence, incidence and risk factors. Crit Care Med. 2005;33:1565-71.
2. Drakulovic MB, Torres A, Bauer TT, Nicolas JM, Nogué S, Ferrer M. Supine body position as a risk factor for nosocomial pneumonia in mechanically ventilated patients: a randomised trial. Lancet. 1999;354(9193):1851-8.
3. Robertson L. Recognizing the critically ill patient. Anesth Int Care Med. 2013;14(1):11-4.
4. Vincent JL. Give your patient a fast hug (at least) once a day. Crit Care Med. 2005;33(6):1225-9.

CHAPTER 2

Community-acquired Pneumonia

Ruchira Wasudeo Khasne, Atul Prabhakar Kulkarni

■ CASE STUDY

A 36-year-old male, with no comorbidities, presented to emergency room (ER) with fever, body ache, cough with expectoration for 5 days, and progressive increase in shortness of breath for 2 days.

On examination, he was confused, dyspneic, febrile (temperature of 101°F), tachycardic (pulse rate 120 beats/min, regular), and hypotensive (BP 70 mm Hg systolic). He was tachypneic [respiratory rate (RR) 35 breaths/min] and his saturation on pulse oximetry was 90% on rebreathing mask with 15 L/min O_2.

On systemic examination, crepitations and bronchial breathing were heard in the lower part of right side of chest. Rest of the examination was unremarkable. X-ray of chest was suggestive of right lower lobe pneumonia.

Q1. Define community-acquired pneumonia (CAP).

Pneumonia is defined as inflammation and consolidation of lung tissue due to infectious agents. Pneumonia, which develops outside the hospital, is considered as CAP.[1] Severe CAP (sCAP) is accepted terminology used to describe intensive care unit (ICU)-admitted patients with CAP as they might require organ support as per European Respiratory Society/European Society of Intensive Care Medicine/European Society of Clinical Microbiology and Infectious Diseases/Latin American Thoracic Association (ERS/ESICM/ESCMID/ALAT) guidelines (ESICM Task force) for the management of severe CAP.[2] CAP has always been a clinical diagnosis, combining features of an acute respiratory infection, and new infiltrates with or without pleural effusion on chest radiograph (CXR).

Q2. What are the differential diagnoses of CAP?

The differential diagnoses of CAP are described in **Table 1**.

Q3. What are the clinical features of CAP?

Clinically, pneumonia is defined as presence of two or more of the following signs and symptoms—productive cough, purulent sputum, dyspnea or tachypnea (RR > 20 breaths/min), fever, chills and rigors, and pleuritic chest pain in conjunction with a new opacity on CXR. Some patients may be hypothermic and this may indicate poor prognosis.[1] It may be associated with nonrespiratory symptoms such as headache, altered sensorium, seizure, nausea, vomiting, abdominal pain, diarrhea, myalgia, and arthralgia. Sometimes, extrapulmonary signs and symptoms may dominate the clinical picture, e.g., encephalitis, meningitis, cranial nerve palsies (e.g., especially with *Mycoplasma pneumoniae* infection), glomerulonephritis, and cerebellar ataxia (e.g., with *Legionella* pneumonia infection). Periodontal disease with foul-smelling sputum can be seen in anaerobic infections. Bacteremia due to *Staphylococcus aureus* and *Streptococcus pneumoniae* can lead to metastatic manifestations such as endocarditis, brain abscess, and meningitis.

Q4. How does the clinical presentation of CAP differ in the elderly patients?

This group may present in a subtler way. They often present with nonrespiratory symptoms such as delirium/acute confusional status, fatigue, lethargy, decreased appetite, and urinary incontinence. Generally, these patients do not cough or produce sputum, do not show rise in white blood counts, and may be afebrile at times. They may present with worsening of a preexisting conditions such as chronic cardiopulmonary diseases or metabolic disorders such as diabetes mellitus. Even radiological diagnosis is often difficult in this group when it is associated with chronic lung disease and if the etiology is of noninfectious origin. Causative agents in elderly patients are similar to those in the younger patients. Besides that, polymicrobial infections and aspirational pneumonia are more frequent.[3]

A trial of bilevel positive airway pressure (BiPAP) [fraction of inspired oxygen (FiO_2): 1.0, inspiratory positive airway pressure (IPAP): 14 cmH_2O, and expiratory positive airway pressure (EPAP): 6 cmH_2O] was given. The arterial blood gas (ABG) showed: pH 7.34, partial pressure of carbon dioxide

TABLE 1: Differential diagnoses of CAP.

	Clinical presentation	Diagnostic test
Respiratory conditions		
Acute bronchitis	Often related to viral upper respiratory tract infection, no wheeze, and no rales	CXR often normal
Acute exacerbation of COPD	Smokers or past smokers, increase in amount of sputum, change in color of sputum, and worsening of cough and dyspnea and wheeze	CXR reveals hyperinflated lung fields, flattened diaphragm with or without infiltrates
Acute exacerbation of asthma	Frequent attacks of dyspnea with bronchospasm, often at night in a known case of allergic asthma, frequent seasonal variations, markedly improvement after the inhalation of a bronchodilator drug, and inhaled steroids	CXR often normal
Acute exacerbation of bronchiectasis	Recurrent infection associated with fever, worsening dyspnea, increased expectoration with purulent sputum, bronchorrhea, and hemoptysis	• CXR suggestive of underlying bronchiectatic changes • HRCT is confirmatory
Aspiration pneumonitis	Seen in patients with reduced level of consciousness with poor cough reflex	CXR shows new infiltrates
Pulmonary embolus or infarction	• Sudden onset of dyspnea, hypoxia, sometimes pleuritic pain, hemoptysis, and syncope (after exclusion of other etiologies) • There is often evidence of a deep venous thrombosis, hypercoagulable condition	• CXR usually normal, abnormal V/Q scan • 2D echo often shows RV dysfunction • CT pulmonary angiogram is gold standard
Interstitial lung disease	• Gradual onset of breathlessness and nonproductive cough • Velcro rales at the bases	• CXR shows interstitial shadows with loss of lung volume • PFT s/o restrictive lung disease • HRCT is diagnostic
Hypersensitivity pneumonitis	Exposure to allergens in sensitized patients, postexposure fever, rigors, and dyspnea	• Positive serum precipitins, serum IgE levels • CXR shows bilateral nodular shadows, hilar lymphadenopathy • HRCT
Pulmonary manifestation of connective tissue disorders	Signs and symptoms similar to ILD with history of underlying collagen vascular disease	• ANA blot test • HRCT
Bronchogenic carcinomas	Smoking is major risk factor. Constitutional symptoms with loss of appetite and loss of weight, hemoptysis	CXR consolidation with cavitation, calcification with or without hilar lymph nodes, and pleural effusion
Radiation pneumonitis	History of radiotherapy	Abnormal CXR
Cardiovascular conditions		
Congestive heart failure	PND followed by orthopnea, with signs of fluid retention. Distention of the neck veins, pedal edema, and cardiomegaly	• Abnormal ECG • 2D echo showing cardiac dysfunction • CXR shows cardiomegaly with bilateral perihilar "batwing" appearance
Acute pulmonary edema	Acute onset of dyspnea, pink frothy sputum, and PND	CXR shows signs of pulmonary edema

(ANA: antinuclear antibody; CAP: community-acquired pneumonia; COPD: chronic obstructive pulmonary disease; CXR: chest radiograph; ECG: electrocardiogram; HRCT: high-resolution computed tomography; IgE: immunoglobulin E; ILD: interstitial lung disease; PFT: pulmonary function test; PND: paroxysmal nocturnal dyspnea)

(pCO_2) 39 mm Hg, partial pressure of oxygen (pO_2) 88.1 mm Hg, HCO_3 23.9 mmol/L, base excess (BE) 2.0 mmol/L, and anion gap (AG) 7.6. After 2 hours of ICU admission, patient was intubated due to continued respiratory distress. Rapid sequence intubation was performed and positive pressure ventilation was commenced.

Q5. What is the current evidence for use of noninvasive ventilation (NIV) and high-flow nasal cannula (HFNC) in management of CAP?

Trial of noninvasive mechanical ventilation (NIV) may be given, with strict and vigilant monitoring, in those who do not require immediate intubation. This may result in lesser need for intubation and better survival. As per ESICM task force[2] for sCAP with acute hypoxemic respiratory failure not needing immediate intubation *suggested use* of HFNC instead of conventional oxygen therapy. But it is a conditional recommendation with very low quality of evidence. NIV might be an option in certain patients with persistent hypoxemic respiratory failure not needing immediate intubation, irrespective of high-flow nasal oxygen (HFNO) (conditional recommendation and low quality of evidence). Early identification of failure of NIV is important, as several trials showed that prolonged NIV before intubation are associated with poor outcome.[4] The precise role of HFNC in the management and prevention of hypoxia is controversial. HFNC can deliver heated and humidified 100% O_2 at a flow rate of up to 60 L/min. It works in various ways as follows:

- Ability to deliver up to 100% O_2 with high-flow ensuring constant oxygen delivery and reduced nasopharyngeal dead space.
- Decreases CO_2 rebreathing and provides O_2 reservoir thus, decreasing work of breathing.
- Prevents supraglottic collapse and decreases nasopharyngeal resistance that creates continuous positive airway pressure (CPAP) effect.
- Prevents drying of nasal mucosa and enhances mucociliary clearance.

High-flow nasal cannula seems more effective than conventional oxygen therapy and is noninferior to NIV. In low-risk hypoxemic patients, HFNC prevents intubation compared to conventional oxygen therapy. The FLORALI study compared HFNC, standard facemask or NIV in patients with acute hypoxemic respiratory failure without hypercapnia. There was no difference in need for intubation in all groups but there was a significant difference in favor of HFNC in terms of 90-day mortality.[5] However, a recent meta-analysis showed that HFNC is well tolerated but there was no difference in intubation or mortality compared to usual care. The precise role of HFNC in this setting is controversial. Further, large randomized controlled trials (RCTs) are required to assess its utility.[6]

Q6. What are the risk factors for the development of CAP?

The risk factors for the development of CAP are given in **Table 2**.

Apart from abovementioned risk factors, individuals with genetic variability are predisposed to the development of pneumonia, e.g., toll-like receptor 6 (TLR6) polymorphism is associated with increased risk of Legionnaires' disease.[7]

TABLE 2: Risk factors for the development of CAP.[12,13]

Immunocompetent patients at risk	
Patient status	• >65 years • Male sex • Malnourished • Dense urbanization • Poor functional status • Genetic variability
Lifestyle	• Smoking and alcoholism
Environmental	• House overcrowding and poor ventilation • Socioeconomic status • Contact with children • Indoor and outdoor pollutions
Comorbidities	• Previous pneumonia • Chronic respiratory disease • COPD • Obstructive sleep apnea • Asthma • Chronic heart disease • Heart failure • Diabetes mellitus • Cerebrovascular disease/stroke • Diabetes • Immunosuppression • Dementia • Cancer • Chronic liver disease • Chronic renal disease
Medications	• Proton pump inhibitors • Benzodiazepines • Inhaled steroids
Other	• Aspiration • Acid suppressing agents, steroids, and immunosuppressants
Immunocompromised patients at risk	
Immunosuppression	• Patients with autoimmune diseases receiving steroids or immunosuppressive therapy or biological therapy • Cancer with immunosuppressive treatment • Waiting list for solid-organ transplantation (with or without immunosuppressive treatment) • Other immunosuppression
Immunocompromised	• Asplenia/splenic dysfunction • Primary immunodeficiencies
HIV	–

(CAP: community-acquired pneumonia; COPD: chronic obstructive pulmonary disease; HIV: human immunodeficiency virus)

Specific variants of the *FER* gene are associated with a reduced risk of death in patients with sepsis due to pneumonia.[8]

Q7. What are the objective criteria for judging severity of CAP?
Objective criteria like pneumonia severity index (PSI) [confusion, urea, RR, blood pressure, and age >65 years (CURB-65)] can help the physician to stratify the patients **(Table 3)** for management. These criteria can supplement clinical judgment but cannot replace it. CURB-65 is used when blood test results are available and CRB-65 is used when blood tests are not readily available. PSI is used to predict 30-day mortality. American Thoracic Society (ATS 2019)[9] guideline has suggested clinicians to use a validated clinical prediction rule for prognosis, preferentially the PSI (strong recommendation, moderate quality of evidence) over the CURB-65 to determine the need for hospitalization in adults diagnosed with CAP in addition to clinical judgement.[9] In patients with sCAP with hypotension requiring vasopressors or respiratory failure requiring mechanical ventilation, direct admission to ICU is strongly recommended.

Q8. Which are the causative microorganisms for CAP?[10]
The microbial etiology of CAP is changing, particularly due to widespread introduction of the pneumococcal conjugate vaccine, and increased recognition of the role of viral pathogens by recently introduced molecular diagnostic methods.

Immunocompetent patients:
- *Common causes*:
  - *Streptococcus pneumoniae*
  - *Haemophilus influenzae*
  - *Staphylococcus aureus*
  - Influenza virus
  - Other respiratory viruses such as parainfluenza virus (PIV) and respiratory syncytial virus (RSV)
  - Virus, adenovirus, coronavirus, human metapneumovirus, and rhinovirus
- *Less common causes:*
  - *Pseudomonas aeruginosa* or other gram-negative rods
  - *Pneumocystis jirovecii*
  - *Moraxella catarrhalis*
  - Mixed microaerophilic and anaerobic oral flora
- *Uncommon causes*:
  - *Mycobacterium tuberculosis*
  - Nontuberculous mycobacteria
  - *Nocardia* species
  - *Legionella, Mycoplasma pneumoniae*, and *Chlamydophila pneumoniae*
  - *Chlamydophila psittaci* and *Coxiella burnetii*
  - *Histoplasma capsulatum, Coccidioides* species, *Blastomyces dermatitidis*, and *Cryptococcus*, and *Aspergillus* species.

Immunocompromised patients: The common differential diagnosis of CAP in immunocompromised patients are opportunistic infections such as *Pneumocystis jiroveci* and *Mycobacterium tuberculosis* and other opportunistic fungal infections such as *Cryptococcus neoformans, Histoplasma capsulatum, Coccidioides immitis*, and viral infections *Cytomegalovirus* (CMV).[11]

Q9. What is the incidence of viruses as a cause of CAP? Enumerate the viruses causing CAP.
Recently, the clinical use of rapid molecular techniques has demonstrated that viruses such as influenza, respiratory syncytial virus, and severe acute respiratory syndrome coronavirus 2 (SARS-CoV-2) constitute the initial cause of sCAP, alongside mixed viral–bacterial infections with *S. pneumoniae* and *S. aureus* (20–30%).[2] Also, bacterial pathogens often coexist with viruses. An observational study by the Centers for Disease Control and Prevention (CDC) in 2015 in 2,259 patients of CAP found that respiratory viruses were a more frequent cause of CAP compared to bacteria. They detected causative organism in 38% of patients, out of which 22% had viral etiology. *S. pneumoniae* (5%) was the third most common causative agent, after rhinovirus (9%) and influenza (6%).[14] Bacteria were the only causative agent in 11%, and bacterial viral codetection was found in 3%, and viral-viral codetection occurred in 2% of patients. Fungal or mycobacterial agents were identified rarely (1%).

Following viruses cause CAP:[15]
- *Immunocompetent host:*
  - Influenza (H1N1)
  - Adenovirus
  - Avian influenza (H5N1)
  - Respiratory syncytial virus
  - Rhinovirus
  - Parainfluenza virus
  - Measles
- *Immunocompromised host:*
  - CMV
  - Herpes simplex virus (HSV)
  - Varicella zoster virus (VZV)
- *Emerging viruses*:
  - Coronavirus
  - Hantavirus

Q10. How will you investigate a patient with CAP?
Recommendations for diagnostic testing remain controversial. Routine diagnostic testing is optional for outpatients as per the Infectious Diseases Society of America

TABLE 3: Criteria to judge severity of CAP.

PSI (ATS) also known as Patient Outcomes Research Team (PORT) developed by Fine et al.	• Consist of 20 variables which are associated with mortality
	• Patients are categorized into five strata (I–V) with increasing risk of mortality:
	  – *Class (I–III):* Mortality is <1%
	  – *Class IV:* 9% mortality
	  – *Class V:* 27% mortality
	• *PSI I–II:* Can be treated at home
	• *PSI III:* Needs to be observed in emergency room till further decision
	• *PSI IV–V group:* Recommended for hospitalization

CRB-65/CURB-65: Proposed by the British Thoracic Society (BTS) to predict mortality • *C:* Confusion • *U:* Urea >7 mmol/L (= BUN >19 mg/dL) • *R:* Respiratory rate ≥30 breaths/min • *Blood pressure*, systolic pressure <90 mm Hg or diastolic pressure ≤60 mm Hg • *65:* age ≥65 years Score range from 0 to 5	*Scores with mortality rate (%):* • *Score 0:* 0.7% • *Score 1:* 3.2% • *Score 2:* 3% • *Score 3:* 17% • *Score 4:* 41.5% • *Score 5:* 57% *Further grouped into three groups:* 1. *Group 1:* 0 or 1 score with mortality low (1.5%) likely suitable for home treatment 2. *Group 2:* 2 score with mortality intermediate (9.2%) hospitalize the patient for treatment 3. *Group 3:* 3 or more score with mortality high (22%) Likely to require ICU admission especially if CURB-65 score = 4 or 5
The CRB-65: Simplified version of CURB-65, without inclusion of blood urea Applicable in outpatient clinics	*Further grouped into three groups:* 1. *Group 1:* 0 score with mortality low (1.2%), likely suitable for home treatment 2. *Group 2:* 1–2 score with mortality intermediate (8.15%), likely need hospital referral and assessment 3. *Group 3:* 3–4 or more score with mortality high (31%), urgent hospital admission

IDSA/ATS criteria for severe CAP includes major and minor criteria:
• *Major criteria:* Dependence on mechanical ventilation and septic shock that requires vasopressors
• *Minor criteria:*
  – Respiratory rate >30 breaths/min PaO_2/FiO_2 ratio <250
  – Multilobar infiltrates
  – Confusion/disorientation
  – Uremia (BUN level >20 mg/dL)
  – Leukopenia (WBC count <4,000 cells/mm^3)
  – Thrombocytopenia (platelet count <100,000 cells/mm^3)
  – Hypothermia (core temperature <36°C)
  – Hypotension requiring aggressive fluid resuscitation
	One major plus three minor signifies patient with severe CAP

SMART-COP:
• Systolic arterial pressure <90 mm Hg
• Multilobar involvement on CXR
• Albumin level <35 g/L
• *Respiratory rate:*
  – 50 years and younger: ≥25 breaths/min
  – Older than 50 years: ≥30 breaths/min
• Tachycardia (≥125 beats/min)
• New-onset confusion
Oxygen level:
• *50 years and younger:* PaO_2 <70 mm Hg, oxygen saturation ≤93%, or $PaO_2 = FiO_2$ ratio <333
• *Older than 50 years:* PaO_2 <60 mm Hg, oxygen saturation ≤90%, or $PaO_2 = FiO_2$ ratio <250, arterial pH <7.35
	• Various variables are described carrying points
	• SMART-COP score of 3 or more points identifies 92% of those who will require intensive respiratory support
	• It guides to assess need for intensive respiratory or vasopressor support
	(*SMART-COP:* Systolic blood pressure, Multilobar chest radiography involvement, Albumin level, Respiratory rate, Tachycardia, Confusion, Oxygenation, and arterial pH)

Many other scoring systems such as CAP-PIRO, A-DROP, and S-CAP can be used to prognosticate CAP outcomes.
(ATS: American Thoracic Society; BUN: blood urea nitrogen; CAP: community-acquired pneumonia; CXR: chest radiograph; FiO_2: fraction of inspired oxygen; ICU: intensive care unit; IDSA: Infectious Diseases Society of America; PaO_2: partial pressure of arterial oxygen; WBC: white blood cell)

(IDSA)/ATS practice guidelines.⁹ Patients hospitalized for severe CAP, Gram stain, and good quality sputum culture should be done. Inpatients with moderate-to-severe pneumonia, apart from blood and sputum culture, urinary antigens for pneumococci and *Legionella* can be done. Invasive respiratory samples are not routinely required. But if the disease is severe and diagnosis is not certain, extensive diagnostic testing such as fungal and tuberculosis cultures, bronchoscopy or nonbronchoscopic bronchoalveolar lavage (BAL), thoracentesis with pleural fluid analysis, and lung biopsy should be considered. In following circumstances, extensive diagnostic tests are required:

- ICU admission
- Failure of outpatient antibiotic therapy
- Cavitary infiltrates
- Leukopenia
- Active alcohol abuse
- Chronic severe liver disease
- Severe obstructive/structural lung disease
- Asplenia (anatomic or functional)
- Pleural effusion.

Testing for viral pathogens is recommended in both outpatient and inpatient settings. Conscious effort should be made toward "pathogen-directed treatment". Though aggressive diagnostic tests yield positive results in only 58% of patients overall, it is higher in sicker patients. The ATS 2019 guidelines suggest that diagnostic testing should be done, whenever the result is likely to change the empiric therapy and when diagnostic yield is expected to be maximum.⁹

Etiological diagnosis of CAP remains a challenge. Even a positive sputum culture does not give definitive diagnosis as it can be due to colonization. Hence, based on certainty of the etiology, CAP is categorized into definite or probable.

It is definite when:
- Positive blood cultures and/or pleural fluid culture for a pathogen
- Presence of *P. jirovecii* in induced sputum or in BAL
- A fourfold or greater rise in antibody titer in serologic testing for atypical pathogens
- Isolation of *Legionella pneumophila* or a fourfold rise in antibody titer or positive urinary antigen test, positive direct fluorescence antibody test plus an antibody titer of ≥1:256, and amplification of nucleic acid of *Legionella* species from a nasopharyngeal swab specimen
- Isolation of *M. tuberculosis* from sputum.

It is probable when:
- Sputum culture yields heavy or moderate growth of a predominant bacterial pathogen with a compatible Gram stain or a light growth of a pathogen in which sputum Gram stain reveals a bacterium compatible with the culture results.
- Amplification of nucleic acid of *M. pneumoniae*; *C. pneumoniae*; influenza viruses A and B; PIVs 1, 2, and 3; adenovirus, RSV; and human metapneumovirus from a nasopharyngeal swab specimen.
- Diagnosed as a case of aspiration pneumonia clinically.

Routine diagnostic workup should always include CXR, complete white blood count, sputum culture, blood culture, electrolytes, creatinine, and pulse oximetry to diagnose moderate or severe CAP. Comprehensive molecular testing significantly improves pathogen detection (87% vs. 39% with culture-based methods) even after antimicrobial administration.¹⁶

Following diagnostic tests should be done:
- *Sputum culture:* Good quality sputum is defined as smear with >25 polymorphonuclear neutrophils and <10 squamous epithelial cells per low-power field. Poor quality sputum can give wrong results. If only one morphologic type of bacteria is in the specimen, then it is the most likely pathogen. It should be reported in semiquantitative manner (1+ to 4+).
- Identify the respiratory colonizers while interpreting sputum culture, e.g., *Candida* species, coagulase-negative staphylococci, enterococci and gram-positive bacteria (except *Nocardia*), and streptococci (except *S. pneumoniae*). Sputum examination before administration of antibiotics and culture within 24 hours yields a correct diagnosis in 80% of cases of pneumococcal pneumonia.¹⁷ ATS 2019 guidelines⁹ recommended sputum culture in patients with severe disease as well as in all inpatients empirically treated for methicillin-resistant Staphylococcus aureus (MRSA) or *P. aeruginosa*.
- *Endotracheal aspirates or BAL:* In hospitalized patient who are intubated or those who are not able to produce adequate sputum, endotracheal aspirates or bronchoscopically obtained samples may be required.
- *Blood culture:* It should be preferably performed before antibiotic administration for all patients with moderate or severe CAP. Positive blood culture yields microbial diagnosis of CAP which provides additional information about antibiotic resistance. Blood culture is especially important in immunodeficient patients with CAP. Utility of blood culture is mainly seen in inpatients with pneumococcal pneumonia (20–25%) and in hematogenous *S. aureus* pneumonia. Very few cases of *H. influenzae*, *P. aeruginosa*, and rarely with *M. catarrhalis* yield positive results. Thus, positive blood culture rarely guides to modify the treatment or narrow the antibiotic

therapy. ATS 2019 guidelines have recommended to obtain blood culture in patients with severe disease as well as in all inpatients empirically treated for MRSA or P. aeruginosa.[9]

- *Urinary antigens:* Urinary antigen test is available for S. pneumoniae and Legionella. S. pneumoniae urinary antigens: All serotypes of S. pneumoniae are detected and it yields results within 15 minutes. Its sensitivity of 74.0% [95% confidence interval (CI) 66.6-82.3] and specificity of 97.2% (92.7-99.8) with bacteremic pneumococcal pneumonia and is considered as gold standard.[18] This test gives positive results even if antibiotics are administered. ATS 2019 guidelines[9] do not support routine testing urine for pneumococcal antigen in adults with CAP except in adults with severe CAP (conditional recommendation, low quality of evidence).
  - *Limitations of urinary antigen testing:*
    - Expensive to perform
    - Does not assess antibiotic susceptibility
    - False-positive results in pediatric patients with nasopharyngeal colonization with S. pneumoniae and those who suffered CAP in the last 4 months.
- *Legionella urinary antigen test:* Serogroup I infection is diagnosed by detection of urinary antigen by radioimmunoassay or enzyme-linked immunosorbent assay. Routine testing for Legionella antigen is not recommended as per ATS guidelines 2019 except in cases of Legionella outbreak or recent travel or in adults with severe CAP.[9] Ordering this test should be based on local epidemiology or in a case of severe pneumonia with no response to empirical β-lactam therapy. Its sensitivity is 74.0% (68.0-81.0) and specificity is 99.1% (98.4-99.7).[18] It gives positive results starting from 1st day of disease and positivity continues for several weeks even if the patient is on antibiotics.
  - *Limitations:*
    - It diagnoses only type 1 serogroup.
    - It does not give any information about antibiotic resistance.
- *Bronchoscopy:* It is most useful in immunocompromised host, diagnosis of tuberculosis with negative sputum samples, P. jirovecii, fungal or viral pathogens, and to diagnose noninfectious etiology.
- *Thoracentesis:* Usually not required in uncomplicated parapneumonic effusion (exudative stage) which resolves with appropriate antimicrobial therapy. If it fails to resolve, it gets infected and develops into fibropurulent stage which requires drainage. Additionally, pleural fluid drainage and analysis play a major role to differentiate conditions which mimic bacterial pneumonia such as tuberculosis, collagen vascular disease.
- *Open lung biopsy:* It remains the last resort in patients who continue to deteriorate and etiology is unclear or in patients with treatment failure.

Q11. What is the latest update on molecular diagnostic testing for CAP?

Molecular diagnostic techniques has a sensitivity of 70-80% and high specificity (99-100%).[19] This modality detects 23.6% more pathogens than traditional culture techniques.[20] It has short turnaround time facilitates to rapidly modify antibiotics quickly.

- This test should be used as an additional diagnostic testing and should be reserved for those selected group of patients in which results can facilitate change in management.
- It also provides information about drug resistance mechanisms (e.g., 20-40% of the isolates causing pneumococcal CAP shows high resistance to macrolides, whereas 3-8% present high resistance to fluoroquinolones based on this technique).
- Theoretically, it is an attractive option to modify treatment. For example, one can safely discontinue empirical β-lactams in patients with sCAP caused by Legionella or Mycoplasma species detected by PCR or can discontinue all antibiotics in case of viral CAP if bacterial multiplex PCR is negative or deescalate to a single agent or to a narrower agent. It identifies multiple isolates from one sample and aids to diagnose bacterial (including atypical) or viral pneumonia. Baudel et al.[21] studied BAL samples of CAP patients by multiplex PCR. He found that PCR-based approach aids to higher degree of etiological diagnosis (66%) compared to nonmolecular techniques, especially in patients who had previously received antibiotics.

Recently published guidelines by ESICM[2] have suggested to send lower respiratory tract sample (either sputum or endotracheal aspirates) for multiplex PCR testing (virus and/or bacterial detection) if the technology is available or whenever nonstandard sCAP antibiotics are prescribed or considered with conditional recommendation having very low quality of evidence. 2019 ATS[9] clinical practice document has recommended molecular assay for influenza whenever influenza viruses are circulating in the community. Influenza nucleic acid amplification test (NAAT) is preferred over a rapid influenza diagnostic test by antigen testing (strong recommendation, moderate quality of evidence). The routine testing of noninfluenza respiratory viruses has not recommended by this guideline, unless identified as having severe CAP and/or various immunocompromising conditions.

Limitation: It is safety concern to modify antibiotic regimen. As there remains the possibility of false positive results and unnecessary escalation antibiotics and emergence of antibiotic-resistant pathogens and its cost which lowers its evidence to support. Its role to de-escalate empirical antibiotic treatment is still uncertain. As PCR of *S. aureus* based on detection of *mecA* gene, it cannot differentiate MRSA colonization from infection and even coagulase-negative staphylococci (CoNS) carry the same gene lead to inadvertent use of vancomycin and linezolid.

Q12. Should SARS-CoV-2 diagnostic testing be done in CAP?

As per Indian Council of Medical Research (ICMR) advisory on purposive testing strategy for SARS-CoV-2 in revised on February 2023,[22] following are advised tests—rapid antigen test (RAT) at home or self-testing and molecular tests real-time reverse transcription–polymerase chain reaction (RT-PCR). ICMR recommends the use of standard Q SARS-CoV-2 Ag detection assay as a point of care diagnostic assay for testing in combination with the gold standard RT-PCR test.

- *Rapid antigen test:* Standard Q SARS-CoV-2 Ag rapid chromatographic immunoassay for qualitative detection of specific antigens to SARS-CoV-2. It has a very high specificity (99.3 to 100% at the two sites) and low sensitivity (50.6–84% in two independent evaluations, depending upon the viral load of the patient). Nasopharyngeal swab needs to be collected and test can be interpreted as positive or negative after 15 minutes.
- *Real time RT-PCR:* WHO recommends for laboratory diagnosis SARS-CoV-2 based on detection of unique sequences of virus RNA by NAAT such as real-time RT-PCR.[13] The Food and Drug Administration/emergency use authorization/conformité européenne marked in vitro diagnostic (FDA EUA/CE-IVD) approved RT-PCR kits are highly specific and detect the presence or absence of SARS-CoV-2 viral nucleic acid and thus directly confirm viral infection in a human sample. The RT-PCR test is the current gold standard diagnostic method and it is advised to use real-time RT-PCR as the frontline test for diagnosis of SARS-CoV-2. Minimum time taken for the test varies between different systems with a minimum of 2–5 hours. Other molecular methods such as virus antigen or serological antibody testing are currently recommended for use only in research settings and not in clinical decision-making.

Q13. What is the role of imaging in patients with CAP?

Imaging is essential for the investigation of diagnosis and management of CAP.

- *Chest X-ray:* Presence of a new infiltrate on CXR aids in diagnosis of CAP. In adults with CAP whose symptoms have resolved within 5–7 days ATS 2019[9] guidelines have suggested that routine follow-up chest imaging is not required.
  - *Limitations:*
    - Low sensitivity
    - Patients admitted with clinical diagnosis of CAP may not show parenchymal opacification. Patients admitted with negative CXR may develop radiographic infiltrates within 48 hours.[23]
    - Diagnostic accuracy is 75% for consolidation and 47% for pleural effusion.
    - Image quality is lower in bedridden patients.
    - Risk of radiation exposure
    - High interobserver variability
    - Less accurate in obese, severely immuno-suppressed patients, and in patients with previous pathologies on CXR.
- *Computed tomography thorax:* It is the gold standard. It provides detailed information about lung parenchyma and mediastinum which helps in diagnosis and management. It gives more accurate information about complications such as pleuritis and pulmonary necrosis in nonresponding pneumonia. It excludes other noninfectious diagnosis such as atelectasis, pulmonary infarction, tumor, and interstitial lung disease that may appear similar to pneumonia on CXR. CT finding identifies fungal pneumonia or pneumonia caused by mycobacteria. A study published in 2015 showed that early CT thorax affect the diagnosis and management in patients visiting in ER with suspected CAP. They found that 30% of patients were reclassified as not having pneumonia.[24]
  - *Limitations:*
    - Expensive
    - It should be reserved for more complex cases where therapeutic failure occurs.
    - Cannot perform at the bedside
    - Risk of exposure to radiation

Q14. What is the role of ultrasound in diagnosis of CAP?

One systemic review and meta-analysis including 16 studies (2,359 patients) showed that lung ultrasound helps in CAP diagnosis and management. It has good sensitivity of 94.0% (95% CI 92.0–96.0) and specificity of 96.0% (94.0–97.0) in the diagnosis of pneumonia in adults.[25]

- It is portable and fast.
- It does not use radiation.
- It can be performed in pregnant woman at bedside.
- It is Easily reproducible.
- It is a real-time scanning, aids in detection of consolidation, and its associated complications such as pleural effusion with or without septations.

Limitations:
- Slow learning curve
- Interoperator variability

Q15. How do you approach a patient with CAP and pleural effusion?

Light's criteria determine presence of exudate based on protein and lactate dehydrogenase (LDH) levels.[26]
- Pleural fluid protein to serum protein ratio > 0.5
- Pleural fluid LDH to serum LDH ratio >0.6
- Pleural fluid level more than two-thirds of upper value for serum LDH.
  Additional criteria confirm exudate if results equivocal.
  Serum albumin—pleural fluid albumin <1.2 g/dL.
  If the fluid is exudative, efforts should be made to find the etiology.

Total and differential cell count: Increase cell count with neutrophilia is usually associated with bacterial infection and empyema. In lymphocytic predominant pleural fluid, tuberculosis should be ruled out. Atypical cells are usually seen in malignancy.
- *Gram stain and culture:* It helps in early identification of causative organisms.
- Low pH, low glucose, and high LDH suggest exudative fluid.
- Lymphocytic predominance is also seen in other nontubercular etiology, adenosine deaminase activity (ADA) should be done to rule out tuberculosis.

  Parapneumonic effusion occurs in 20–40% of CAP. Most of the times, pleural effusion resolves with appropriate antimicrobial therapy. Ultrasound-guided fluid aspiration and its analysis should be considered when diagnosis is uncertain. It helps to identify exact etiology as well as it can differentiate other conditions such as tuberculosis, tumor, collagen vascular disease, and pulmonary emboli. Tube thoracostomy and drainage of the effusion should be considered if diagnostic aspiration yields exudates, pleural fluid with a pH <7.2, or a positive Gram stain or culture.

Q16. What is empiric choice of antibiotics in treating CAP?

Empirical antibiotic therapy is the cornerstone in management of CAP.[9] Early administration of antibiotics within 4 hours of presentation should be encouraged in unstable patients with septic shock. Whereas in stable patients, early therapy does not offer any advantage in lowering the mortality, but leads to increased risk of misdiagnosis and adverse effects.[27] The standard antibiotic regimens for CAP are the combination of a β-lactam (usually a cephalosporin) and a macrolide or monotherapy with a respiratory fluoroquinolone. ATS guideline 2019[9] suggests that stronger evidence favors the use of β-lactam/macrolide combination. ESICM task force has also supported the addition of macrolides and not the fluoroquinolones, to β-lactam as an empirical antibiotic therapy. Use of respiratory fluoroquinolones as empirical antibiotics must be avoided in situations where tuberculosis cannot be excluded. Fluoroquinolones should be judiciously used in tuberculous endemic area.[28]

Q17. What is the treatment of CAP as per the ATS/IDSA guidelines?

Antimicrobial treatment is empirical as the exact causative organism is not identified in many patients with CAP.[9] First line of treatment should vary from region to region as per local epidemiology. Most guidelines recommend that antibiotic treatment should be based on the severity of disease at the time of presentation **(Table 4)**.

Q18. Describe the role of monotherapy versus combination antibiotic therapy in CAP?

In patients with mild to moderate pneumonia without suspicion of atypical infection, β-lactam monotherapy is not inferior to β-lactam plus macrolide combination therapy which is a conditional recommendation for outpatients based on resistance levels as per ATS 2019 guidelines.[9] However, in severe pneumonia (PSI >IV) or with clinical suspicion of atypical pneumonia showed delayed achievement in clinical stability with monotherapy.[29,30] Combination therapy compared with β-lactam therapy alone is significantly associated with less 30 days' mortality rate in patients with moderate to severe CAP. Combination therapy is superior due to broader coverage of unidentified atypical pathogens and macrolide-specific immunomodulatory, quorum sensing, or alveolar epithelial effects.[31]

Q19. In suspected viral pneumonia, which antivirals should be used and for how many days?

As per the World Health Organization (WHO) recommendations,[32] currently circulating H1N1 2009 virus is susceptible to neuraminidase inhibitor (NAI) (oseltamivir). In suspected case of viral pneumonia, early antiviral therapy with NAI within 48 hours of onset of influenza is recommended without waiting for laboratory results. Early antivirals reduce viral shedding, duration, and severity of symptoms, thereby decreasing complications and mortality. ATS 2019 guidelines[9] have strongly recommended to prescribe oseltamivir for adults with CAP who test positive for influenza in the inpatient setting, independent of duration of illness before diagnosis. Patients with severe progressive illness requiring hospitalization, doubling the dose to 75 mg twice a day for 10 days is recommended.[33] Considering the beneficial effects of early initiation of oseltamivir (within 48 hours) in reducing the symptoms and further progression to lower respiratory

TABLE 4: Antimicrobial treatment of CAP as per the ATS/IDSA guidelines.

Outpatients/low severity

Healthy patient with no use of antimicrobials within last 3 months	Macrolide (strong recommendation) Doxycycline (weak recommendation)	• Amoxicillin 1 g three times daily (strong recommendation, moderate quality of evidence) • Doxycycline 100 mg twice daily (conditional recommendation, low quality of evidence) or • Macrolide (azithromycin 500 mg on first day then 250 mg daily) or • Clarithromycin 500 mg twice daily or • Clarithromycin extended release 1,000 mg daily only in areas with pneumococcal resistance to macrolides <25% (conditional recommendation, moderate quality of evidence) • Levofloxacin 750 mg daily • Moxifloxacin 400 mg daily, or • Gemifloxacin 320 mg daily
Presence of comorbidities such as chronic heart, lung, liver, or renal disease; diabetes mellitus; alcoholism; malignancies; asplenia; immunosuppressing conditions or use of immunosuppressing drugs; or use of antimicrobials within the previous 3 months	• Respiratory fluoroquinolone (strong recommendation) Or • A β-lactam plus a macrolide (strong recommendation) Or • High-dose amoxicillin (1 g three times daily) or amoxicillin-clavulanate (2 g two times daily) is preferred Or • β-lactam plus doxycycline is preferred	

Inpatients

Inpatients nonsevere pneumonia	• β-lactam plus a macrolide (strong recommendation) Or • Respiratory fluoroquinolone monotherapy (strong recommendation, high quality of evidence) • If prior history MRSA/pseudomonas: MRSA/pseudomonas coverage and send culture and PCR • β-lactam and doxycycline (conditional recommendation, low quality of evidence)	• β-lactam (ampicillin 1 sulbactam 1.5–3 g every 6 h, cefotaxime 1–2 g every 8 h, ceftriaxone 1–2 g daily, or ceftaroline 600 mg every 12 h) and • Macrolide (azithromycin 500 mg daily or clarithromycin 500 mg twice daily) (strong recommendation, high quality of evidence), or • Monotherapy with a respiratory fluoroquinolone (levofloxacin 750 mg daily, moxifloxacin 400 mg daily) (strong recommendation, high quality of evidence) • CAP with contraindications to macrolides and • Fluoroquinolones (combination therapy with a β-lactam and Doxycycline 100 mg twice daily)

Inpatients severe pneumonia	• β-lactam plus macrolide (strong recommendation, high quality of evidence)
	Or
	• β-lactam respiratory plus fluoroquinolone (strong recommendation) if prior history MRSA/ pseudomonas: MRSA/ pseudomonas coverage and send culture and PCR
		β-lactam:
		• Ampicillin 1 sulbactam 1.5–3 g every 6 hours,
		• Cefotaxime 1–2 g every 8 hours,
		• Ceftriaxone 1–2 g daily, or
		• Ceftaroline 600 mg every 12 hours
		Macrolide: Azithromycin 500 mg daily or clarithromycin 500 mg twice daily.
		Fluoroquinolone:
		• Levofloxacin 705 mg once a day
		• Moxifloxacin 400 mg once a day
		• *MRSA:* Vancomycin 15 mg/kg 12 hourly
		  – Linezolid 600 mg 12 hourly
		• *Pseudomonas:* Piperacillin-tazobactam
		  – 4.5 gm 6 hourly
		  – Cefepime 2 g 8 hourly
		  – Ceftazidime 2 g 8 hourly
		  – Imipenem 500 6 hourly
		  – Meropenem 1 g 8 hourly
		  – Aztreonam 2 g 8 hourly

(ATS: American Thoracic Society; CAP: community-acquired pneumonia; CA-MRSA: community-acquired methicillin-resistant *Staphylococcus aureus*; ICU: intensive care unit; IDSA: Infectious Diseases Society of America)

tract complications, guideline has suggested to initiate anti-influenza treatment who is positive for influenza in the outpatient setting as well. ESICM task force[2] suggested to use oseltamivir to sCAP in PCR-based influenza confirmed cased but even if PCR is not available to confirm diagnosis, guideline has suggested to use oseltamivir during the period of influenza season. Intravenous (IV) peramivir (NAI), inhaled laninamivir (NAI), and favipiravir (T-705) are newer antivirals.

Q20. What is mixed viral and bacterial pneumonia?

Seasonal and pandemic influenza are frequently complicated by bacterial superinfections most commonly due to *S. pneumoniae, S. aureus,* and *H. influenzae,* which lead to increase in hospitalization and mortality. They are subdivided into combined viral/bacterial and postinfluenza pneumonia.[34] In combined viral/bacterial pneumonia, viruses, bacteria, and the host, all interact with each other. Postinfluenza pneumonia is less complicated as virus has been cleared. It is due to virus-induced changes to the host that affect the course of bacterial infection. It is still unclear whether viral organism is the primary causative agent or it has predisposed the patient to secondary bacterial infection. The severity of the disease is due to influenza-induced damage to the airway epithelium, which leads to increased colonization of bacteria at the basal membrane and impaired host defense against secondary infection. Clinically, it is difficult to differentiate bacterial and viral pneumonia early in the course of disease and the markers of inflammation are also not specific. But microbiological and/or molecular techniques may help to guide the treatment. Thus, ATS 2019[9] guidelines have recommended to prescribe initial standard antibacterial treatment for adults with clinical and radiographic evidence of CAP who test positive for influenza in the inpatient. Once early clinical stability is achieved and there is no evidence of a bacterial pathogen, earlier discontinuation of antibiotic treatment at 48–72 hours should be considered. Treatment is similar to viral and bacterial pneumonia.

Q21. Do patients with sCAP with aspiration risk factors should be treated with a risk-based therapy regimen or standard sCAP antibiotics?

The ATS 2019 and ESICM task force suggested to prescribe standard CAP therapy regimen instead of therapy targeting anaerobic bacteria.[2,9]

Q22. What are the complications of CAP?

- *Severe CAP with multiorgan failure [multiple organ dysfunction syndrome (MODS)]:* Presents with septic shock leading to multiorgan involvement causing respiratory, renal, hepatic failure, coagulopathy, encephalopathy, and meningitis.
- *Parapneumonic effusions and empyema:* Seen in up to 60% of patients with severe CAP.
- Acute respiratory distress syndrome (ARDS).
- *Necrotizing pneumonia:* Lung cavitation and abscess formation, predominantly seen with *S. aureus*, gram-negative bacilli, *Aspergillus, Mycobacterium*, and *Nocardia* species.
- *Cardiac complications:* Myocardial infarction, arrhythmias, and decompensated cardiac failure mainly associated with bacterial infections and influenza.

Q23. Does CAP increase the risk of development of subsequent acute cardiovascular events? What is the evidence for this?

Community-acquired pneumonia is associated with significant increase in acute cardiovascular events and early as well as late mortality. In a recent study, 30% of patients admitted to hospital for CAP developed acute cardiovascular complications and the incidence remained high up to 10 years after the CAP episode. These patients develop new or worsening heart failure, arrhythmias and myocardial infarctions, and strokes. There is a complex interaction between preexisting conditions leading to hypoxia, relative ischemia, and upregulation of the sympathetic system. Systemic inflammation leads to release of cytokines, endotoxin-mediated activation of platelets generating a procoagulant state, direct pathogen-mediated reduce inotropism and plaque instability leading to risk of plaque rupture, and acute coronary syndrome. Further evidence is required to identify potential therapeutic and preventative strategies to reduce the complications.[35,36] Macrolide is an important therapeutic agent used for CAP but it should be used cautiously particularly in elderly patients due to increased risk of QT prolongation and life-threatening arrhythmias.

Q24. What is the supportive treatment for CAP?

Those who are admitted with CAP with hypoxemia should receive O_2 therapy initially. Respiratory failure despite of high O_2 therapy should be managed with NIV or invasive ventilation. NIV is particularly beneficial in those patients who are immunocompromised, underlying chronic lung disease including obstructive and restrictive lung disease—*P. jirovecii* infection. Vigilant monitoring is required when patient is on NIV and prompt detection of NIV failure is warranted which mandates immediate intubation and ventilation with low-tidal volume lung protective ventilation strategy (6 mL/kg of ideal body weight). If patient is in shock, early use of vasopressors (noradrenaline) is recommended after optimizing fluid status by assessing dynamic measures of fluid responsiveness. Further, management of sepsis should be done as per surviving sepsis campaign guidelines.[37,38] Other supportive management includes nutritional support, deep venous thrombosis and stress ulcer prophylaxis, and chest physiotherapy.

Aerosolized antibiotics in severe CAP: Use of aerosolized antibiotics is based on a sound physiological rationale that has potential to deliver a high concentration of the drug at the site of infection without much systemic adverse effects.

A global survey conducted in 2017 revealed that 63.4% of 261 ICUs used inhaled antibiotics, mainly for infection with MDR organisms causing ventilator-associated pneumonia (VAP) and ventilator-associated tracheobronchitis (VAT)[38] but not in case of CAP. Most guidelines recommend inhaled antibiotics only as a last resort in intractable cases with MDR infections as evidence on this topic gives conflicting results.

Q25. What are other adjunctive therapies for CAP? What is the role of steroids in management of CAP?
Agents with anti-inflammatory properties are being studied as adjunctive therapy to achieve balance between proinflammatory and anti-inflammatory mediators. Statins with its anti-inflammatory property and its ability to reduce cardiovascular events have been studied, but the results are controversial.[39] The use of steroids in CAP has been contentious till date. Various society guidelines having differing recommendations. ATS and IDSA are against the use of steroids in CAP[9] whereas ERS, ESICM, ESCMID, and ALAT supports use of steroids in CAP.[2,19]

- ATS 2019 has "not recommended" routine use of steroids with nonsevere CAP (strong recommendation, high quality of evidence).
- In sCAP, guideline has "suggested" not to use steroids routinely (conditional recommendation with moderate quality of evidence.[9]
- In case of severe influenza pneumonia, ATS guideline does not support use of steroids.

In contrast to ATS guidelines, ESICM guidelines favor steroid use and methylprednisolone (0.5 mg·kg⁻¹ every 12 h for 5 days) is a reasonable option if shock is present. But it is with conditional recommendation and low quality of evidence.[2] This recommendation does not apply to patients with sCAP caused by influenza[40] SARS, in case of uncontrolled diabetes and on corticosteroid treatment for other reasons.

There have been several systematic reviews and metanalysis which explored the efficacy of steroids in sCAP. In 2017, the Cochrane published metanalysis[41] including 17 RCTs (n = 2,264) and found that mortality and morbidity were low with steroid use in sCAP (RR 0.58, 95% CI 0.40–0.84; moderate-quality evidence) and not in case of nonsevere CAP (RR 0.95, 95% CI 0.45–2.00). But hyperglycemia was more common with steroid therapy as an adverse effect (RR 1.72, 95% CI 1.38–2.14). Recently, role of steroids (methylprednisolone) in sCAP has been studied in terms of mortality benefit in 2022 by Meduri et al.[42] It is a double-blind placebo-controlled RCT (n = 584) on using low-dose methylprednisolone treatment in critically ill patients with sCAP as per ATS/IDSA criteria. They used methylprednisolone for 21 days (40 mg methylprednisolone for 7 days, 20 mg for 7 days, 12 mg for 7 days). There is significant difference (16 vs. 18%; adjusted OR 0.9, 95% CI 0.57–1.4) in 60-day mortality between the methylprednisolone and placebo arms. But associated editorial suggested to have larger scale RCTs before strong recommendations are made on this aspect. Use of hydrocortisone in early sCAP has been evaluated by Dequin PF et al.[43] They found hydrocortisone is beneficial in terms of reduced 28-day mortality. It is a multicenter, double blind, placebo-controlled trial with balanced baseline characteristics, minimum selection bias and high level of adherence to protocol. Hydrocortisone (200 mg/day for 4 days) is initiated within ~20 hours from hospital admission. They observed reduction in 28-day mortality in hydrocortisone group by 6.2% compared to placebo which is 11.9% with difference of −5.6% (−9.6 to −1.7%), $p = 0.006$. There is no significant difference in cumulative 28-day incidence of hospital acquired infection (9.8 vs. 11.1%) and cumulative incidence of GI bleeding (2.2 vs. 3.3%). But intervention group has shown significantly more requirement of insulin day 7 (35.5 vs. 20.0 IU/day). The cumulative incidence of endotracheal intubation is significantly less in intervention group (18.0 vs. 29.5%), and there is less incidence of new initiation of vasopressor in the intervention group (15.3 vs. 25.0%).

Although prednisolone or methylprednisolone is preferred steroid over hydrocortisone in patients with sCAP yet we need to determine which corticosteroid (hydrocortisone or methylprednisolone) shows a better profile based on different type of pathogens, outweighing potential adverse effects. One metanalysis[44] showed benefits of prednisolone or methylprednisolone in terms of mortality, length of ICU stay and need for mechanical ventilation. In subgroup analysis, they showed that prednisolone or methylprednisolone therapy (OR 0.37, 95% CI 0.19–0.72) reduced total mortality, whereas hydrocortisone use did not (OR 0.90, 95% CI 0.54–1.49) as per this metanalysis. It is still unclear which phenotype would benefit the most with steroids and any biomarker to predict the response with steroid treatment. Results of REMAP-CAP study, a nonpandemic steroid domain would definitely throw better clarity on this practice.

Q26. How long should the antibiotics be given to this patient?
Patient with CAP usually achieves clinical stability within 5–7 days of appropriate antimicrobial therapy. Patient should be treated for a minimum of 5 days provided that the patient is afebrile for last 48–72 hours, and should not have more than one CAP-associated sign of clinical instability, before discontinuation of therapy.[9] Following are the criteria for clinical stability:[45]

- Temperature <37.8°C
- Heart rate <100 beats/min

- Respiratory rate <24 breaths/min
- Systolic blood pressure >90 mm Hg
- Arterial oxygen saturation >90% or pO_2 >60 mm Hg on room air
- Ability to maintain oral intake
- Normal mental status

When 7 days or less duration of antibiotic therapy was compared to a duration of 8 days or more, there was no difference in outcome.[46]

Longer duration of therapy may be required in the event of inappropriate initial empiric therapy or CAP complicated by extrapulmonary manifestations (such as cavities, tissue necrosis, meningitis, or endocarditis). The variation in duration will depend on the following:

- *Etiology:* For example, *Legionella* pneumonia must be treated for at least 14 days.
- *Virulence of pathogen:* Organisms like *S. aureus*, enteric gram-negative bacteria require longer course. Particularly, *S. aureus* pneumonia mandates treatment for at least 4 weeks since shorter duration may be suboptimal and has associated risk of endocarditis and deep-seated infections patient's age, accompanying comorbidities, immune status, and response to treatment.
- *Choice of antibiotics:* Antibiotics like azithromycin with longer half-lives can be given for shorter duration (3–5 days).
- Infection with rare pathogens, e.g., *Burkholderia pseudomallei* or endemic fungi.

Q27. When will you change over to oral antibiotics?

Once patient achieves clinical stability, he should be switched over to oral antibiotics of the same class and discharge day. Discharging patients earlier may lead to more readmissions and deaths.

Q28. What is the role of biomarkers in patients with CAP? What is the role of procalcitonin (PCT) in management of CAP?

Various biomarkers are available for use in patients with sepsis. A systematic review[47] studied sensitivity and specificity of biomarkers. They found that biomarkers can predict the mortality with moderate accuracy but offer no additional advantage over the CAP-specific score. The area under the curve (AUC) values in descending manner were seen with proadrenomedullin (0.80) and prohormone forms of atrial natriuretic peptide (0.79). It is followed by cortisol (0.78), PCT (0.75), copeptin (0.71), and C-reactive protein (CRP) (0.62). Though CRP is a widely used biomarker, its predictive ability for mortality is considerably poor.

Procalcitonin is a biomarker that has been extensively studied. In response to bacterial infections, PCT levels increase. PCT has a reasonably high predictive value.[48] It has high sensitivity but moderate specificity to differentiate bacterial and viral infections. PCT level ≥0.25 ng/mL is a predictor of bacterial infection. ATS 2019 guidelines[9] strongly recommend that regardless of initial serum PCT level, empiric antibiotic therapy should be initiated in adults with clinically suspected and radiographically confirmed CAP. Recent ESICM task force guidelines also support PCT-guided therapy to reduce the duration of antibiotics.

Based on PCT levels:
- *PCT higher than 0.5 µg/L:* Antibiotics use is strongly encouraged.
- *PCT higher than 0.25 µg/L:* For outpatients, patients in emergency departments/inpatients antibiotic are encouraged.
- *PCT lower than 0.10 µg/L:* Antibiotics use is discouraged.[49]

A recent multicenter trial demonstrated that using PCT-guided antibiotic therapy did not result in lower use of antibiotics when compared to usual care in patients who presented to the emergency department with suspected lower respiratory tract infection.[50] PCT often normal in the setting of *Legionella* and *Mycoplasma* infections and it has a poor sensitivity in the presence of mixed bacterial and viral infections.[51] However, a meta-analysis including 14 trials with 4,221 participants reported that the use of PCT to guide antibiotic treatment resulted in a reduction in the exposure to antibiotics from median 8 days to 4 days. PCT guidance is not associated with increased mortality or treatment failure in any clinical setting.[52] Recently, host gene expression molecular classifiers discriminate noninfectious from infectious illness as well as bacterial from viral causes of acute respiratory infection. These classifiers developed are externally validated in five publicly available datasets with AUC, 0.90–0.99. Its overall accuracy is (87%) better than PCT (78%) with p less than 0.03.[53]

Q29. What is "nonresponding pneumonia (NRP)" and what are the causes of nonresponding pneumonia?

It is a situation with inadequate clinical response despite antibiotic treatment. Inadequate host response can be either due to mismatch between the susceptibility of a common causative organism, unexpected microorganisms, or nosocomial superinfection in CAP. As many as 15% of patients with CAP may not respond appropriately to initial antibiotic therapy. Following patterns are observed in NRP:

- *Progressive NRP:* There is clinical deterioration of patient leading to acute respiratory failure and/or septic shock, within the first 72 hours of admission. If it occurs after 72 hours, it is often related to intercurrent complications, worsening of underlying disease, or superadded nosocomial infection.

- *Persistent NRP:* Absence of or delay in achieving clinical criteria of stability which is seen in patients with high PSI scores.

Nonresolving or slow resolving pneumonia: Those who present with persistence of pulmonary infiltrates for >30 days after initial pneumonia is referred to as nonresolving or slow resolving pneumonia.

Q30. How do you approach a patient with nonresponding pneumonia?

Assess the risk factors for delayed resolution, e.g., age, comorbidities, severity of pneumonia, and specific pathogens. If the rate of resolution is appropriate, then continue the same therapy and observe but if it is getting delayed then review the history, get clues for unusual pathogens, identify complications with aggressive diagnostic approach, and search for other noninfectious causes.

When pneumonia fails to resolve, following considerations should be kept in mind:[1]
- Incorrect identification of causative organism
- Correct organism but inappropriate dose and antibiotic choice
- Correct organism and correct antibiotic but infection is loculated (empyema)
- No identification of causative organism and empirical therapy directed toward wrong organism
- *Resistant organisms:* Resistant *S. pneumoniae*, nosocomial Legionnaires' disease from contaminated water source
- Newly developed nosocomial pneumonia
- *Reconsider the etiology:* Tuberculosis, *Actinomyces*, or *Nocardia* species, polymicrobial (10% of cases of pneumonia)
- *Metastatic infection:* Persistent bacteremia leads to endocarditis, meningitis, septic arthritis, or deep abscess such as splenic or renal abscess.
- Obstruction (lung cancer, foreign body) and postobstructive pneumonia
- Always consider drug fever
- Noninfectious causes
- *Unrecognized, concurrent infection:* Intravascular catheter, urinary, abdominal, and skin infections particularly in ICU patients.

Q31. How do you investigate a patient with NRP?
- Repeat blood cultures
- Repeat respiratory cultures (cautious interpretation of gram-negative bacilli as early colonization is more common than superinfection)
- Perform CT thorax (additional information about parenchymal lesions, mediastinal, or prebronchial lymphadenopathy, and noninfectious disease such as bronchiolitis obliterans organizing pneumonia)
- Perform diagnostic thoracentesis (if pleural fluid is present, drain after pleural fluid analysis)
- Perform bronchoscopy with BAL with or without transbronchial biopsy (to diagnose infectious and/or noninfectious conditions)
- Consider endobronchial ultrasound (EBUS)-guided fine-needle aspiration (FNA) or transbronchial biopsy or consider surgical lung biopsy and/or video-assisted thoracoscopic surgery if diagnosis is not apparent.

Q32. When will you suspect community-acquired MRSA (CA-MRSA)?

Two distinct types of MRSA pneumonia are observed:[54]
1. Traditional nosocomial pneumonia with hospital-acquired strains
2. True community-acquired strain associated with exotoxin production which leads to life-threatening necrotizing pneumonia.

Despite a low frequency, CA-MRSA is an important cause of CAP with high mortality if not suspected early. It usually occurs in outbreaks affecting previously healthy young patients with preceding influenza infection. It is often lethal cause of CAP and is resistant to standard antimicrobial treatment.[55] CA-MRSA carries Panton–Valentine leukocidin (PVL) gene which is responsible for exotoxin production that promotes invasiveness and rapid progression of disease. It is preceded by "flu-like" illness or necrotizing skin infection like household history of PVL-*S. aureus* skin sepsis. Patient presents with hemoptysis, hypotension, diarrhea, vomiting, tachycardia, tachypnea, and often complicated by severe necrotizing pneumonia, staphylococcal shock syndrome. Complications such as cavitation, pneumothorax, jaundice, empyema, acute renal failure, and pericarditis are common in post-MRSA pneumonia. On investigations, these patients show multilobar infiltrates on CXR, effusions, and cavitation. They show markedly elevated CRP, leukopenia, increased creatinine kinase, and multiple gram-positive cocci on sputum Gram stain.

Q33. Which drugs are active against CA-MRSA?

Whenever CA-MRSA is a concern, inappropriate antibiotic therapy may lead to increase in mortality. Hospitalized patients with severe CAP are defined as those requiring ICU admission, necrotizing or cavitary infiltrates, and empyema. If any one of these conditions are present, empirical therapy for MRSA is recommended till sputum and/or blood culture results.[56]

Current evidence favors linezolid as a drug of choice for CA-MRSA pneumonia as it suppresses exotoxin production in in vitro models.¹ Antibiotics that suppress toxin production may warrant consideration for treatment of CA-MRSA pneumonia over vancomycin as later does not decrease toxin production. However, an emergence of resistance to clindamycin has been reported and instead of monotherapy, clindamycin, or rifampin may be added with other anti-CA-MRSA drugs. Daptomycin should not be used for CA-MRSA pneumonia because its effectiveness is reduced in presence of lung surfactants. There is no evidence for tigecycline to treat CA-MRSA pneumonia.

Newer drugs such as ceftaroline (a fifth-generation cephalosporin) and ceftobiprole are active against CA-MRSA in treatment of CAP with PSI III-IV in Asian patients.[57] Quinupristin-dalfopristin is newer antibiotics for CA-MRSA but evidence is scarce. MRSA pneumonia complicated by empyema and drainage procedures along with antibiotics are advised.

In case of methicillin-sensitive *S. aureus* (MSSA), empirical combination therapy is recommended with β-lactam and a respiratory fluoroquinolone until susceptibility results are available. Avoid use of linezolid and vancomycin in MSSA infection. Depending upon the extent of infection, duration of treatment varies from 7 to 21 days. *S. aureus* infection causing segmental pneumonia may be treated for 2 weeks depending on the extent of infection. Hematogenous spread mandates treatment for 4 weeks. *S. aureus* causing cavitating pneumonia and lung abscess needs treatment for several weeks.[56]

Q34. What is the role of tigecycline in treatment of CAP?
Tigecycline has emerged as an attractive option for treatment of severe CAP who requires hospitalization; however, limited data is available about its effectiveness.[58] It should be reserved for the patients who are allergic to β-lactam or quinolone, infection caused by resistant organism, or previous treatment failure with routine antimicrobials for CAP. Though tigecycline has potent in vitro activity against CA-MRSA, data of efficacy of MRSA pneumonias are somewhat limited.[59]

Q35. What is atypical pneumonia?
Bacteria including *M. pneumoniae, Chlamydia pneumoniae, Chlamydia psittaci, L. pneumophila,* and respiratory viruses are recognized to cause "atypical pneumonia". Other agents such as *C. psittaci* (formerly *C. psittaci*), *Francisella tularensis, M. tuberculosis, C. burnetii* and in patients with acquired immunodeficiency syndrome (AIDS), *Pneumocystis,* and nontuberculous mycobacteria are also known to cause atypical pneumonia.[3] Pneumonia caused by these agents might have slightly "atypical" presentation, e.g., *Legionella* species can present with headache, confusion, diarrhea, and clinical manifestations of hyponatremia. *M. pneumoniae* can be associated with upper respiratory involvement (otitis and pharyngitis), skin changes (Stevens–Johnson syndrome), and hemolytic anemia. Extrapulmonary manifestations such as arthritis, endocarditis, and meningitis are seen in immunocompromised patients but are rare. However, clinical or radiological differentiation between typical or atypical pneumonia is not reliable to guide antibiotic treatment. *M. pneumoniae* is susceptible to macrolides, tetracyclines, quinolones, streptomycin, pristinamycin, and ketolides. Erythromycin-resistant strains of *M. pneumoniae* have been isolated due to point mutations in *23rRNA* gene.

Q36. What are the management concerns in patients with *Legionella* pneumonia (Legionnaire's disease)?
Pneumonia occurring due to *Legionella* infection is termed as Legionnaire's disease. It is often mild, self-limited flu-like illness called "Pontiac fever" often diagnosed clinically during outbreaks. It is mainly due to exposure to contaminated water and its subsequent aspiration leading to pneumonia. High-risk group includes old age, male gender, tobacco smoking, diabetes, hematological malignancy, cancer, end-stage renal disease, human immunodeficiency virus (HIV) infections, and patients with immunosuppression. Clinically and radiologically, *Legionella* pneumonia is similar to other forms of CAP but fails to respond to routine β-lactam monotherapy. Choice of antibiotic is quinolone which are superior to macrolides as per current evidence. Quinolones lowers mortality rate and there is significant decrease in length of hospital stay.[60] Apart from this, doxycycline can be used. Duration of treatment in mild-to-moderate disease lasts for 7–10 days whereas in severe disease or immunocompromised host, it is to be continued till 21 days.

Q37. How will you treat a patient with SARS-CoV-2 who has CAP?
As per the clinical practice guidelines for management of adult COVID-19 patients by ICMR—COVID-19 national task force /joint monitoring group,[61] the treatment strategies are as per **Flowchart 1**.

Q38. What are the newer antibiotics under development to treat CAP?
- *New macrolide:* EDP-788 has activity against many bacterial organisms, including the macrolide-resistant isolates of *S. pneumoniae, Streptococcus pyogenes*, and MRSA.
- *New tetracyclines:* TP-271 is a promising new fluorocycline antibiotic active against community-acquired respiratory gram-positive and gram-negative bacteria including atypical pathogens.
- *Ketolide:* Known as nafithromycin (WCK-4873) and it acts against MDR pneumococci.

Community-acquired Pneumonia

Flowchart 1: Clinical practice guidelines for management of adult COVID-19 patients.

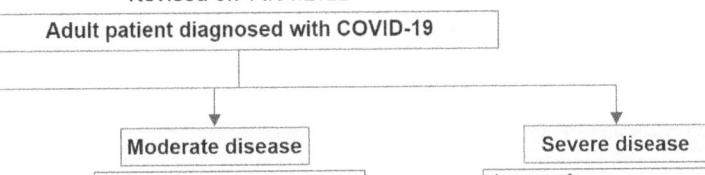

AIIMS/ICMR-COVID-19 National Task Force/Joint Monitoring Group (Dte.GHS)
Ministry of Health & Family Welfare, Government of India
CLINICAL GUIDANCE FOR MANAGEMENT OF ADULT COVID-19 PATIENTS
Revised on 14/01/2022

Adult patient diagnosed with COVID-19

Mild disease
Upper respiratory tract symptoms and/or fever WITHOUT shortness of breath or hypoxia

Home isolation and care
(Refer to relevant guideline)

MUST DOs
- Physical distancing, indoor mask use, strict hand hygiene
- Symptomatic management (hydration, anti-pyretics, anti-tussive)
- Monitor temperature and oxygen saturation (by applying a SpO_2 probe to fingers)
- Stay in contact with treating physician

Seek immediate medical attention if:
- Difficulty in breathing or SpO_2 ≤93%
- High grade fever/severe cough, particularly if lasting for >5 days
- A low threshold to be kept for those with any of the high-risk features

High-risk for severe disease or mortality
- Age > 60 years
- Cardiovascular disease, and CAD
- Diabetes mellitus and other immunocompromised states (such as HIV)
- Active tuberculosis
- Chronic lung/kidney/liver disease
- Cerebrovascular disease
- Obesity
- Unvaccinated

- Antibiotics should not be used unless there is clinical suspicion of bacterial infection
- Possibility of coinfection of COVID-19 with other endemic infections must be considered
- Systemic corticosteroids are not indicated in mild disease

Do not use in COVID-19
- Lopinavir-ritonavir
- Hydroxychloroquine
- Ivermectin
- Neutralizing monoclonal antibody
- Convalescent plasma
- Molnupiravir
- Favipiravir
- Azithromycin
- Doxycycline

Moderate disease
Any one of:
1. Respiratory rate ≥24/min, breathlessness
2. SpO_2: 90% to ≤ 93% on room air

ADMIT IN WARD

Oxygen support:
- Target SpO_2: 92–96% (88–92% in patients with COPD)
- Preferred devices for oxygenation: non-rebreathing face mask
- Awake proning encouraged in all patients requiring supplemental oxygen therapy (sequential position changes every 2 hours)

Anti-inflammatory or immunomodulatory therapy:
- Dexamethasone 6 mg/day or equivalent dose of methylprednisolone (32 mg in 4 divided doses) usually for 5 to 10 days or until discharge, whichever is earlier.
- Patients may be initiated or switched to oral route if stable and/or improving
- There is no evidence for benefit for systemic steroids in those NOT requiring oxygen supplementation, or on continuation after discharge
- Anti-inflammatory or immunomodulatory therapy (such as steroids) can have risk of secondary infection such as invasive mucormycosis when used at higher dose or for longer than required

Anticoagulation:
- Prophylactic dose of unfractionated heparin or low molecular weight heparin (weight based e.g., enoxaparin 0.5, mg/kg per day SC) There should be no contraindication or high risk of bleeding

Monitoring:
- *Clinical monitoring:* Respiratory rate, hemodynamic instability, change in oxygen requirement
- Serial CXR; HRCT chest to be done ONLY if there is worsening
- *Lab monitoring:* CRP, D-dimer, blood sugar 48 to 72 hrly, CBC, KFT, LFT 24 to 48 hrly

Severe disease
Any one of:
1. Respiratory rate >30/min, breathlessness
2. SpO_2 < 90% on room air

ADMIT IN HDU/ICU

Respiratory and cardiovascular support:
- Consider use of NIV (Helmet or face mask interface depending on availability) in patients with increasing oxygen requirement, if work of breathing is LOW
- Consider use of HFNC in patients with increasing oxygen requirement
- Intubation should be prioritized in patients with high work of breathing /if NIV is not tolerated
- Use institutional protocol for ventilatory management when required
- Need for vasopressors to be considered based on clinical situation

Anti-inflammatory or immunomodulatory therapy:
- Dexamethasone 6 mg/day or equivalent dose of methylprednisolone (32 mg in 4 divided doses) usually for 5 to 10 days or until discharge, whichever is earlier. No evidence for benefit in higher doses
- Anti-inflammatory or immunomodulatory therapy (such as steroids) can have risk of secondary infection such as invasive mucormycosis when used at higher dose or for longer than required

Anticoagulation:
- Prophylactic dose of unfractionated heparin or low molecular weight heparin (weight based e.g., enoxaparin 0.5 mg/kg per day SC). There should be no contraindication or high risk of bleeding

Supportive measures:
- Maintain euvolemia (if available, use dynamic measures for assessing fluid responsiveness)
- If sepsis/septic shock: Manage as per existing protocol and local antibiogram

Monitoring:
- *Clinical monitoring:* Work of breathing, hemodynamic instability, change in oxygen requirement
- Serial CXR; HRCT chest to be done only if there is worsening
- *Lab monitoring:* CRP, D-dimer, blood sugar 48 to 72 hrly; CBC, KFT, LFT 24 to 48 hrly

→ After clinical improvement, discharge as per revised discharge criteria

Additionally in moderate or severe disease at high risk of progression
Consider Remdesivir for up to 5 days (200 mg IV on day 1 followed by 100 mg IV OD for next 4 days)
- To be started within 10 days of onset of symptoms, in those having moderate to severe disease with high risk of progression (requiring supplemental oxygen), but who are NOT on IMV or ECMO
- No evidence of benefit for treatment more than 5 days
- NOT to be used in patients who are NOT on oxygen support or in home setting
- Monitor for RFT and LFT (remdesivir not recommended if eGFR <30 mL/min/m² AST/ALT >5 times UNL) (not an absolute contraindication)

Additionally in rapidly progressing moderate or severe disease
Consider Tocilizumab preferably within 24–48 hours of onset of severe disease/ICU admission [4 to 6 mg/kg (400 mg in 60 kg adult) in 100 mL NS over 1 hour] if the following conditions are met:
- Rapidly progressing COVID-19 not responding adequately to steroids and needing oxygen supplementation or IMV
- Preferably to be given with steroids
- Significantly raised inflammatory markers (CRP and/or IL-6)
- Rule out active TB, fungal, systemic bacterial infection
- Long term follow up for secondary infections (such as reactivation of TB, flaring of Herpes)

- *New quinolone:* ACH-702, WCK-771 acts against many MDR organisms. WCK-2349 is an oral amino-acidic ester, a prodrug of levonadifloxacin with remarkably high oral bioavailability. WCK-771, KPI-10, JNJ-Q2, and gepotidacin have sufficient penetration to respiratory tissues, improved activity against resistant respiratory pathogens, including MRSA. Avarofloxacin appears to be one of the most potent fluoroquinolones currently under clinical development. Gepotidacin (GSK2140944) is a novel broad-spectrum fluoroquinolone.
- *Glycopeptide-cephalosporin heterodimer antibiotic:* TD-1607 is the most potent among daptomycin, vancomycin, teicoplanin, linezolid, and ceftaroline which acts against gram-positive organisms.
- *Oxazolidinones:* Radezolid, a more potent oral antibiotic than linezolid, also showed excellent activity against CAP pathogens. Delpazolid, radezolid, and MRX-1 are promising agents for difficult CAP.
- Further research is warranted in order to assess potential superiority of newer antibiotics.[62]

Q39. What is the role of immunization in prevention of pneumonia?

Vaccination against influenza and to some extent *S. pneumoniae* have definitive role in preventing pneumonia.

Currently, two types of influenza vaccines have been proposed:
1. Inactivated influenza vaccine (IIV)
2. Intranasal live attenuated influenza vaccine (LAIV4)

Role of pneumococcal vaccine has not been clearly defined. Currently, two types of pneumococcal vaccines are available:
1. Polysaccharide vaccine
2. Conjugate vaccine

Q40. What are the isolation practices in patients with MRSA pneumonia in ICU?

Standards precautions, contact precautions, and additional precautions should be implemented to prevent spread of MRSA in healthcare facility as per the CDC.

Q41. What is the CAP bundle?[63]

A pilot program in Britain, involving 16 hospitals, had implemented a quality improvement program referred as "CAP bundle". They analyzed 2,118 adults and showed that there is significant reduction in 30-day mortality (13.6–8.8%) after implementation of CAP bundle. Also, they observed that there is better adherence to early administration of antibiotics within 4 hours of admission. There are four elements of CAP bundle (acronym COST):
1. *Chest radiograph*: To be obtained within 4 hours of hospital admission in all adults with suspected CAP
2. Oxygen assessment and prescription in keeping with the British Thoracic Society oxygen guidelines
3. Severity assessment supported by the CURB-65 score
4. Timely and targeted antibiotics given according to CAP severity within 4 hours of admission.

REFERENCES

1. Fishman JA, Grippi MA, Elias JA. Fishman's Pulmonary Diseases and Disorders, 5th edition. New York: McGraw-Hill Education; 2015. pp. 4181-211.
2. Martin-Loeches I, Torres A, Nagavci B. Aliberti S, Antonelli M, Bassetti M, et al. ERS/ESICM/ESCMID/ALAT guidelines for the management of severe community-acquired pneumonia. Intensive Care Med. 2023;49:615-32.
3. Mandell GL, Dolin RB. Principles and Practices of Infectious Diseases, 7th edition. Philadelphia: Elsevier; 2010. pp. 891-916.
4. Carrillo A, Gonzalez-Diaz G, Ferrer M, Martinez-Quintana ME, Lopez-Martinez A, Llamas N, et al. Non-invasive ventilation in community-acquired pneumonia and severe acute respiratory failure. Intensive Care Med. 2012;38:458-66.
5. Frat JP, Thille AW, Mercat A, Girault C, Ragot S, Perbet S, et al. High-flow oxygen through nasal cannula in acute hypoxemic respiratory failure. N Engl J Med. 2015;372:2185-96.
6. Monro-Somerville T, Sim M, Ruddy J, Vilas M, Gillies MA. The effect of high-flow nasal cannula oxygen therapy on mortality and intubation rate in acute respiratory failure: A Systematic review and meta-analysis. Crit Care Med. 2017;45:e449-56.
7. Misch EA, Verbon A, Prins JM, Skerrett SJ, Hawn TR. A TLR6 polymorphism is associated with increased risk of Legionnaires' disease. Genes Immun. 2013;14:420-6.
8. Rautanen A, Mills TC, Gordon AC, Hutton P, Steffens M, Nuamah R, et al. Genome-wide association study of survival from sepsis due to pneumonia: an observational cohort study. Lancet Respir Med. 2015;3:53-60.
9. Metlay JP, Waterer GW, Long AC, Anzueto A, Brozek J, Crothers K, et al. Diagnosis and treatment of adults with community-acquired pneumonia. An Official Clinical Practice Guideline of the American Thoracic Society and Infectious Diseases Society of America. Am J Respir Crit Care Med. 2019;200:e45-e67.
10. Musher DM, Thorner AR. Community-Acquired Pneumonia. N Engl J Med. 2014;371:1619-28.
11. Apisarnthanarak A, Mundy LM. Etiology of community-acquired pneumonia. Clin Chest Med. 2005;26:47-55.
12. Torres A, Peetermans WE, Viegi G, Blasi F. Risk factors for community-acquired pneumonia in adults in Europe: A literature review. Thorax. 2013;68:1057-65.
13. Prina E, Ranzani OT, Torres A. Community-acquired pneumonia. Lancet. 2015;386:1097-108.
14. Jain S, Self WH, Wunderink RG, Fakhran S, Balk R, Bramley AM, et al. Community-Acquired Pneumonia Requiring Hospitalization among U.S. Adults. N Engl J Med. 2015;373: 415-27.
15. Falsey A, Walsh E. Viral pneumonia in older adults. Clin Infect Dis. 2006;42:518-24.
16. Gadsby NJ, Russell CD, Mchugh MP, Mark H, Conway Morris A, Laurenson IF, et al. Comprehensive molecular testing for

respiratory pathogens in community-acquired pneumonia. Clin Infect Dis. 2016;62:817-23.
17. Musher DM, Montoya R, Wanahita A. Diagnostic value of microscopic examination of gram-stained sputum and sputum cultures in patients with bacteremic pneumococcal pneumonia. Clin Infect Dis. 2004;39:165-9.
18. Gutiérrez F, Masiá M, Rodríguez JC, Ayelo A, Soldán B, Cebrián L, et al. Evaluation of the immunochromatographic Binax NOW assay for detection of Streptococcus pneumoniae urinary antigen in a prospective study of community-acquired pneumonia in Spain. Clin Infect Dis. 2003;36:286-92.
19. Martin-Loeches I, Torres A. New guidelines for severe community-acquired pneumonia. Curr Opin Pulm Med. 2021;27(3):210-5.
20. Lin WH, Chiu HC, Chen KF, Tsao KC, Chen YY, Li TH, et al. Molecular detection of respiratory pathogens in community-acquired pneumonia involving adults. J Microbiol Immunol Infect. 2022;55(5):829-37.
21. Baudel JL, Tankovic J, Dahoumane R, Carrat F, Galbois A, Ait-Oufella H, et al. Multiplex PCR performed of bronchoalveolar lavage fluid increases pathogen identification rate in critically ill patients with pneumonia: A pilot study. Ann Intensive Care. 2014;4:35.
22. ICMR. (2023). Advisory on Purposive Testing Strategy for COVID-19 in India. [online] Available from: https://www.icmr.gov.in/pdf/covid/strategy/Advisory_COVID_Testing_08022023.pdf [last accessed August, 2023].
23. Hagaman JT, Panos RJ, Rouan GW, Shipley RT. Admission chest radiograph lacks sensitivity in the diagnosis of community-acquired pneumonia. Am J Med Sci. 2009;337:236-40.
24. Claessens YE, Debray MP, Tubach F, Brun AL, Rammaert B, Hausfater P, et al. Early chest computed tomography scan to assist diagnosis and guide treatment decision for suspected community-acquired pneumonia. Am J Respir Crit Care Med. 2015;192:974-82.
25. Chavez MA, Shams N, Ellington LE, Naithani N, Gilman RH, Steinhoff MC, et al. Lung ultrasound for the diagnosis of pneumonia in adults: a systematic review and meta-analysis. Respir Res. 2014;15(1):50.
26. Light RW. The light criteria: the beginning and why they are useful 40 years later. Clin Chest Med. 2013;34:21-6.
27. Welker JA, Huston M, McCue JD. Antibiotic timing and errors in diagnosing pneumonia. Arch Intern Med. 2008;168:351-6.
28. Lee MS, Oh JY, Kang CI, Kim ES, Park S, Rhee CK, et al. Guidelines for antibiotic use in adults with community-acquired pneumonia. Infect Chemother. 2018;50:160-98.
29. Garin N, Genné D, Carballo S, Chuard C, Eich G, Hugli O, et al. β-lactam monotherapy vs β-lactam-macrolide combination treatment in moderately severe community-acquired pneumonia: A randomized noninferiority trial. JAMA Intern Med. 2014;174:1-8.
30. Mandell LA, Waterer GW. Empirical therapy of community-acquired pneumonia: advancing evidence or just more doubt? JAMA. 2015;314:396-7.
31. Rodrigo C, Mckeever TM, Woodhead M, Lim WS, British Thoracic Society. Single versus combination antibiotic therapy in adults hospitalised with community-acquired pneumonia. Thorax. 2013;68:493-5.
32. World Health Organization. (2010). WHO Guidelines for Pharmacological Management of Pandemic Influenza A (H1N1) 2009 and Other Influenza Viruses: Part I Recommendations. [online] Available from: https://www.who.int/csr/resources/ publications/swineflu/h1n1_guidelines_pharmaceutical_ mngt.pdf. [Last Accessed August, 2023].
33. Fiore AE, Fry A, Shay D, Gubareva L, Bresee JS, Uyeki TM, et al. Antiviral agents for the treatment and chemoprophylaxis of influenza—recommendations of the Advisory Committee on Immunization Practices (ACIP). MMWR Recomm Rep. 2011;60:1-24.
34. van der Sluijs KF, van der Poll T, Lutter R, Juffermans NP, Schultz MJ. Bench-to-bedside review: bacterial pneumonia with influenza—pathogenesis and clinical implications. Crit Care. 2010;14:219.
35. Corrales-Medina VF, Alvarez KN, Weissfeld LA, Angus DC, Chirinos JA, Chang CC, et al. Association between hospitalization for pneumonia and subsequent risk of cardiovascular disease. JAMA. 2015;313:264-74.
36. Restrepo MI, Reyes LF. Pneumonia as a cardiovascular disease. Respirology. 2018;23:250-9.
37. Rhodes A, Evans LE, Alhazzani W, Levy MM, Antonelli M, Ferrer R, et al. Surviving Sepsis Campaign: International Guidelines for Management of Sepsis and Septic Shock: 2016. Intensive Care Med. 2017;43:304-77.
38. Alves J, Alp E, Koulenti D, Zhang Z, Ehrmann S, Blot S, et al. Nebulization of antimicrobial agents in mechanically ventilated adults in 2017: an international cross-sectional survey. Eur J Clin Microbiol Infect Dis. 2018;37(4):785-94.
39. Khan AR, Riaz M, Bin Abdulhak AA, Al-Tannir MA, Garbati MA, Erwin PJ, et al. The role of statins in prevention and treatment of community-acquired pneumonia: a systematic review and meta-analysis. PLoS One. 2013;8:e52929.
40. Ni YN, Chen G, Sun J, Liang BM, Liang ZA. The effect of corticosteroids on mortality of && patients with influenza pneumonia: a systematic review and meta-analysis. Crit Care 2019;23:99.
41. Stern A, Skalsky K, Avni T, Carrara E, Leibovici L, Paul M. Corticosteroids for pneumonia. Cochrane database Syst Rev. 2017;12:CD007720.
42. Meduri GU, Shih M-C, Bridges L, Martin TJ, El-Solh A, Seam N, et al. Low-dose methylprednisolone treatment in critically ill patients with severe community-acquired pneumonia. Intensive Care Med. 2022;48:1009-23.
43. Dequin PF, Meziani F, Quenot JP, Kamel T, Ricard JD, Badie J, et al; CRICS-TriGGERSep Network. Hydrocortisone in severe community-acquired pneumonia. N Engl J Med. 2023;388(21):1931-41.
44. Huang J, Guo J, Li H, Huang W, Zhang T. Efficacy and safety of adjunctive corticosteroids therapy for patients with severe community-acquired pneumonia. Medicine. 2019;98:e14636.
45. Halm EA, Fine MJ, Marrie TJ, Coley CM, Kapoor WN, Obrosky DS, et al. Time to clinical stability in patients hospitalized with

community-acquired pneumonia: implications for practice guidelines. JAMA. 1998;279:1452-7.
46. Li JZ, Winston LG, Moore DH, Bent S. Efficacy of short-course antibiotic regimens for community-acquired pneumonia: A meta-analysis. Am J Med. 2007;120:783-90.
47. Viasus D, Del Rio-Pertuz G, Simonetti AF, Garcia-Vidal C, Acost- Reyes J, Garavito A, et al. Biomarkers for predicting short-term mortality in community-acquired pneumonia : A systematic review and meta-analysis. J Infect. 2016;72:273-82.
48. Pfister R, Kochanek M, Leygeber T, Brun-Buisson C, Cuquemelle E, Machado MB, et al. Procalcitonin for diagnosis of bacterial pneumonia in critically ill patients during 2009 H1N1 influenza pandemic: a prospective cohort study, systematic review and individual patient data meta-analysis. Crit Care. 2014;18:R44.
49. Christ-Crain M, Stolz D, Bingisser R, Müller C, Miedinger D, Huber PR, et al. Procalcitonin guidance of antibiotic therapy in community-acquired pneumonia: A randomized trial. Am J Respir Crit Care Med. 2006;174(1):84-93.
50. Huang DT, Yealy DM, Filbin MR, Brown AM, Chang CC, Doi Y, et al. Procalcitonin-Guided Use of Antibiotics for Lower Respiratory Tract Infection. N Engl J Med. 2018;379:236-49.
51. Wunderink RG, Waterer G. Advances in the causes and management of community-acquired pneumonia in adults. BMJ. 2017;358:j2471.
52. Schuetz P, Wirz Y, Sager R, Stolz D, Tamm M, Bouadma L, et al. Procalcitonin to initiate or discontinue antibiotics in acute respiratory tract infections (Review). Cochrane Database Syst Rev. 2017;10:CD007498.
53. Tsalik EL, Henao R, Nichols M, Burke T, Ko ER, Mcclain MT, et al. Host gene expression classifiers diagnose acute respiratory illness etiology. Sci Transl Med. 2016;8:322-11.
54. Defres S, Marwick C, Nathwani D. MRSA as a cause of lung infection including airway infection, community-acquired pneumonia and hospital-acquired pneumonia. Eur Respir J. 2009;34:1470-6.
55. Kallen AJ, Brunkard J, Moore Z, Budge P, Arnold KE, Fosheim G, et al. Staphylococcus aureus Community-Acquired Pneumonia During the 2006 to 2007 Influenza Season. Ann Emerg Med. 2009;53:358-65.
56. Liu C, Bayer A, Cosgrove SE, Daum RS, Fridkin SK, Gorwitz RJ, et al. Clinical practice guidelines by the Infectious Diseases Society of America for the treatment of methicillin-resistant Staphylococcus aureus infections in adults and children. Clin Infect Dis. 2011;52:e18-55.
57. Zhong NS, Sun T, Zhuo C, D'Souza G, Lee SH, Lan NH, et al. Ceftaroline fosamil versus ceftriaxone for the treatment of Asian patients with community-acquired pneumonia: a randomised, controlled, double-blind, phase 3, non-inferiority with nested superiority trial. Lancet Infect Dis. 2015;15:161-71.
58. Falagas M, Karageorgopoulos D, Dimopoulos G. Clinical significance of the pharmacokinetic and pharmacodynamic characteristics of tigecycline. Curr Drug Metab. 2009;10:13-21.
59. Falagas ME, Metaxas EI. Tigecycline for the treatment of patients with community-acquired pneumonia requiring hospitalization. Expert Rev Anti Infect Ther. 2009;7:913-23.
60. Burdet C, Lepeule R, Duval X, Caseris M, Rioux C, Lucet JC, et al. Quinolones versus macrolides in the treatment of legionellosis: a systematic review and meta-analysis. J Antimicrob Chemother. 2014;69:2354-60.
61. ICMR. (2023). Adult patient diagnosed with COVID-19. [online] Available from: https://www.icmr.gov.in/pdf/covid/techdoc/COVID_Clinical_Management_19032023.pdf [Last accessed August, 2023].
62. Liapikou A, Cillóniz C, Torres A. Investigational drugs in phase I and phase II clinical trials for the treatment of community-acquired pneumonia. Expert Opin Investig Drugs. 2017;26:1239-48.
63. Lim WS, Rodrigo C, Turner AM, Welham S, Calvert JM. British Thoracic Society community-acquired pneumonia care bundle: Results of a national implementation project. Thorax. 2016;71:288-90.

CHAPTER 3

Liberation from Mechanical Ventilation, Ventilator-associated Pneumonia, and ICU-acquired Weakness

Jacob George Pulinilkunnathil, Vijaya Patil

CASE STUDY

A 36-year-old gentleman with fat embolism syndrome following a road traffic accident was being ventilated for type 1 respiratory failure for the past 7 days. He was not on any antibiotics and seemed to be improving with improved gas exchange over the past 48 hours. On day 7, the sedation was stopped and the patient was calm and comfortable, on pressure support ventilation (PSV) with a pressure support of 12 cmH$_2$O, positive end-expiratory pressure (PEEP) of 6 cmH$_2$O and fraction of inspired oxygen (FiO$_2$) 0.4. He was generating tidal volume between 6 and 8 mL/kg. A plan to liberate the patient from mechanical ventilation was made, and a spontaneous breathing trial (SBT) with T-piece was given. 20 minutes into the breathing trial, the patient became diaphoretic, tachypneic (respiratory rate 40 breaths/min), tachycardic (heart rate 130 beats/min), and seemed to be in respiratory distress. He was put back on PSV for the day.

Q1. When will you assess the patient for liberation from mechanical ventilation?

As early as 1987, Hall et al. had suggested to replace the term weaning from mechanical ventilation by the more appropriate term "liberation from mechanical ventilation".[1] The intensivist should plan for liberation from mechanical ventilation from the moment the patient is initiated on mechanical ventilation. Once the primary pathology is resolved (or resolving), and the patient remains hemodynamically stable or is on a minimal dose of vasopressors, with FiO$_2$ requirement <0.4, the patient should be considered for a weaning trial.[2,3]

The decision to liberate the patient from mechanical ventilation is facilitated by the use of nurse/respiratory therapist driven protocolized weaning strategies. Weaning protocols are developed on the basis of the best available scientific evidence and are not biased by human decisions. Apart from a subset of neurosurgical patients, weaning protocols significantly reduce the duration of ventilation among all patient subsets.[4,5] Although not fully supported by evidence, the American Thoracic Society (ATS) guidelines suggest the use of weaning protocols in those who are mechanically ventilated for >24 hours.[6]

In protocolized weaning, the bedside nurse or technician assesses the patient for the possibility of successful weaning as per the criteria as suggested by a collective task force in 2001.[7]

- Hemodynamic stability, i.e., absence of any ongoing vasopressors or only a minimal dose of vasopressors (norepinephrine ≤2 µg/kg/min, or dopamine or dobutamine ≤5 µg/kg/min)
- Adequate oxygenation, i.e., a PaO$_2$/FiO$_2$ (PF) ratio >150–200 on FiO$_2$ ≤0.4–0.5 and PEEP of 5–8 cmH$_2$O, and pH >7.25
- Resolution of the primary pathology
- No evidence of a new infection or myocardial ischemia. After ensuring that these criteria are fulfilled, the sedation is stopped, and the patient is allowed to wake up and trigger the ventilator. Once the patient is awake, generating adequate minute volume and obeying commands, a SBT is carried out.

Q2. What is automatic tube compensation (ATC) and what is its role in weaning?

Some modern ventilators offer ATC or tube compensation (TC) which is supposed to facilitate better patient-ventilator synchrony and reduce the work of breathing. While breathing through a narrow endotracheal tube, there is a nonlinear gas flow across the tube that depends upon the inspiratory flow rate. This results in dissipation of pressure at the carinal end of endotracheal tube and the airway pressure that is set may not reach the carinal end of the endotracheal tube. This pressure drop results in inadequate pressure support and increased work of breathing, especially when the inspiratory demand and inspiratory flows are high. Patients undergoing SBT with pressure support mode or continuous positive airway pressure (CPAP) can have either an overcompensation or undercompensation for this pressure drop—both leading to patient-ventilator dyssynchrony. ATC compensates for this by continuously monitoring the intratracheal pressure based on the patient's inspiratory flow, the circuit pressure, and properties of the endotracheal tube in a closed loop manner. Similarly, the expiratory pressure at the tracheal end of the endotracheal tube is also measured, and in the case of expiratory resistance or dynamic hyperinflation, the expiratory airway pressure is reduced so that gas flow occurs, and the set PEEP is maintained at the carinal end of endotracheal tube. The effect of this auto-setting the intrinsic PEEP to extrinsic PEEP in patients who might be dependent on auto-PEEP for keeping alveoli open [chronic obstructive pulmonary disease (COPD)] is not clear. Altogether, by maintaining the set PEEP and reducing the pressure drop across the endotracheal tube, ATC may provide better comfort, thereby reducing ventilator dyssynchrony and requirement of sedatives and neuromuscular blockade. ATC controller incorporates several variables into the ventilator system, such as the type of tube, internal diameter, and additional general settings including the percentage of support that is to be given. With these input variables, the ATC controller in the ventilator calculates the support that is to be given and adjusts the support in a closed loop manner. Extreme care must be taken to ensure that these details are entered correctly, and patient is continually monitored for adverse effects and increased work of breathing. Apart from ATC, adequate ventilatory support should be given as per the patient's disease status. Even for the given inner diameter of the tube, because of crusting of secretions, tube kinks and secretions inside the tube, adequate compensation may not be attained with ATC. Hence, all patients on ATC need vigilant and continuous monitoring. Multiple trials on the effect of ATC on weaning have not revealed a positive result as compared to other weaning modes.[8-10]

Automated weaning systems: Over the recent years, there has been an increased interest in the use of automated closed loop systems for weaning. These automated closed loop systems have a system of continuous monitoring with real-time interventions to adapt to the patient's ventilatory needs. They are able to recognize a patient's ability to breathe spontaneously, reducing avoidable delays of clinician recognition of the patient's weaning status, clinician expertise, and his workload. Depending on the inherent programming, some systems can switch automatically from controlled modes to spontaneous ones while others rely on clinician activation for the same. Cochrane reviews suggest that automated systems reduce ventilation duration and intensive care unit (ICU) length of stay although there was no influence on mortality, reintubation, or hospital length of stay. However, more homogeneous good quality trials are required before they can be recommended for routine use in ICU.[4,11-13]

Table 1 summarizes the available closed loop systems for automated weaning.

Q3. How does liberation from mechanical ventilation affect cardiac function and oxygen consumption?
Mechanical ventilation reduces the venous return to the heart and thereby reduces the preload to both ventricles. By an increase in the pleural pressure, mechanical ventilation reduces the transmural pressure, resulting in an overall improved left ventricular function. During resumption of spontaneous breathing, as this positive pressure is reduced or removed, the preload to the heart increases, the afterload of the left ventricle increases (as the transmural pressure increases), and consequently, the stress on the left ventricle

TABLE 1: Available closed loop systems for automated weaning.

Trade name of closed loop system	Description
Adaptive support ventilation (ASV)	• Closed loop monitoring of inspiratory pressure, respiratory rate, and minute ventilation. It can automatically adjust pressure support according to spontaneous respiratory rate to maintain minute ventilation set by clinician • IntelliVent-ASV® uses similar monitoring, adjust minute ventilation but also monitors end-tidal carbon dioxide, positive end-expiratory pressure, and the fraction of inspired oxygen
Proportional assist ventilation	• Maintains a preset clinician determined support throughout inspiration • Augments inspiratory support based on changes in compliance and resistance (based on patient demand)
SmartCare pressure support by Drager	• Closed loop monitoring of pressure support based on respiratory rate, tidal volume, and end-tidal carbon dioxide • Provides automatic protocolized weaning
Neurally adjusted ventilatory assist (NAVA)	Measures the electrical diaphragmatic activity via a catheter inserted in the esophagus and delivers breath in time with and proportional to diaphragmatic activity to maintain adequate tidal volume
Mandatory minute ventilation (MMV)	Maintains a predetermined minute ventilation based on closed loop control of the mandatory breaths rate and spontaneous breaths

increases. This can precipitate myocardial ischemia and pulmonary edema in vulnerable patients, which initiates a vicious spiral eventually causing a failure to wean.[14] At the bedside, weaning-induced cardiac failure can be readily assessed by simple tests such as measurement of brain-type natriuretic peptide (BNP), N-terminal pro-BNP (NT-proBNP), plasma-protein concentration, and by bedside echocardiography. Patients at risk of failing a SBT may be identified by measuring the plasma BNP level. Dessap and colleagues showed that the baseline plasma BNP level was higher in patients who failed a SBT as compared to those who successfully passed SBT.[15] However, baseline BNP levels are not specific for weaning-induced cardiac dysfunction and could be elevated in other conditions such as elderly patients, those with sepsis, renal dysfunction, and pulmonary hypertension.[16]

Grasso and colleagues in a cohort of COPD patients found that the elevation of NT-proBNP during a SBT from baseline values before a SBT accurately predicted weaning-induced cardiac dysfunction in a cohort of COPD patients.[17] Similarly, an increase in plasma-protein concentration by 6% from baseline after a SBT was also shown to correlate with weaning-induced pulmonary edema.[18]

Weaning-induced cardiac dysfunction can be readily assessed at bedside noninvasively using echocardiography and lung ultrasound. Doppler measurement of early (E) and late (A) peak diastolic velocities across the mitral valve and tissue Doppler mitral annulus (Ea) in combination can accurately predict weaning-induced pulmonary artery occlusion pressure elevation.[19] Lung ultrasound will reveal the appearance of "B" lines in those patients who develop pulmonary edema after SBT, induced by liberation from mechanical ventilation.[20]

Spontaneous breathing trial increases the oxygen consumption and oxygen demand by about 15%. This is due to the mechanical load on the respiratory muscles, as it takes over the work of breathing. Unless this increased oxygen demand is met, redistribution of blood flow occurs and tissue hypoxia and lactic acidosis ensue.[21]

Q4. How will you carry out a SBT?
To carry out SBT, switch over from a controlled mode to pressure support mode and monitor for the patient for signs of respiratory distress such as tachypnea, tachycardia, diaphoresis, and use of accessory muscles. If the patient does not show signs of increased work of breathing and the minute volume generated is adequate, the pressure support then can be gradually reduced. If the patient does not develop respiratory distress even on pressure support of 7–10 cmH_2O, or CPAP of 5 cmH_2O,[22] the patient can be extubated. PSV with pressure support of 5–10 cmH_2O reduces the work of inspiration by 30–60%. Hence, these patients might experience a proportional increase in work of breathing after extubation. Usually, this increase in work of breathing is well tolerated although it may result in a failure to be liberated from mechanical ventilation in borderline patients.[23]

One can also use a direct T-piece trial for liberation from mechanical ventilation, especially in patients with short-term ventilation and in those whom occult cardiac failure is suspected and needs assessment before extubation.

In centers where synchronized intermittent mandatory ventilation (SIMV) is still considered as a weaning mode, one should gradually decrease the rate of mandatory breaths and observe for signs of respiratory distress. However, current evidence discourages use of SIMV alone as a weaning mode.[24]

All these methods—T-piece trial, PSV, and SIMV alone were compared by Brochard et al. and they found that PSV fared better as a weaning mode compared to others.[25] Esteban and colleagues found that the time to liberation from mechanical ventilation was significantly higher for patients on SIMV alone than PSV or T-piece alone.[26]

In 2008, the Awakening and Breathing Controlled (ABC) trial suggested that the combined approach of daily interruption of sedation along with a SBT results in faster liberation from mechanical ventilation than routine care and SBT.[27]

Q5. What is the optimal duration of SBT?
Spontaneous breathing trial of 30-minute duration has the same predictive ability for liberation from mechanical ventilation failures as that of a 120-minute SBT, with the majority of the failures occurring within 20 minutes.[28] Hence, the current practice is to carry out a 30-minute SBT with the probable exceptions of those who are at high risk of weaning failures such as COPD or those who had a very prolonged duration of mechanical ventilation. The data on SBT for these high-risk groups is lacking, and these patients might benefit from a longer liberation trial (not backed by strong evidence) or may be extubated and put electively on noninvasive ventilation (NIV).

Q6. Discuss the liberation from mechanical ventilation and extubation in neurological patients.
Liberation from mechanical ventilation in patients with neurological injury poses a clinical dilemma to the intensivist. It is not clear whether all clinical features including a level of consciousness compatible with successful extubation are required to extubate these patients. Doctors will be skeptical to extubate those with low Glasgow Coma Scale (GCS), even if they otherwise meet the criterion for SBT. These patients will have delayed extubation, increased risk

for pneumonia, increased mortality, increased ICU length of stay, and increased treatment costs. In a prospective study of 136 patients, early extubation of the patients who passed SBT, irrespective of their GCS, was associated with reduced pneumonia rates, reduced ICU length of stay, and reduced hospital length of stay. This suggests that liberation from mechanical ventilation in patients with neurological injury should be approached differently, and the patients who pass SBT may be extubated safely irrespective of their GCS score.[29,30]

Q7. Should we do a cuff leak test in all patients before extubation?

The cuff leak test was initially proposed by Miller and Cole as a method to diagnose patients who fail extubation due to upper airway edema. Here, exhaled volumes are measured before and after deflation of the endotracheal tube cuff, while the patient is still on mechanical ventilation. Various studies have suggested various cutoffs to diagnose laryngeal edema. A difference of 10% (10–24%) between inspired and expired tidal volume or 110 mL (88–283 mL) absolute differences in the volumes, rules out significant laryngeal edema.[6,31] However, there are many reports of the test being falsely positive, unnecessary prolonging extubation in many patients.[32] The guidelines suggest performing the leak test only in high-risk cases such as those who had traumatic intubation, ventilation for >6 days, female sex, and those who were reintubated after an unplanned extubation.[6]

For patients who are at high risk for postextubation laryngeal edema, systemic steroids administered prior to extubation seemed to reduce the inflammatory markers and the incidence of laryngeal edema. Methylprednisolone (20 mg) started 12 hours prior to planned extubation and repeated every 4 hours has shown to substantially reduce the reintubation due to laryngeal edema, the last dose being given immediately before extubation.[33] Similar results were also found in another two trials that used a single bolus of 40 mg methylprednisolone 4 hours before extubation.[34,35] The guidelines recommend that in patients who are at high risk of laryngeal edema, if the cuff leak is minimal/absent, systemic steroids (methylprednisolone) should be administered at least 4 hours prior to extubation. There is no role of repeating a cuff leak test after the administration of steroids.[6]

Q8. How frequently should SBT be done and why?

It is very important to detect failure of SBT early so that patient fatigue can be avoided. Diaphragmatic fatigue is one of the major causes for weaning failure and prolonged mechanical ventilation. Weaning failure due to other causes such as cardiac failure and dyselectrolytemia can also contribute to diaphragmatic fatigue prolonging the duration of mechanical ventilation.

It is proposed that any skeletal muscle when subjected to excessive load undergoes either a high-frequency contractile fatigue due to accumulation of inorganic phosphate or a low-frequency contractile fatigue due to development of muscle injury or combination of both. Laghi et al. in a study on healthy volunteers showed that induction of diaphragmatic fatigue produced a significant reduction in contractility that persisted for a period of at least 24 hours.[36] In animal models, it has been shown that low-frequency fatigue that develops due to breathing against a load causes a muscle injury that peaks after 72 hours resulting in a chronic reduction in the force-generating capacity of the diaphragm.[37] Laghi et al. failed to prove the role of low-frequency fatigue in causing weaning failure immediately after a SBT and proposed that other abnormalities such as diaphragmatic weakness, atrophy, high-frequency fatigue, and hyperinflation may be contributory factors.[38] It seems that although we cannot attribute weaning failure to the low-frequency fatigue, it might be still important as it may lead to respiratory muscle injury that peaks at 72 hours.[39,40] Trials have explored the possibility of further improving the chance of extubation success by eliminating the high-frequency contractile fatigue after SBT. The results of the RECONNECT trial though seemingly encouraging, need further validation.[41]

The optimum time for a repeat SBT in case of prior SBT failure is a matter of debate. Most clinicians prefer to perform the next SBT only after 24 hours of rest, although twice daily SBTs have also been conducted.[42,43] Trials have looked into the benefit of twice daily SBT versus single SBT and results are awaited.[44] Till the evidence is strong, the current practice is in favor of a once daily SBT.

Q9. What is difficult weaning and weaning failure?

Weaning failure is defined as "the failure to pass an initial trial of spontaneous breathing or requirement of reintubation within 48 hours of extubation". Some authors consider up to 72 hours for defining weaning failure.[45] Extubation failure of any cause will also be included as weaning failure. Weaning failure has been classified as per the definitions of the International Consensus Conference in 2005 and is summarized in **Flowchart 1**.[24]

Simple weaning: Patients who are successfully extubated after the first SBT.

Difficult weaning: Patients who fail the initial SBT and require up to three SBTs, or up to 7 days from the first or initial SBT for liberation from mechanical ventilation.

Prolonged weaning: Patients who require more than three SBTs or >7 days from the initial SBT.

Liberation from Mechanical Ventilation, Ventilator-associated Pneumonia, and ICU-acquired Weakness

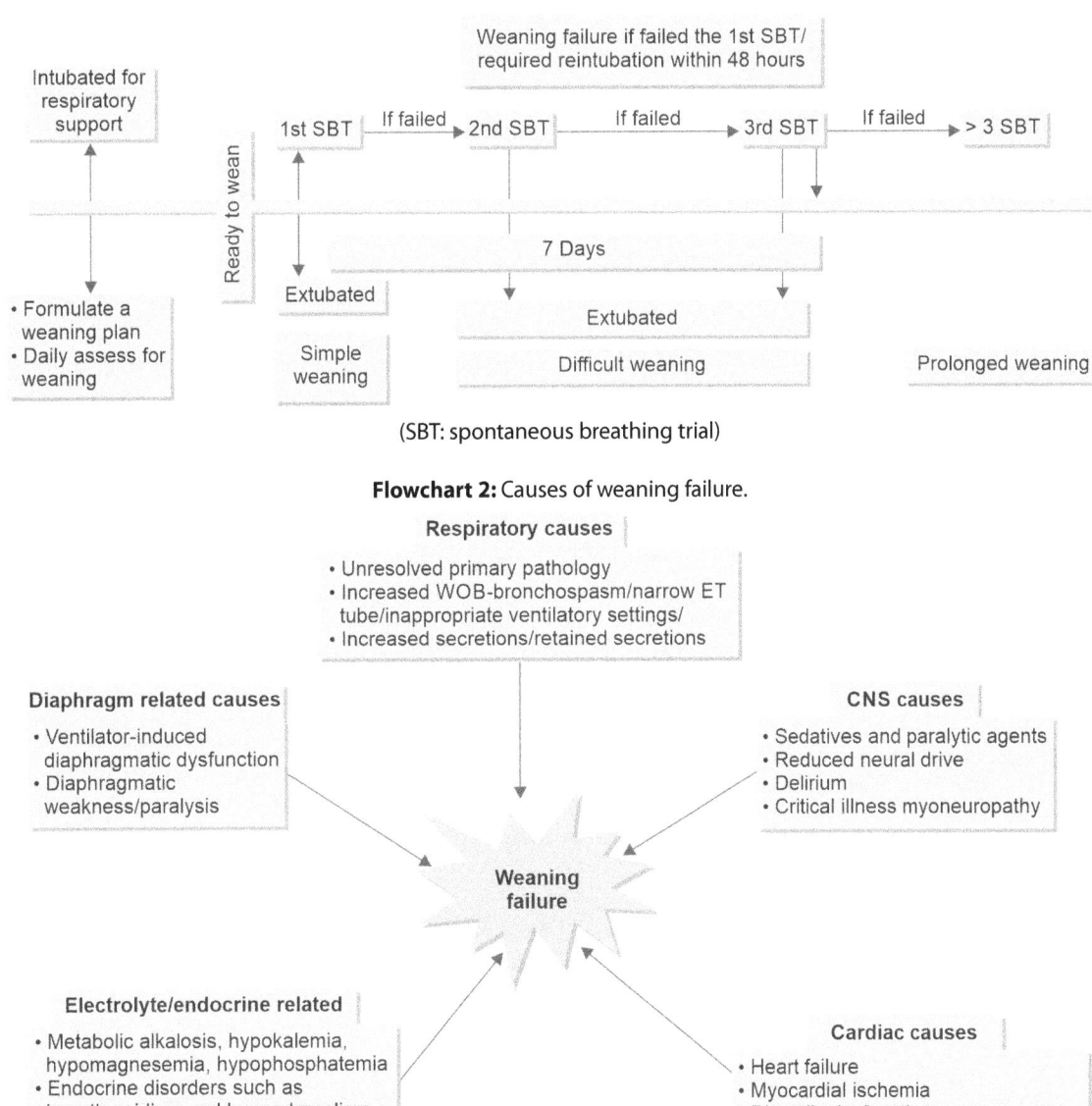

Flowchart 1: Classification of weaning.

(SBT: spontaneous breathing trial)

Flowchart 2: Causes of weaning failure.

(CNS: central nervous system; ET: endotracheal tube; WOB: work of breathing)

Q10. How will you approach a case of weaning failure? What is the ABCDE approach?

In case of a prior weaning failure, one should try to find out cause of failure and optimize patient's condition before the next weaning attempt. There are various causes of weaning failure and a structured algorithm may help in ruling out these causes. The important causes can be clubbed together and remembered with the aid of mnemonic—ABCDE—Airway (respiratory), Brain, Cardiac, Diaphragm, and Endocrine-related causes as shown in **Flowchart 2**.[46]

Q11. How can you predict weaning failure at the bedside?

For successful liberation from ventilatory support, the patient needs to have a good general condition with the ability to protect his airway. The ventilatory capacity of the patient needs to be assessed objectively. The success of liberation from mechanical ventilation can be predicted by measuring the ventilatory demand and the ventilatory capacity with the help of simple weaning indices or integrated weaning indices. Patients who are at a high risk of laryngeal edema should be evaluated by a cuff leak test (mentioned earlier).

Patients at high risk for weaning failure need to be identified early and monitored closely. The risk factors for weaning failure include:[47]

- Elderly, age ≥ 65 years
- Cardiac failure
- The presence of other comorbidities than cardiac failure
- The primary indication for intubation being pneumonia

- Patents who have already failed two or more consecutive SBTs
- Those who have a baseline partial pressure of arterial carbon dioxide ($PaCO_2$) >45 mm Hg at extubation
- An APACHE II score >12 on the day of extubation
- Poor cough reflex
- Stridor or upper airway obstruction at extubation.

Among the various variables assessed, eight have been found to have a reasonable ability to predict weaning failure **(Table 2)**.

Q12. How will you prepare the patient prior to the next SBT?

- Encourage passive and active limb movements when feasible and assess for myopathy and neuropathy.
- Sedations should be stopped, and the patient should be fully awake. Assess for the presence of delirium using standard screening tools.
- The patient should be conscious, co-operative, pain-free, comfortable, and preferably in a propped-up position so that he can take deep breaths, optimize his functional residual capacity (FRC) and gas exchange.
- Address any increased airway secretions and bronchospasm.
- Review the chart for assessing cumulative fluid balance/net fluid gain. If possible, ensure a negative or at least a neutral fluid balance over the last 24–48 hours.
- Optimize other factors such as anemia, fever, and pain.
- Maintain adequate nutrition and avoid overfeeding. Avoid gastric distention, decompress the stomach in case of significant gastric distention.
- Correct acid-base abnormalities and dyselectrolytemia.
- Assess the cardiac function to rule out diastolic dysfunction and weaning-induced pulmonary edema. In indicated cases, optimize the preload and afterload and consider extubation to NIV. Prolonged T-piece trials should be discouraged in these borderline patients and pressure support/CPAP may be preferred over T-piece as SBT.
- In case the patient has failed the previous SBT on T-piece, SBT with CPAP or pressure support may be tried.[24]

The patient was put back on PSV. Bedside transthoracic echocardiography did not reveal any systolic/diastolic dysfunction or pleural effusion. Consolidation was seen on lung ultrasound on the right side. Overnight his FiO_2 requirement increased to 0.6 to maintain a saturation of 94%. He was febrile overnight (103°F). A repeat chest X-ray (CXR) confirmed the presence of a new patch on the right side of the chest.

Q13. How will you approach this patient?

Fever in the ICU is defined by the Society of Critical Care Medicine (SCCM) as a temperature >38.3°C, i.e., 101°F.[48,49] Common sources for infections in critically ill patients include sinusitis, dental infections, pneumonia, bloodstream infections, infective endocarditis, meningitis or central nervous system (CNS) infections, renal and urinary tract infections, intra-abdominal infections such as diverticulitis, *Clostridium difficile* infections and skin infections such as necrotizing fasciitis, cellulitis, etc. Noninfectious causes for fever include subarachnoid hemorrhage, fat embolism, deep vein thrombosis (DVT), thrombophlebitis, malignancy, drugs, acalculous cholecystitis, pancreatitis, acute respiratory distress syndrome (ARDS), thyrotoxicosis, ovulation, etc.

Hyperthermia (temperature >106°F) is usually caused by noninfectious etiologies such as malignant hyperthermia and neuroleptic malignant syndrome. These conditions, therefore, do not warrant investigations or antibiotics. On the contrary, fever >102°F is usually caused by infectious causes, warranting active investigation for source and treatment with antimicrobials as per the clinical picture. However, it has to be kept in mind that fever of this magnitude can be rarely caused by noninfectious etiologies such as acute

TABLE 2: Weaning indices.

Parameters assessed	Normal range of value
Tidal volume (unassisted)	At least 5–6 mL/kg of body weight
Respiration (unassisted)	Regular, without periods of apnea, and respiratory rate <35 breaths/min
Minute ventilation (unassisted)	<10 L/min (exclude apnea and hypoventilation also). Hyperventilation of >15–20 L/min has a high chance of weaning failure
RR/VT (liter)—the RSBI index on room air, with T-piece	<105
Diaphragm strength as assessed by maximum inspiratory pressure after 20–25 seconds tube occlusion with a one-way valve (PI_{max})	≤20 cmH$_2$O
Neural drive $P_{0.1}/P_{Imax}$	<0.3
Integrative index (CROP)	>13 mL/breaths/min

(CROP: compliance (dynamic), respiratory rate, oxygenation, maximum inspiratory pressure; $P_{0.1}$: occlusion pressure at initial 100 milliseconds of inspiration; P_{Imax}: maximum inspiratory pressure after 20 seconds of endotracheal tube occlusion; RR: respiratory rate; RSBI: rapid shallow breathing index; VT: tidal volume in liters)

adrenal insufficiency and drug fever. Fever <102°F can be due to numerous reasons, including both infectious and noninfectious etiologies, and a judicious approach regarding investigations and antibiotics is required.[50]

Evaluation of patients with fever will include a complete hemogram, culture of blood, urine and sputum/bronchoalveolar lavage (BAL), imaging (thorax, abdomen, and lower limb veins), and biomarkers. If a diagnosis of pneumonia is confirmed on imaging, then further evaluation depends on the microbiology of the respiratory tract samples. The Infectious Diseases Society of America (IDSA) guidelines suggest noninvasive sampling [nondirect bronchoalveolar lavage (NDBAL)] to diagnose ventilator-associated pneumonia (VAP), while the European guidelines suggest invasive sampling.[51-53] Although, the sampling method does not affect the mortality or length of stay, noninvasive sampling techniques have a risk of falsely identifying VAP thus prolonging antibiotic exposure.[52,53] The currently available data do not suggest any significant difference between the two modalities of sampling.[54,55] Blood cultures may yield an organism different from the organism causing the VAP or may be sterile. Numerous markers for diagnosis of infection/inflammation have been proposed such as erythrocyte sedimentation rate (ESR), C-reactive protein (CRP), procalcitonin, proadrenomedullin, lipopolysaccharide (LPS)-binding protein, soluble triggering receptor expressed on myeloid cells-1 (sTREM-1), and presepsin. ESR, CRP, and procalcitonin are routinely available while the others are not.[56]

Q14. Discuss the common biomarkers for sepsis.

Procalcitonin: Procalcitonin is released into circulation by activated monocytes circulating in blood during episodes of sepsis and trauma. The level rises within 2 hours of infection and peaks up at 6 hours identifying infections; earlier than conventional blood culture.[57,58] Procalcitonin is also elevated in noninfective conditions such as burns, major surgery, and end-stage renal failure.[59] There have been numerous trials evaluating the role of procalcitonin in various scenarios such as to differentiating between infective and noninfective conditions, de-escalating and stopping antibiotics, predicting the efficacy of initial empirical therapy, and also in predicting the mortality of patients admitted in ICU.[60-62] The current guidelines recommend using procalcitonin only to aid a decision regarding de-escalation or stopping antibiotics and suggest against the use of procalcitonin to rule out bacterial infection or to defer initiation of antibiotics.[59,63] For the same reasons, the current IDSA guidelines recommend the use of only clinical criteria over the use of serum procalcitonin for diagnosing VAP.[53]

Q15. How will you classify VAP?

Earlier, VAP was classified into early-onset VAP that occurred within 4 days of ventilation and late-onset VAP that occurred after 5 days of ventilation. This difference was initially considered to be clinically significant as early-onset VAP was considered to be caused by bacteria similar to those causing community-acquired pneumonia, e.g., *Streptococcus pneumoniae*, *Haemophilus influenzae*, methicillin-sensitive *Staphylococcus aureus* (MSSA), susceptible *Enterobacteriaceae,* and late-onset VAP by multidrug-resistant (MDR) bacteria from the hospital environment such as *Klebsiella*, *Pseudomonas*, *Acinetobacter*, *Enterobacter*, *Escherichia coli*, and methicillin-resistant *S. aureus* (MRSA).[64-66] Currently, there are increasing reports of lack of difference in microbiology across both groups and patients who are in contact with the healthcare environment or who are immunosuppressed are prone for MDR infections irrespective of the onset of VAP.[38,39] This patient has a new onset of high-grade fever with worsening oxygenation. The CXR showed a new patch which is likely to be of infective origin (VAP, as it has developed after 48 hours of intubation). The current management will warrant a hike in antibiotics directed against the possible pathogens, after collection of BAL/NDBAL for culture and sensitivity. It might be reasonable to send a blood culture and procalcitonin also if the drawbacks of these investigations are clearly understood.

Q16. What makes patients on mechanical ventilation susceptible to VAP?

- Bypassing anatomical barrier namely larynx and glottis
- Suppression of cough and mucociliary clearance
- Suppression of local humoral and cellular immunity
- Aspiration of pathogens during intubation
- Translocation of pathogens during orotracheal intubation or through aspiration of supraglottic secretions
- Improper aseptic precaution during bronchoscopy or tracheal suctioning

Q17. What is the differential diagnosis of a patch on CXR in ICU?

The differential diagnosis of a patch on CXR in ICU is summarized in **Table 3**.

Q18. What antibiotics will you prescribe for this patient?

A reasonable approach toward empiric antibiotic selection in VAP is given in **Flowchart 3**.[53]

Among the newer antibiotics, daptomycin cannot be used for MRSA infections (as it is inactivated in the lungs), tigecycline (in normal doses) is not recommended for hospital-acquired or VAP (higher doses may be required). The use of high-dose tigecycline and parenteral fosfomycin

TABLE 3: Radiological differentials for a patch on chest X-ray.

Diagnosis	Radiologic features
Consolidation/pneumonia	• Unilateral or bilateral parenchymal opacity, with air bronchogram following the lobar anatomy in case of lobar pneumonia • Diffuse distribution of opacities in case of bronchopneumonia
Collapse	• Complete opacification of airspace, associated with features of volume loss such as rib crowding, lobar opacification without air bronchogram, mediastinal shift to the same side, and elevation of the diaphragm
Pulmonary embolism	• Nonspecific atelectasis with an elevation of the hemidiaphragm, peripheral wedge-shaped pulmonary infarct (see chapter on pulmonary embolism) • These may be accompanied by a dilation of the pulmonary artery and small-to-moderate, unilateral pleural effusion
Pulmonary edema	Bilateral interstitial and alveolar edema, spreading from the center to the periphery, cardiomegaly, prominent upper zone markings, Kerley B lines, and bilateral symmetrical pleural effusion which can be mild-to-moderate
Re-expansion pulmonary edema	Interstitial edema involving the affected hemithorax. Cardiomegaly will be absent, and signs of cardiac failure also will be absent
Pleural effusion	Unilateral or bilateral, uniform opacity, with no air bronchogram mediastinal shift may be present to the opposite side. In case of supine film, the effusion will seep uniformly throughout producing uniform haziness on the same side
Parenchymal fibrosis	Interstitial thickening with associated volume loss, unilateral or bilateral, apicobasal gradient need not be maintained. History of any specific medical drugs, irradiation, or comparison with previous radiology will help to diagnose this condition
Bronchiolitis obliterans organizing pneumonia (BOOP), pulmonary hemorrhage, eosinophilic pneumonia, drug-induced parenchymal disease	• Nonspecific, diffuse patchy alveolar infiltrates not limited to the lobar anatomy. Eosinophilic pneumonia—reverse pulmonary edema • BOOP—usually peripheral patchy consolidation

Flowchart 3: Selection of antibiotics for ventilator-associated pneumonia.

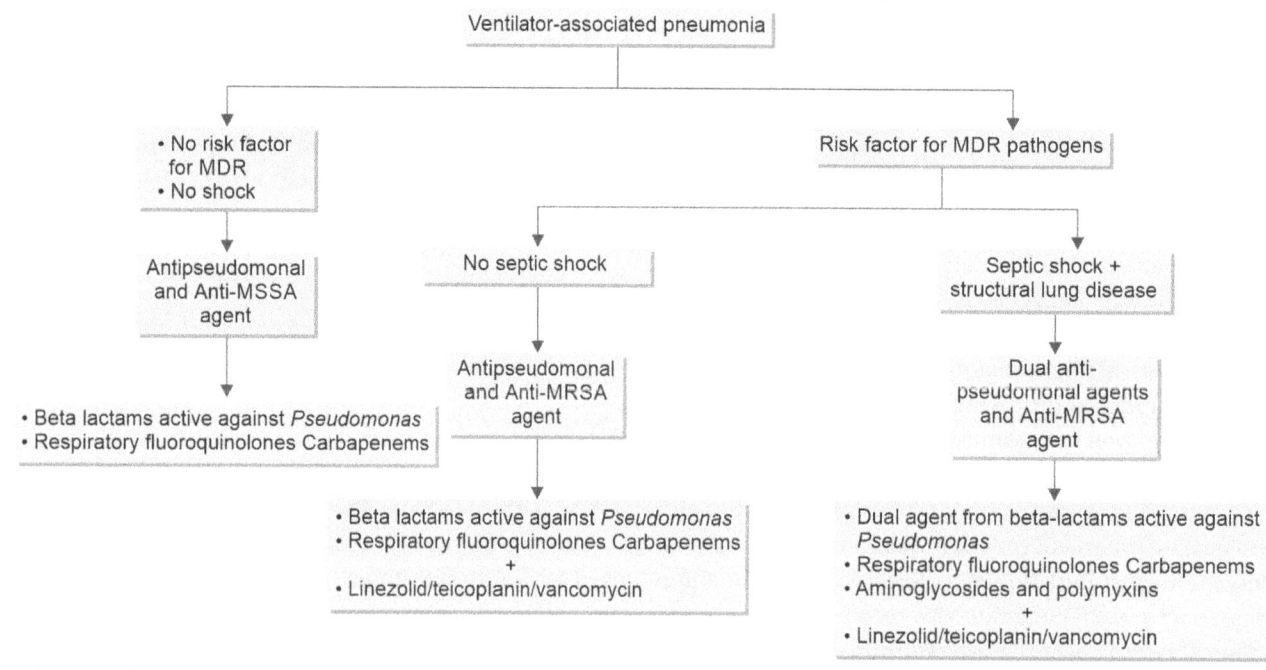

(MDR: multidrug-resistant; MRSA: methicillin-resistant *Staphylococcus aureus*; MSSA: methicillin-sensitive *Staphylococcus aureus*)

for MDR pathogens, although they appear to be promising, cannot be recommended currently.[67-69] Antibiotics need to be changed according to culture and sensitivity reports and may be administered for a duration of 7 days or less, if guided by clinical response and procalcitonin levels. Longer durations of treatment will be required for patients who develop complications of VAP such as empyema or lung abscess, patients in whom the VAP is caused *Pseudomonas*, carbapenem-resistant *Enterobacteriaceae* and *Acinetobacter*, and also in those patients who are immunocompromised.[53]

Taking all of these into consideration, the recommended empirical antibiotics for this patient will include either beta-lactams (cephalosporins with antipseudomonal activity such as ceftazidime, cefepime, and antipseudomonal penicillin such as piperacillin-tazobactam), respiratory fluoroquinolones (levofloxacin and moxifloxacin), or carbapenems (meropenem or imipenem) **(Flowchart 4)**.

Q19. What is clinical pulmonary infection score (CPIS)?

A consensus on the diagnosis of VAP in ICU is difficult to attain in view of numerous confounders such as ventilator-associated tracheobronchitis (VAT) and nonspecific findings in the CXR. It was suggested that an integrated clinicoradiological approach with the help of CPIS could help to identify the patients who have VAP. An increasing CPIS suggests a worsening infection and warrants a change in antibiotics as per clinical judgment.

Clinical pulmonary infection score **(Table 4)** consists of six clinical and laboratory parameters with total score ranging from 0 to 12. A score of ≥6 has a good correlation with the diagnosis of VAP.[70] CPIS of >6 has a sensitivity of 72% and a specificity of 85%, for the presence of VAP.[55] Although the calculation of CPIS seems relatively simple and straightforward, there can be substantial interobserver variability in calculating CPIS, limiting its routine use in clinical trials.[70] The current IDSA guidelines suggest the use of clinical criteria than CPIS for initiating and stopping of antibiotics.[53]

Q20. What are ventilator-associated events (VAEs)?

Diagnosing VAP solely based on clinical criteria or radiologic criteria leads to either overdiagnosis or underdiagnosis of VAP. At times it will be difficult to differentiate VAP from noninfectious conditions such as pulmonary edema or ARDS. This leads to difficulties in VAP surveillance. To overcome this, the Centers for Disease Control and Prevention (CDC) has put forward a set of epidemiological definitions called VAEs with VAP being one of them.[71] VAEs are the complications occurring in mechanically ventilated patients that need to be reported, irrespective of its nature or mechanism of origin.

TABLE 4: Clinical pulmonary infection score.

Measured parameter	Score
Temperature (°C):	
• 36.5–38.4°C	0
• 38.5–38.9°C	1
• ≤36°C or ≥39°C	2
Leukocytes in the blood (cells/mm^3):	
• 4,000–11,000/mm^3	0
• <4,000/mm^3 or >11,000/mm^3	1
• >50% band cells	2
Tracheal secretions (subjective visual scale):	
• Absent	0
• Present, but not purulent	1
• Purulent	2
Radiographic findings (on chest radiography, excluding CHF and ARDS):	
• Absent infiltrates	0
• Diffuse/patchy infiltrate	1
• Localized infiltrate	2
Culture results (endotracheal aspirate):	
• No or mild growth	0
• Moderate or florid growth	1
• Moderate or florid growth and pathogen consistent with Gram stain	2
Oxygenation status (defined by PaO$_2$: FiO$_2$):	
• >240 or ARDS	0
• ≤240 and absence of ARDS	2

(ARDS: acute respiratory distress syndrome; CHF: congestive heart failure; FiO$_2$: fraction of inspired oxygen; PaO$_2$: partial pressure of arterial oxygen)

To be assessed for VAE, patients should be ventilated for a minimum of 4 calendar days, with at least 2 days of clinical stability. Each VAE is defined for a period of 14 days. Hence, a patient can have only one VAE per fortnight. The classification of VAE is shown in **Flowchart 4**.

Organisms such as *Candida* species, coagulase-negative *Staphylococcus* (CoNS), and *Enterococcus* species can be identified as a positive microbiological result only if isolated from pleural fluid or lung tissue and not from sputum, endotracheal aspirates, BAL, or protected specimen brushings. Positive microbiological test of normal/respiratory flora should be ignored.[71]

As mentioned earlier, these are surveillance definitions and are not supposed to be used for treatment decisions.[71]

Q21. What is the VAP bundle?

"Bundles" in critical care are a group of practice points; each supported by a high level of evidence and produces a greater effect on outcomes when performed together. Bundles of care encourage the consistent delivery of each element, thereby avoiding individual preferences, practices, and conflicts of interests.[72]

Flowchart 4: Ventilator-associated events.

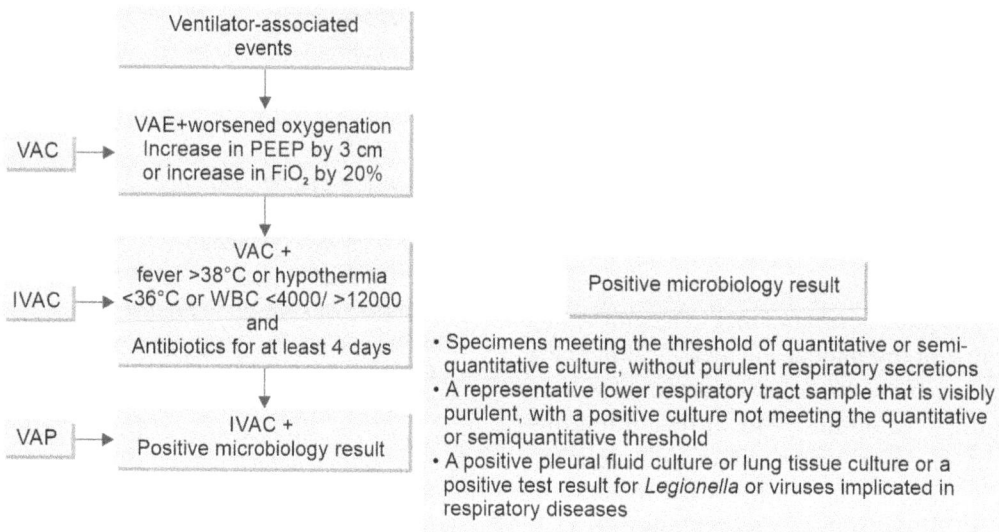

(FiO$_2$: fraction of inspired oxygen; IVAC: infection-related ventilator-associated condition; PEEP: positive end-expiratory pressure; VAC: ventilator-associated condition; VAEs: ventilator-associated events; VAP: ventilator-associated pneumonia; WBC: white blood cell)

Ventilator-associated pneumonia bundle may be adopted from international/national societies and then modified according to local hospital policies or current infection control practices prevalent in those hospitals. The Institute for Healthcare Improvement (IHI) initially proposed the concept of bundles of care and VAP bundles. The initial VAP bundle consisted of hand hygiene, head-end elevation of bed, oral care with chlorhexidine, stress ulcer, and DVT prophylaxis.[73] **Table 5** represents the suggested practice with evidence statement from Scottish Intensive Care Society.[74] They differ from the classical IHI VAP bundle[73] by not suggesting peptic ulcer prophylaxis or DVT prophylaxis as they have no direct relation in reducing VAP rates.

The use of VAP bundle has been shown to reduce VAP rates consistently across the world. Implementation of a VAP bundle across Spain resulted in a successful reduction of VAP rates to more than half.[75] The bundle used by this group had seven mandatory recommendations, viz., (1) staff training in airway management, (2) hand hygiene, (3) ensuring endotracheal tube cuff pressure above 20 cmH$_2$O, (4) oral care with chlorhexidine, (5) head-end elevation of bed, (6) steps to reduce ventilator days, and (7) discouraging scheduled changes of ventilator circuits. Apart from these, they added three "highly recommended measures" such as (1) selective decontamination of the digestive tract, (2) subglottic suctioning, and (3) short-course antibiotics for trauma patients with altered sensorium.

The latest update by SHEA/IDSA/APIC in 2022 continues to put emphasis on bundled care approach.[76] However, there are substantial changes in the practices of care. The guidelines advocate:
- Usage of high-flow nasal oxygen or noninvasive positive pressure ventilation to avoid intubation or to minimize the duration and prevent reintubations
- Usage of spontaneous awakening trials or sedation protocols to minimize sedation
- Oral hygiene by "daily toothbrushing"

The guidelines also propose additional measures such as to reduce infectious complications, which are as follows:
- Use of endotracheal tubes with subglottic secretion drainage and early tracheostomy
- Postpyloric feeding in those who are at high risk of aspiration

Contrary to the previous guidelines, the current update strongly recommend against the use of chlorhexidine for oral care, probiotics, polyurethane endotracheal tube cuffs, tapered endotracheal tube cuffs, automated control of endotracheal cuff pressures, and frequent endotracheal cuff pressure monitoring as none of these measures have proven benefit albeit an increased risk.

A provisional diagnosis of VAP was made and antibiotics were escalated to piperacillin-tazobactam. The patient initially had an increase in patch size but later became afebrile and gradually oxygen requirement came down. After further 7 days of ICU stay, liberation from mechanical ventilation was attempted again. The patient was mobilized in the bed and the physiotherapist noticed severe weakness of the thigh

TABLE 5: Ventilator-associated pneumonia (VAP) bundle.

Sr. No.	Intervention	Rationale	Caution	Level of evidence
1.	Avoid intubation in selected populations such as COPD exacerbation, postoperative respiratory failure, pulmonary edema, and in immunosuppressed patients	NIV and HFNC can be used to avoid intubation in select populations, thereby reducing the need for endotracheal intubation, resulting in low VAP rates	Failure of NIV is associated with high mortality rates	High
2.	Daily sedation interruption, maintaining a light sedation, daily awakening, and daily spontaneous breathing trials	Daily interruption of sedatives avoids accumulation of sedatives in the body, promoting easy arousal and thereby early liberation from mechanical ventilation	• Analgesia and patient-ventilator synchrony should be maintained • Sedation holidays may be avoided in patients who are paralyzed, patients with raised intracranial pressure, severe acute respiratory distress syndrome, ongoing therapeutic hypothermia, and in those on end-of-life care	High
3.	Continuous subglottic aspiration of secretions	Subglottic aspiration of oropharyngeal secretions reduces microaspiration across the cuff and thereby reduce the incidence of VAP, ventilator days, and ICU length of stay	Reintubation for those who are already intubated with endotracheal tubes without subglottic suction is not recommended	Moderate
4.	Head of the bed elevated to 30–45°	Head-end elevation of bed prevents reflux of esophageal contents and may decrease VAP rates	May not be applicable in hemodynamically unstable patients, those with spinal trauma and pelvic injuries	Low
5.	Daily oral care with chlorhexidine (0.12–2%) solution	Reduces the colonization of the oropharynx with hospital-acquired pathogens	• Careless use can contaminate chlorhexidine A time gap between chlorhexidine mouth care and brushing should be maintained as toothpaste inactivates chlorhexidine. Avoid in patients with a breach of the oral mucosa • Can cause chemical pneumonitis and ARDS, if aspirated	Low

(ARDS: acute respiratory distress syndrome; COPD: chronic obstructive pulmonary disease; HFNC: high-flow nasal cannula; ICU: intensive care unit; NIV: noninvasive ventilation)

muscles and shoulder muscles with a grade of power 3/5 in all four limbs in these muscles.

Q22. Discuss about ICU-acquired weakness (ICUAW)?

Intensive care unit-acquired weakness is a common occurrence in ICU with an incidence of around 25–65% of patients undergoing mechanical ventilation for at least 5 days.[77] Apart from residual paralysis from diseases that resulted in ICU admission [such as Guillain–Barré syndrome (GBS), myasthenia gravis, and stroke], ICUAW entity is due to an alteration in the structure and function of muscles and nerves termed as critical illness neuropathy, critical illness myopathy (CIM), and a combination of both.

Q23. How will you evaluate a case of ICUAW?

Intensive care unit-acquired weakness may result from weakness predominantly due to muscle problems (CIM), due to nerve damage [critical illness polyneuropathy (CIP)], or a combination of both. A definitive diagnosis is made from history of having a critical illness, clinical examination eliciting muscle weakness [modified Medical Research Council (mMRC) score < 48/60], and electrophysiological criteria as well as a muscle biopsy.[78] Clinical examination will reveal the presence of symmetrical weakness, more in the proximal muscles than the distal muscles, or may be revealed during evaluation of a difficult-to-wean patient. Deep tendon reflexes although preserved, may be reduced. Eliciting muscle weakness via mMRC score may not be applicable in sedated patients, in patients with delirium, and also in uncooperative patients. In a conscious cooperative patient, mMRC is tested in all four limbs (muscle groups tested in the upper limb include abduction at shoulder, flexion at elbow, and extension at wrist extension. Similarly in lower limb, the muscle groups tested are the hip flexors, knee extensors, and ankle dorsiflexors) with a maximum score of 60. Handgrip dynamometry can be used as a quick diagnostic test, as it is easy to perform and facilitates early identification of patients with significant weakness.

In all suspected cases, the use of electrophysiological testing is advocated, and characteristic abnormalities may be seen in cases of CIP and CIM, although there is a significant overlap and inconclusive results, CIP is mainly an axonal defect with both sensory and motor neuropathy. Nerve conduction studies reveal normal latency, nerve conduction velocities, reduced amplitude of sensory nerve action potential (SNAP), and reduced compound muscle action potential (CMAP). CIM affects only the muscle and is characterized by a CMAP which is prolonged and reduced amplitude, with normal SNAP **(Table 6)**.

Muscle biopsy can be done via open biopsy or fine-needle biopsy. Myosin loss or myosin:actin ratio < 1.7 has been reported as abnormal.

Excessive adrenergic stimuli can result in muscle apoptosis and muscle damage. This concept seems to be strengthened when we look at a recently published retrospective study. They found that patients with sepsis, high APACHE II score, and requiring prolonged ventilation and vasopressors had a significantly higher incidence of ICUAW (73.8% vs. 33.7%, $p < 0.0001$). The dose and duration of vasopressors also seemed to be an independent cause for ICUAW in multivariate analysis. Whether the use of vasopressors is a cause of ICUAW or whether the use of vasopressors represented a severe illness with severe inflammation needs to be confirmed in future trials. This study opens up an area of conflict whether it is the inflammation associated with severe illness or the use of adrenergic drugs that result in ICUAW.[79]

Risk factors for ICUAW have been shown in **Box 1**.

Intensive care unit-acquired weakness usually presents after 1 week of ICU stay, although there have been reports of earlier onset also. The sensory system, higher mental function, cranial nerve function, and autonomic nervous system function is preserved. In contrast to other conditions such as GBS, reflexes are also preserved. Lumbar puncture with cerebrospinal fluid (CSF) examination is seldom required as temperature and higher mental functions will be normal. If done, CSF findings will be normal.

Q24. How will you investigate a patient with ICUAW?

Laboratory investigations: Creatine kinase is nonspecific but may be raised. The magnitude of its rise will depend on the myositis. In case of very high elevations, rhabdomyolysis should be suspected rather than ICUAW. Nerve conduction studies demonstrate normal conduction velocity but decreased CMAPs, prolonged CMAP duration (in case of predominant muscle involvement), and reduced compound motor and SNAP in case of predominant neural involvement. In case of persisting dilemma, muscle or/and nerve biopsy will help in the diagnosis.

Q25. What are the strategies to reduce the incidence of ICUAW?

Simple steps such as strictly avoiding hyperglycemia, aggressive management of sepsis, early mobilization, preventing muscle mass breakdown by maintaining adequate nutritional intake, correction of dyselectrolytemia, minimal use of neuromuscular blockade and steroids, and early rehabilitation or passive mobilization may help to reduce the severity of ICUAW.[77,79]

TABLE 6: Distinguishing features of critical illness polyneuropathy and critical illness myopathy.

Critical illness polyneuropathy	Critical illness myopathy
History of critical illness	History of critical illness
Demonstrated clinical weakness with mMRC <48/60 or difficult weaning from ventilator	Demonstrated clinical weakness with mMRC <48/60 or difficult weaning from ventilator
Exclusion of other neuromuscular disorder	Exclusion of other neuromuscular disorder
Nerve conduction studies—normal latency and nerve conduction velocities with reduced SNAP amplitude and CMAP action potential	Electrophysiological studies—prolonged CMAP with reduced amplitude (<80% of normal), normal SNAP, normal nerve conduction with no conduction block
Nerve biopsy: Early days—normal Late days—axonal loss	Muscle biopsy with evidence of myopathy (e.g., myosin or muscle necrosis)

(CMAP: compound muscle action potential; mMRC: modified Medical Research Council; SNAP: sensory nerve action potential)

BOX 1: Risk factors for intensive care unit-acquired weakness.

- Sepsis
- Multiorgan dysfunction syndrome (increased organ dysfunction scores)
- Systemic inflammatory response syndrome
- Hyperglycemia
- Older age
- Female sex
- Immobilization
- Malnutrition
- Corticosteroids
- Neuromuscular blockade
- Adrenergic vasopressors

Q26. Discuss the recovery from ICUAW.

Recovery from ICUAW depends upon whether it is the group of muscles or nerves that are predominantly involved. The recovery is significantly slowed in cases of nerve involvement.[80] ICUAW has a slow recovery, requiring weeks or months for recovery. Persisting ICUAW significantly impairs the quality of life, the physical function, and also contributes toward the mortality at the end of 1 year.[77]

Q27. What are the long-term outcomes in patients who need long-term ventilatory support? Which patients develop chronic critical illness? What are their outcomes?

About 5–10% of patients who survive an episode of critical illness remain dependent on organ support, without showing any signs of recovery. These patients repeatedly fail to wean from ventilatory support, develop profound weakness, cachexia, and edema and infections from MDR organisms. The neuroendocrine changes such as hormonal disturbances, delirium, and coma also persist well beyond the acute phase of critical illness. With specialized care and protocolized weaning in dedicated centers, about 50% of them are liberated successfully from ventilatory support by 30–45 days. Patients who remain ventilator dependent, even after about 2 months, are unlikely to get extubated at any point of time in their life. Patients with chronic critical illness have a high mortality, mostly within 2–3 months. The 1-year survival is only about 50%, with only 10% being discharged home without functional disability.[81,82]

Cognitive dysfunction after critical illness: Critical illness and ICU stay also affect the cognitive function of the survivors adversely. In a study of a mixed population of critically ill patients, with normal cognitive function before ICU admission, it was found that almost 40% patients had cognitive impairment, resembling patients with moderate head injury or mild Alzheimer's disease, at 3 months. There was some improvement in cognition such that the incidence reduced to 24–34% after 1 year of follow-up. The duration of delirium was independently associated with a worse cognitive function although age and total dosage of sedatives did not correlate with the outcome.[83,84]

The patient had a prolonged weaning due to severe ICUAW. Measures for infection control were actively pursued and the patient was actively mobilized. Tracheostomy was deemed unnecessary at this point as he was improving steadily. After a week, he was successfully extubated and discharged to the ward.

REFERENCES

1. Hall JB, Wood LD. Liberation of the patient from mechanical ventilation. JAMA. 1987;257(12):1621-8.
2. Peñuelas Ó, Thille AW, Esteban A. Discontinuation of ventilatory support: new solutions to old dilemmas. Curr Opin Crit Care. 2015;21(1):74-81.
3. El-Khatib MF, Bou-Khalil P. Clinical review: liberation from mechanical ventilation. Crit Care. 2008;12(4):221.
4. Blackwood B, Alderdice F, Burns KE, Cardwell CR, Lavery G, O'Halloran P. Protocolized versus non-protocolized weaning for reducing the duration of mechanical ventilation in critically ill adult patients. Cochrane Database Syst Rev. 2010;(5):CD006904.
5. Girard TD, Ely EW. Protocol-driven ventilator weaning: reviewing the evidence. Clin Chest Med. 2008;29:241-52.
6. Girard TD, Alhazzani W, Kress JP, Ouellette DR, Schmidt GA, Truwit JD, et al. An Official American Thoracic Society/American College of Chest Physicians Clinical Practice guideline: liberation from mechanical ventilation in critically ill adults. Rehabilitation protocols, ventilator liberation protocols, and cuff leak tests. Am J Respir Crit Care Med. 2017;195:120-33.
7. MacIntyre NR, Cook DJ, Ely EW Jr, Epstein SK, Fink JB, Heffner JE, et al. Evidence-based guidelines for weaning and discontinuing ventilatory support: a collective task force facilitated by the American College of Chest Physicians; the American Association for Respiratory Care; and the American College of Critical Care Medicine. Chest. 2001;120:375S-95S.
8. Guttmann J, Haberthür C, Mols G, Lichtwarck-Aschoff M. Automatic tube compensation (ATC). Minerva Anestesiol. 2002;68:369-77.
9. Unoki T, Serita A, Grap MJ. Automatic tube compensation during weaning from mechanical ventilation: evidence and clinical implications. Crit Care Nurse. 2008;28:34-42.
10. Oto J, Imanaka H, Nakataki E, Ono R, Nishimura M. Potential inadequacy of automatic tube compensation to decrease inspiratory work load after at least 48 hours of endotracheal tube use in the clinical setting. Respir Care. 2012;57:697-703.
11. Belliato M. Automated weaning from mechanical ventilation. World J Respirol. 2016;6:49-53.
12. Burns KE, Lellouche F, Lessard MR. Automating the weaning process with advanced closed-loop systems. Intensive Care Med. 2008;34:1757-65.
13. Rose L, Schultz MJ, Cardwell CR, Jouvet P, McAuley DF, Blackwood B. Automated versus non-automated weaning for reducing the duration of mechanical ventilation for critically ill adults and children. Cochrane Database Syst Rev. 2014;(6):CD009235.
14. Gomez H, Pinsky MR. Effect of mechanical ventilation on heart-lung interactions. In: Tobin MJ (Ed). Principles and Practice of Mechanical Ventilation, 3rd edition. Columbus: McGraw-Hill Education; 2013.
15. Mekontso-Dessap A, de Prost N, Girou E, Braconnier F, Lemaire F, Brun-Buisson C, et al. B-type natriuretic peptide and weaning from mechanical ventilation. Intensive Care Med. 2006;32:1529-36.
16. McLean AS, Huang SJ, Salter M. Bench-to-bedside review: the value of cardiac biomarkers in the intensive care patient. Crit Care. 2008;12:215.

17. Grasso S, Leone A, De Michele M, Anaclerio R, Cafarelli A, Ancona G, et al. Use of N-terminal pro-brain natriuretic peptide to detect acute cardiac dysfunction during weaning failure in difficult-to-wean patients with chronic obstructive pulmonary disease. Crit Care Med. 2007;35:96-105.
18. Anguel N, Monnet X, Osman D, Castelain V, Richard C, Teboul JL. Increase in plasma protein concentration for diagnosing weaning-induced pulmonary oedema. Intensive Care Med. 2008;34:1231-8.
19. Lamia B, Maizel J, Ochagavia A, Chemla D, Osman D, Richard C, et al. Echocardiographic diagnosis of pulmonary artery occlusion pressure elevation during weaning from mechanical ventilation. Crit Care Med. 2009;37:1696-701.
20. Mongodi S, Via G, Bouhemad B, Storti E, Mojoli F, Braschi A. Usefulness of combined bedside lung ultrasound and echocardiography to assess weaning failure from mechanical ventilation. Crit Care Med. 2013;41:e182-5.
21. Mohsenifar Z, Hay A, Hay J, Lewis MI, Koerner SK. Gastric intramural pH as a predictor of success or failure in weaning patients from mechanical ventilation. Ann Intern Med. 1993;119:794-8.
22. Dres M, Teboul JL, Anguel N, Guerin L, Richard C, Monnet X. Extravascular lung water, B-type natriuretic peptide, and blood volume contraction enable diagnosis of weaning-induced pulmonary edema. Crit Care Med. 2014;42:1882-9.
23. Tobin MJ. Extubation and the myth of "minimal ventilator settings". Am J Respir Crit Care Med. 2012;185:349-50.
24. Boles JM, Bion J, Connors A, Herridge M, Marsh B, Melot C, et al. Weaning from mechanical ventilation. Eur Respir J. 2007;29:1033-56.
25. Brochard L, Rauss A, Benito S, Conti G, Mancebo J, Rekik N, et al. Comparison of three methods of gradual withdrawal from ventilatory support during weaning from mechanical ventilation. Am J Respir Crit Care Med. 1994;150:896-903.
26. Esteban A, Frutos F, Tobin MJ, Alia I, Solsona JF, Valverdu I, et al. A comparison of four methods of weaning patients from mechanical ventilation. Spanish Lung Failure Collaborative Group. N Engl J Med. 1995;332:345-50.
27. Girard TD, Kress JP, Fuchs BD, Thomason JW, Schweickert WD, Pun BT, et al. Efficacy and safety of a paired sedation and ventilator weaning protocol for mechanically ventilated patients in intensive care (Awakening and Breathing Controlled trial): a randomised controlled trial. Lancet. 2008;371:126-34.
28. Esteban A, Alía I, Tobin Mj, Gil A, Gordo F, Vallverdú I, et al. Effect of spontaneous breathing trial duration on outcome of attempts to discontinue mechanical ventilation. Am J Respir Crit Care Med. 1999;159:512-8.
29. Coplin WM, Pierson DJ, Cooley KD, Newell DW, Rubenfeld GD. Implications of extubation delay in brain-injured patients meeting standard weaning criteria. Am J Respir Crit Care Med. 2000;161:1530-6.
30. Hsieh AH, Bishop MJ, Kubilis PS, Newell DW, Pierson DJ. Pneumonia following closed head injury. Am Rev Respir Dis. 1992;146:290-4.
31. Miller RL, Cole RP. Association between reduced cuff leak volume and postextubation stridor. Chest. 1996;110:1035-40.
32. De Backer D. The cuff-leak test: what are we measuring? Crit Care. 2005;9:31-3.
33. François B, Bellissant E, Gissot V, Desachy A, Normand S, Boulain T, et al. 12-h pretreatment with methylprednisolone versus placebo for prevention of postextubation laryngeal oedema: a randomised double-blind trial. Lancet. 2007;369(9567):1083-9.
34. Cheng KC, Chen CM, Tan CK, Chen HM, Lu CL, Zhang H. Methylprednisolone reduces the rates of postextubation stridor and reintubation associated with attenuated cytokine responses in critically ill patients. Minerva Anestesiol. 2011;77:503-9.
35. Cheng KC, Hou CC, Huang HC, Lin SC, Zhang H. Intravenous injection of methylprednisolone reduces the incidence of postextubation stridor in intensive care unit patients. Crit Care Med. 2006;34:1345-50.
36. Laghi F, D'Alfonso N, Tobin MJ. Pattern of recovery from diaphragmatic fatigue over 24 hours. J Appl Physiol. 1995;79:539-46.
37. Jiang TX, Reid WD, Road JD. Free radical scavengers and diaphragm injury following inspiratory resistive loading. Am J Respir Crit Care Med. 2001;164:1288-94.
38. Laghi F, Cattapan SE, Jubran A, Parthasarathy S, Warshawsky P, Choi YS, et al. Is weaning failure caused by low-frequency fatigue of the diaphragm? Am J Respir Crit Care Med. 2003;167:120-7.
39. Road J, Jiang TX, Reid WD. Weaning failure, muscle injury, and fatigue. Am J Respir Crit Care Med. 2003;168:1539-40.
40. Vassilakopoulos T, Zakynthinos S, Roussos C. Bench-to-bedside review: weaning failure—should we rest the respiratory muscles with controlled mechanical ventilation? Crit Care. 2006;10:204.
41. Fernandez MM, González-Castro A, Magret M, Bouza MT, Ibañez M, García C, et al. Reconnection to mechanical ventilation for 1 h after a successful spontaneous breathing trial reduces reintubation in critically ill patients: a multicenter randomized controlled trial. Intensive Care Med. 2017;43:1660-7.
42. Marelich GP, Murin S, Battistella F, Inciardi J, Vierra T, Roby M. Protocol weaning of mechanical ventilation in medical and surgical patients by respiratory care practitioners and nurses: effect on weaning time and incidence of ventilator-associated pneumonia. Chest. 2000;118:459-67.
43. Burns KE, Raptis S, Bakshi J, Cook DJ, Jones A, Epstein SK, et al. Practice variation in weaning critically ill adults from invasive mechanical ventilation: preliminary results of an international survey. Am J Respir Crit Care Med. 2011;183:A6247.
44. ClinicalTrials.gov. (2018). The frequency of screening and SBT technique trial: the FAST Trial. (2018). [online] Available from: https://clinicaltrials.gov/ct2/show/NCT02969226. [Last accessed August, 2023].
45. MacIntyre NR, Epstein SK, Carson S, Scheinhorn D, Christopher K, Muldoon S. Management of patients requiring prolonged mechanical ventilation. Chest. 2005;128:3937-54.

46. Heunks LM, van der Hoeven JG. Clinical review: the ABC of weaning failure—a structured approach. Crit Care. 2010;14:245.
47. Mcconville JF, Kress JP. Weaning patients from the ventilator. N Engl J Med. 2012;367:2233-9.
48. O'Grady NP, Barie PS, Bartlett JG, Bleck T, Carroll K, Kalil AC, et al. Guidelines for evaluation of new fever in critically ill adult patients: 2008 update from the American College of Critical Care Medicine and the Infectious Diseases Society of America. Crit Care Med. 2008;36:1330-49.
49. Marik PE. Fever in the ICU. Chest. 2000;117:855-69.
50. Cunha BA. Fever in the intensive care unit. Intensive Care Med. 1999;25:648-51.
51. Torres A, Niederman MS, Chastre J, Ewig S, Fernandez-Vandellos P, Hanberger H, et al. Summary of the international clinical guidelines for the management of hospital-acquired and ventilator-acquired pneumonia. ERJ Open Res. 2018;4:00028-2018.
52. Torres A, Niederman MS, Chastre J, Ewig S, Fernandez-Vandellos P, Hanberger H, et al. International ERS/ESICM/ESCMID/ALAT guidelines for the management of hospital-acquired pneumonia and ventilator-associated pneumonia: guidelines for the management of hospital-acquired pneumonia (HAP)/ventilator-associated pneumonia (VAP) of the European Respiratory Society (ERS), European Society of Intensive Care Medicine (ESICM), European Society of Clinical Microbiology and Infectious Diseases (ESCMID) and Asociación Latinoamericana del Tórax (ALAT). Eur Respir J. 2017;50(3):1700582.
53. Kalil AC, Metersky ML, Klompas M, Muscedere J, Sweeney DA, Palmer LB, et al. Management of adults with hospital-acquired and ventilator-associated pneumonia: 2016 clinical practice guidelines by the Infectious Diseases Society of America and the American Thoracic Society. Clin Infect Dis. 2016;63:e61-111.
54. Canadian Critical Care Trials Group. A randomized trial of diagnostic techniques for ventilator-associated pneumonia. N Engl J Med. 2006;355:2619-30.
55. Papazian L, Thomas P, Garbe L, Guignon I, Thirion X, Charrel J, et al. Bronchoscopic or blind sampling techniques for the diagnosis of ventilator-associated pneumonia. Am J Respir Crit Care Med. 1995;152:1982-91.
56. Singer M. Biomarkers in sepsis. Curr Opin Pulm Med. 2013;19:305-9.
57. Reinhart K, Meisner M. Biomarkers in the critically ill patient: procalcitonin. Crit Care Clin. 2011;27:253-63.
58. Meisner M. Update on procalcitonin measurements. Ann Lab Med. 2014;34:263-73.
59. Wacker C, Prkno A, Brunkhorst FM, Schlattmann P. Procalcitonin as a diagnostic marker for sepsis: a systematic review and meta-analysis. Lancet Infect Dis. 2013;13:426-35.
60. Tanrıverdi H, Tor MM, Kart L, Altın R, Atalay F, SumbSümbüloğlu V. Prognostic value of serum procalcitonin and C-reactive protein levels in critically ill patients who developed ventilator-associated pneumonia. Ann Thorac Med. 2015;10:137-42.
61. Stolz D, Smyrnios N, Eggimann P, Pargger H, Thakkar N, Siegemund M, et al. Procalcitonin for reduced antibiotic exposure in ventilator-associated pneumonia: a randomised study. Eur Respir J. 2009;34:1364-75.
62. Sotillo-Díaz JC, Bermejo-López E, García-Olivares P, Peral-Gutiérrez JA, Sancho-González M, Guerrero-Sanz JE. Role of plasma procalcitonin in the diagnosis of ventilator-associated pneumonia: systematic review and meta-analysis. Med Intensiva. 2014;38:337-46.
63. Bouadma L, Luyt CE, Tubach F, Cracco C, Alvarez A, Schwebel C, et al. Use of procalcitonin to reduce patients' exposure to antibiotics in intensive care units (PRORATA trial): a multicentre randomised controlled trial. Lancet. 2010;375(9713):463-74.
64. Langer M, Cigada M, Mandelli M, Mosconi P, Tognoni G. Early onset pneumonia: a multicenter study in intensive care units. Intensive Care Med. 1987;13:342-6.
65. Golia S, Sangeetha KT, Vasudha CL. Microbial profile of early and late onset ventilator associated pneumonia in the intensive care unit of a tertiary care hospital in Bengaluru, India. J Clin Diagn Res. 2013;7:2462-6.
66. Dias M, Marçal P, Amaro P. Ventilator-associated pneumonia (VAP)—Early and late-onset differences. Eur Respir J. 2013;42(Suppl 57):P2457.
67. Silverman JA, Mortin LI, Vanpraagh AD, Li T, Alder J. Inhibition of daptomycin by pulmonary surfactant: in vitro modeling and clinical impact. J Infect Dis. 2005;191:2149-52.
68. Ramirez J, Dartois N, Gandjini H, Yan JL, Korth-Bradley J, McGovern PC. Randomized phase 2 trial to evaluate the clinical efficacy of two high-dosage tigecycline regimens versus imipenem-cilastatin for treatment of hospital-acquired pneumonia. Antimicrob Agents Chemother. 2013;57:1756-62.
69. Hawkey PM, Warren RE, Livermore DM, McNulty CA, Enoch DA, Otter JA, et al. Treatment of infections caused by multidrug- resistant Gram-negative bacteria: report of the British Society for Antimicrobial Chemotherapy/Healthcare Infection Society/British Infection Association Joint Working Party. J Antimicrob Chemother. 2018;73(Suppl 3):iii2-iii78.
70. Zilberberg MD, Shorr AF. Ventilator-associated pneumonia: the clinical pulmonary infection score as a surrogate for diagnostics and outcome. Clin Infect Dis. 2010;51:S131-5.
71. CDC. (2019). Ventilator-associated event (VAE). [online] Available from: https://www.cdc.gov/nhsn/pdfs/pscmanual/10-vae_final.pdf. [Last accessed August, 2023].
72. Khan P, Divatia JV. Severe sepsis bundles. Indian J Crit Care Med. 2010;14(1):8-13.
73. Institute for Healthcare Improvement. (2012). How-to guide: prevent ventilator-associated pneumonia. [online] Available from: http://www.ihi.org/resources/Pages/Tools/HowtoGuidePreventVAP.aspx. [Last accessed August, 2023].
74. Health Protection Scotland. (2017). Preventing ventilator associated pneumonia (VAP). [online] Available from: http://www.hps.scot.nhs.uk/haiic/ic/resourcedetail.aspx?id=987. [Last accessed August, 2019].

75. Álvarez-Lerma F, Palomar-Martínez M, Sánchez-García M, Martínez-Alonso M, Álvarez-Rodríguez J, Lorente L, et al. Prevention of ventilator-associated pneumonia. Crit Care Med. 2018;46:181-8.
76. Glowicz J, Landon E, Sickbert-Bennett E, Aiello A, DeKay K, Hoffmann K, et al. (2023). SHEA/IDSA/APIC Practice Recommendation: Strategies to prevent healthcare-associated infections through hand hygiene: 2022 Update. Infect Control Hosp Epidemiol. 2023;44(3):355-76.
77. Hermans G, Van den Berghe G. Clinical review: intensive care unit acquired weakness. Crit Care. 2015;19:274.
78. Jolley SE, Bunnell AE, Hough CL. ICU-acquired weakness. Chest. 2016;150:1129-40.
79. Kress JP, Hall JB. ICU-acquired weakness and recovery from critical illness. N Engl J Med. 2014;370:1626-35.
80. Wolfe KS, Patel BK, MacKenzie EL, Giovanni SP, Pohlman AS, Churpek MM, et al. Impact of vasoactive medications on ICU-acquired weakness in mechanically ventilated patients. Chest. 2018;154(4):781-7.
81. Koch S, Wollersheim T, Bierbrauer J, Haas K, Mörgeli R, Deja M, et al. Long-term recovery in critical illness myopathy is complete, contrary to polyneuropathy. Muscle Nerve. 2014;50:431-6.
82. Carson SS. Definitions and epidemiology of the chronically critically ill. Respir Care. 2012;57:848-56.
83. Nelson JE, Cox CE, Hope AA, Carson SS. Chronic critical illness. Am J Respir Crit Care Med. 2010;182:446-54.
84. Pandharipande PP, Girard TD, Jackson JC, Morandi A, Thompson JL, Pun BT, et al. Long-term cognitive impairment after critical illness. N Engl J Med. 2013;369:1306-16.

CHAPTER 4

Acute Exacerbation of Chronic Obstructive Pulmonary Disease

Gautam Gondal, Jacob George Pulinilkunnathil, Kapil Gangadhar Zirpe, Atul Prabhakar Kulkarni

CASE STUDY

A 72-year-old male, a known case of chronic obstructive pulmonary disease (COPD), coronary artery disease (CAD), and heart failure (HF), was admitted to the intensive care unit (ICU) with breathlessness, high-grade fever, and cough with mucopurulent expectoration. On admission to the ICU, he was diaphoretic, febrile (temperature 38°C), with sinus tachycardia [heart rate (HR) 106 beats/min], normotensive [blood pressure (BP) 110/78 mm Hg], and tachypneic [respiratory rate (RR) 30 breaths/min]. The oxygen saturation on room air was 60% that improved to 80% with oxygen supplementation. An arterial blood gas (ABG) collected at the time of ICU admission showed a pH of 7.26, with a partial pressure of carbon dioxide (PCO_2) 88 mm Hg, partial pressure of oxygen (PO_2) 45 mm Hg, HCO_3 30 mmol/L, and lactate 3.5 mmol/L.

Q1. What are the differential diagnoses from the history? How will you approach the case?

The differential diagnosis for dyspnea progressing over a period of hours to days includes acute exacerbation of pre-existing obstructive airway diseases, pneumonia with respiratory failure and sepsis, congestive cardiac failure (CCF), pulmonary embolism, acute exacerbation of an underlying interstitial lung disease (ILD), pneumothorax, acute respiratory distress syndrome (ARDS), etc. In an autopsy study of patients who died within 24 hours of admission for presumptive COPD exacerbation, the most common causes of death were HF (37%), pneumonia (28%), and pulmonary thromboembolism (21%), while only 14% had a primary cause of death as COPD.[1] Hence, a rapid diagnosis and exclusion of the differential diagnosis is important in these patients.

Appropriate initial investigations in these patients include an ABG, chest X-ray, electrocardiograph, complete hemogram, renal functions, and serum electrolytes, including phosphate and potassium. Brain natriuretic peptide (BNP), echocardiography, and cardiac troponins may also be useful in identifying underlying cardiac stretch and ischemia. If there is a change in sputum characteristics with an increased purulence, a sample should be sent for Gram stain, microscopy, and culture sensitivity. In the presence of sepsis or septic shock, or associated pneumonia, it is good practice to take blood cultures prior to antibiotics, without causing a delay in antibiotic administration.

In the emergency room (ER) or ICU, a rapid ultrasound examination as per the Bedside Lung Ultrasound in Emergency (BLUE) protocol has a sensitivity and specificity for identifying respiratory pathologies as shown in **Table 1**. The appropriate protocolized use of ultrasound can thus correctly identify the diagnosis in 90.5% of cases (*see* **Flowchart 1** for a schematic representation of BLUE protocol).[2-5] Interpretation of the common radiology signs and the possible differentials are discussed in **Table 2**.

Q2. How will you manage this patient with acute exacerbation of chronic obstructive pulmonary disease (AECOPD)?

Chronic obstructive pulmonary disease exacerbation is defined as "an acute event in the natural disease course, characterized by a variation from the patient's baseline symptoms, beyond normal day-to-day variation that requires treatment with oral corticosteroids or antibiotics, or both, in a patient with underlying COPD."[6,7] Once the diagnosis of AECOPD is confirmed, the risk factors and etiology of

TABLE 1: Sensitivity and specificity of lung ultrasound in patients presenting with acute respiratory failure (ARF).

Cause of ARF identified on USG	Sensitivity	Specificity
Obstructive airway disease	85–89%	88–97%
Pulmonary edema	85–97%	87–100%
Pneumonia	89–94%	90–94%
Pneumothorax	80–88%	100%

(USG: ultrasonography)

Flowchart 1: Schematic representation of Bedside Lung Ultrasound in Emergency (BLUE) protocol for acute respiratory emergencies.[2]

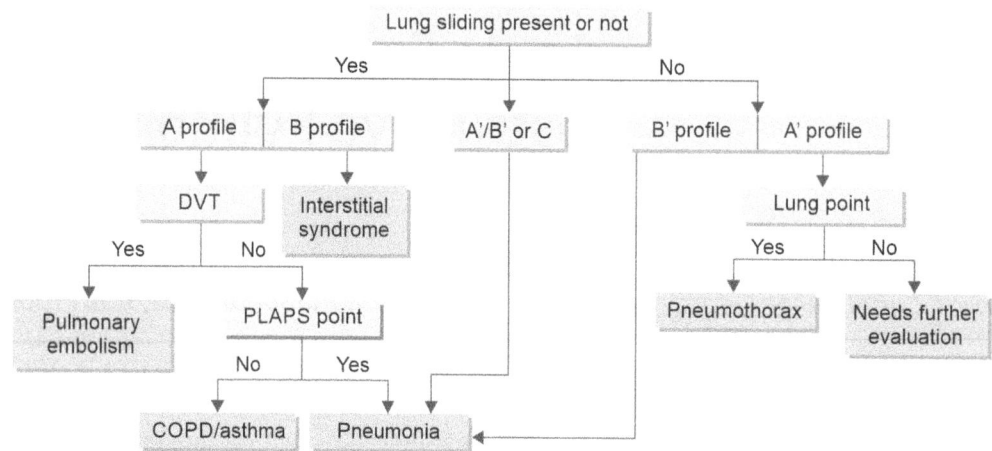

(COPD: chronic obstructive pulmonary disease; DVT: deep vein thrombosis; PLAPS: posterolateral alveolar and/or pleural syndrome)

TABLE 2: Radiology findings and possible cause of acute respiratory failure.

Ultrasound finding	Diagnosis	Other corroborative evidence	Caveats for a trainee
Lung sliding	• Absent lung sliding with the identification of lung point indicates pneumothorax • Presence of B-lines/presence of lung pulse rules out pneumothorax	"Stratosphere sign"	Need caution regarding the presence of bullae, fibrosis, or a mainstem intubation
Hypoechoic space	A hypoechoic space above the diaphragm indicates pleural effusion	"Quad sign" and "sinusoid sign"	• Can be mimicked by intraparenchymal fluid (lung abscess) • Should not be confused with ascites
Loss of pleural line	Tissue-like sign indicates the presence of consolidated lung	"Shred sign" and dynamic air bronchograms	Tissue signs can also be seen with malignancy, atelectasis, contusion, and infarction
Noncompressible veins	Deep vein thrombosis and pulmonary embolism	Presence of echogenic thrombus within the vein, absence of color Doppler signal, loss of respiratory flow phasicity, and loss of response to augmentation	Patients with normally compressible veins can still have DVT and pulmonary embolism from the pelvic veins
B-lines	Pulmonary edema and interstitial lung disease (ILD)	Echo might show features of cardiac failure or raised pulmonary artery wedge pressure	Can mimic ARDS, pneumonia, interstitial lung disease and fibrosis, lymphangitis, focal contusion, and noncardiogenic pulmonary edema

(ARDS: acute respiratory distress syndrome; DVT: deep vein thrombosis)

AECOPD should be ascertained. The common risk factors and etiologies for AECOPD are given in **Table 3**.

Typically, patients with AECOPD will present with an acute worsening of cough, breathlessness, increased sputum volume, and purulence. Fever and pedal edema are also common due to associated infections and cardiac failure. In all patients with AECOPD, a thorough initial assessment of severity will help to decide location of treatment. Initial clinical evaluation will involve looking for signs of respiratory failure such as respiratory distress, altered sensorium, presence of flaps, elevated jugular venous pressure, pedal edema, and other signs of right HF. In addition to evaluation of the symptoms, the history of previous episodes of exacerbations and hospitalizations is important to assess the patient's risk. Low-risk patients are those with no more than one exacerbation and no hospitalization for exacerbations in the previous year, while patients with increased risk have more than or equal to two exacerbations or require

TABLE 3: Risk factors and etiology for chronic obstructive pulmonary disease (COPD) exacerbation.

Risk factors for AECOPD	History of prior exacerbations, history of hospitalizations for prior AECOPD, elderly, duration of underlying COPD, mucous hypersecretion, presence of other comorbidities such as cardiac disease, diabetes mellitus, and pulmonary hypertension
Infectious etiologies for AECOPD	*Respiratory viral infections:* Rhinovirus, respiratory syncytial virus (especially in elderly adults with chronic lung and heart illness), influenza, parainfluenza, adenovirus, coronavirus, and human metapneumovirus *Bacterial infections: Haemophilus influenzae, Moraxella, Streptococcus pneumoniae,* etc.[8]
Noninfectious etiologies	Myocardial ischemia, congestive heart failure, aspiration, or pulmonary embolism, etc.[6]

(AECOPD: acute exacerbation of chronic obstructive pulmonary disease)

TABLE 4: Classification of acute exacerbation of chronic obstructive pulmonary disease (AECOPD) based on clinical signs, response to treatment, and arterial blood gas (ABG).

Severity	Clinical sign	Response to treatment
No respiratory failure	Respiratory rate 20–30 breaths/min, with no change in mental status or active use of accessory muscles	Hypoxemia improves with supplemental oxygen (28–35%) and no increase in $PaCO_2$
ARF: Not life-threatening	Tachypnea >30/min, use of accessory muscles, and stable mental status	Hypoxemia improves with supplemental oxygen (28–30%) but mild increase in $PaCO_2$ to 50–60 mm Hg
ARF: Life-threatening	Tachypnea >30/min, use of accessory muscles, and associated acute change in mental status	Hypoxemia requiring an FiO_2 >0.4 and associated increase in $PaCO_2$ >60 mm Hg or presence of acidosis

(ARF: acute respiratory failure; FiO_2: fraction of inspired oxygen; $PaCO_2$: partial pressure of arterial carbon dioxide)

hospitalization for COPD exacerbation in the previous year.[9,10] After risk assessment, AECOPD is classified on the basis of signs of respiratory failure, sensorium, oxygen requirement, and presence of hypercarbia and acidosis **(Table 4)**.

Criteria that would necessitate hospitalization for patients with acute exacerbation include acute respiratory failure (ARF), presence of cyanosis or pedal edema, presence of comorbidities, advanced age, those who have inadequate support at home, and those who fail to respond to the initial management. These patients will require close monitoring for identifying signs of worsening of respiratory failure, increasing respiratory distress, and also the response to therapy. The Dyspnea, Eosinopenia, Consolidation, Acidemia, and Atrial Fibrillation (DECAF) score and blood urea nitrogen, altered mental status, and pulse (BAP)-65 are robust predictors of mortality and can stratify patients into low risk and high risk, aiding in deciding treatment location, treatment escalation, and early palliation **(Table 5)**.[11-14]

TABLE 5: DECAF score and BAP-65 score.

DECAF score variables and score	BAP-65 score
Dyspnea—housebound but independent: 1 point	Blood urea nitrogen >25
Dyspnea—housebound but dependent: 2 points	
Eosinopenia <0.05 × 10⁹/L: 1 point	Altered mental status
Consolidation: 1 point	Tachycardia (pulse >109 beats/min)
Acidemia (pH <7.3): 1 point	Age >65 years
Atrial fibrillation: 1 point	
DECAF 0–1: Low risk DECAF 3–6: High risk	BAP-65 score of 0 or 1: Low risk Score of 2: Intermediate risk Score of 3 or 4: High risk

(BAP: blood urea nitrogen, altered mental status, pulse; DECAF: Dyspnea, Eosinopenia, Consolidation, Acidemia, and Atrial Fibrillation)

Q3. What is the pathophysiology of AECOPD?

Chronic obstructive pulmonary disease patients have resting expiratory flow limitation (EFL) due to airway inflammation and airway narrowing that leads to insufficient time for expiration and causes air trapping. The end-expiratory lung volumes (EELVs) fluctuate widely and are influenced by the extent of EFL and the ventilatory demand. During exercise or in any situation of increased demand, as the inspired tidal volume increases, EFL causes an increase in the EELV from the baseline, which is called dynamic hyperinflation (DH). AECOPD is associated with an abrupt increase in airway resistance due to bronchospasm and mucosal edema that worsens EFL and DH. DH reduces the compliance of the respiratory system, limiting the tidal volume despite an increasing inspiratory effort. The patient becomes tachypneic and adopts a rapid shallow breathing pattern, which further worsens the DH. Due to EFL and DH, intrapulmonary pressures remain positive even at the end of expiration, which is termed auto-positive end-expiratory pressure (auto-PEEP). This acts as an inspiratory load and can be significantly high in AECOPD, adding to the work of breathing.[15]

Q4. What are the phenotypes in COPD?

A COPD phenotype[16,17] refers to characteristics or a combination of characteristics that describe differences in COPD patients based on parameters such as clinical symptoms, exacerbations, and response to treatment. The widely accepted phenotypes are:

- *Chronic bronchitis (CB):* This means the presence of productive cough for >3 months per year in 2 or more consecutive years. A process in which mucus is overproduced in response to inflammatory signals, known as "mucus metaplasia," is the pathologic foundation for CB 5.

  The primary mechanisms responsible for excessive mucus in COPD are overproduction and hypersecretion by goblet cells and decreased elimination of mucus. Mucus hypersecretion develops as a consequence of cigarette smoke exposure, acute and chronic viral infection, bacterial infection, or inflammatory cell activation of mucin gene transcription via activation of the epidermal growth factor receptor. This leads to overproduction of mucus and hypersecretion from increased degranulation by neutrophil-mediated elastase. This is compounded by difficulty in clearing secretions because of poor ciliary function, distal airway occlusion, and ineffective cough secondary to respiratory muscle weakness and reduced peak expiratory flow.

- *Emphysematous:* It is a pathological diagnosis that affects the air spaces distal to the terminal bronchiole and is characterized by abnormal permanent enlargement of lung air spaces with the destruction of their walls. There is destruction of lung parenchyma with loss of elastic recoil, leading to hyperinflation and air trapping.

- *Asthma–COPD overlap:* Persistent airflow limitation with several features usually associated with asthma and several features usually associated with COPD (typically is asthmatic smoker)

- *Frequent exacerbator:* Presence of frequent exacerbations (two or more per year)

- *Rare exacerbator:* Presence of rare exacerbations (no or just one exacerbation)

Emerging COPD phenotypes[18] are as follows:

- *Pulmonary cachexia phenotype:* Body mass index (BMI) lower than 21 kg/m^2
- *Overlap COPD and bronchiectasis:* High-resolution computed tomography (HRCT) confirmation of bronchiectasis and definite COPD diagnosis
- *Upper lobe-predominant emphysema phenotype:* Computed tomography (CT) findings consistent of predominant upper lobe emphysema
- *Fast decliner phenotype:* Rapid decline of lung function
- *Comorbidities or systemic phenotype:* High comorbidities burden, predominantly cardiovascular and metabolic
- *Alpha1 antitrypsin deficiency:* Genetic condition caused by deficiency of alpha1 antitrypsin induced by biomass
- *No smoking COPD:* Induced by biomass exposure

Traditionally, COPD has been understood as a single disease caused by smoking, but there are a number of risk factors beyond tobacco and other forms of smoking. The Global Initiative for Chronic Obstructive Lung Disease (GOLD) 2023[19] document proposes a new taxonomy of COPD and suggests six etiotypes on the origin of COPD:

1. *Genetically determined COPD (COPD-G):* Alpha1 antitrypsin deficiency, other genetic variants
2. *COPD due to abnormal lung development (COPD-D):* Early life events including premature birth, low birth weight, etc.
3. *Environmental COPD:*
   a. Cigarette smoking COPD (COPD-C): Exposure to tobacco smoke, passive smoking, vaping, e-cigarettes, and cannabis smoking
   b. Biomass and pollution exposure (COPD-P): Exposure to household pollution, air pollution, occupational hazards, and wildfire smoke
4. *COPD due to infections (COPD-I):* Childhood infections, tuberculosis-associated infections, HIV-associated infections
5. *COPD and asthma (COPD-A):* Particularly associated with childhood asthma
6. COPD of unknown cause (COPD-U)

Q5. What are the endotypes of COPD?

An endotype is a subtype of a health condition defined by a distinct pathophysiological mechanism. The endotypes of COPD include the following:

- *Eosinophilic COPD:* Eosinophilic COPD patients may have more reversibility to bronchodilators and a better response to corticosteroid therapy in reducing exacerbations than patients without blood or sputum eosinophils and comprise 10–15% of COPD patients.[20] These patients show an increase in sputum and blood eosinophils and an increased fractional exhaled nitric oxide (FeNO), which are characteristic features of asthma and may also have a history of previous asthma or allergies. Eosinophilic COPD patients may also have more frequent exacerbations, although this has not been confirmed in other studies in which increased blood eosinophil counts were not related to exacerbation frequency. The underlying mechanisms of eosinophilia in COPD are uncertain.

Increased concentrations of interleukin (IL)-5 in induced sputum have been reported in COPD patients with sputum eosinophilia.[21] There is an increase in granulocyte-macrophage colony-stimulating factor (GM-CSF), which is important for maintaining eosinophil survival in lungs, and of CCL5 (RANTES), which is important in recruitment of eosinophils. Both of these factors are secreted by airway epithelial cells. There is now convincing evidence from post hoc analysis and prospective studies to show that increased blood eosinophil counts predict a clinically useful reduction in exacerbations with the addition of inhaled corticosteroids (ICS) in COPD.

- *Neutrophilic COPD:* Neutrophilic COPD patients may have inflammatory cells in sputum with a predominance of neutrophils and macrophages and usually few eosinophils. Circulating neutrophils are not useful in defining sputum neutrophilia or the neutrophilic phenotype of COPD, but they may be predictive of which patients may be more likely to develop pneumonia. It is induced by cigarette or biomass smoke, colonizing bacteria (especially *Haemophilus influenzae*), and oxidative stress, which release neutrophil chemotactic factors from airway epithelial cells and macrophages in the lung to recruit neutrophils from the circulation.[22]

The neutrophilic inflammation in COPD is unresponsive to corticosteroids, even in high doses, and may reflect the marked reduction in histone deacetylase-2 (HDAC2) seen in COPD lungs, which is secondary to oxidative stress. This indicates the need for more specific anti-neutrophilic therapies in COPD. Neutrophilic inflammation may be reduced by other anti-neutrophilic drugs, including anti-tumor necrosis factor (TNF), anti-CXCR, anti-IL-1β blocking antibodies, and p38 mitogen-activated-protein kinase (MAPK) inhibitors, but disappointingly, these approaches have been clinically ineffective. Roflumilast, an oral phosphodiesterase-4 inhibitor, reduces neutrophilic (and eosinophilic) inflammation in COPD patients and does reduce exacerbations when added to other treatments.

Q6. How will you manage a patient presenting with AECOPD?

Initial management of a patient presenting with AECOPD involves assessment and stabilization of airway, maintaining breathing, and assisting circulation as needed. A summary of the advantages and limitations of commonly done investigations in AECOPD is summarized in **Table 6**.

Monitoring of oxygen saturation with pulse oximetry should be initiated immediately, in addition to monitoring other vital signs. An ABG is warranted in this patient to assess the ventilatory and metabolic status. These patients need to be started on nebulized bronchodilators, oxygen titrated to arterial saturation of 88–92%, corticosteroids, antibiotics, and at times on noninvasive ventilation (NIV) also. Fluids and electrolyte balance need to be monitored on a patient-to-patient basis as circulatory insufficiency may be present in spite of patients being edematous, and diuretics in these patients could be counterproductive. On the other hand, the venous filling pressures might be high due to salt and water retention, and excessive fluids might be harmful. The heart–lung interaction might be altered in the case of right ventricular (RV) dysfunction, and these patients might have a raised value of pulse pressure variation (PPV) and stroke volume variation (SVV) secondary to RV dysfunction. Hence, the presence of high PPV or SVV may not be useful indices at the bedside to guide fluid administration.[23] Drugs used for medical therapy in AECOPD and the current recommendations are summarized in **Table 7**.

Q7. What is the role of systemic steroids in AECOPD?

Glucocorticoids in AECOPD are associated with many positive benefits such as rapid improvement in symptoms, improvement in lung function, reduction in hospital stay, and reduced risk of treatment failure and relapse at 1 month.[24] As oral glucocorticoids are well absorbed and have good oral bioavailability, the oral route is recommended for managing AECOPD. Intravenous glucocorticoids should be administered to those patients who are either too sick to take oral steroids, retain them, or absorb oral medications, such as those in shock or having severe vomiting or in periarrest situations. The GOLD guidelines suggest oral prednisolone 40 mg once daily for the majority of AECOPD.[25] In cases where intravenous methylprednisolone is required, trials have shown no benefit for doses > 240 mg/day.[26] A 5–7-day course of oral steroids is recommended for most patients as evidence suggests that a 5-day steroid course is comparable to 14 days of steroid therapy for the majority of patients.[27] Once the patient has improved, glucocorticoid therapy may be abruptly discontinued as adrenal suppression does not develop with short-course steroid treatment unless the treatment duration of therapy is >3 weeks.

Q8. What is the role of procalcitonin in initiation and continuation of antibiotics in AECOPD?

Procalcitonin is a marker of inflammation that is more specific than C-reactive protein (CRP) and erythrocyte sedimentation rate (ESR) for bacterial infections. It is commonly used in clinical practice in conjunction with clinical judgment

TABLE 6: Investigations in patients with acute exacerbation of chronic obstructive pulmonary disease (AECOPD).

Investigation	Advantage	Limitation
Full blood count	WBC count and differential count can help to differentiate between an infective cause and a noninfective cause of AECOPD. Eosinophil count can also help in prognostication	• Not available at the bedside • Severe sepsis may be associated with leukopenia and neutropenia apart from leukocytosis
Sputum for culture and sensitivity and viral studies	For suspected infections, it helps to identify those requiring antibiotics and antivirals	Cannot differentiate colonization from infection leading to overtreatment
Serum biochemistry	Dyselectrolytemia is associated with hypoxia and hypercapnia and worse outcome. Most of the patients will have hyponatremia, hypokalemia, hypomagnesemia, and hypophosphatemia	The mechanism of dyselectrolytemia might not be evident and treating the same may be difficult
Arterial blood gases	To characterize the type of respiratory failure, ventilatory status, severity of the exacerbation, and ongoing monitoring of the patient	Invasive and costly
CRP and procalcitonin	To assess the inflammation, may be able to differentiate bacterial causes from others	• Not to be used to decide on initiating antibiotics • Costly • False-positive and false-negative results are common
CXR	Can assess cardiac size, pulmonary edema, pneumonia, pleural effusions, and pneumothorax	• Hyperinflation and bullae are common • Increased bronchovascular markings in chronic bronchitis might mimic edema or pneumonia
ECG	Identifies old-/new-onset myocardial ischemia, ventricular hypertrophy, and arrhythmias	• Frequently has features of right heart strain • Multifocal atrial tachycardia • Sinus tachycardia and ST-T changes are common
Echocardiography	Can be used to assess biventricular function, right heart dysfunction, and regional wall motion abnormality	• Limited by poor acoustic window • Observer-dependent Doppler measurements
Troponin/BNP	A rise is suggestive of cardiac injury/cardiac stretch	Limited by other factors such as renal impairment and old age
CT scan	• Can assess parenchymal as well as pleural pathologies well • Delineates cardiac structures and pulmonary vasculature	• Still a research tool • Exposure to dye and contrast

(BNP: brain natriuretic peptide; CRP: C-reactive protein; CT: computed tomography; CXR: chest X-ray; ECG: electrocardiography; WBC: white blood cell)

TABLE 7: Medical treatment for acute exacerbation of chronic obstructive pulmonary disease (AECOPD).

Drug class	Examples	Special comments	Recommendations
Aerosolized short-acting β-agonists (SABA)	Salbutamol and levosalbutamol	Caution in patients with coronary insufficiency and arrhythmias	• SABA with or without SAMA are recommended as initial bronchodilators • Maintenance therapy with either long-acting β-agonists or long-acting muscarinic antagonists or their combinations should be initiated before discharge
Short-acting muscarinic antagonist (SAMA)	Ipratropium bromide	Caution in patient with glaucoma, urinary retention	
• Inhaled corticosteroids (ICS) • Oral steroids	• Budesonide • Fluticasone propionate • Beclomethasone dipropionate • Prednisolone (oral)	• ICS associated with oral candidiasis • Systemic corticosteroids associated with risk of GI ulceration, hyperglycemia, hypertension, HPA suppression, increased risk of infections	• Single-agent ICS are not recommended as monotherapy although nebulized budesonide alone has been used in some patients • Systemic corticosteroid use is associated with improved oxygenation, faster recovery, and shorter hospitalization. Not recommended for duration of >5–7 days[17,18]
Methylxanthines	• Theophylline • Aminophylline	Narrow therapeutic index, cardiac arrhythmias, CNS excitation	Not recommended due to side effect profile
Antibiotics		Choice depends on the presence of risk factors for adverse outcomes and for resistant organisms	• Indicated in the presence of worsened dyspnea, increased purulence of sputum, and increased volume of sputum • Antibiotics reduce the risk of short-term mortality by almost 77%, treatment failure, relapse, and hospitalization duration[30]

(CNS: central nervous system; GI: gastrointestinal; HPA: hypothalamic–pituitary–adrenal)

to decide upon continuing and stopping antibiotics in patients with sepsis. Available literature suggests that a procalcitonin-guided algorithm for management reduces the antibiotic exposure and treatment side effects without any decrease in same clinical efficacy.[28] In a recent trial, to guide the initial antibiotic therapy in patients admitted to the ICU with AECOPD, the use of a 5-day procalcitonin algorithm was associated with a nonsignificant trend toward overall increased mortality. Among those patients who were not started on antibiotics at the time of trial enrollment, mortality was significantly higher in the procalcitonin arm. In contrast to the previous trials on procalcitonin, this trial failed to reduce the antibiotic exposure in the ICU and in the hospital also. Before refuting the role of procalcitonin in de-escalation of antibiotics in patients with AECOPD, based on this trial, it has to be remembered that this was an open-label study prone to treatment bias. Antibiotics administered prior to trial inclusion may have underestimated the probability of infection, and till now, no society or guidelines recommend procalcitonin levels to initiate antibiotics in patients with suspected infection.[29]

Examination of the previous medical records of the patient revealed that he had been admitted thrice to the hospital in a span of 12 months for similar complaints. He had recently visited his specialist for worsening of breathing difficulty 3 days back. A spirometry done showed forced expiratory volume in 1 second/forced vital capacity (FEV_1/FVC) of 57% and FEV_1 of 40%. Prior to admission, even when he was at his physical best, he reported that he had to stop for breath while walking about 100 meters. A COPD assessment test (CAT) score was handed out, and he was identified to have a CAT score of 15. How will you classify his disease condition?

Chronic obstructive pulmonary disease is considered as a systemic disease, and the impact of the disease is assessed based upon the risk of exacerbations, combined with assessment of symptoms and spirometry classification. The new GOLD guidelines separate spirometry grading from symptoms and exacerbation risks.[25] This is clinically relevant as it correlates with important comorbidities and provides information regarding diagnosis and prognosis along with therapeutic interventions required for managing the patient. Severe exacerbations of COPD have an independent and negative impact on survival in patients with COPD.[31]

The new classification of COPD, adopted from GOLD 2019, is summarized in **Flowchart 2**.

Our patient is an elderly gentleman with cardiac comorbidities and life-threatening respiratory failure. His disease will classify as GOLD grade 3 group D. He will require hospital admission, close monitoring, and probably ICU care *also. In view of his condition, he was admitted to the medical ward for initiation of medical management.*

Q9. What are the implications of his cardiac status in managing COPD?

COPD/cardiovascular disease (CVD) relationship
Chronic obstructive pulmonary disease is a chronic disease and can be frequently associated with or coexists with other acute or chronic medical conditions, including CVDs. Both COPD and CVD are usually diseases of the elderly and share similar predisposing factors such as cigarette smoking and atherosclerosis. CVD is present in >50% of patients admitted with AECOPD, and around 20% of AECOPD admissions are due to an acute decompensated cardiac condition.[32,33] Associated comorbid cardiac illness has been associated with reduced survival from AECOPD, particularly with early inpatient mortality, and the underlying cardiac cause is often the cause of death in mild and moderate COPD as compared to advanced COPD where there will be a respiratory cause for the majority of deaths. Cardiac dysfunction during COPD exacerbations is characterized by a raised level of cardiac troponins and serum BNP and N-terminal pro-BNP (NT-proBNP) in the blood. The exact pathophysiology of this relationship (COPD and cardiac dysfunction) is unclear, and respiratory infections, hypoxia, tachycardia, and autonomic dysfunction have been suggested. The management of AECOPD in the presence of CAD does not differ much from the routine management of AECOPD. Inhaled anticholinergic medications–inhaled anticholinergic agent either alone or in combination with a short-acting β-agonists (SABA) are safely used for managing the acute symptoms of AECOPD. The inhaled β-2 agonists (salbutamol and levosalbutamol) preferentially act on β-2 receptors and do not increase the risk of myocardial infarction. These agents can cause arrhythmias, peripheral vasodilation, and hypokalemia, although the incidence of fatal arrhythmias remains low. Theophylline in low doses may have the potential to reverse steroid resistance and aid in limiting inflammation by activating histone deacetylase. Theophylline's use is particularly common as a third-line bronchodilator as the treatment is relatively cheap. Theophyllines have a narrow therapeutic index and are frequently associated with anxiety, dyspepsia, muscle spasms, tachycardia, arrhythmias, gastrointestinal (GI) symptoms, etc. in approximately 40% of patients. Due to their propensity for tachycardia and narrow therapeutic index, this group of drugs may be needed to be avoided in patients with COPD exacerbations and underlying CVD.[34] Cardioselective β-blockers may be continued in AECOPD, as these patients have tachycardia and autonomic dysfunction, which will be accentuated during exacerbations. Evidence suggests that

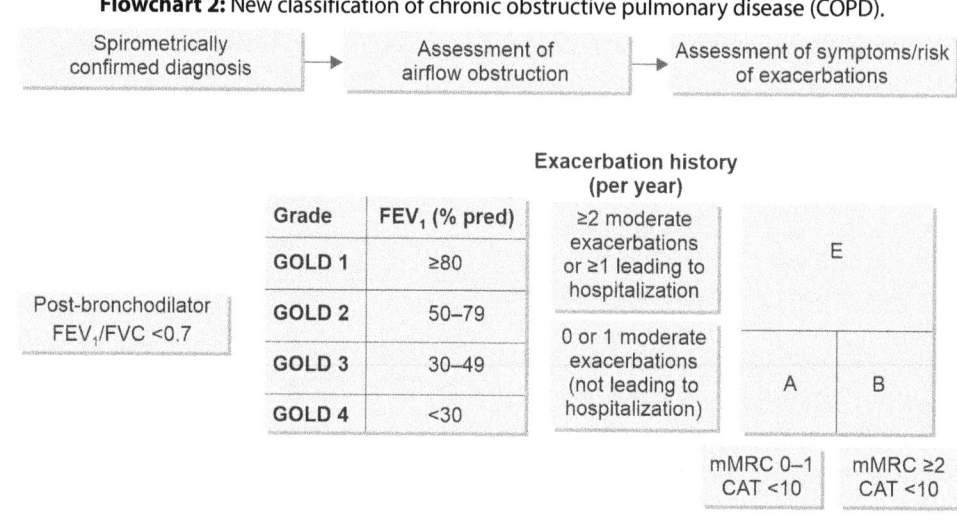

Flowchart 2: New classification of chronic obstructive pulmonary disease (COPD).

(CAT: chronic obstructive pulmonary disease assessment test; FEV$_1$: forced expiratory volume in 1 second; FVC: forced vital capacity; GOLD: Global Initiative for Chronic Obstructive Lung Disease; mMRC: modified Medical Research Council)
Source: Adapted from GOLD 2023 report.

mortality is lower in patients with AECOPD who are taking β-blockers at the time of an exacerbation than in those who are not. Other commonly used cardiac medications such as aspirin, statins, and angiotensin receptor blockers (ARBs) have a plausible role to ameliorate the inflammation associated with AECOPD and need not be stopped.[34]

The patient was started on oxygen therapy in the ward while a call was sent seeking ICU admission. He was started on oxygen at a flow rate of 6 L/min via simple face mask and maintained a saturation of 96%. However, after 1 hour, the dyspnea and tachypnea did not settle, and an ABG revealed worsening of CO$_2$ levels.

Q10. How is oxygen therapy titrated in COPD patients?
Oxygen therapy in COPD
All patients with AECOPD who are hypoxic will require titrated oxygen administration targeting an oxygen saturation of 88–92% as evidence suggests a significantly lower mortality in patients with titrated oxygen therapy.[37] Injudicious and unmonitored administration of oxygen in COPD patients can lead to worsening hypercapnia and respiratory acidosis by mechanisms explained in **Box 1**. For patients at risk for developing hypercapnic acidosis (those in whom initial ABG shows raised PCO$_2$ with normal pH and/or a high bicarbonate level), even lower oxygen saturation in the range of 85–88% is acceptable.

The hypoxia in COPD exacerbation is usually amenable to low flow of oxygen, and fraction of inspired oxygen (FiO$_2$) >0.4 is seldom required. To start off, oxygen therapy with low concentration venturi mask (24–28%) or low-flow nasal cannula (1–2 L/min) with saturation monitoring

BOX 1: Proposed mechanism of worsening of type II respiratory failure due to oxygen therapy.[35,36]
- Worsening of the ventilation–perfusion mismatch due to the loss of hypoxic pulmonary vasoconstriction
- A rightward shift of the CO$_2$ dissociation curve because of the reduced affinity of oxygenated hemoglobin to CO$_2$ (Haldane effect) leading to an increased partial pressure of CO$_2$ in arterial blood (PaCO$_2$)
- Increased resorption atelectasis due to higher oxygen concentration in the lungs
- A reduction in ventilation due to an inhibition of hypoxic drive

is recommended. An ABG should be repeated after 30–60 minutes to check for pH and PCO$_2$.[38] If a patient develops hypercapnic respiratory failure during oxygen therapy, the oxygen therapy must be gradually stepped down to the lowest FiO$_2$ level required to maintain a saturation in the range of 88–92%. Such patients should be initiated on NIV to support ventilation along with titrated oxygenation as sudden withdrawal of supplementary oxygen therapy can cause life-threatening rebound hypoxemia. An approach to oxygen therapy in AECOPD is shown in **Flowchart 3**.

Q11. What are the indications of home oxygen therapy in COPD?
The indications for home oxygen therapy in COPD[19] are as follows:
- Partial pressure of arterial oxygen (PaO$_2$) at or below 55 mm Hg or arterial oxygen saturation (SaO$_2$) at or below 88%, with or without hypercapnia confirmed twice over a 3-week period, *or*

Flowchart 3: Oxygen therapy in acute exacerbation of chronic obstructive pulmonary disease (AECOPD).

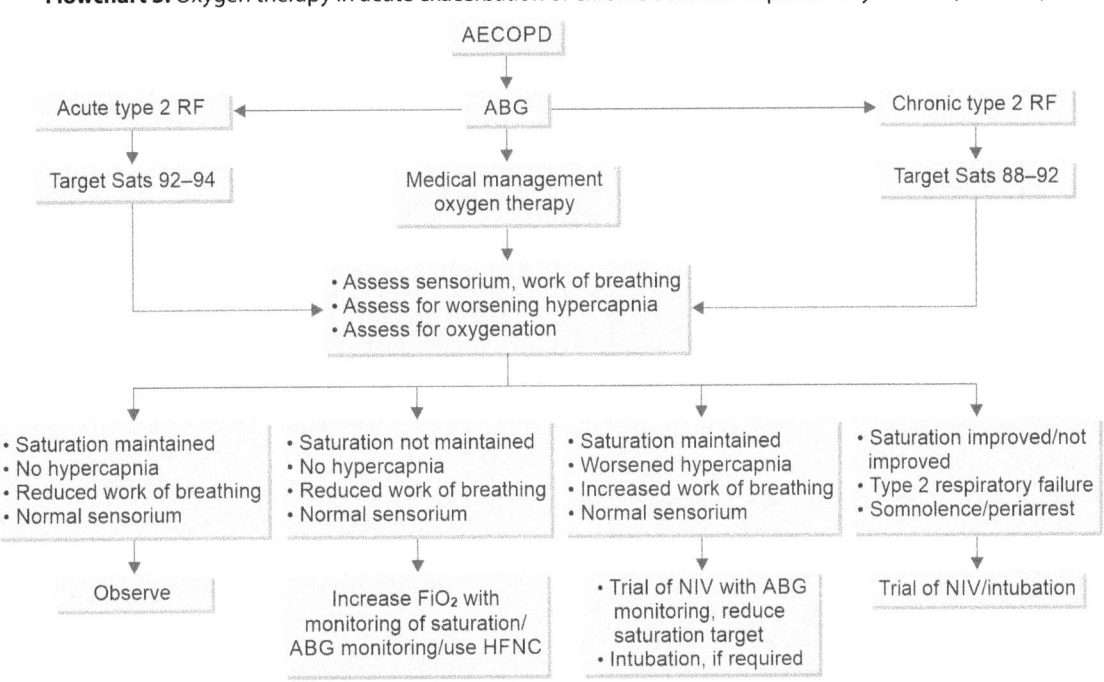

(ABG: arterial blood gas; FiO$_2$: fraction of inspired oxygen; NIV: noninvasive ventilation; RF: respiratory failure)

- PaO$_2$ below 60 mm Hg or SaO$_2$ below 88% if there is evidence of pulmonary hypertension, pulmonary edema suggesting CCF, or polycythemia (hematocrit > 55%).

All patients on long-term oxygen therapy (LTOT) should be reviewed in the outpatient department (OPD) after 60–90 days with a repeat ABG or oxygen saturation at room air.

Q12. What is the role of high-flow nasal cannula oxygenation (HFNCO) in AECOPD?

High-flow nasal cannula (HFNC) generates a gas flow of up to 60 L/min, which is heated and humidified before being delivered to the patient. Its advantages lie in the fact that the HFNC interface is better tolerated than a facemask/NIV, and the oxygen being humidified causes fewer side effects of the high flow of oxygen and air. The humidified oxygen is delivered at prespecified flow rates that match the peak inspiratory flow rates of patients (up to 60 L/min). This high flow maintains a small amount of PEEP (0.7 cm for every 10 L of flow with mouth closed and 0.35 cm if the mouth open).[39] HFNCO reduces the inspiratory time fraction, allows the respiratory muscles to be rested, and reduces the RR, thereby reducing alveolar dead space and wasted ventilation. HFNCO also helps in producing a washout of nasopharyngeal dead space and reduces the anatomical dead space.[39-42]

A recent study showed small reductions in transcutaneous carbon dioxide tensions after short-term therapy with HFNC when compared to titrated oxygen in patients with AECOPD.[43] Another study showed a trend toward lower 30 days mortality and lower need for intubation with HFNC as compared to NIV.[44] However, these results could not be reproduced in later studies.[45] Though some studies comparing HFNCO and conventional oxygen therapy for long-term oxygen supplementation in COPD patients show physiological benefits and reduced incidence of AECOPD, hospital admissions, and symptoms in AECPOD, the efficacy in treating AECOPD as compared to NIV has not been established without doubt.[46,47]

Q13. What is the role of NIV in respiratory failure in patients with AECOPD?

Noninvasive ventilation is considered to be the gold standard in managing patients with AECOPD and in those with severe respiratory failure or who fail to respond to initial medical treatment with oxygen therapy.[48] Use of NIV for AECOPD is a class I indication.[49,50] The European Respiratory Society/American Thoracic Society (ERS/ATS) guidelines recommend NIV for AECOPD in three clinical settings:[51]

1. To prevent acute respiratory acidosis, i.e., when the arterial CO$_2$ is normal or elevated but pH is normal (although NIV may not be tolerated)
2. To prevent clinical deterioration in patients with borderline respiratory acidosis (pH: 7.25–7.35)
3. As an alternative to invasive ventilation

Despite the evidence regarding the efficacy of NIV in AECOPD, a recent audit found that the use of NIV in many centers still remains inappropriate with regard to patient selection. Not surprisingly, the mortality was higher in those who received NIV, stressing the fact that proper patient selection and vigilant patient monitoring are important for the success of NIV.[52]

Q14. What are the general contraindications for the use of NIV?

Contraindications for the use of NIV[50] are mentioned in **Box 2**.

Q15. How will you initiate NIV?[50]

A stepwise approach to the initiation of NIV is given below:

Pre-requisites: Explain the procedure to the patient, ensure appropriate indication for NIV, select appropriate interface (oral, nasal, full facemask, or helmet), select machine—either NIV or ICU ventilator, institute appropriate monitoring, and have adequately trained personnel. Preliminary data suggest that dedicated NIV ventilators outperform ICU ventilators and transport ventilators by allowing better patient-ventilator synchrony by minimizing the leak and also compensating for any leak.[53,54]

Depending on whether conventional or NIV ventilator is used, initial settings are done. On NIV ventilator, spontaneous or spontaneous/timed mode is selected. On conventional ventilators, dedicated NIV mode (pressure preset) is used. Inspiratory positive airway pressure (IPAP) and expiratory positive airway pressure (EPAP) settings are titrated to effect. Start with low settings, IPAP of 6–8 cmH_2O and EPAP of 2–4 cmH_2O. The difference between IPAP and EPAP should be at least 4 cmH_2O initially and titrated according to tidal volume. In ICU ventilators, PEEP is equal to the selected EPAP, and pressure support is selected over PEEP (PS = IPAP – EPAP).

Increase EPAP by 1–2 cmH_2O till all inspiratory efforts are sensed by the machine and a breath is triggered. Inability of the machine to sense patient effort in the absence of major leak indicates the presence of auto-PEEP in patients with AECOPD.

Fraction of inspired oxygen is set directly on some NIV ventilators. Supplemental O_2 is provided in others titrated to saturation goal. IPAP is increased stepwise by 1–2 cmH_2O till adequate tidal volume and minute ventilation are achieved with no major leak. Pressure points on the nasal bridge and paranasal regions are padded up to prevent sores, and the mask is held on the face once the settings are accepted. After the patient gets accustomed to the flow, the mask is then strapped on with harness.

Monitoring for safety and therapeutic response should include vital signs such as pulse, BP, electrocardiography (ECG), oxygen saturation, sensorium, RR, patient–ventilator asynchrony, leaks, respiratory distress, use of accessory muscles, tolerance to NIV, and mask. ABGs are required initially at 1–2 hours to check for gas exchange.

Noninvasive ventilation therapy, nebulization and monitoring with ECG, and pulse oximetry were started. Chest X-ray showed a dense consolidation on the right side. He continued to be tachypneic with RR increasing to 40 breaths/min, HR 130 beats/min, BP 160/100 mm Hg, and SpO_2 80% despite NIV and FiO_2 at 40%. He was becoming drowsy but remained arousable.

Q16. What seems to be happening? How will you proceed?

Certain factors are associated with NIV failure **(Table 8)**.

Apart from these factors **(Table 8)**, NIV failure should be recognized appropriately by combination of clinical and ABG parameters, and these patients should be intubated immediately as NIV failure is associated with increased mortality **(Box 3)**.[55]

The criteria **(Box 3)** for admitting patients with AECOPD to the ICU include severe dyspnea that fails to respond to the best medical management and a trial of NIV, diminished mental status (confusion, lethargy, and coma), presence of community-acquired pneumonia, presence of cardiovascular instability, pulmonary embolism, need for invasive mechanical ventilation, lack of proper monitoring

---

BOX 2: General contraindications for noninvasive ventilation (NIV) use.

- *Inability to protect the airway:* Coma, CVA with bulbar involvement, and upper airway obstruction
- *Hemodynamic instability:* Uncontrolled arrhythmia and high doses of vasoactive medications
- *Inability to fix the NIV interface:* Facial abnormalities, facial burns, facial trauma, and facial anomaly
- Life-threatening hypoxemia
- *Severe GI symptoms:* Vomiting, upper GI bleed, and recent upper GI surgery
- Copious secretions
- Nonavailability of trained medical personnel

(CVA: cerebrovascular accident; GI: gastrointestinal)

TABLE 8: Factors associated with noninvasive ventilation (NIV) failure.

Patient factors	• Presence of pneumonia as a cause of AECOPD • Copious secretions • Poor respiratory muscle strength as assessed as poor nutritional status (NRS-2002 score >3) • Apache score >20.5
Intervention factors	• Not tolerating NIV • Absence of proper interface
Treatment response	Failure to improve in the first hour of therapy

(AECOPD: acute exacerbation of chronic obstructive pulmonary disease; NRS: nutritional risk screening)

BOX 3: Criteria for identifying failed noninvasive ventilation (NIV) in acute exacerbation of chronic obstructive pulmonary disease (AECOPD).

Clinical parameters:
- Life-threatening hypoxemia
- Tachypnea >35 breaths/min
- Impaired mental status

ABG parameters:
- Worsening of arterial blood gases pH in 1–2 hours
- Lack of improvement in arterial blood gases and/or pH after 4 hours
- Severe acidosis (pH <7.25) and hypercapnia ($PaCO_2$ >60 mm Hg)

(ABG: arterial blood gas; $PaCO_2$: partial pressure of arterial carbon dioxide)

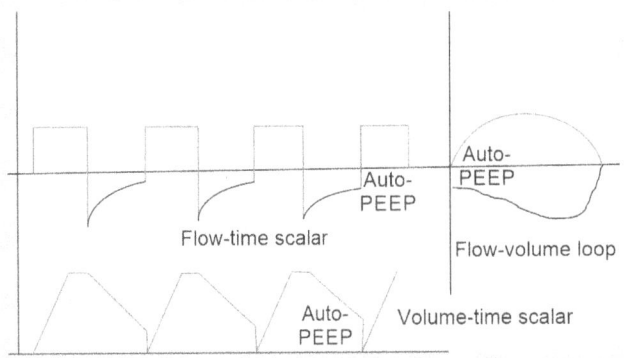

Fig. 1: Detection of auto-PEEP from ventilator graphics.
(PEEP: positive end-expiratory pressure)

of NIV in ER/wards, periarrest situation, etc. Our patient with RR >30 breaths/min, saturation of 80% on oxygen therapy, and $PaCO_2$ of 88 mm Hg fits into the AECOPD category of life-threatening ARF.

Q17. What are the indications for initiating invasive mechanical ventilation in AECOPD patients?

Mechanical ventilation in AECOPD is initiated in patients who have failed NIV or have contraindications to NIV. Proper monitoring and early identification of worsening patient condition on NIV are essential to prevent acute decompensation as it is associated with higher mortality. In AECOPD due to expiratory airflow limitation, expiration is prolonged, and as the next breath is initiated, some amount of air remains trapped in alveoli. This results in the development of auto-PEEP or intrinsic PEEP, which further worsens the breathing difficulty and work of breathing. Auto-PEEP results in increased EELV and pushes the diaphragm down. The diaphragm has to generate enough negative pressure to overcome both the auto-PEEP and produce further negative pressure to cause airflow. A flattened diaphragm is at anatomical disadvantage for effective contraction and reduces the effective inspiratory strength. With auto-PEEP, the intrathoracic pressure increases, leading to a reduction in venous return increase in RV afterload, which also reduces the left ventricular (LV) preload in series and in parallel (ventricular interdependence). These exaggerated hemodynamic effects of auto-PEEP can contribute to hypotension, pulseless electrical activity (PEA), and cardiac arrest.

Q18. How do you detect the presence of auto-PEEP in patients on invasive mechanical ventilation?

Bedside observation of the ventilator graphics provides clues to the presence of auto-PEEP.

On flow–time scalar, the inspiration will start even before expiration is completed, and the flow reaches the baseline.

Also, the volume–time curve will not touch the baseline during expiration, indicating that expiration is not being completed as the next breath is initiated. The flow–volume loop will show the amount of volume at the end of expiration as the next breath is initiated **(Fig. 1)**.[56]

Measuring auto-PEEP

Auto-PEEP can be measured in patients in whom the spontaneous breathing has been abolished. The airway is occluded at the end of exhalation by an expiratory hold maneuver, thereby terminating the flow in expiration and allowing equilibration of alveolar pressure with the airway pressure. The resulting airway pressure thus represents the average PEEP present within the lung at the end of expiration (total PEEP). Auto-PEEP is calculated by subtracting the set external PEEP from total PEEP. In a spontaneously breathing patient, determination of auto-PEEP requires insertion of esophageal balloon. A negative deflection in esophageal pressure from the start of inspiratory effort to the onset of inspiratory flow denotes auto-PEEP.

Q19. What ventilator settings do you start with in patients with AECOPD?

In addition to airflow limitation, inappropriate ventilator settings resulting in shorter expiratory time may precipitate or worsen auto-PEEP. Thus, during mechanical ventilation, care should be taken so that the expiration is complete and auto-PEEP is minimized.

Appropriate initial ventilator settings would be as follows to start with:

- Volume-assist control (with alarm settings for high peak pressures) or pressure assist-control (with alarm limits for minute ventilation)
- Tidal volume 6–8 mL/kg predicted body weight
- Initial RR 10–12 breaths/min
- *PEEP:* Initially, 0 cmH_2O, when the patient is paralyzed and ventilated. Later, once the patient starts breathing

spontaneously, we can start with 5 cmH$_2$O, later titrated to approximately 80% of auto-PEEP.
- FiO$_2$ titrated to obtain SpO$_2$ 90-92%
- Short inspiratory time and high peak flow 60-90 L/min
- Prolonged inspiration to expiration (I:E) ratio 1:4 or more while checking that the expiration is complete.
- By reducing set RR, inspiratory time and increasing the peak inspiratory flow rate, the absolute expiratory time is increased, preventing development or worsening of auto-PEEP. Currently, setting very high flow rates are also not advisable and are suggested to cause ventilator-induced lung injury.[57]
- Treatment of the auto-PEEP includes optimal medical treatment for the airflow limitation and adjusting ventilator settings, thereby allowing enough expiratory time by reducing the RR and decreasing tidal volume. The patient's ventilatory requirements can be reduced by treating anxiety, pain, and fever. The use of endotracheal tubes with large internal diameter (ID) and clearing secretions from the endotracheal tube will also help to reduce flow resistance. In cases of acute severe airflow limitation leading to auto-PEEP, the patient will require sedation and paralysis.[58,59]

Q20. Discuss aerosolized therapy in a mechanically ventilated patient and strategies to improve aerosol drug therapy.

Aerosolized drugs form a significant route of drug delivery in the ICU and are commonly used in cases of airway inflammation or alveolar inflammation, such as in patients with obstructive airway diseases, ventilator-associated tracheobronchitis, and pneumonia. The effectiveness of nebulization depends upon the generator of aerosol particles, the size of the aerosolized particles, ventilatory settings, positioning of the nebulizer in the ventilatory circuit, the dose and formulation of the drug to be administered, patient factors (which are often not modifiable) such as the anatomy of airway and lungs, the presence of inflammation and mucous plugging in the lung, the permeability of drug across the mucosal membranes, and clearance of the drug in the lung.[60]

A comparison of the various aerosol delivery devices is shown in **Table 9**.

Drug delivery via aerosols occurs mainly by three principles: (1) Inertial impaction, (2) gravitational sedimentation, and (3) diffusion or Brownian motion. Inertial impaction is the target for aerosol therapy for airway diseases such as COPD, asthma, and ventilator-associated tracheobronchitis, while drug delivery depends upon sedimentation in the distal airways and diffusion at the alveolar level. For adequate drug delivery, the size of the generated aerosols is important, and if the particle size is >3 µm, the majority of the aerosols will be trapped in the circuit and upper airway. A size of 1-3 µm is the target size for aerosol therapy, and particles <0.5 µm remain suspended in the airways and are expelled during expiration.[60-62]

Q21. How will you optimize the ventilator settings during aerosol therapy?

Ventilator settings for ensuring drug delivery during aerosol therapy should be modified as follows:[61]
- *Mode:* Prefer a volume-controlled mode over pressure-controlled mode
- *Higher tidal volume:* 8 mL/kg with a prolonged inspiratory time
- Preferring a constant inspiratory flow pattern over a decelerating or ramp pattern
- Selecting lower inspiratory flow rates, as tolerated by the patient
- Avoiding both heated humidifiers and heat and moisture exchangers during nebulization. Heated humidity decreases the amount of drug delivered by increasing the size of the aerosols. Heat/moisture exchangers must be repositioned at the expiratory end of the circuit to avoid contamination of the environment and need to be replaced to avoid obstruction of the filter and expiratory circuit.

The patient was ventilated and required a PEEP of 10 cmH2O and 60% FiO$_2$ to maintain a an SO$_2$ of 94%. Gradually, the patient improved, and the PEEP was reduced to 5 cmH$_2$O and FiO$_2$ 40% while maintaining saturation of 95% by day 3. The patient became hemodynamically stable and afebrile by day 3. It was decided to try to liberate the patient from mechanical ventilation, and the patient was placed on a T-piece. Within 10 minutes, he became diaphoretic, tachycardic (HR 130 beats/min), and tachypneic (>40 breaths/min).

Q22. How long do you do a weaning trial?

Weaning or liberation from mechanical ventilation includes the process of discontinuation of the patient from ventilator support and removal of the endotracheal tube. The weaning process can be divided into three steps:

Step 1: Daily sedation holidays and permitting spontaneous breaths (once the clinician thinks that the primary pathology has resolved and the patient is hemodynamically stable)

Step 2: Spontaneous breathing trial (SBT)

Step 3: Extubation

All patients should have their sedation stopped daily and allowed to wake up. Combining an awakening trial along with an SBT has been shown to hasten the weaning process and reduce ventilator days.[63] Once the primary

TABLE 9: Comparison of various aerosol delivery routes in intensive care unit (ICU).

Type of nebulizer	Jet nebulizer	Ultrasonic nebulizer	Vibrating mesh nebulizer	Metered dose inhalers
Mechanism of action	Uses air or oxygen under high pressure to generate aerosols	Uses piezoelectric crystal to generate aerosols	The drug is pumped through a vibrating mesh that creates the aerosol. The size of the droplets depends directly on the diameter of the mesh	Contains solution of the drug with propellants delivered through an atomization nozzle
Performance	Highly variable. Depends upon pressure of gas flow and position in ventilator circuit. Can cause circuit contamination, increased work of triggering, alter tidal volume and airway pressure during spontaneous breathing	Low variability. Particle size and efficacy depend on the vibration frequency and amplitude of crystal	Very low variability	Low variability. Requires priming and shaking of the MDI before actuation when it has not been used for 24 hours
Noise and temperature	Noisy. Low temperature of aerosols	No noise. Significant heating up to 10–15° occurs. Can lead to denaturation and inactivation of the drugs	No noise. Aerosols are of ambient temperature	No noise. Aerosols are of ambient temperature
Combination therapy	Possible	Possible	Possible	Impossible
Treatment time	High	Low	Low	Low
Contamination chance	High	Low	Low	Impossible
Cost	Low	High	Very high	Intermediate
Residual volume	High	Intermediate	Very less	Not applicable
Position in circuit	Proximal to the ventilator	15–40 cm from the Y-piece in the inspiratory limb	15–40 cm from the Y-piece in the inspiratory limb	15 cm from the Y-piece, used with a collapsible in line spacer

(MDI: metered-dose inhaler)

pathology requiring ventilation resolves and the patient is hemodynamically stable, the patient may be assessed for his ability to breathe independently. Weaning trials can be done either with a T-piece or pressure support. A weaning trial of half an hour is as good as a weaning trial of 120 minutes, and prolonged SBT is not usually required. No advantage could be demonstrated for attempting multiple SBT per day, and currently, only one weaning trial is done every 24 hours. For a detailed discussion on weaning, please refer to the chapter on weaning and ventilator-associated pneumonia (Chapter 3).

Q23. How will you approach the patient if he fails weaning?

Weaning failure occurs when the patient is unable to pass a weaning test (SBT) or has to be reintubated within 48 hours of extubation. Most of the patients fall into the category of simple weaning, i.e., successful extubation after the first SBT **(Table 10)**.

TABLE 10: Classification of weaning.

Type	Feature
Simple weaning (up to 60%)	Extubated successfully after first SBT
Difficult weaning (30–40% of patients)	Extubated successfully but requiring up to 3 attempts of SBT within 7 days after first SBT
Prolonged weaning (6–15% of patients)	Extubation after 3 SBTs or requiring >7 days of SBT

(SBT: spontaneous breathing trial)

Failure of the first SBT puts this patient in the difficult weaning group.

Approach to a patient with weaning failure includes the following components:
- Identification of possible causal factors
- Therapeutic strategies to address the cause
- Reattempt weaning

Identification of possible causal factors

Various factors contribute to weaning failure, and identification of the root causal factor is not possible in most cases. The most common cause of weaning failure is nonresolution of the primary illness for which the patient required ventilatory support. Along with this, there are various reasons that can be attributed to weaning failure—these factors may have developed during the course of illness, or they may have coexisted at admission but were missed. Malnutrition and hypothyroidism are strong predictors of weaning failure along with other factors such as myocardial ischemia, delirium, dyselectrolytemia, and pneumonia.[64] **Table 11** gives an overview of the various possible causes.

Q24. How will you diagnose weaning-induced pulmonary edema?

Understanding the heart–lung interactions during mechanical ventilation and weaning is important for recognizing and treating weaning-induced pulmonary edema.[65,66]

- During mechanical ventilation, the positive intrapleural pressure reduces the venous return to the heart. This

TABLE 11: Causes of weaning failure.

System affected	Cause	Evaluation
Respiratory (airway/lung)	*Increased resistance: Endotracheal tube:* • Small diameter • Thick secretions • Tube kinking *Ventilator circuit:* • Dead space of circuit • Expiratory valve dysfunction • Circuit compliance *Airways:* Bronchospasm	*Clinical examination:* • Auscultation of chest • Check equipment for condensation and exhalation valve block • Ventilator graphics
	Reduced compliance *Lung:* • Dynamic hyperinflation • Pneumonia and ARDS • Pulmonary edema • Atelectasis *Chest wall:* • Large pleural effusions • Morbid obesity • Intra-abdominal hypertension • Anasarca	*Clinical examination:* • Auscultation • Ventilator graphics • Ultrasonography and echo • Chest X-ray
Brain dysfunction	• Delirium • Depression • Anxiety • Oversedation	• Assess for delirium and daily awakening from sedation • Control of pain and anxiety • Family involvement
Cardiovascular dysfunction	• Myocardial ischemia • Acute pulmonary edema • Fluid overload	• Echocardiography • NT-proBNP and troponin • ECG
Diaphragm and respiratory muscle weakness	• Phrenic nerve dysfunction • Ventilator-induced diaphragmatic dysfunction (VIDD) • Critical illness polyneuropathy (CIPN) • Critical illness myopathy • Dynamic hyperinflation	• Assess neural drive by measuring the airway occlusion pressure at 100 ms (P0.1) • Measurement of maximal inspiratory pressure • Assessment of muscle power • Mobilizing patients early in their ICU stay • Avoiding hyperglycemia
Endocrine and electrolyte disturbances	• Hypokalemia • Hypophosphatemia • Hypomagnesemia • Adrenal insufficiency • Hypothyroidism	Biochemistry reports of serum electrolytes and endocrine results

(ARDS: acute respiratory distress syndrome; ECG: electrocardiography; ICU: intensive care unit; NT-proBNP: N-terminal pro-brain natriuretic peptide)

results in a reduced preload of RV and a sequentially reduced preload of LV, and a reduction in the total intrathoracic blood volume. The positive intrapleural pressure reduces the transmural pressure and the afterload of left ventricle, thereby reducing the work of the left ventricle, facilitating LV ejection.
- During spontaneous breathing, the intrathoracic pressure falls, and the venous return to the heart increases. The transmural pressure increases, and the afterload of the left ventricle increases. Due to an increased venous return and a simultaneously increased afterload of LV, the intrathoracic blood volume increases.
- The increased work of the left ventricle, together with increased thoracic blood volume, can precipitate LV myocardial ischemia and pulmonary edema in vulnerable patients.
- Additionally, weaning trials increase the oxygen consumption and oxygen demand by about 15% as the mechanical load on the respiratory muscles increases as it takes over the work of breathing.

Diagnosis of weaning-induced pulmonary edema
As already mentioned, removal of the positive pressure facilitates venous return and increases RV preload. A volume-overloaded RV encroaches onto the LV during diastole due to the phenomenon of "ventricular interdependence," thereby reducing the LV end-diastolic volume and increasing the LV end-diastolic pressures.

In a COPD patient, RV dilatation can also result from an increased afterload due to hypoxemia, hypercapnia, and the presence of DH. As the work of breathing increases, adrenergic tone increases, which can result in an increased LV afterload. Along with an increased preload, diminished cardiac contractility from an increased LV afterload can also worsen the LV function. This is further worsened by deep inspiratory efforts, which raise the transmural LV and aortic pressure and increase the LV and aortic afterload.

Diastolic dysfunction is also an important cause of weaning failure as noted by Moschietto et al. They found that patients who failed SBT had echocardiographic features of poor LV relaxation in contrast to those who passed SBT.[67]

At the bedside, weaning-induced cardiac failure can be readily assessed by simple tests such as measurement of BNP, NT-proBNP, and plasma-protein concentration and by bedside echocardiography. ECG might show tachycardia, arrhythmias, ST-T changes, or frank ischemia. Doppler measurement of early (E) and late (A) peak diastolic velocities across the mitral valve and tissue Doppler mitral annulus (Ea) in combination can accurately predict weaning-induced pulmonary artery occlusion pressure elevation. Lung ultrasound will reveal the appearance of "B-lines" in those patients who develop pulmonary edema after SBT induced by liberation from mechanical ventilation.[65,68] Liu et al. found that more than half of the weaning failures were associated with weaning-induced pulmonary edema, and COPD was one of the independent predictors of weaning-induced pulmonary edema.[69]

Management of weaning-induced pulmonary edema will depend on the hemodynamic response and the underlying mechanism responsible for the weaning failure. In patients with increased preload, diuretic administration will be useful. Empirical therapy with diuretics in all patients is not justified and, in fact, may be deleterious. An increase in afterload is usually manifested as a hypertensive response during SBT. Vasodilators such as nitroglycerin (NTG) reduce the preload by systemic venous dilatation and improve myocardial oxygenation by coronary vasodilatation apart from reducing the afterload by arterial vasodilatation. There has been no specific advantage for any particular ventilatory strategy in patients who are at risk for weaning-induced cardiac dysfunction. These patients should be put back on controlled positive-pressure ventilation, maintaining adequate PEEP. Once the underlying cause for cardiac dysfunction has been identified and treated, SBT may be repeated again. Patients at high risk for cardiac dysfunction who tolerate SBT may be extubated to NIV and maintained on NIV postextubation.[68]

Q25. What is the role of NIV in patients with postextubation respiratory failure (PERF)?
Development of respiratory failure after extubation, followed by reintubation, is associated with increased mortality and morbidity. NIV can be utilized for the prevention and treatment of PERF. Patients who are at high risk of extubation failure (COPD) benefit from early and prophylactic application of NIV in preventing extubation failure and reducing reintubation rates.[70] These patients should be closely monitored to identify NIV failure. However, in cases of established PERF, NIV has been shown to be ineffective and might be associated with increased mortality rates due to delay in intubation.[71] The ERS/ATS clinical practice guidelines suggest not to use NIV for the treatment of PERF.[51]

Q26. What are the criteria for defining patients at high risk of extubation failure?
The criteria for defining patients at high risk of extubation failure are described in **Table 12**.

Q27. What is the role of HFNC in PERF?
The indications of HFNC are being explored for many uses, including postextubation management where the prevention of reintubation is the primary goal without delaying appropriate reintubation. As compared to regular oxygen

TABLE 12: Risk factors for extubation failure.

Criteria for defining patients at high risk of extubation failure—at least one among the following should be present:

1	Age >65 years
2	Congestive heart failure
3	Moderate or severe chronic obstructive pulmonary disease
4	APACHE II score higher than 12
5	Body mass index above 30 kg/m^2
6	Weak cough with abundant secretions
7	More than one SBT failure
8	Mechanical ventilation >7 days

(SBT: spontaneous breathing trial)

therapy, HFNC is associated with lower rates of reintubation in patients with low risk for reintubation and is noninferior to NIV in patients at high risk for reintubation.[72,73] Available data suggest that HFNC is an effective method of delivering oxygen after extubation and might improve outcomes in hypoxemic respiratory failure. However, till date, there are no recommendations for the routine use of HFNC in the ICU in cases of PERF.

The patient was extubated the next day to NIV, and he successfully tolerated the extubation. His nebulized medications were converted to inhalers, as per the suggestion from the pulmonologist. He was actively enrolled in limb and chest physiotherapy. Prior to discharge from the ICU, the patient asks counsel from you regarding his disease status and future.

Q28. What suggestions will you give to reduce the incidence of further AECOPD?

Patients requiring hospitalization for AECOPD have poor prognosis and a low 5-year survival rate (about 50%).[74] Patient factors such as older age, malnutrition, presence of comorbidities, and history of previous hospitalizations for COPD exacerbations are poor prognostic markers. Similarly, those with increased respiratory symptoms, worse lung function, and lower exercise capacity have an increased mortality following an AECOPD. Pulmonary rehabilitation is shown to be effective in preventing episodes of AECOPD and reducing the frequency and duration of hospitalization.[75] Vaccination against both the influenza virus and pneumococci might reduce the incidence of AECOPD, pneumonia, and other serious illness and death and is currently recommended by the guidelines.[9] Regimens of prophylactic antibiotics, including macrolides and fluoroquinolones, should be weighed against the adverse drug reactions and the risk of antibiotic resistance.

Q29. What is the role of surgery in COPD?

Lung volume reduction surgery (LVRS)[76] is performed for patients with end-stage COPD to improve their quality of life. The NETT trial carried out in 2003, was a multicentric, randomized controlled trial that enrolled over 1,000 patients to determine the effect of optimal medical therapy as compared to a combination of optimal medical therapy plus LVRS. Inclusion criteria for this trial included:
- BMI <32 kg/m^2
- FEV_1 of <45% predicted
- $PaCO_2$ of <60 mm Hg
- PaO_2 of >45 mm Hg
- 6-minute walk test distance of >140 m
- No smoking for at least 4 months before initial screening

The trial demonstrated that heterogeneous distribution of upper lobe-predominant emphysema and low baseline exercise capacity had a better outcome with LVRS. A subgroup of LVRS patients with FEV_1 or diffusing capacity of the lungs for carbon monoxide (DLCO) <20% and homogenous emphysema on CT scans were more likely to be harmed than to benefit from surgical intervention.

The surgical options for the treatment of COPD[4] are as follows:
- *Bullectomy:* Giant bullae are indicated for surgical resection that occupies more than one third of the hemithorax and compresses adjacent viable lung tissue. Reductions in dyspnea; improvements in lung, respiratory muscle, and cardiac performance; and exercise tolerance have been reported.[77]
- *LVRS:* It improves survival in severe emphysema patients with an upper-lobe emphysema and low post-rehabilitation exercise capacity.
- *Bronchogenic lung reduction:* In select patients with advanced emphysema, bronchoscopic interventions reduce EELV and improve exercise tolerance, health status, and lung function at 6–12 months following treatment. Endoscopic lung volume reduction (ELVR) includes airway bypass stents, endobronchial one-way valves (EBV), self-activating coils, sealants, and thermal ablative techniques.
- *Lung transplantation:* In appropriately selected patients with very severe COPD, lung transplantation has been shown to improve the quality of life and functional capacity.[78]

Q30. What are the indications for referral for lung transplantation?

The International Society for Heart and Lung Transplantation (ISHLT) consensus document recommends referral to a lung transplant center for a COPD patient with BODE (BMI, obstruction, dyspnea, and exercise capacity) score of 5 or

higher with additional factors suggestive of increased risk of mortality such as:
- Progressive disease despite maximal treatment and frequent acute exacerbations
- Increase in BODE score >1 over the past 24 months
- Pulmonary artery to aorta diameter >1 on CT scan
- FEV_1 <25% predicted
- Resting hypoxemia (resting PaO_2 <60 mm Hg) or hypercapnia ($PaCO_2$ >50 mm Hg)

Q31. What are the indications for listing for lung transplantation?

The ISHLT consensus document recommends admitting a COPD patient to the waiting list for lung transplant in case of any one of the following criteria:
- BODE score of 7–10
- FEV_1 of <20% predicted
- Presence of moderate-to-severe pulmonary hypertension
- Three or more exacerbations (requiring hospitalizations) in the preceding year

REFERENCES

1. Zvezdin B, Milutinov S, Kojicic M, Hadnadjev M, Hromis S, Markovic M, et al. A postmortem analysis of major causes of early death in patients hospitalized with COPD exacerbation. Chest. 2009;136:376-80.
2. Lichtenstein DA, Mezière GA. Relevance of lung ultrasound in the diagnosis of acute respiratory failure: the BLUE protocol. Chest. 2008;134:117-25.
3. Wallbridge P, Steinfort D, Tay TR, Irvinng L, Hew M. Diagnostic chest ultrasound for acute respiratory failure. Respir Med. 2018;141:26-36.
4. Patel CJ, Bhatt HB, Parikh SN, Jhaveri BN, Puranik JH. Bedside lung ultrasound in emergency protocol as a diagnostic tool in patients of acute respiratory distress presenting to emergency department. J Emerg Trauma Shock. 2018;11:125-9.
5. Hew M, Tay T. The efficacy of bedside chest ultrasound: from accuracy to outcomes. Eur Respir Rev. 2016;25:230-46.
6. Anzueto A, Sethi S, Martinez FJ. Exacerbations of chronic obstructive pulmonary disease. Proc Am Thorac Soc. 2007;4(7):554-64.
7. Celli BR, MacNee W, ATS/ERS Task Force. Standards for the diagnosis and treatment of patients with COPD: a summary of the ATS/ERS position paper. Eur Respir J. 2004;23:932-46.
8. Wilkinson TMA, Aris E, Bourne S, Clarke SC, Peeters M, Pascal TG, et al. A prospective, observational cohort study of the seasonal dynamics of airway pathogens in the aetiology of exacerbations in COPD. Thorax. 2017;72:919-27.
9. Vogelmeier CF, Criner GJ, Martínez FJ, Anzueto A, Barnes PJ, Bourbeau J, et al. Global Strategy for the Diagnosis, Management, and Prevention of Chronic Obstructive Lung Disease 2017 report: GOLD executive summary. Arch Bronconeumol. 2017;53:128-49.
10. Celli BR, Barnes PJ. Exacerbations of chronic obstructive pulmonary disease. Eur Respir J. 2007;29:1224-38.
11. Steer J, Gibson J, Bourke SC. The DECAF score: predicting hospital mortality in exacerbations of chronic obstructive pulmonary disease. Thorax. 2012;67:970-6.
12. Echevarria C, Steer J, Heslop-Marshall K, Stenton SC, Hickey PM, Hughes R, et al. Validation of the DECAF score to predict hospital mortality in acute exacerbations of COPD. Thorax. 2016;71:133-40.
13. Tabet R, Ardo C, Makhlouf P, Hosry J. Application of BAP-65: a new score for risk stratification in acute exacerbation of chronic obstructive pulmonary disease. J Clin Respir Dis Care. 2016;2:1-4.
14. Sangwan V, Chaudhry D, Malik R. Dyspnea, Eosinopenia, Consolidation, Acidemia and Atrial Fibrillation score and BAP-65 score, tools for prediction of mortality in acute exacerbations of chronic obstructive pulmonary disease: a comparative pilot study. Indian J Crit Care Med. 2017;21:671-7.
15. O'Donnell DE, Parker CM. COPD exacerbations 3: pathophysiology. Thorax. 2006;61:354-61.
16. Vestbo J. COPD: definition and phenotypes. Clin Chest Med. 2014;35(1):1-6.
17. Weatherall M, Travers J, Shirtcliffe PM, Marsh SE, Williams MV, Nowitz MR, et al. Distinct clinical phenotypes of airways disease defined by cluster analysis. Eur Respir J. 2009;34(4):812-8.
18. Corlateanu A, Mendez Y, Wang Y, Garnica RJA, Botnaru V, Siafakas N. Chronic obstructive pulmonary disease and phenotypes: a state-of-the-art. Pulmonology. 2020;26(2):95-100.
19. Global Initiative for Chronic Obstructive Lung Disease. Gold guidelines 2023. [online] Available from: https://goldcopd.org/2023-gold-report-2/ [Last accessed August, 2023]
20. Oshagbemi OA, Burden AM, Braeken DCW, Henskens Y, Wouters EFM, Driessen JHM, et al. Stability of blood eosinophils in patients with chronic obstructive pulmonary disease and in control subjects, and the impact of sex, age, smoking, and baseline counts. Am J Respir Crit Care Med. 2017;195:1402-4.
21. Criner GJ, Celli BR, Singh D, Agusti A, Papi A, Jison M, et al. Predicting response to benralizumab in chronic obstructive pulmonary disease: analyses of GALATHEA and TERRANOVA studies. Lancet Resp Med. 2020;8:158-70.
22. Gross NJ, Barnes PJ. New therapies for asthma and chronic obstructive pulmonary disease. Am J Respir Crit Care Med. 2017;195:159-66.
23. de Leeuw PW, Dees A. Fluid homeostasis in chronic obstructive lung disease. Eur Respir J Suppl. 2003;46:33s-40s.
24. Viniol C, Vogelmeier CF. Exacerbations of COPD. Eur Respir Rev. 2018;27:170103.
25. Global Initiative for Chronic Obstructive Lung Disease. (2018). Gold Report: 2019 New Gold Reports for Personal Use. [online] Available from: www.goldcopd.org. [Last accessed August, 2019].
26. Kiser TH, Allen RR, Valuck RJ, Moss M, Vandivier RW. Outcomes associated with corticosteroid dosage in critically ill patients with acute exacerbations of chronic obstructive pulmonary disease. Am J Respir Crit Care Med. 2014;189:1052-64.
27. Leuppi JD, Schuetz P, Bingisser R, Bodmer M, Briel M, Drescher T, et al. Short-term vs conventional glucocorticoid

therapy in acute exacerbations of chronic obstructive pulmonary disease: the REDUCE randomized clinical trial. JAMA. 2013;309:2223-31.
28. Mathioudakis AG, Chatzimavridou-Grigoriadou V, Corlateanu A, Vestbo J. Procalcitonin to guide antibiotic administration in COPD exacerbations: a meta-analysis. Eur Respir Rev. 2017;26:160073.
29. Daubin C, Valette X, Thiollière F, Mira JP, Hazera P, Annane D, et al. Procalcitonin algorithm to guide initial antibiotic therapy in acute exacerbations of COPD admitted to the ICU: a randomized multicenter study. Intensive Care Med. 2018;44:428-37.
30. Ram FS, Rodriguez-Roisin R, Granados-Navarrete A, Garcia-Aymerich J, Barnes NC. Antibiotics for exacerbations of chronic obstructive pulmonary disease. Cochrane Database Syst Rev. 2006;(2):CD004403.
31. Kahnert K, Alter P, Young D, Lucke T, Heinrich J, Huber RM, et al. The revised GOLD 2017 COPD categorization in relation to comorbidities. Respir Med. 2018;134:79-85.
32. Agabiti N, Belleudi V, Davoli M, Forastiere F, Faustini A, Pistelli R, et al. Profiling hospital performance to monitor the quality of care: the case of COPD. Eur Respir J. 2010;35:1031-8.
33. MacDonald MI, Shafuddin E, King PT, Chang CL, Bardin PG, Hancox RJ. Cardiac dysfunction during exacerbations of chronic obstructive pulmonary disease. Lancet Respir Med. 2016;4:138-48.
34. Roversi S, Fabbri LM, Sin DD, Hawkins NM, Agustí A. Chronic obstructive pulmonary disease and cardiac diseases. An urgent need for integrated care. Am J Respir Crit Care Med. 2016;194:1319-36.
35. Abdo WF, Heunks LM. Oxygen-induced hypercapnia in COPD: myths and facts. Crit Care. 2012;16:323.
36. Cornet AD, Kooter AJ, Peters MJ, Smulders YM. The potential harm of oxygen therapy in medical emergencies. Crit Care. 2013;17:313.
37. Austin MA, Wills KE, Blizzard L, Walters EH, Wood-Baker R. Effect of high flow oxygen on mortality in chronic obstructive pulmonary disease patients in prehospital setting: randomised controlled trial. BMJ. 2010;341:c5462.
38. O'Driscoll BR, Howard LS, Earis J, Mak V. BTS guideline for oxygen use in adults in healthcare and emergency settings. Thorax. 2017;72:498-9.
39. Parke RL, Eccleston ML, McGuinness SP. The effects of flow on airway pressure during nasal high-flow oxygen therapy. Respir Care. 2011;56:1151-5.
40. Mauri T, Turrini C, Eronia N, Grasselli G, Volta CA, Bellani G, et al. Physiologic effects of high-flow nasal cannula in acute hypoxemic respiratory failure. Am J Respir Crit Care Med. 2017;195(9):1207-15.
41. Hernández G, Roca O, Colinas L. High-flow nasal cannula support therapy: new insights and improving performance. Crit Care. 2017;21:62.
42. Helviz Y, Einav S. A systematic review of the high-flow nasal cannula for adult patients. Crit Care. 2018;22:71.
43. Pilcher J, Eastlake L, Richards M, Power S, Cripps T, Bibby S, et al. Physiological effects of titrated oxygen via nasal high-flow cannulae in COPD exacerbations: a randomized controlled cross-over trial. Respirology. 2017;22:1149-55.
44. Lee MK, Kim SH, Lee WY, Yong SJ, Lee SJ, Jung YR, et al. The efficacy of high-flow nasal cannulae oxygen therapy in severe acute exacerbation of chronic obstructive pulmonary disease: a randomized controlled trial. Eur Respir J. 2016;48:PA3058.
45. Lee MK, Choi J, Park B, Kim B, Lee SJ, Kim SH, et al. High flow nasal cannulae oxygen therapy in acute-moderate hypercapnic respiratory failure. Clin Respir J. 2018;12:2046-56.
46. Storgaard LH, Hockey HU, Laursen BS, Weinreich UM. Long-term effects of oxygen-enriched high-flow nasal cannula treatment in COPD patients with chronic hypoxemic respiratory failure. Int J Chron Obstruct Pulmon Dis. 2018;13:1195-205.
47. Vogelsinger H, Halank M, Braun S, Wilkens H, Geiser T, Ott S, et al. Efficacy and safety of nasal high-flow oxygen in COPD patients. BMC Pulm Med. 2017;17:143.
48. Davidson AC, Banham S, Elliott M, Kennedy D, Gelder C, Glossop A, et al. BTS/ICS guideline for the ventilatory management of acute hypercapnic respiratory failure in adults. Thorax. 2016;71:ii1-35.
49. Chawla R, Khilnani GC, Suri JC, Ramakrishnan N, Mani RK, Prayag S, et al. Guidelines for noninvasive ventilation in acute respiratory failure. Indian J Crit Care Med. 2006;10:117-47.
50. Chawla R, Chaudhry D, Kansal S, Khilnani GC, Mani RK, Nasa P, et al. Guidelines for noninvasive ventilation in acute respiratory failure. Indian J Crit Care Med. 2013;17:42-70.
51. Rochwerg B, Brochard L, Elliott MW, Hess D, Hill NS, Nava S, et al. Official ERS/ATS clinical practice guidelines: noninvasive ventilation for acute respiratory failure. Eur Respir J. 2017;50:1602426.
52. Roberts CM, Stone RA, Buckingham RJ, Pursey NA, Lowe D. Acidosis, non-invasive ventilation and mortality in hospitalised COPD exacerbations. Thorax. 2011;66:43-8.
53. Hess DR, Branson RD. Know your ventilator to beat the leak. Chest. 2012;142:274-5.
54. Carteaux G, Lyazidi A, Cordoba-Izquierdo A, Vignaux L, Jolliet P, Thille AW, et al. Patient ventilator asynchrony during noninvasive ventilation: a bench and clinical study. Chest. 2012;142:367-76.
55. Shah NM, D'Cruz RF, Murphy PB. Update: non-invasive ventilation in chronic obstructive pulmonary disease. J Thorac Dis. 2018;10(Suppl. 1):S71-9.
56. Majid MM, Culver DA, Minai OA, Arroliga AC. Auto-positive end-expiratory pressure: mechanisms and treatment. Cleve Clin J Med. 2005;72:801-9.
57. Gattinoni L, Marini JJ, Collino F, Maiolo G, Rapetti F, Tonetti T, et al. The future of mechanical ventilation: lessons from the present and the past. Crit Care. 2017;21:183.
58. Davidson AC. The pulmonary physician in critical care. 11: critical care management of respiratory failure resulting from COPD. Thorax. 2002;57:1079-84.
59. Ahmed SM, Manazir A. Mechanical ventilation in patients with chronic obstructive pulmonary disease and bronchial asthma. Indian J Anaesth. 2015;59:589-98.
60. Ari A. Aerosol therapy in pulmonary critical care. Respir Care. 2015;60:858-74.

61. Luyt CE, Hékimian G, Bréchot N, Chastre J. Aerosol therapy for pneumonia in the intensive care unit. Clin Chest Med. 2018;39:823-36.
62. Dhanani J, Fraser JF, Chan HK, Rello J, Cohen J, Roberts JA. Fundamentals of aerosol therapy in critical care. Crit Care. 2016;20:269.
63. Girard TD, Kress JP, Fuchs BD, Thomason JWW, Schweickert WD, Pun BT, et al. Efficacy and safety of a paired sedation and ventilator weaning protocol for mechanically ventilated patients in intensive care (Awakening and Breathing Controlled Trial): a randomised controlled trial. Lancet. 2008;371(9607):126-34.
64. Ghoneim AHA, El-Komy HM, Gad DM, Abbas AM. Assessment of weaning failure in chronic obstructive pulmonary disease patients under mechanical ventilation in Zagazig University Hospitals. Egypt J Chest Dis Tuberc. 2017;66:65-74.
65. Richard C, Teboul JL. Weaning failure from cardiovascular origin. Intensive Care Med. 2005;31:1605-7.
66. Vignon P. Cardiovascular failure and weaning. Ann Transl Med. 2018;6:354.
67. Moschietto S, Doyen D, Grech L, Dellamonica J, Hyvernat H, Bernardin G. Transthoracic echocardiography with Doppler tissue imaging predicts weaning failure from mechanical ventilation: evolution of the left ventricle relaxation rate during a spontaneous breathing trial is the key factor in weaning outcome. Crit Care. 2012;16:R81.
68. Teboul JL. Weaning-induced cardiac dysfunction: where are we today? Intensive Care Med. 2014;40:1069-79.
69. Liu J, Shen F, Teboul JL, Anguel N, Beurton A, Bezaz N, et al. Cardiac dysfunction induced by weaning from mechanical ventilation: incidence, risk factors, and effects of fluid removal. Crit Care. 2016;20:369.
70. Nava S, Gregoretti C, Fanfulla F, Squadrone E, Grassi M, Carlucci A, et al. Noninvasive ventilation to prevent respiratory failure after extubation in high-risk patients. Crit Care Med. 2005;33:2465-70.
71. Esteban A, Frutos-Vivar F, Ferguson ND, Arabi Y, Apezteguía C, González M, et al. Noninvasive positive-pressure ventilation for respiratory failure after extubation. N Engl J Med. 2004;350:2452-60.
72. Hernández G, Vaquero C, González P, Subira C, Frutos-Vivar F, Rialp G, et al. Effect of postextubation high-flow nasal cannula vs conventional oxygen therapy on reintubation in low-risk patients: a randomized clinical trial. JAMA. 2016;315:1354-61.
73. Hernández G, Vaquero C, Colinas L, Cuena R, González P, Canabal A, et al. Effect of postextubation high-flow nasal cannula vs noninvasive ventilation on reintubation and postextubation respiratory failure in high-risk patients. JAMA. 2016;316:1565-74.
74. Hoogendoorn M, Hoogenveen RT, Rutten-van Molken MP, Vestbo J, Feenstra TL. Case fatality of COPD exacerbations: a meta-analysis and statistical modelling approach. Eur Respir J. 2011;37:508-15.
75. Puhan MA, Gimeno-Santos E, Scharplatz M, Troosters T, Walters EH, Steurer J. Pulmonary rehabilitation following exacerbations of chronic obstructive pulmonary disease. Cochrane Database Syst Rev. 2011;(10):CD005305.
76. Horwood CR, Mansour D, Abdel-Rasoul M, Metzger G, Han J, Aggarwal R, et al. Long-term results after lung volume reduction surgery: a single institution's experience. Ann Thorac Surg. 2019;107(4):1068-73.
77. Marchetti N, Criner GJ. Surgical approaches to treating emphysema: lung volume reduction surgery, bullectomy, and lung transplantation. Semin Respir Crit Care Med. 2015;36(4):592-608.
78. Verleden GM, Gottlieb J. Lung transplantation for COPD/pulmonary emphysema. Eur Respir Rev. 2023;32:220116.

Acute Severe Asthma

Babu K Abraham, Meghena Mathew

CASE STUDY

A 40-year-old gentleman with an ideal body weight of 70 kg comes to the emergency department with wheezing and breathlessness of 3 days' duration, which has worsened over the past 1 day. He is a known asthmatic on treatment with inhaled fluticasone and salmeterol (corticosteroid and long-acting β-2 agonist). On arrival, he is diaphoretic, tachypneic, tachycardic, and unable to speak in sentences. His saturation is 81% on room air. His vital parameters are heart rate of 140 beats/min, respiratory rate of 35 breaths/min, and blood pressure of 100/70 mm Hg. On auscultation, he has bilateral rhonchi.

Q1. What are the signs of acute severe asthma? What is the differential diagnosis that needs to be considered in this scenario?

Signs of acute severe asthma are a respiratory rate >30 breaths/min, use of accessory muscles of respiration, a pulse rate >120 beats/min, an oxygen saturation (SpO_2) on air that is <90%, inability to talk in sentences, a hunched posture, agitated appearance, and a peak expiratory flow rate (PEFR) ≤50% of predicted or best.[1] Some patients, with chronic asthma, may not be able to get their PEFR ever to that predicted for their height and weight. In such patients, we accept their best PEFR as normal for them and a reduction of 5% from their best PEFR is considered a sign of acute severe exacerbation.

The differential diagnosis for this clinical scenario should include pulmonary edema, viral pneumonia, chronic obstructive pulmonary disease (COPD) exacerbation, anaphylaxis, foreign body inhalation, and airway neoplasm compromising the airway.

Q1a. How is acute severe asthma different from uncontrolled asthma, difficult-to-treat asthma, and severe asthma?

Acute severe asthma is a different entity as compared to the other mentioned conditions. Both uncontrolled asthma and difficult-to-treat asthma will not have respiratory failure in their definition and will be more of an outpatient practice presentation.

Uncontrolled asthma[1] is a reason for persistent symptoms and exacerbations. It is defined by the presence of one of the following features—poor symptom control (defined as frequent symptoms or need for frequent reliever use, limitation of activity by asthma symptoms, and night waking due to asthma symptoms), frequent exacerbations (≥2/year) requiring oral steroids, or serious exacerbations (≥1/year) requiring hospitalization.

Difficult-to-treat asthma[1] is one that is uncontrolled despite the usage of medium or high-dose inhalational corticosteroid (ICS) with a second controller drug (e.g., long-acting β-2 agonist) or that requires oral steroid or that requires high-dose treatment to maintain good symptom control to reduce the risk of exacerbations.

Severe asthma[1] is a type of difficult-to-treat asthma where symptoms are uncontrolled despite adherence with high-dose inhalational steroids and long-acting β-2 agonist treatment and management of contributory factors or that can potentially worsen if the high-dose treatment is reduced.

Q1b. Does identifying asthma phenotypes help in improved management of patients with difficult-to-treat category?

Asthma phenotypes are patients with recognizable clusters of similar demographic, clinical, and/or pathophysiological characteristics.

Some of the most common asthma phenotypes described include allergic asthma, nonallergic asthma, adult-onset asthma seen in women predominantly, asthma with incomplete reversibility to bronchodilators, and asthma with obesity.

The other phenotypic classification of asthma is inflammatory phenotyping—type 2 or non-type 2. Type 2 is characterized by increased eosinophils and non-type 2 is characterized by elevated neutrophils. Eosinophilic inflammation is steroid responsive. Hence, type 2 patients with acute exacerbation will benefit with ICSs started at the earliest. However, during severe exacerbation, they might be refractory to even high-dose ICSs and they might benefit with oral corticosteroids.

Q1c. Describe the severity classification of asthma exacerbation.

Asthma severity is classified into mild, moderate, or severe.

The features of mild to moderate exacerbations include the ability to talk in phrases, absence of agitation, tachypnea, preference for a sitting position, pulse rate of 100-120 beats/min, absence of use of accessory muscles of respiration, SpO_2 on room air of 93-95%, and PEF > 50% predicted or the best value.

Severe exacerbation refers to when a patient is able to talk only in words, sits hunched forward, is agitated, respiratory rate of >30 breaths/min, pulse rate of >120 beats/min, accessory muscles are being used, SpO_2 on air is <90%, and PEF ≤ 50% predicted or best.

Q1d. Discuss the immediate management of this patient.

The immediate management of this patient should begin with an assessment of A (airway), B (breathing), and C (circulation). Look for altered mentation and a silent chest. Place a transcutaneous pulse oximetry and start oxygen via nasal cannulae or face mask to maintain SpO_2 around 93-95%. It may be difficult to do a PEFR monitoring in this situation and hence an arterial blood gas (ABG) analysis can be done. During an asthma exacerbation, partial pressure of arterial carbon dioxide ($PaCO_2$) is often <40 mm Hg. A $PaCO_2$ >40 mm Hg should be taken as an indication for respiratory fatigue.

The mainstay of acute severe asthma treatment is bronchodilator and steroid therapy. Start a short-acting β-2 agonist (SABA), a short-acting antimuscarinic agent (SAMA), and oral or intravenous corticosteroid. Salbutamol (2.5-5 mg) by nebulization every 20 minutes for three doses is a good choice for a SABA.[2] Evidence for pressurized metered-dose inhaler with a spacer during a severe and near-fatal asthma is less robust. After the initial repeated doses of nebulization, salbutamol (2.5-5 mg) should be continued every 1-4 hours, based on the clinical response to the initial therapy.[1-3] Effectiveness of salbutamol therapy is inversely proportional to the severity of bronchospasm.[4] There is a lot of evidence evolving now on the use of combination inhalational steroids—formoterol as an alternative to high-dose salbutamol demonstrating similar efficacy and safety profile. However, currently, challenges would be in terms of the availability of this combination as a nebulized solution and probably more data would be required to demonstrate better efficacy. Systemic steroids should be started early, especially when the response to initial bronchodilator therapy is poor. Both oral and intravenous steroids are equally effective. The doses recommended are either 1 mg/kg of prednisolone, 100 mg every 6th hourly[1,2] of hydrocortisone, or 0.5-1 g/kg of methylprednisolone in once-daily or divided doses. Their average duration of onset of action is 6-12 hours. Hence, the earlier the steroid is administered, the better the outcome[5] and less the relapse.[6] Intravenous route should be reserved for patients with impending respiratory arrest or for those who are already in respiratory arrest. High-dose ICSs should be given within the first hour after the presentation in patients not receiving systemic steroids.[1] In case of poor response to initial therapy, or persistent hypoxemia, or in those with forced expiratory volume in 1 second (FEV1) <25-30% done at the time of admission, intravenous magnesium is the next drug to be considered. Magnesium sulfate 2 g given intravenously over 20 minutes is the recommended dose.[1,2] It should be used with caution in patients with hypermagnesemia and renal failure.

Antibiotics are not routinely recommended unless there is a strong suspicion or evidence of lung infection as the trigger for asthma exacerbation.[1]

Frequent reassessment of the patient's response to therapy is absolutely essential. Failure to respond to medical therapy and respiratory fatigue warrants intensive care observation and early intubation and ventilation.[7] The decision to intubate and ventilate is purely based on clinical signs and must be made by an experienced physician without much delay.

This patient on admission has all features of acute severe asthma. The ideal strategy in the immediate management of acute severe asthma exacerbation is early recognition and timely intervention before the attack becomes life-threatening. The goal of management of asthma exacerbation is reversal of airflow limitation.

Arterial blood gas (room air) done shows pH—7.48, PCO_2—26 mm Hg, PO_2—50 mm Hg, HCO_3—28 mEq/L, and lactate—1.24.

Q2. Is there a role for noninvasive ventilation (NIV) or oxygen by high-flow nasal cannula (HFNC) in the management of acute severe asthma management?

The role of NIV in acute severe asthma, unlike in COPD, is not well proven.[8,9] If attempted, patients have to be carefully selected and closely monitored. NIV can probably be tried in patients who are not in impending respiratory failure, are hemodynamically stable, are neurologically intact, have no secretions, and are able to cooperate. A number of studies show potential benefit[8,10] in carefully selected groups, but larger clinical trials will be required before NIV can be recommended for all asthma patients.

Similarly, the evidence for the use of HFNC in this setting is still debatable. The available data at this point of time is more in patients who present to the emergency room with acute dyspnea and hypoxemia of variable etiology. Compared to NIV, HFNC has shown to improve the sensation of dyspnea and comfort in this group of patients[11] with no difference in the intubation rate. At this point of time, no recommendation can be made on the use of HFNC in acute severe asthma in adults. There is emerging evidence for the safety and efficacy of HFNC in acute severe asthma in the pediatric population.[12]

Q2a. What is asthma–COPD overlap syndrome?

Patients with features of both asthma and COPD are characterized under this umbrella. Typically seen in the elderly population. They can have frequent exacerbations. Lung function studies will show persistent expiratory airway limitation. These patients will benefit from ICSs along with long-acting β agonist and long-acting muscarinic agonist as their maintenance therapy.[1] The management of this phenotype, when presenting with acute exacerbation, will be very similar to as mentioned earlier.

Despite having been initiated on intravenous steroids, nebulized SABA, nebulized SAMA, and intravenous magnesium patient shows no signs of symptomatic improvement. An ABG taken 1 hour into therapy shows pH—7.35, PCO_2—40 mm Hg, PO_2—64 mm Hg, and lactate of 3.5.

Q3. What are the indications for intensive care unit (ICU) admission in a patient with acute severe asthma? When would intubation and mechanical ventilation be considered? What are the rescue therapies that have been tried to prevent intubation and ventilation?

Indications for ICU admission in acute severe asthma exacerbations are lack of response to initial medical management, deteriorating PEF despite therapy, worsening oxygenation (<92%), worsening respiratory distress, respiratory fatigue with rising PCO_2, and anticipated need for mechanical ventilation.

The indications for intubation and ventilation are impending respiratory arrest from fatigue with altered sensorium that interferes with appropriate therapy, cardiac arrest, and respiratory arrest.

This patient warrants intubation as he is showing early signs of physical exhaustion with a rising trend of PCO_2 (from PCO_2 of 26 in the first ABG to PCO_2 of 40 in the second ABG) and lactic acidosis. Rising CO_2 is a sign of alveolar hypoventilation and in acute severe asthma, a normal PCO_2 is indicative of hypoventilation. The pathogenesis of lactic acidosis in acute severe asthma is unclear and multiple mechanisms have been proposed, including increased lactic acid production from anaerobic metabolism of the respiratory muscles that are under stress of increased work and decreased lactate clearance by the liver due to hypoperfusion/hypoxia and use of β-2 agonist.[4]

Many rescue therapies have been tried to avert intubation and break the bronchospasm in patients with acute severe asthma and they include the following:

Heliox
Heliox is a mixture of helium (He) and oxygen (O_2) mixed in a ratio of He:O_2—70:30 for medical use. Its density is less than that of air and it improves ventilation by reducing frictional resistance in the gas flow, encouraging laminar flow, and thus decreasing the work of breathing.[13] The low fraction of inspired oxygen (FiO_2) in the mixture limits its application in a hypoxic patient. In studies involving both intubated and nonintubated patients with both adult and pediatric population, the use of Heliox showed no significant difference in the recovery of bronchospasm.[14,15]

Intravenous ketamine
Ketamine has been tried in the treatment of refractory acute severe asthma both in children and adults[16] with mixed results. It is administered as a bolus dose of 0.5–1 mg/kg followed by infusion of 2 mg/kg/h under intensive care monitoring. Multiple case reports are available on the use of ketamine in severe asthma.[16,17]

Adrenaline
In addition to the β-2 agonist property, adrenaline through its action on other catecholamine receptors provides additional favorable effects in acute severe asthma. It reduces bronchial mucosal edema by its potent microvascular vasoconstrictive action. It causes further bronchodilation by decreasing the parasympathetic tone. It has also been shown to improve the partial pressure of arterial oxygen (PaO_2). Adrenaline given subcutaneously is the preferable route in asthma and can be tried in patients who do not tolerate or respond to nebulized medications. Use this drug with caution in patients >40 years of age, with known cardiac disease, and in pregnant women.

Intravenous leukotriene inhibitors
A randomized study comparing montelukast with placebo showed significant improvement in FEV1 in the montelukast group.[18] However, this study has been criticized for its methodology. The role of leukotriene antagonist is probably more applicable in asthma exacerbation secondary to aspirin or nonsteroidal anti-inflammatory drugs (NSAIDs). The recommended dose is montelukast as a single 7–14 mg infusion over 5 minutes.

Inhalational anesthetic agents

Halothane, isoflurane, and sevoflurane exert bronchodilatory properties by direct action on bronchial smooth muscle via calcium-dependent channels and by attenuating cholinergic tone. They reduce peak airway pressure within minutes of application and decrease pulmonary artery pressure. The dose of inhalational agents administrated needs to be titrated to clinical response. There are multiple case reports detailing the effects of isoflurane and sevoflurane in acute severe asthma.[19-21] But there are no randomized controlled trials (RCTs) to confirm their efficacy. Significant hypotension and myocardial depression are the most common side effects. Their use in the ICU is limited by cost, need for specialized equipment, need for intensive monitoring, and need for a scavenging system.

The use of intravenous β-2 agonist as a rescue therapy is no longer recommended.[1,2] Other therapies that have been reported in the literature are intravenous glucagon, nebulized clonidine, nebulized calcium channel blockers, and nebulized lidocaine.

Clinically, the patient has not responded to medical therapy and has progressed into a state of impending respiratory failure. A decision has been taken to intubate and ventilate him.

Q4. Describe the preparation required for intubating this patient. Mention the choice of sedation and premedications that are used.

Pathophysiology of asthma exacerbation includes increasing bronchospasm, increasing air trapping with worsening dynamic hyperinflation (DHI), depletion of catecholamines, and dehydration due to insensible losses. This leads to a patient who is exhausted with little physiological reserve. Post intubation there can be devastating consequences resulting from rapid fall in blood pressure and SpO_2. Anticipation and preparation are the keys to preventing or dealing with this deterioration.

Intubation should be planned and achieved as early as possible. Anticipate rapid desaturation in patients whose SpO_2 is ≤93%. Preoxygenate using a bag-valve-mask ventilation system or NIV. It may be difficult to achieve adequate preoxygenation due to their high residual volume and functional residual capacity.[22] When bagging, make sure that small tidal volumes, high-flow rates, and prolonged expiratory phase are used in an attempt to prevent breath stacking and generation of auto-positive end-expiratory pressure (PEEP). Place a couple of wide-bore intravenous cannulae and load them with intravenous fluid in anticipation of postintubation hypotension. Have inopressors kept ready for use if necessary. Have large-size endotracheal tubes (ETTs) (size 8 and above) and all the drugs required for modified rapid sequence intubation (RSI) ready.

Nasotracheal intubation is to be avoided as nasal polyps are common in asthmatics. Orotracheal intubation with larger diameter ETT helps with the decrease in airway resistance, toileting of airways, and therapeutic bronchoscopy if needed.

The preferred approach of intubation would be modified RSI. Pretreatment with lidocaine may be indicated in patients who have not received any bronchodilators. Opioid and barbiturates help to blunt sympathetic response secondary to intubation; however, there is a small risk of histamine release. Ketamine and propofol are considered the drugs of choice for induction.[23] Ketamine is the preferred drug as it does not cause hypotension (dose: 1-2 mg/kg intravenous bolus followed by an infusion at 0.5-0.75 mg/kg/h). It may be contraindicated in patients with hypertension, ischemic heart disease, raised intracranial pressure (ICP), and preeclampsia. Propofol too has been shown to have bronchodilator effect. However, its greatest drawback is hypotension. Other drugs such as midazolam and etomidate have been used as induction agents.

There is no difference between using succinylcholine or a nondepolarizing agent for paralysis.[7]

The patient has been successfully intubated and is being hand ventilated. Arrangements are being made to connect him to mechanical ventilation (Flowchart 1).

Q5. Discuss the management of sedation and paralytic agents post intubation and describe the initial ventilator settings in this patient.

Once intubated, sedation is essential to improve patient comfort, decrease tissue oxygen consumption, control respiratory rate, decrease air trapping, and provide better patient–ventilator synchrony. To provide adequate analgesia with amnesia and adequate suppression of respiratory rate, a combination of an opioid (fentanyl: 1-2 μg/kg/h) with a benzodiazepine (midazolam: 2-10 mg/h) can be used. The use of neuromuscular blocker should be reserved for patients who cannot be adequately ventilated with deep sedation alone and if used, it should be restricted to <24 h. The drug of choice would be cisatracurium in a dose of 1-2 μg/kg/min due to its better cardiorespiratory effects and nonhepatic or renal elimination.[7]

The objectives of setting a ventilator in a patient with acute severe asthma are to prevent breath stacking and reduce DHI. This is achieved by keeping a low tidal volume, a low respiratory rate, higher inspiratory flows, and a short inspiratory time (Ti). The occurrence of hypotension immediately after initiation of mechanical ventilation can be due to a combination of DHI, hypovolemia, vasodilatory effect of induction drugs, and tension pneumothorax.

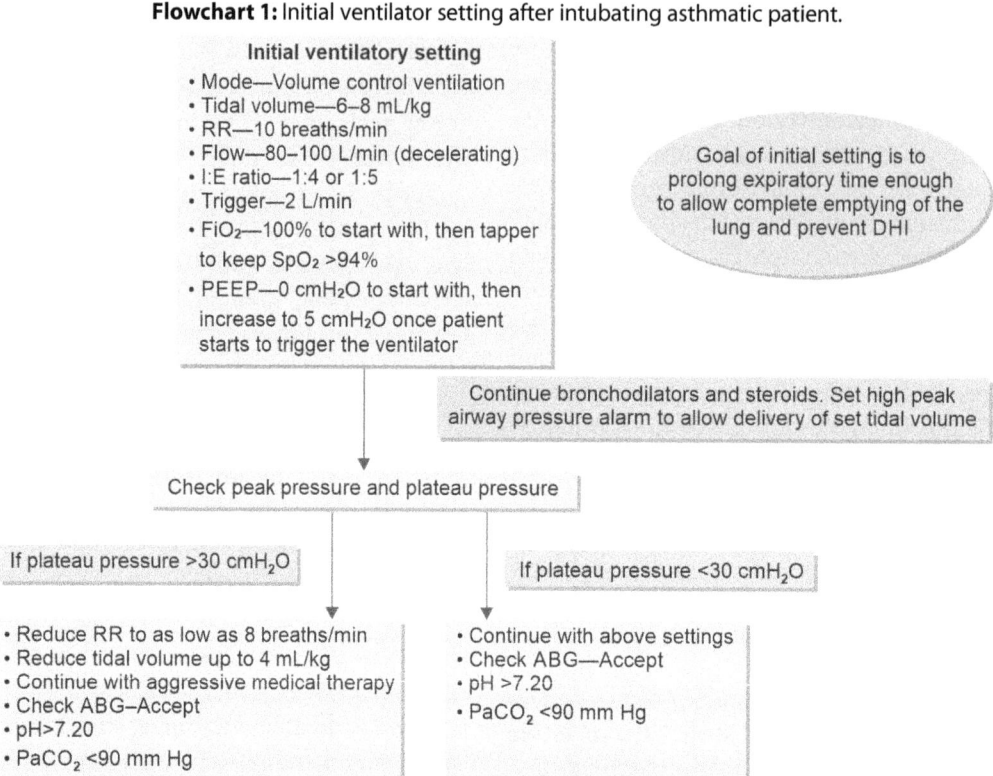

Flowchart 1: Initial ventilator setting after intubating asthmatic patient.

(ABG: arterial blood gas; DHI: dynamic hyperinflation; FiO_2: fraction of inspired oxygen; $PaCO_2$: partial pressure of arterial carbon dioxide; PEEP: positive end-expiratory pressure; RR: respiratory rate)

First, choose the mode in which the patient should be ventilated. There is no single preferred mode of ventilation for these patients. Outcomes have been similar with both volume preset and pressure preset modes.[24] However, volume preset mode is preferred as it has been most studied. The suggested initial ventilator settings in a volume-controlled ventilation are a tidal volume of 6–8 mL/kg of ideal body weight, respiratory rate of 10 breaths/min, peak inspiratory flow of 60 L/min with constant flow pattern or 80–90 L/min with decelerating flow pattern, an inspiratory to expiratory ratio (I:E ratio) of 1:4 to 1:5, FiO_2 of 100%, and a PEEP of 0 cm Hg, as long as the patient is sedated and paralyzed.

The FiO_2 has to be gradually reduced from 100% with the goal to maintain saturation >94%. As the sedation is lightened and the patient starts to trigger the ventilator, the trigger sensitivity should be kept at 2 L/min. Monitor the plateau pressure closely and keep it <30 cmH_2O. Set the peak pressure alarm above the patient's peak pressure seen on the ventilator to avoid hypoventilation. The low respiratory rate and tidal volume (6 mL/kg) used for preventing DHI in asthma ventilation can cause hypercapnia. It is acceptable to allow hypercapnia with a safe limit set at pH above 7.2 and PCO_2 at 90 mm Hg.[25,26] "Permissive hypercapnic ventilation" is the terminology used for this type of ventilator setting.

After initiating mechanical ventilation, always do a quick bedside examination looking for symmetrical chest rise, bilateral equal air entry, and evaluation of vital parameters looking for hypotension and hypoxia.

After a couple of hours of setting the ventilator, the high-pressure alarm starts to go off frequently.

Q6. Explain how to troubleshoot high-pressure alarms in this patient.

A peak inspiratory pressure of >80–100 cmH_2O is not unusual in patients with severe asthma. Set the high-pressure alarm limit at 100 cmH_2O to facilitate delivery of the set tidal volume. The most common cause for high-pressure alarm would be worsening bronchospasm. However, other causes such as decreased lung/pleural compliance (e.g., hyperinflation, pneumonia, pneumothorax) and patient-ventilator dyssynchrony need to be looked for.

To troubleshoot high peak airway pressure alarm, it is essential to differentiate between an airway resistance problem and a lung compliance issue. Peak pressure is the sum of airway resistance pressure, PEEP, and lung elastic pressure, while plateau pressure, obtained by applying an inspiratory pause, reflects alveolar pressure. When both peak pressure and plateau pressure increase, it is indicative of a compliance problem. Evaluate the patient for a lung

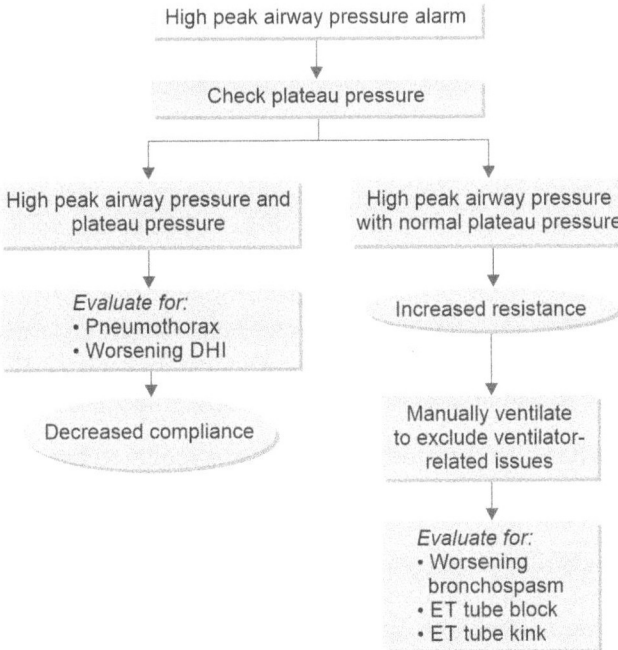

Flowchart 2: Evaluating high peak airway pressure alarm.

(DHI: dynamic hyperinflation; ET: endotracheal)

parenchymal, pleural, and chest wall or a diaphragmatic problem. An elevated peak airway pressure with a normal plateau indicates an airway resistance problem.

Then evaluate the patient for worsening bronchospasm, ETT block or kink **(Flowchart 2)**.

All of a sudden, he develops hypotension (80/50 mm Hg) with worsening hypoxia, which rapidly deteriorates into a pulseless electrical activity (PEA).

Q7. Enumerate the possible causes for this sudden setback and discuss how the cardiac arrest can be managed.

Advanced cardiac life support (ACLS) algorithm needs to be initiated for the PEA cardiac arrest while simultaneously looking for a reversible cause.

The cause for PEA cardiac arrest that is specific for patients with acute severe asthma on mechanical ventilation is DHI, which is accentuated by positive pressure ventilation. DHI happens in asthma due to incomplete exhalation leading to air trapping. This further worsens if the ventilator is not set properly giving sufficient expiratory time for the lung to empty.

Positive pressure ventilation by virtue of creating a change in heart–lung interaction can cause cardiac arrest by decreasing the preload to the right ventricle, increasing pericardial pressure, and increasing total pulmonary vascular resistance and right ventricular strain. The change in transpulmonary pressure can predispose to tension pneumothorax. The other factors that worsen hemodynamic instability are sedation-induced vasodilatation and preexisting hypovolemia.

If DHI is suspected, a trial of hypoventilation (delivering 2–3 breaths/min of 100% oxygen for a few minutes) can be done both as a diagnostic and therapeutic intervention. Tension pneumothorax could be a cause for PEA arrest and if clinically suspected, a needle thoracostomy followed by intercostal drainage needs to be done. Other causes of PEA cardiac arrest include electrolyte abnormalities (including lethal hyperkalemia if succinylcholine was used for intubation of a patient with respiratory acidosis), severe acidosis, myocardial ischemia (particularly if high-dose β-2 agonists were used systemically), and ETT displacement, kinking, or plugging should be recognized and treated appropriately.

The patient has been successfully resuscitated out of PEA with a return of spontaneous circulation (ROSC) of <2 minutes. However, he continues to require a FiO_2 of 1 to maintain an SpO_2 >88%.

Q8. What are the possible causes of postintubation hypoxia and how can they be managed?

The common causes for postintubation hypoxia are right main stem intubation, ETT displacement, ETT blockage, leakage of air around the ETT, pneumothorax, gastric distension decreasing respiratory system compliance, mechanical malfunction of the ventilator apparatus, aspiration, and worsening bronchospasm. Identification of these complications is essential as management differs and the initial assessment includes clinical examination, chest X-ray, and use of bedside ultrasonogram.

Right main stem intubation

Clinical examination usually clinches the diagnosis. Diminished chest movement of the left hemithorax and auscultation revealing asymmetrical breath sounds with absent air entry on the left is usually diagnostic. Postintubation chest X-ray will confirm the diagnosis.

Pneumothorax

There should be a high level of suspicion for a pneumothorax. Look for increased airway pressures and unilateral absent breath sound with hyperresonant percussion note. Bedside ultrasonography (USG) examination can be helpful. An emergent needle thoracostomy followed by intercostal drainage should be performed immediately as this could progress to tension pneumothorax if left unattended.

Endotracheal tube displacement

Assess the position of the tube at the lip level. A chest X-ray or direct visualization with a laryngoscope can be done to evaluate any displacement. Once identified, direct visualization and repositioning under sedation are advised.

Endotracheal tube blockage
Decreased bilateral air entry, difficulty to deliver set tidal volume, and a rising peak pressure should alert one with the possibility of a tube block. This condition also warrants replacement with a new tube.

Endotracheal tube cuff leak
A cuff leak can be diagnosed by an audible air leak and inability of the ventilator to deliver the set tidal volume. If there is a cuff leak, replace the tube.

Gastric distension
Gastric distension can decrease respiratory compliance and usually occurs following the application of NIV or vigorous bag-valve-mask ventilation prior to intubation. It can be diagnosed by clinical examination and is treated by decompressing the stomach by placing a nasogastric tube.

Pneumonia
Suspect pneumonia if the patient has a fever and thick purulent sputum. A chest X-ray will usually help with the diagnosis. Antibiotics need to be initiated if pneumonia is suspected.

Finally, a quick check of the ventilator by placing a test lung will help in evaluating the functioning of the ventilator.

The patient's hypoxia improves with therapy but he continues to be deeply sedated and paralyzed to facilitate mechanical ventilation. On performing an end-inspiratory hold and end-expiratory hold, the plateau pressure is recorded to be 40 cmH_2O with a peak pressure of 80 cmH_2O, and intrinsic PEEP of 18 cmH_2O.

Q9. What do the above pressure measurements mean and could this patient have DHI?
This patient has both elevated plateau pressure and peak airway pressure, which is a sign of decreased lung compliance (*see* Q6). In a patient with pure asthma, decreased lung compliance could be an indicator of impending DHI.

Dynamic hyperinflation happens when inadequate expiratory time leads to incomplete emptying of alveoli with associated trapping of some amount of the delivered tidal volume in the alveoli at the end of expiration. With every breath, more and more air is entrapped in the alveoli, thus making the pressure within the alveoli to go up and the compliance of the lung to come down. This can be assessed at the bedside by measuring the plateau pressure which is a surrogate of alveolar pressure, intrinsic PEEP which is the measure of auto-PEEP, and end exhalation volume which tells us about the amount of gas trapped in the alveoli.

Measuring plateau pressure helps in assessing for DHI[27,28] and a pressure >30 cmH_2O is associated with increased lung complication.[29] Measuring the intrinsic PEEP by doing an expiratory pause maneuver has no definite cutoff value, which has been associated with increased risk for DHI since it can be falsely low in patients with severe airway obstruction due to airway closure.[30] A flow time scalar with an expiratory flow limb that fails to return to baseline before the initiation of subsequent breath is indicative of presence of an auto-PEEP. DHI can also be monitored by looking at the total exhaled volume of gas during a 20-40 seconds apnea (end-inspiratory lung volume, i.e., VEI). A VEI >20 mL/kg has been associated with barotrauma and adverse heart-lung interactions. Since this technique cannot be done easily at the bedside, it is not used routinely.[7] Many experts agree that complications are rare when plateau pressure is <30 cmH_2O and intrinsic/auto-PEEP is <15 cmH_2O.[31]

Q10. How can the ventilator settings be modified based on these findings (given above)?
Three ventilator strategies that can be employed to reduce DHI are (1) reduction of respiratory rate to 8-10 breaths/min, (2) reduction of tidal volume to 4 mL/kg, and (3) shortening of inspiratory time to allow greater time for exhalation.

Reduction of respiratory rate has the greatest impact on the reduction of DHI. However, setting a respiratory rate of <10 breaths/min would require deep sedation and may be even paralytic agents. The reduction of tidal volume is limited by the inverse relation it has with dead space. The impact of reducing minute ventilation below 10 L/min on DHI is very minimal.[32] The aim is to achieve sufficient expiratory time (I:E ratio of 1:4 to 1:5) to allow the lungs to empty. This can be monitored by observing the flow time scalar and allowing the expiratory flow wave to touch the baseline before the initiation of the next breath. If a decelerating flow pattern is being used, in volume control ventilation, changing to a square wave flow pattern would increase the flow rates further and prolong the expiratory time further.

These interventions need to be monitored closely. A plateau pressure decreasing below 30 cmH_2O and a flow time scalar showing expiratory flow touching baseline are signs of resolving hyperinflation. Despite optimizing these maneuvers, if DHI does not settle, it clearly indicates that there is severe bronchospasm and this can be overcome only with aggressive bronchodilator therapy and steroids.

Q11. What is the role of extrinsic PEEP in this patient?
Extrinsic PEEP has no role in patients with acute severe asthma who are sedated/paralyzed and have no spontaneous efforts. The application of external PEEP in such patients has to be done with caution as it can worsen lung compliance and exacerbate the DHI. A low level of PEEP (5 cmH_2O), in patients who are triggering the ventilator or are spontaneously breathing, can decrease the inspiratory work of breathing and help improve ventilator triggering by

decreasing the pressure gradient needed to overcome auto-PEEP.[33] Every time extrinsic PEEP is added or increased, the plateau pressure needs to be checked to make sure there is no worsening of air trapping and lung compliance.

After optimizing the ventilator settings, an ABG is repeated and shows a pH—7.28, PCO$_2$—67 mm Hg, PO$_2$—75 mm Hg, and HCO$_3$—29 mEq/L.

Q12. What are the contraindications to permissive hypercapnia?

Contraindications to permissive hypercapnia are recent myocardial infarction, pregnancy, and raised ICP.

Despite the direct myocardial depressant effect, hypercapnia can cause an increase in heart rate by inducing sympathetic hyperactivity. This can predispose to arrhythmias, which are poorly tolerated in acute myocardial infarction. It can also cause pulmonary artery vasoconstriction and lead to hemodynamic instability in patients with right heart dysfunction.

Hypercapnia causes increased ICP by its direct cerebral arteriolar vasodilatory effect, which leads to increased cerebral blood flow.

In pregnancy, high CO$_2$ can cross the placental barrier and cause fetal acidosis, shifting the oxygen dissociation curve to the right, and decreasing the fetal hemoglobin affinity for oxygen.

Despite optimizing the mechanical ventilator settings and aggressive bronchodilator therapy, the patient continues to have severe bronchospasm and is difficult to ventilate.

Q13. Discuss the management of refractory bronchospasm.

Unfortunately, despite aggressive bronchodilator therapy, some patients continue to have refractory bronchospasm, hypoxia, and can be difficult to ventilate. In such patients, the following therapies can be tried.

Heliox
See Q3

Inhaled general anesthetic agents
See Q3

Ketamine infusion
See Q3

Bronchoscopic removal of impacted mucus
This technique has been anecdotally reported to decrease airway pressures and improve gas exchange.[34] It may be considered in patients with persistent high peak airway pressure and difficulty in weaning from a mechanical ventilator. The concern with this technique is worsening bronchospasm.

Extracorporeal life support
Extracorporeal life support (ECLS) has been attempted in the management of severe asthma. Venovenous ECLS has been used for extracorporeal CO$_2$ removal. Probably an ideal situation for its use may be patients with severe hyperinflation, profound respiratory acidosis, and hemodynamic instability who have not responded to maximum medical therapy. Evidence for routine ECLS use in acute severe asthma is still lacking.[35]

Methylxanthines
Drugs in this group were once the first line in the management of acute severe asthma. However, they have been shown to have no additional benefits when used along with β-2 agonist in an acute setting.[1-3] They are not very potent bronchodilators and have an increased incidence of adverse effects when used in combination with SABA.[36] However, patients who are on long-term oral theophylline can be continued on the same dose after checking baseline serum theophylline levels.

Intravenous β-2 agonist
Routine use of parenteral β-2 agonist is no longer a part of treatment for adult asthma exacerbation guidelines.[1] Use has been associated with increased adverse effects such as tachycardia, myocardial injury, and lactic acidosis.

After 24 hours of aggressive bronchodilator therapy and optimized mechanical ventilation, the patient's bronchospasm has settled. He is weaned off paralytic agents and sedation. He wakes up appropriately.

Q14. What criteria need to be met before he can be weaned off mechanical ventilation and extubated?

There are no guidelines for weaning and extubating patients specifically recovering from acute severe asthma. One safe approach is to perform a spontaneous breathing trial once the patient is awake, bronchospasm has settled, and PaCO$_2$ has normalized. Once airway resistance is <20 cmH$_2$O, auto-PEEP is <10 cmH$_2$O, and there is no evidence of neuromuscular weakness, extubation should be attempted.[7] Post extubation, observation for 12–24 hours in ICU would be prudent.

On attempting a trial of spontaneous breathing, he goes into respiratory distress and needs to be placed back on the control mode of ventilation.

Q15. Discuss the causes of failure to wean from mechanical ventilation.

Factors that cause weaning failure are persistent bronchospasm, impaired respiratory mechanics, cardiac dysfunction, neuromuscular weakness, electrolyte imbalance, metabolic and endocrine factors, and cognitive dysfunction. These need to be looked for and treated appropriately. Persistent bronchospasm is a very common cause for weaning failure and probably needs revaluation of medical therapy. Severe muscle weakness is seen in up to 15% of patients who undergo mechanical ventilation for severe asthma.[37] The pathogenesis of this myopathy is unclear and has been attributed to the combined use of steroids and neuromuscular paralytic agents.[37,38] Use of deep sedation alone can also lead to muscle inactivity that results in myopathy, which is generally reversible.

Q16. Is there a role for extracorporeal membrane oxygenation (ECMO) if he fails multiple attempts at weaning in asthma?

Evidence for the use of ECMO in acute severe asthma is limited.[39] It can be considered when the severe bronchospasm is refractory to maximal medical therapy and ventilation becomes difficult with significant hypercapnia and hemodynamic instability. ECMO can also be considered to prevent complications of mechanical ventilation such as DHI, pneumothorax, and in situations of ventilator-related complications such as severe air leaks and ventilator-induced lung injury. At this point of time, due to the lack of strong evidence, the need for intensive monitoring, the financial implications, and the complications associated with its use, ECMO can only be recommended as a rescue therapy for acute severe asthma. Multiple case reports are available showing good success rates with ECMO therapy in asthma.[40,41] A recent retrospective observational cohort study[42] evaluated patients with asthma exacerbations and respiratory failure, who were intubated after medical management. These patients were treated in an ECMO-capable hospital. This study compared patients who received ECMO with patients who did not get ECMO showed decreased mortality, at the expense of higher hospital costs and suggested that ECMO could be an important salvage therapy. However, well-defined clinical trials only can better answer this question.

REFERENCES

1. Global Initiative for Asthma. (2023). Global strategy for asthma management and prevention. [online] Available from: www.ginasthma.org. [Last accessed July, 2023].
2. British Thoracic Society, Scottish Intercollegiate Guidelines Network. British guideline on the management of asthma. [online] Available from: www.brit-thoracic.org.uk. [Last accessed July, 2023].
3. National Heart, Lung, and Blood Institute. (2007). National Asthma Education and Prevention Program: Expert Panel Report III: Guidelines for the diagnosis and management of asthma. (NIH publication no. 08-4051). [online] Available from: www.nhlbi.nih.gov/guidelines/asthma/asthgdln.htm. [Last accessed July, 2023].
4. Corbridge TC, Hall JB. The assessment and management of adults with status asthmaticus. Am J Respir Crit Care Med. 1995;151:1296-316.
5. Chapman KR, Verbeek PR, White JG, Rebuck AS. Effect of a short course of prednisone in the prevention of early relapse after the emergency room treatment of acute asthma. N Engl J Med. 1991;324:788-94.
6. Rowe BH, Spooner C, Ducharme F, Bretzlaff J, Bota G. Corticosteroids for preventing relapse following acute exacerbations of asthma. Cochrane Database Syst Rev. 2001;1:CD000195.
7. Brenner B, Corbridge T, Kazzi A. Intubation and mechanical ventilation of the asthmatic patient in respiratory failure. Proc Am Thorac Soc. 2009;6(4):371-9.
8. Gupta D, Nath A, Agarwal R, Behera D. A prospective randomized controlled trial on the efficacy of noninvasive ventilation in severe acute asthma. Respir Care. 2010;55:536-43.
9. Scala R. Noninvasive ventilation in severe acute asthma? Still far from the truth. Respir Care. 2010;55:630-7.
10. Allison MG, Winters ME. Noninvasive ventilation for the emergency physician. Emerg Med Clin North Am. 2016;34:51-62.
11. Rittayamai N, Tscheikuna J, Praphruetkit N, Kijpinyochai S. Use of high-flow nasal cannula for acute dyspnea and hypoxemia in the emergency department. Respir Care. 2015;60:1377-82.
12. Alcock A, Thompson C, Robertson R, Ali T. G500(P) An examination of the safety and efficacy of high flow nasal cannula therapy for acute severe asthma and viral induced wheeze in paediatric critical care. Arch Dis Child. 2016;101:A296-7.
13. Kass JE, Terregino CA. The effect of heliox in acute severe asthma: a randomized controlled trial. Chest. 1999;116:296-300.
14. Ho AM, Lee A, Karmakar MK, Dion PW, Chung DC, Contardi LH. Heliox vs air-oxygen mixtures for the treatment of patients with acute asthma: a systematic overview. Chest. 2003;123:882-90.
15. Kass JE, Castriotta RJ. Heliox therapy in acute severe asthma. Chest. 1995;107:757-60.
16. Shlamovitz GZ, Hawthorne T. Intravenous ketamine in a dissociating dose as a temporizing measure to avoid mechanical ventilation in adult patient with severe asthma exacerbation. J Emerg Med. 2011;41:492-4.
17. Denmark TK, Crane HA, Brown L. Ketamine to avoid mechanical ventilation in severe pediatric asthma. J Emerg Med. 2006;30:163-6.
18. Camargo Jr CA, Smithline HA, Malice MP, Green SA, Reiss TF. A randomized controlled trial of intravenous montelukast in acute asthma. Am J Respir Crit Care Med. 2003;167:528-33.
19. Masuda Y, Tatsumi H, Goto K, Imaizumi H, Yoshida SI, Kimijima T, et al. Treatment of life-threatening hypercapnia with isoflurane in an infant with status asthmaticus. J Anesth. 2014;28:610-2.
20. Schutte D, Zwitserloot AM, Houmes R, de Hoog M, Draaisma JM, Lemson J. Sevoflurane therapy for life-threatening asthma in children. Br J Anaesth. 2013;111:967-70.

21. Shankar V, Churchwell KB, Deshpande JK. Isoflurane therapy for severe refractory status asthmaticus in children. Intensive Care Med. 2006;32:927-33.
22. McFadden ER. Acute severe asthma. Am J Respir Crit Care Med. 2003;168:740-59.
23. Brown RH, Wagner EM. Mechanisms of bronchoprotection by anesthetic induction agents: propofol versus ketamine. Anesthesiology. 1999;90:822-8.
24. Williams TJ, Tuxen DV, Scheinkestel CD, Czarny D, Bowes G. Risk factors for morbidity in mechanically ventilated patients with acute severe asthma. Am Rev Respir Dis. 1992;146(3):607-15.
25. Feihl F, Perret C. Permissive hypercapnia. How permissive should we be? Am J Respir Crit Care Med. 1994;150(6 Pt 1):1722-37.
26. Rodrigo GJ, Rodrigo C, Hall JB. Acute asthma in adults: a review. Chest. 2004;125:1081-102.
27. Oddo M, Feihl F, Schaller MD, Perret C. Management of mechanical ventilation in acute severe asthma: practical aspects. Intensive Care Med. 2006;32:501-10.
28. Leatherman JW. Mechanical ventilation for severe asthma. In: Tobin MJ (Ed). Principles and Practice of Mechanical Ventilation, 3rd edition. New York: McGraw-Hill; 2013. pp. 727-39.
29. Leatherman J. Life-threatening asthma. Clin Chest Med. 1994;15:453-79.
30. Leatherman JW, Ravenscraft SA. Low measured auto-positive end-expiratory pressure during mechanical ventilation of patients with severe asthma: hidden auto-positive end-expiratory pressure. Crit Care Med. 1996;24:541-6.
31. Corbridge T, Corbridge S. Severe asthma exacerbation. In: Fink M, Abraham E, Vincent JL, Kochanek PM (Eds). Textbook of Critical Care, 5th edition. Philadelphia: Elsevier Saunders; 2005. pp. 587-97.
32. Leatherman JW, McArthur C, Shapiro RS. Effect of prolongation of expiratory time on dynamic hyperinflation in mechanically ventilated patients with severe asthma. Crit Care Med. 2004;32:1542-5.
33. Tobin MJ. Advances in mechanical ventilation. N Engl J Med. 2001;344:1986-96.
34. Khan MF, Al Otair HA, Elgishy AF, Alzeer AH. Bronchoscopy as a rescue therapy in patients with status asthmaticus: two case reports and review of literature. Saudi J Anaesth. 2013;7(3):327-30.
35. Mikkelsen ME, Woo YJ, Sager JS, Fuchs BD, Christie JD. Outcomes using extracorporeal life support for adult respiratory failure due to status asthmaticus. ASAIO J. 2009;55:47-52.
36. Nair P, Milan SJ, Rowe BH. Addition of intravenous aminophylline to inhaled beta(2)-agonists in adults with acute asthma. Cochrane Database Syst Rev. 2012;12: CD002742.
37. Kesler SM, Sprenkle MD, David WS, Leatherman JW. Severe weakness complicating status asthmaticus despite minimal duration of neuromuscular paralysis. Intensive Care Med. 2009;35:157-60.
38. Leatherman JW, Fleugel WW, David WS, Davies SF, Iber C. Muscle weakness in mechanically ventilated patients with severe asthma. Am J Respir Crit Care Med. 1996;153: 1686-90.
39. Alzeer AH, Al Otair HA, Khurshid SM, Badrawy SEI, Bakir BM. A case of near fatal asthma: the role of ECMO as rescue therapy. Ann Thorac Med. 2015;10:143-5.
40. Hebbar KB, Petrillo-Albarano T, Coto-Puckett W, Heard M, Rycus PT, Fortenberry JD. Experience with use of extracorporeal life support for severe refractory status asthmaticus in children. Crit Care. 2009;13:R29.
41. Ju MH, Park JJ, Jhang WK, Park SJ, Shin HJ. Extracorporeal membrane oxygenation support in a patient with status asthmaticus. Korean J Thorac Cardiovasc Surg. 2012;45(3):186-8.
42. Zakrajsek JK, Min SJ, Ho PM, Kiser TH, Kannappan A, Sottile PD, et al. Extracorporeal membrane oxygenation for refractory asthma exacerbations with respiratory failure. Chest. 2023;163(1):38-51.

Pulmonary Embolism

Jacob George Pulinilkunnathil, Shilpushp Jagannath Bhosale, Atul Prabhakar Kulkarni

CASE STUDY

A 36-year-old female presented to casualty with breathing difficulty of 1-hour duration. She had just landed at the airport after an 18-hour flight when she started to feel breathlessness. She was wheeled into the emergency where the saturation was 76%, and she had tachycardia [heart rate (HR)—108 beats/min] and hypotension [blood pressure (BP)—90/70 mm Hg]. There were no added sounds on chest auscultation. A 12-lead electrocardiogram (ECG) showed sinus tachycardia with a right-axis deviation. Echo showed normal right-sided chambers, but mild-to-moderate tricuspid regurgitation. Her chest X-ray was normal. She has been taking oral contraceptives for the past 6 months. How will you approach the case?

This woman with no significant past medical history presented with acute-onset dyspnea after a prolonged flight during which probably she was not ambulatory. This prolonged duration of flight might have predisposed her to deep venous thrombosis (DVT) of leg veins and subsequent pulmonary embolism (PE). The differential diagnosis of acute-onset dyspnea is given in **Table 1**.

Q1. What are the common risk factors for PE?

In the human body, the pathways of coagulation, anticoagulation, and thrombolysis are interrelated and tightly regulated. In conditions where the regulation is altered, such as endothelial injury, in the presence of hypercoagulability and stasis (Virchow's triad of venous thrombosis), venous clots develop. These clots in the venous system get carried to the lungs via the right heart, causing PE.

The risk is higher for larger clots originating in the veins of the thighs or pelvis, although clots in the veins of the calves or arms may also be associated with PE. Although one or more risk factors can be easily identified in most patients who present with venous thromboembolism (VTE), about 12% of patients with PE lack a known risk factor.[1]

TABLE 1: Differential diagnosis of acute-onset dyspnea.

Clinical signs	Common differential diagnoses
Normal vesicular breath sounds	Pulmonary embolism, pericardial tamponade, metabolic acidosis, panic attack, and severe anemia
Reduced breath sounds	Acute severe asthma, acute exacerbation of COPD, pneumothorax, and pleural effusion
Bilateral crepitations	ARDS, bilateral pneumonia, congestive cardiac failure, and chronic bronchitis
Bilateral wheeze	Asthma exacerbation, COPD exacerbation, anaphylaxis, and cardiogenic pulmonary edema
Stridor	Foreign body, laryngitis, and anaphylaxis

(ARDS: acute respiratory distress syndrome; COPD: chronic obstructive pulmonary disease)

Major surgery, such as joint replacements, or major trauma, such as lower-limb fractures or spinal cord injury, are strong risk factors for VTE.[2,3] Cancers such as lung cancer, stomach, pancreas, or hematological cancers remain a major predisposing factor for VTE.[4-6]

Oral contraceptives or hormonal therapies are also predisposed to a higher risk of VTE in females.[7,8]

The European Society of Cardiology (ESC) in 2019 suggested that major trauma, spine injury, fracture of the lower limb, hospitalization for myocardial infarction, heart failure, or atrial fibrillation within the last 3 months or history of VTE had the highest odds ratio (>10 OR) for development of VTE.[2,3]

The various other risk factors for VTE are given in **Table 2**.

Q2. What are the common presenting features of PE?

Pulmonary embolism presents with vague symptoms such as pleuritic pain, hemoptysis, acute circulatory collapse, and acute-onset dyspnea. Contrary to the common belief, dyspnea may be present only on exertion and absent during

TABLE 2: Risk factors for venous thromboembolism.	
Immobilization	• History of recent travel for a duration of >4 hours • A history of recent surgery, trauma to lower limb or pelvis or spinal cord • A history of stroke
Malignancy	• Hematological malignancies • Lung cancer • Gastrointestinal cancer • Pancreatic cancer • Brain cancer
Medications	• Oral contraceptive pills • Antipsychotic drugs
Inherited causes	• Factor V mutation (Leiden) • Antithrombin III deficiency • Protein C deficiency • Protein S deficiency • Antiphospholipid antibody syndrome • Prothrombin gene mutation • Dysfibrinogenemia • Hyperhomocysteinemia[10,11]
Miscellaneous	• History of thrombophlebitis or prior pulmonary embolism, heart failure, or chronic obstructive pulmonary disease • Recent hospitalization within 3 months of heart failure or atrial fibrillation • Recent hospitalization within 3 months for myocardial infarction • History of autoimmune diseases • History of receiving blood transfusion or agents stimulating erythropoiesis • Recent infections such as pneumonia, urinary tract infections (UTIs) • Other conditions such as inflammatory bowel disease, superficial venous thrombosis, diabetes mellitus, and hypertension[12]

rest. Patients may also present with orthopnea, while some present with features of DVT only.[9]

This patient is in respiratory distress with severe desaturation, tachypnea, and tachycardia. The BP is stable, and there are no clinical findings suggestive of myocardial infarction, chronic obstructive pulmonary disease (COPD), asthma, effusion, or tamponade. Her history of oral contraceptive medication is a predisposing factor for PE, and PE seems to be the likely diagnosis. How do you assess the severity of PE and why?

The severity of PE is classified according to the short-term mortality risk: Low (<1%), intermediate (<3–15%), and high (>15%). Intermediate- and high-risk patients are clinically identified by the presence of hypotension [systolic blood pressure (SBP) <90 mm Hg or a drop in SBP >40 mm Hg, not fully explained by sepsis, hypovolemia, or arrhythmia] or biochemical and echocardiography features of right ventricular (RV) strain.[11,13]

High-risk PE can have clinical manifestations ranging from cardiac arrest to features of obstructive shock such as SBP <90 mm Hg or the need for vasopressors to maintain BP >90 mm Hg with features of persistent end-organ hypoperfusion.[14]

The Pulmonary Embolism Severity Index (PESI) score is used to categorize the severity and associated risk of mortality after PE.[15,16] For rapid bedside application, a simplified version was proposed and has been most extensively validated.[17-20]

The simplified PESI score contains six variables: (1) *A*ge, (2) *C*ancer, (3) *C*hronic cardiopulmonary disease, (4) *P*ulse rate >110 beats/min, (5) *S*BP <100 mm Hg, and (6) *O*xygen saturation <90% (these variables can be remembered by the aid of mnemonic—*ACCPSO*). Each variable is assigned a value of 1, and the presence of any one variable is associated with an increased risk of mortality.[21]

Q3. Describe the pathophysiology of acute PE.
Acute PE causes failure of both circulation and gas exchange. RV failure due to acute pressure overload is the primary cause of death in massive PE. Clots in the pulmonary circulation lead to an increase in the pulmonary vascular resistance (PVR) and afterload of the RV. This increase in PVR is mainly due to the release of thromboxane A2 and serotonin.[22] The thin-walled RV is unable to handle acute pressure overload and cannot acutely generate a mean pulmonary artery pressure (PAP) >40 mm Hg.

When as much as 30–50% of the pulmonary circulation is occluded, hemodynamic effects of PE start to manifest. The RV initially dilates, resulting in increased myocyte stretch, the interventricular septum bulges into the left ventricle (LV), and the LV compliance and end-diastolic volume reduce. This results in a reduced LV filling, reduced stroke volume, systemic hypotension, and hemodynamic instability. It is suggested that there are massive infiltrates of inflammatory cells in RV myocardium, partly explained by high levels of epinephrine released as a result of the PE-induced "myocarditis" causing RV ischemia.[23,24] The forward flow may still be maintained by the associated inotropic and chronotropic stimulation.

Respiratory failure in PE is a consequence of hemodynamic instability. Hypoxemia occurs due to a ventilation–perfusion (V/Q) mismatch, although reduced venous saturation secondary to a reduced cardiac output, reopening of a physiologically closed foramen ovale, pulmonary hemorrhage, pleural effusion, and pulmonary infarct may also contribute. Hypoxia is also a potent pulmonary vasoconstrictor, and PVR increases as the degree of hypoxia increases **(Flowchart 1)**.[11,25,26]

Q4. How do you diagnose PE, and what are the prediction rules for PE?

Pulmonary embolism is commonly suspected in a patient with dyspnea, chest pain, syncope, or hemoptysis.[27-29]

Chest pain is usually caused by pleural irritation due to distal emboli causing pulmonary infarction.

A chest X-ray and electrocardiographic changes are usually nonspecific in PE but may be useful for excluding other causes of dyspnea or chest pain.[30,31]

Assessment of the clinical probability of PE is an important step in the workup for a suspected case of PE. The pretest probability of PE determines the need for further diagnostic investigations. For example, while a normal D-dimer assay can safely rule out PE in patients with a low or intermediate clinical probability of PE, without further workup, the same value might lead to missing out as much as 10% and 20% of patients at high risk.[11]

The first prediction rule for PE contained eight variables and was validated in a small sample by Hoellerich et al. in 1986.[32] The commonly used scores are the Wells rule, the Geneva score, and the Charlotte and Miniati rules. Recently, most rules were simplified to increase their acceptance and usefulness for clinicians. The three levels of clinical probability (low, intermediate, or high) were modified to classify patients in two categories ("PE likely/unlikely" for the Wells score or "safe/unsafe" for the Charlotte rule) **(Table 3)**. All rules have been validated in outpatients, with the exception of the Wells rule and the Miniati rule. Hence, these two are the preferred tools to be used in hospitalized patients.

With most of the prediction scores, the proportion of patients with confirmed PE can be expected to be 10% in the low-probability category, around 30% in the moderate-probability category, and around 65% in the high-probability category.[32]

Q5. How will you approach a case of suspected PE?

The symptomatology of PE is vague and nonspecific, ranging from being asymptomatic to being fatal. Hence, it is important that a high level of suspicion can be maintained so that these cases are not missed. A pragmatic approach to a suspected case of PE is given in **Flowchart 2**.

The first step in assessing a patient with suspected PE is to assess the risk of PE with one of the scoring systems, as subsequent investigations are guided by these.

The presenting signs and symptoms are nonspecific, and thus, any patient with dyspnea or chest pain can lead to suspicion of PE and thus lead to overzealous investigations, causing high costs of unnecessary tests and related complications.

The pulmonary embolism rule-out criteria (PERC) was developed with the purpose of selecting, on clinical grounds, patients whose likelihood of having PE is so low that diagnostic workup may not even be initiated **(Table 4)**.[33] Carpenter et al. suggested that the negative likelihood ratio for the PERC rule is 0.17.[34] The post-test probability of diagnosing PE depends both on the characteristics of the diagnostic test and on the pretest probability, and in patients at low (<15%) risk for PE, the workup for PE can be as harmful as the PE itself.[33]

PERC

The PERC was developed in 2004 by Kline et al. and later prospectively validated (after excluding patient groups such as those in whom dyspnea was not the chief presenting complaint, cancer patients, patients having thrombophilia or family history of thrombophilia, patients on beta-blockers, patients with transient tachycardia, amputees, obese patients in whom leg swelling cannot be reliably ascertained, and those with baseline chronic hypoxia). The PERC consist of eight variables, including the patient's age, tachycardia

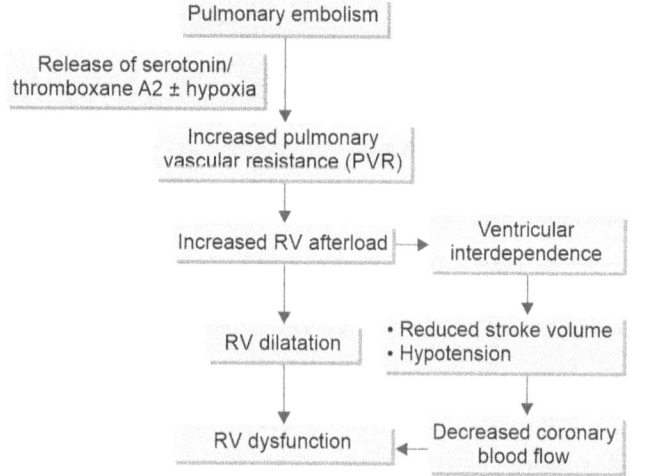

Flowchart 1: Pathophysiology of right ventricular (RV) dysfunction in pulmonary embolism.

TABLE 3: Modified Wells score (mnemonic—ABCDEFG).

Well's criteria	Simplified score
Alternative diagnosis is less likely than PE	1
Bed rest (immobilization) for >3 days or surgery in past 4 weeks	1
Cancer (active disease on treatment or palliation or received treatment in the recent 6 months)	1
Diagnosis of DVT: Leg swelling and pain	1
Embolism (DVT/PE) in the past	1
Frank blood in sputum (hemoptysis)	1
Greater than 100 heartbeats/min	1
PE likely	More than one point
PE unlikely	One point or less

(DVT: deep venous thrombosis; PE: pulmonary embolism)

Flowchart 2: Approach to a suspected case of pulmonary embolism (PE).

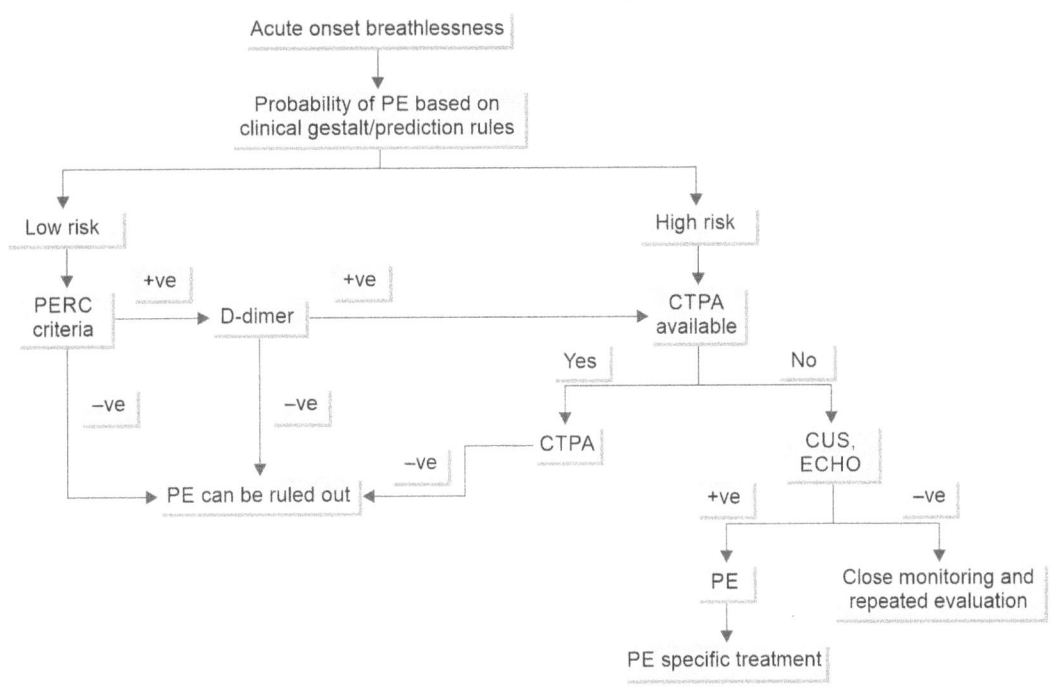

(CTPA: computed tomography pulmonary angiography; CUS: compression ultrasonography; PERC: pulmonary embolism rule-out criteria)

TABLE 4: Pulmonary embolism rule-out criteria (PERC).		
Variables	**Cutoff**	**Comments**
Age	<50 years	
Heart rate	<100 beats/min	Not valid if on beta-blockers, transient tachycardia
Arterial oxygen saturation	≥95%	Not valid in cases of chronic hypoxia
Hemoptysis	Absent	
Oral contraceptives	Absent	Not valid in high-risk cases such as cancer patients, patients having thrombophilia, or family history of thrombophilia
Immobilization within 4 weeks	Absent	
History of prior venous thromboembolism (VTE)	Absent	Not valid in high-risk cases such as cancer patients, patients having thrombophilia, or family history of thrombophilia
Unilateral leg swelling	Absent	Not valid if amputee or obese, interfering with the assessment of leg swelling

at presentation, arterial oxygen saturation, other symptoms such as hemoptysis, leg swelling, and past history of estrogen use, and prior venous thrombosis or surgery or trauma within the previous 1 month (mnemonic *STEAL THAT*—*S*urgery or *T*rauma, *E*strogen use, *A*rterial saturation <95%, *L*eg swelling, *T*achycardia, *H*emoptysis, *A*ge >50 years, and *T*hrombosis—either a PE/DVT in the past or current suspicion of a DVT).[33]

Various diagnostic modalities are routinely used to diagnose PE or, rather, to rule out other causes of breathlessness. Given the limitations of all investigations and the potentially life-threatening impact of underdiagnosing PE, the algorithm for investigating a case of PE is complex and at times expensive. Common laboratory tests, such as routine blood investigations, may help in ruling out infections or anemia as the cause for acute-onset dyspnea. In cases where thrombolysis or heparinization is contemplated, the platelet count and coagulation parameters are important to rule out thrombocytopenia or coagulopathy, which may preclude it.

Arterial blood gas (ABG) may reveal respiratory alkalosis, hypoxia, and a widened A-a gradient, although approximately (30-35% of patients) may have normoxia and normal A-a gradient on ABG. ECG findings are nonspecific, with sinus tachycardia, T-wave inversion in leads V1-V4, a QR pattern in V1, an S1Q3T3 pattern, new-onset right bundle branch block, right axis deviation, and features of RV strain being the most common. In patients with hemodynamic instability, a bedside echocardiography may reveal RV dysfunction or, more importantly, rule out other causes of hypotension apart from PE. A normal echocardiography in the absence of hemodynamic instability cannot rule out PE. Hence, in hemodynamically stable patients, the diagnosis needs to be proved or disproved with further investigations and imaging (*see* **Table 3**).

Q6. What is the role of lower limb ultrasound in patients with suspected PE?

Another useful investigation in patients with suspected PE is lower limb ultrasound (Doppler scans) of the lower limb. It has been observed that generally PE originates from DVT in a lower limb and very rarely from that in upper limb. Thus, lower-limb compression ultrasound (CUS) has replaced venography for diagnosing DVT. CUS has a high sensitivity and specificity for proximal symptomatic DVT.

A proximal DVT in patients suspected of having PE is enough to warrant treatment.

Bilateral CUS of the proximal veins in the groin and popliteal regions, i.e., on the femoral vein and popliteal vein—four-point compression, can identify DVT in 30–50% of patients, sufficient to warrant initiating treatment without further investigation. Inability to compress the vein completely indicates the presence of a clot and is the validated method to diagnose DVT. Complete CUS across the entire length of the lower limb veins might pick up more venous thrombosis, although the specificity for PE is lower. In contrast, a positive proximal CUS result has a 39% sensitivity for diagnosing PE with a specificity of 99%.[20] Thus, identification of a DVT by CUS in a patient with suspected PE reduces the need for further investigation, and exposure to radiation and contrast dye can be safely avoided.

Q7. What is the role of D-dimer in patients with suspected PE?

D-dimer is produced by the degradation of clots by plasmin and consists of adjacent fibrin monomers cross-linked by activated factor XIII. An increased concentration of D-dimer suggests active fibrinolysis with or without ongoing coagulation. D-dimer is also elevated in other conditions such as malignancy, trauma, surgery, infection, or ongoing inflammation. It is measured in plasma by quantitative enzyme-linked immunosorbent assay (ELISA) or ELISA-derived assays or with quantitative latex-derived assays or whole-blood agglutination. A negative result of highly specific D-dimer can safely rule out PE in patients with low risk for PE, but it cannot rule out PE in patients at high risk for PE. False-negative D-dimer assay is obtained in cases where the symptoms are persisting for >3 days, if the PE is small, and in cases where D-dimer is measured using qualitative latex fixation tests. In elderly patients, the D-dimer assay was found to be less specific, with a specificity of 35%. The ESC in 2019 suggested the usage of age-adjusted cutoffs to improve the performance of D-dimer testing, with the cutoff being a value of age ×10 mg/L for those aged above 50 years.[35]

The point-of-care D-dimer assays may be used in patients with a low pretest probability, but the sensitivity is found to be lower than the laboratory D-dimer values.[36]

Plasma D-dimer measurement using a highly sensitive assay is recommended in patients with low or intermediate clinical probability or in those patients where PE seems unlikely to reduce the need for unnecessary imaging.[37]

Q8. What other biomarkers of RV strain are useful in patients with suspected PE?

Biomarkers of RV strain, such as brain natriuretic peptide (BNP), N-terminal proBNP (NT-proBNP), and troponin, have been shown to be associated with a worse prognosis, irrespective of the Simplified Pulmonary Embolism Severity Index (sPESI) score. Those with normal biomarkers and an elevated sPESI ≥ 1 had an estimated mortality of 2.5%, while the mortality increased to 5.8% in patients with elevated NT-proBNP ≥ 600 pg/mL. Patients having both RV dysfunction on echocardiography and an elevated NT-proBNP have an even higher mortality (10.8%) **(Flowchart 3)**.[11]

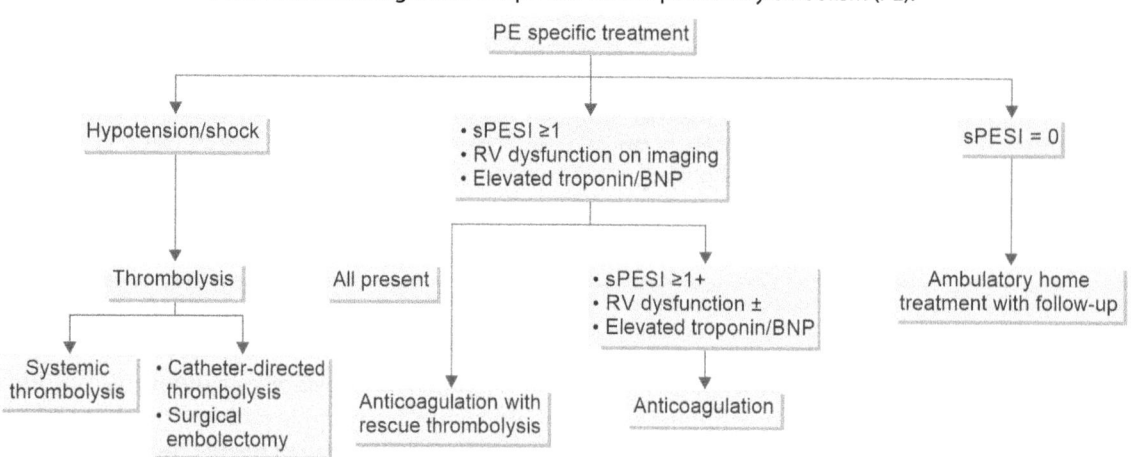

Flowchart 3: Management of a proven case of pulmonary embolism (PE).

(BNP: brain natriuretic peptide; RV: right ventricular; sPESI: Simplified Pulmonary Embolism Severity Index)

Q9. What are the general recommendations for the diagnosis of PE?

In suspected high-risk PE with hemodynamic instability, bedside echocardiography or emergency computed tomography pulmonary angiography (CTPA) (depending on availability and clinical circumstances) is strongly recommended for diagnosis.[37]

It is recommended that the diagnostic strategy be based on clinical probability, assessed either by clinical judgment or by a validated prediction rule in patients with suspected PE without hemodynamic instability. It is recommended to rule out PE as diagnosis if the perfusion lung scan is normal.[37]

In a patient with clinical suspicion of PE, it is recommended to accept the diagnosis of PE if a CUS shows a proximal DVT. However, if CUS shows only a distal DVT, further testing should be considered to confirm the diagnosis of PE.[37]

Table 5 summarizes the investigations commonly used in the diagnosis of PE.

Q10. What will be the diagnostic algorithm in pregnancy?

The commonly used clinical prediction rules are not validated for use in pregnancy. Although pregnancy-specific scoring system (the "LEFt" rule) has been suggested, it has not been validated in large cohorts. The LEFt rule assigns points for each of the three variables, namely left leg presentation (L), edema resulting in ≥2 cm calf circumference difference (E), and first-trimester presentation (Ft).

The negative predictive value is 100%, although the proportion of patients with none of the LEFt criteria is significantly low, and the positive predictive value of the test is low (12%). Pending validation, this rule cannot be used to exclude DVT in pregnancy, though a negative LEFt rule might identify patients at low risk for DVT.[47,48]

D-dimer levels are elevated in normal pregnancy, particularly in the late third trimester and early puerperium, ruling out its use in pregnancy.[49,50]

A chest X-ray can rule out common pathologies such as pneumonia, pleural effusion, or pneumothorax that may mimic PE. Bedside echocardiography will help to diagnose peripartum cardiomyopathy and other cardiac causes of breathlessness. Doppler scan of lower limb veins or a CUS can avoid unnecessary exposure to irradiation, as the management of DVT (if present) is the same as that of PE. Both CTPA and V/Q scans have been suggested as a diagnostic method in pregnancy, with each having its own advantages and disadvantages **(Table 5)**.

In pregnancy, CTPA has a lesser sensitivity due to the hyperdynamic circulation of pregnancy but is still preferred over a V/Q scan if the chest radiography is abnormal. CTPA increases the risk of breast cancer in the mother by 13.6% and may affect the fetal and neonatal thyroid function due to the use of iodinated contrast. On the other hand, fetal radiation is slightly higher with V/Q scan when compared to CTPA unless the ventilation testing is omitted in patients with normal chest X-ray. If the initial scan findings are negative or inconclusive, anticoagulation needs to be started until a PE is excluded on further imaging or testing.

Q11. How do you approach the prognostic strategy of PE?

As discussed earlier, the presence of hemodynamic instability is an independent predictor or poor outcome. PESI has been the most extensively validated score to predict mortality in acute PE.

The presence of concomitant DVT has been identified as an independent prognostic marker associated with death within the first 3 months of acute PE.

Elevation of laboratory biomarkers, such as NT-proBNP >600 ng/L, H-FABP >6 ng/mL, or copeptin >24 pmol/L, may provide further prognostic value in identifying poor outcomes.[51-53]

Pulmonary Embolism Severity Index (classes I and II) has shown to reliably identify patients at low risk of mortality.

The presence of hemodynamic instability with evidence of RV dysfunction on echo along with confirmation of PE on CTPA is enough to define high-risk PE without the need for biomarkers.

Patients who present with clinical parameters suggestive of PE along with echo/CTPA evidence of RV dysfunction and elevated cardiac biomarker levels (positive cardiac troponin test) are classified into the intermediate-high-risk category. Patients in whom the RV appears normal on echocardiography or CTPA and/or have normal cardiac biomarker levels belong to the intermediate-low-risk category.[37,54]

Q12. What is the initial treatment of PE?

The initial management of any patient with suspected PE is as per general intensive care unit (ICU) protocols. All patients should have continuous ECG, BP, and oxygen saturation monitoring. Peripheral intravenous access has to be secured, and intravenous fluids may be started guardedly. The hemodynamic management of a patient with PE is complex and not clearly understood. Clinical features of hypoperfusion, such as cold peripheries and altered sensorium, need to be actively searched for. In cases of hypoperfusion, guarded fluids are advocated. Studies have shown that although small volumes of intravenous fluids increase the cardiac index, aggressive fluid resuscitation results in RV dilatation and RV dysfunction.

TABLE 5: Investigations for pulmonary embolism.[37-39]

Investigations	Findings	Advantages	Limitations and disadvantages
ECG	• Sinus tachycardia RV strain • Right-axis deviation • S1Q3T3 pattern • McGinn–White sign • Complete or incomplete RBBB	• Available readily • Low cost • Rules out myocardial infarction immediately • ECG score >8 as proposed by Daniel et al. predicted poor clinical outcomes	• Highly nonspecific • Low sensitivity
Transthoracic echocardiography	• In patients with an angiographic Miller index >30%, echocardiography demonstrates an RV dilatation (the right-to-left ventricular end-diastolic area ratio higher than 0.6 in apical four-chamber view) • RV hypokinesia/dysfunction (McConnell's sign) or elevated PA pressures • Paradoxical septal wall motion (D-shaped left ventricle) • Visualization of a free-floating right-heart thrombus • In hemodynamically unstable patients, it can identify RV dysfunction or RV failure or other causes for hemodynamic instability • Tricuspid annular plane systolic excursion (TAPSE) is a superior marker as compared to RV/LV ratio to predict 30-day mortality in hemodynamically stable patients. In this group, a value of ≤15 mm is associated with an increased risk of 30-day mortality[40] • 60/60 sign is a combination of a pulmonary ejection acceleration time (measured in the RV outflow tract) <60 ms and a peak systolic tricuspid valve gradient <60 mm Hg suggesting PE • It needs to be mentioned that due to its negative predictive value, the echo findings are around 50%; a negative result cannot exclude PE[41,42]	• Noninvasive, bedside test • Repeatable • No contrast or radiation exposure	• Need to get a good window for image acquisition and interpretation • Highly dependent on skills of performer • A normal echocardiography alone cannot exclude PE in hemodynamically stable patients
Chest X-ray	• Focal oligemia (*Westermark sign*) • Dilated descending pulmonary artery (*Palla's sign*) • Enlarged pulmonary artery (*Fleischner's sign*) • Dilated right descending pulmonary artery with sudden cutoff (*Chang sign*) • Peripheral wedge of airspace opacity and implies lung infarction (*Hampton's hump*)[39]	Chest X-ray is mainly used at bedside to rule out other causes of respiratory distress such as pneumonia, pneumothorax, pericardial effusion, heart failure, and aortic dissection	Very low sensitivity and specificity

Contd...

Contd...

Investigations	Findings	Advantages	Limitations and disadvantages
CTPA	• Multidetector CTPA is the modality of choice for imaging patients with suspected PE. It allows adequate visualization of the pulmonary arteries down to the subsegmental level[43,44] • Filling defects in the pulmonary arteries • Qanadli index describes the clot burden score with a maximum obstruction score for each lung being 20[45]	• Investigation of choice • Rapid and accurate • Other underlying pathologies are also picked up	• Not available at bedside • Not a modality of choice for repeated evaluation or follow-ups • Associated contrast and radiation exposure
Lung scintigraphy (V/Q scan)	The planar V/Q scans with multiple tracers such as xenon-133 gas, krypton-81 gas, technetium-99m-labeled aerosols, or technetium-99m-labeled carbon microparticles can be used. In acute PE, ventilation is expected to be normal in hypoperfused segments	Lesser radiation than CTPA	• Not available everywhere and needs expertise • Can miss out small embolus in the distal branches • Indeterminate images will need further evaluation, delaying diagnosis
Pulmonary angiography	Thrombus can be directly visualized	• Gold standard for diagnosis • Can perform catheter-directed therapies simultaneously • Excellent for peripheral small emboli and those who cannot hold breath	• Invasive, with contrast exposure • Radiation exposure • Mortality due to hemodynamic or respiratory compromise (mortality rates of 0.5–5%)
Magnetic resonance angiography	Thrombus in pulmonary artery	No radiation	• Not available everywhere • Low sensitivity • Not validated in large trials
D-dimer	• Elevated in cases of DVT and PE • For age >50 years, age ×10 is taken as the upper limit for cutoff[46]	• Can easily rule out PE in patients at low risk for PE • Relatively inexpensive test • Rapid assay	• Low specificity • Elevated in other conditions • Cannot exclude PE in high-risk cases • Depends upon assay technique also
Troponin, BNP	Elevated in cases of right ventricular strain	Helps to identify patients with increased risk of PE-related complications, including death	• Low specificity • Cheap

(BNP: brain natriuretic peptide; CTPA: computed tomography pulmonary angiography; DVT: deep venous thrombosis; ECG: electrocardiogram; LV: left ventricle; PE: pulmonary embolism; RBBB: right bundle branch block; RV: right ventricle; V/Q: ventilation–perfusion)

Q13. Discuss the treatment of acute RV failure in high-risk PE.

Volume optimization—cautious volume loading may be appropriate if low arterial pressure is combined with the absence of elevated filling pressures.

The major concern is that volume loading may overdistend the RV and ultimately cause a reduction in cardiac output.[55]

Mercat et al. in 1999 described the effects of fluid loading in patients with submassive PE with a cardiac index <2 and found that only those patients with lower right ventricular end-diastolic volume (RVEDV) to begin with benefitted from fluid.[56] In another retrospective nonrandomized study, Ternacle et al. studied the effect of furosemide versus fluids in submassive PE and showed that patients who received diuretics had improvements in hemodynamic parameters than those who received volume.[57]

Vasopressors and inotropes
After a cautious attempt of fluid bolus, vasopressors should be started without attempting to give further fluids.[58,59] The ideal vasopressor in cardiogenic shock due to PE is unknown, and noradrenaline is generally the preferred vasopressor. Noradrenaline improves the RV function by its inotropic effect and by an improved RV coronary perfusion.[60]

Pure inodilators, such as dobutamine, can result in worsening of hypotension due to associated vasodilation. Nitric oxide administered via an endotracheal tube or face mask can be a safe alternative to reduce the PVR and RV afterload, thereby improving hemodynamics.[61]

Finally, venoarterial extracorporeal membrane oxygenation (VA-ECMO) may be helpful in patients with high-risk PE and circulatory collapse or as rescue in patients who develop cardiac arrest.

In a cardiac arrest situation, thrombolytic therapy should be considered, and cardiopulmonary resuscitation (CPR) should be continued for at least 60–90 minutes before terminating resuscitation attempts.

Although hypoxemia, transient hypercapnia, and positive end-expiratory pressure (PEEP) can affect the patient's hemodynamics adversely, maneuvering the airway will not address this problem but rather may aggravate the hemodynamic collapse. Therefore, it is a good clinical practice to initiate thrombolysis urgently in patients with shock but without contraindications for thrombolysis. High-flow nasal cannula or other high-flow oxygen systems may be judiciously and watchfully used while awaiting the effects of thrombolysis to set in.[62] Severe hypoxia or respiratory distress, unconsciousness, cardiac arrest or pericardiac arrest situations, and all medical emergencies warrant intubation and mechanical ventilation. Ventilation in these patients is better done by avoiding high PEEP and large tidal volumes as positive pressures might be deleterious to a failing RV.

Empiric anticoagulation needs to be started for all patients with suspected or proven PE based on their hemodynamic stability, anticipated need for thrombolysis, presence of renal dysfunction, other comorbidities, etc. Unfractionated heparin (UFH) is started at a dose of 80 IU/kg followed by 18 IU/kg/h and further titrated according to activated partial thromboplastin time (aPTT). It has the advantage of rapid reversal if needed, although frequent aPTT monitoring is cumbersome and costly. Low-molecular-weight heparin (LMWH) is associated with early attainment of therapeutic anticoagulation within 4 hours and may be used in patients who are at low risk of developing hemodynamic instability and also do not have another organ dysfunction including renal dysfunction. LMWH and fondaparinux are generally preferred over UFH as they have a lower risk of causing major bleeding and heparin-induced thrombocytopenia.[63]

After initial therapeutic anticoagulation, further anticoagulation is continued with vitamin K antagonists (VKAs) or nonvitamin K antagonist oral anticoagulant (NOAC). VKAs (warfarin, etc.) are started with heparin overlap, monitoring by prothrombin time.

Alternatively, newer oral anticoagulant agents can be started in hemodynamically stable patients who do not require thrombolysis. Evidence with NOAC (dabigatran, rivaroxaban, apixaban, or edoxaban) in the treatment of VTE suggests that they are at least noninferior with a possible mild reduction in side effects than the standard regimens. Guidelines recommend NOAC as an alternative to heparin/vitamin K regimen in the absence of hemodynamic instability and other contraindications. Dabigatran or edoxaban may be initiated instead of warfarin with an overlap with heparin. Rivaroxaban is approved as an oral monotherapy for acute PE at low or moderate risk for bleeding. It is given as a loading dose of 15 mg twice daily for 3 weeks followed by 20 mg daily.

The EINSTEIN–PE trial suggested that rivaroxaban is associated with statistical therapeutic noninferiority and superior safety with less incidence of major bleeding. These newer oral anticoagulant drugs have not been studied in patients with hypotension nor in patients who have been initially treated with thrombolytic treatment.[64]

Management of PE in pregnancy
Management of PE in pregnancy involves anticoagulation for at least 3 months, and it is continued for 6 weeks in the postnatal period. LMWH is the preferred drug as trials show a lower mortality, lower risk of bleeding as compared with UFH, lesser incidence of heparin-induced thrombocytopenia, and need of lesser monitoring and safety as it does not cross the placenta or enter breast milk. Monitoring of anti-Xa levels is recommended only in high-risk groups such as extremes of body weight or the presence of high-risk factors such as renal impairment or recurrent VTE. Vitamin K analogs are teratogenic and are avoided during the entire course of pregnancy, although they can be used during lactation. The newer oral anticoagulants are also avoided in pregnancy and lactation.[65]

The patient was admitted to the ICU as she remained dyspneic. She was initiated on UFH infusion. A CT pulmonary angiogram was asked for. However, before shifting, the ICU registrar noted that the SBP had fallen to 80 mm Hg, and the peripheries were cold and clammy. The patient now complained of orthopnea. Examination revealed an elevated jugular venous pressure (JVP) tracing, although chest examination was still normal. The relatives wanted to know about the risks and benefits of thrombolysis.

Q14. Describe the role of thrombolytic therapy in PE and the risks involved in thrombolysis.
Patients presenting with PE and hypotension have an increased risk of mortality when receiving anticoagulation alone. In these patients, thrombolysis reduces the mortality rates, irrespective of the risk of bleeding. A comparison of various thrombolytic agents is given in **Table 6**. Various guidelines recommend urgent thrombolysis in PE with shock as meta-analysis[66] has shown better outcomes with thrombolysis.[67-69] However, the same benefit cannot be

TABLE 6: Drugs used for the treatment of pulmonary embolism (PE).

Criteria	Streptokinase	Urokinase	Alteplase	Reteplase	Tenecteplase
Generation	First	First	Second	Third	Third
Clot specific or not	No	No	Yes	Yes	Yes
Half-life (minutes)	12	7–20	4–10	11–19	15–24
Dosage	250,000 units intravenously (IV) over 0.5 hours, followed by 100,000 units/h for 24 hours	4,400 units/kg IV over 10 minutes, followed by 4,400 units/kg/h for 12 hours	100 mg over 2 hours	10 mg bolus, repeated after 30 minutes	Bolus dose: <60 kg: 30 mg 60–70 kg: 35 mg 70–80 kg: 40 mg 80–90 kg: 45 mg ≥90 kg: 50 mg
Food and Drug Administration (FDA) approved for PE	Yes	Yes	Yes	No	No

extrapolated to those with low- or intermediate-risk PE as confirmed from trials in patients with submassive PE (RV dysfunction and elevated troponins). Although there was an improvement in hemodynamics, these patients suffered from a significantly high number of bleeding complications, especially in patients aged >75 years. Long-term follow-up of these patients revealed that thrombolysis did not reduce mortality, functional disability, pulmonary hypertension, RV dysfunction, or incidence of chronic thromboembolic pulmonary hypertension (CTEPH).[70,71]

In intermediate-risk, PE patients without hemodynamic instability but with the presence of RV dysfunction and elevated troponin levels, the impact of thrombolytic treatment was investigated in the Pulmonary Embolism Thrombolysis (PEITHO) trial. Thrombolytic therapy was associated with a significant reduction in the risk of hemodynamic decompensation or collapse, but there was an increased risk of severe extracranial and intracranial bleeding.[72]

The ESC guidelines suggest the initiation of anticoagulation in these patients, with the addition of reperfusion therapy later if they become hemodynamically unstable. The management algorithm for a proven case of PE is shown in **Flowchart 2**.

The patient was started on noradrenaline, and transfer to the computed tomography (CT) console was temporarily withheld. A four-point CUS was done at the bedside by the resident, which showed noncompressibility of the right femoral vein. What is the role of thrombolysis and CPR in cardiac arrest secondary to PE?

In a patient with suspected PE who has a cardiac arrest, CPR may be continued as per protocol. Although CPR along with thrombolysis is associated with increased bleeding, thrombolysis can increase the return of spontaneous circulation and survival to discharge in patients.[73]

CPR may be continued for prolonged periods, with the help of automatic CPR machines if needed. It has to be remembered that CPR is not a contraindication for thrombolysis if the cause of cardiac arrest is suspected to be PE. The guidelines recommend for alteplase (bolus dose of 50 mg with a repeat bolus after 15 minutes) or a single weight-based dose of tenecteplase in these cases with ongoing CPR and suggest calling off futile CPR only after 60–90 minutes (weak recommendation).[74,75] However, if PE is not suspected or if PE is unlikely, thrombolysis should not be administered as it may be associated with worse outcome.[76]

Q15. Discuss the current status of low-dose thrombolysis in patients with PE.
A trial looking at the benefits of a low-dose thrombolysis (compared to conventional thrombolysis) suggested that a lower dose of thrombolytic agent [tissue plasminogen activator (tPA)] could result in faster resolution of pulmonary hypertension as assessed by echocardiography, with no significant increase in bleeding rates. This trial was criticized for its small sample size and the technicality of using echocardiography to assess pulmonary hypertension.[77] A recent study of the retrospective data of patients with PE, a propensity-matched analysis, showed an increased need for escalation of treatment among those patients who received half-dose therapy with alteplase, although there was no significant difference in vasopressor requirement, mechanical ventilation, CPR, mortality, or clinically significant bleeding.[78]

The main trials about therapy of PE are summarized in **Table 7**.

It was decided to thrombolyze the patient in view of hemodynamic instability. The relatives, however, remained skeptical and are enquiring regarding options other than thrombolysis. What other options are available in place of

TABLE 7: Clinical trials on the use of thrombolytic agents in pulmonary embolism (PE).

Trials	Comparisons	Result
UPET[79]	Urokinase versus anticoagulation	Urokinase significantly improved pulmonary perfusion immediately; however, the difference was not sustained at 5 days or more, up to 1 year
USPET[80]	12-hour urokinase versus 24-hour urokinase versus 24-hour streptokinase	• 12 hours of urokinase therapy was equal to 24 hours of urokinase with respect to clot resolution • 24 hours of urokinase was associated with better improvement than streptokinase therapy
Tebbe et al.[81]	Double bolus of reteplase versus 2-hour alteplase infusion	Double bolus of 10 mg reteplase was as effective as 2-hour infusion of 100 mg alteplase in reducing pulmonary vascular resistance
MAPPET-3[26]	Heparin + alteplase versus heparin + placebo	Reduced rate of in-hospital mortality or clinical deterioration requiring treatment escalation was significantly lower with heparin + alteplase than with heparin + placebo. Bleeding incidence was similar in both groups
TIPES[82]	Weight-adjusted, single-bolus tenecteplase + heparin versus placebo + heparin	In hemodynamically stable patients, the reduction of right-to-left ventricle end-diastolic dimension ratio at 24 hours was higher for tenecteplase versus placebo. Two major nonfatal bleeds with tenecteplase versus one with placebo
TOPCOAT[78]	Weight-adjusted, single-bolus tenecteplase or placebo both with heparin in submassive PE	Patients with submassive PE treated with tenecteplase and heparin had an increased probability of a favorable composite outcome
PEITHO[72]	Tenecteplase + heparin versus placebo + heparin	Nonsignificant reduction in mortality in tenecteplase group. Significantly high extracranial bleed in the tenecteplase group. Increased incidence of stroke among age >75 years

(MAPPET-3: Management Strategies and Prognosis of Pulmonary Embolism Trial-3; PEITHO: Pulmonary Embolism Thrombolysis; TIPES: Tenecteplase Italian Pulmonary Embolism Study; TOPCOAT: Tenecteplase or Placebo: Cardiopulmonary Outcomes at Three Months; UPET: Urokinase Pulmonary Embolism Trial; USPET: Urokinase-streptokinase Pulmonary Embolism Trial)

thrombolysis? Discuss the pros and cons of these alternative methods.

Catheter-directed therapies in PE

With progress in technology and experience, intervention radiology is playing an important role in managing massive and submassive PE. Evidence suggests that catheter-directed therapies are reasonable alternatives for patients with massive PE and have contraindications to fibrinolysis or in those who remain unstable after receiving fibrinolysis.[83]

ULTIMA was an industry-sponsored randomized controlled trial (RCT) of UFH versus UFH plus catheter-directed thrombolysis (CDT) with ultrasound-assisted thrombolysis (USAT) and a tPA dose of 10–20 mg over 15 hours in submassive PE. The trial showed that USAT was superior to stand-alone anticoagulation in reversing RV dilation with no increase in bleeding rates. The trial had a high exclusion rate and was not designed to assess the long-term outcomes of CDT, such as CTEPH.[84]

The SEATTLE II trial was an industry-sponsored trial for acute massive and submassive PE that looked into the safety of ultrasound-facilitated, catheter-directed, and low-dose fibrinolysis. The authors suggested that low-dose CDT fibrinolysis improves RV function, decreases pulmonary artery occlusion, and reduces PAP. However, the trial had a high rate of major bleeding and access site complications.[85]

The Pulmonary Embolism Response to Fragmentation, Embolectomy, and Catheter Thrombolysis (PERFECT) was a multicenter PE registry that enrolled patients with both submassive and massive PE and had patients in whom systemic thrombolysis was contraindicated. They concluded that CDT improves RV strain and PAP in patients with no major increase in adverse effects.[86] A brief summary of the various catheter-directed therapies is given in **Table 8**.

Rescue strategies—surgical embolectomy

Surgical embolectomy is performed in hemodynamically unstable cases where thrombolysis has failed or is contraindicated. It has a high mortality, particularly in the elderly (2–46%), and is better reserved for centers with great experience and experienced surgeons. Complications include those associated with cardiac surgery and anesthesia, as well as embolectomy-specific complications such as perforation of the pulmonary artery and cardiac arrest. Over the recent years, with a better patient selection and better perioperative care, there has been a reduction in the early perioperative mortality with rates as low as 6%. Studies have shown that early mortality and late mortality were lower in the surgical group than in the medical group.[87]

A similar US study comparing patients who underwent thrombolysis or surgical embolectomy as first-line therapy did not show difference in mortality, but the thrombolysis group had a higher incidence of stroke and recurrent PE.[88]

TABLE 8: Catheter-directed therapies in pulmonary embolism.

Management	Techniques	Advantages	Disadvantages
Catheter-directed thrombolysis	Direct administration of low-dose thrombolytic agent into the clot	Requires a lower dose of thrombolytic agent and is effective for distal clots. Patients with severe right ventricle dysfunction and are hemodynamically unstable and those who are at high risk of bleeding may benefit from this[39,83]	Associated with a higher chance of bleeding
Ultrasound-assisted thrombolysis	Catheter-directed high-frequency ultrasound is used to break down the clot and simultaneously administer local thrombolysis	• Ultrasound-assisted catheter-directed thrombolysis followed by intravenous heparin might help to attain hemodynamic stability rapidly than conventional thrombolysis[39,83] • It requires lower doses of thrombolytic when compared to catheter-directed thrombolysis	Cost
Rheolytic thrombectomy	Uses saline jet at high velocities to macerate the thrombus and suctions the thrombus via Venturi effect	Useful for removing thrombus in main pulmonary arteries	Prone for arrhythmias, bronchospasm, etc.
Suction thrombectomy	Direct aspiration of thrombus	Useful in cases of thrombus in the main branches of pulmonary artery	Requires surgical cut-down and cardiopulmonary bypass
Rotational thrombectomy and aspiration	Involves the use of a high-speed rotating screw that creates negative pressure within the catheter, resulting in aspiration of thrombus from the catheter tip into the lumen	Effective thrombus removal	Limited experience

Q16. What is the role of a vena cava filter in patients with PE?

Vena cava filter is recommended only if there is a contraindication to anticoagulant treatment in patients with PE or proximal DVT. The results from the available trials do not support the use of vena cava filter in patients with PE when anticoagulant treatment can still be done.[11]

The ESC 2019 recommends no routine use of IVC filters and further suggests that IVC filters should be considered in patients with acute PE and absolute contraindications to anticoagulation and in cases of PE recurrence despite therapeutic anticoagulation.[37]

Q17. What is the role of ECMO in PE?

In the setting of massive PE and hemodynamic failure, ECMO helps in optimizing the RV preload, reducing the hypoxia-induced raised pulmonary vasoconstriction, and helps in maintaining systemic BP and RV coronary perfusion by optimizing afterload, resulting in an overall improvement in biventricular function. In massive PE, VA-ECMO is an important therapeutic option for the hemodynamic stabilization of the patient before pulmonary embolectomy.[89]

The patient underwent systemic thrombolysis with alteplase and improved rapidly. Her hemodynamic parameters and oxygenation status were also improved. She was weaned off oxygen and started ambulation. How long will you advocate follow-up and treatment for PE?

Long-term treatment of PE

The duration of treatment in PE depends on the identification of risk factors. Long-term anticoagulation is essential for patients with PE. A treatment of at least 3 months of anticoagulation is associated with significant reduction in recurrences and a net positive benefit. Guidelines recommend long-term anticoagulation for 3 months after an initial episode of provoked VTE and for ≥3 months after unprovoked VTE.

Oral anticoagulant treatment of indefinite duration is recommended for patients presenting with recurrent VTE not related to a reversible risk factor or in cases of antiphospholipid antibody (APLA) syndrome.

For an extended oral anticoagulation after PE in a patient without cancer, a reduced dose of the NOACs such as apixaban (2.5 mg b.i.d.) or rivaroxaban (10 mg o.d.) should be considered after 6 months of therapeutic anticoagulation.[90,91]

For patients with PE and cancer, weight-adjusted subcutaneous LMWH should be considered for the first 6 months over VKAs and may be continued till the cancer is cured.[92,93]

The patient remained stable throughout, with improvement in oxygenation parameters. She was initiated on oral warfarin with international normalized ratio (INR) monitoring. After 12 weeks, warfarin was stopped, and the patient was asked to remain under clinical follow-up.

REFERENCES

1. Morgenthaler TI, Ryu JH. Clinical characteristics of fatal pulmonary embolism in a referral hospital. Mayo Clin Proc. 1995;70:417-24.
2. Rogers MA, Levine DA, Blumberg N, Flanders SA, Chopra V, Langa KM. Triggers of hospitalization for venous thromboembolism. Circulation. 2012;125:2092-9.
3. Anderson Jr FA, Spencer FA. Risk factors for venous thromboembolism. Circulation. 2003;107:I9-16.
4. Blom JW, Doggen CJ, Osanto S, Rosendaal FR. Malignancies, prothrombotic mutations, and the risk of venous thrombosis. JAMA. 2005;293:715-22.
5. Chew HK, Wun T, Harvey D, Zhou H, White RH. Incidence of venous thromboembolism and its effect on survival among patients with common cancers. Arch Intern Med. 2006;166:458-64.
6. Ku GH, White RH, Chew HK, Harvey DJ, Zhou H, Wun T. Venous thromboembolism in patients with acute leukemia: incidence, risk factors, and effect on survival. Blood. 2009;113:3911-7.
7. van Hylckama Vlieg A, Middeldorp S. Hormone therapies and venous thromboembolism: where are we now? J Thromb Haemost. 2011;9:257-66.
8. de Bastos M, Stegeman BH, Rosendaal FR, Van Hylckama Vlieg A, Helmerhorst FM, Stijnen T, et al. Combined oral contraceptives: venous thrombosis. Cochrane Database Syst Rev. 2014;3:CD010813.
9. Stein PD, Beemath A, Matta F, Weg JG, Yusen RD, Hales CA, et al. Clinical characteristics of patients with acute pulmonary embolism: data from PIOPED II. Am J Med. 2007;120:871-9.
10. Ouellette DW, Patocka C. Pulmonary embolism. Emerg Med Clin North Am. 2012;30:329-75.
11. Konstantinides SV, Torbicki A, Agnelli G, Danchin N, Fitzmaurice D, Galiè N, et al. 2014 ESC guidelines on the diagnosis and management of acute pulmonary embolism. Eur Heart J. 2014;35:3033-69.
12. Aschermann M, Sen JW. Comparison of ESC guidelines 2008 and 2014—diagnostic and treatment of acute pulmonary embolism. Cor Vasa. 2015;57:e270-4.
13. Torbicki A, Perrier A, Konstantinides S, Agnelli G, Galiè N, Pruszczyk P, et al. Guidelines on the diagnosis and management of acute pulmonary embolism. Eur Heart J. 2008;29:2276-315.
14. Harjola VP, Mebazaa A, Celutkiene J, Bettex D, Bueno H, Chioncel O, et al. Contemporary management of acute right ventricular failure: a statement from the Heart Failure Association and the Working Group on pulmonary circulation and right ventricular function of the European Society of Cardiology. Eur J Heart Fail. 2016;18:226-41.
15. Aujesky D, Roy PM, Le Manach CP, Verschuren F, Meyer G, Obrosky DS, et al. Validation of a model to predict adverse outcomes in patients with pulmonary embolism. Eur Heart J. 2006;27:476-81.
16. Aujesky D, Scott OD, Stone RA, Auble TE, Perrier A, Cornuz J, et al. Derivation and validation of a prognostic model for pulmonary embolism. Am J Respir Crit Care Med. 2005;172:1041-6.
17. Jiménez D, Aujesky D, Moores L, Gómez V, Lobo JL, Uresandi F, et al. Simplification of the pulmonary embolism severity index for prognostication in patients with acute symptomatic pulmonary embolism. Arch Intern Med. 2010;170:1383-9.
18. Donze J, Le Gal G, Fine MJ, Roy PM, Sanchez O, Verschuren F, et al. Prospective validation of the Pulmonary Embolism Severity Index. A clinical prognostic model for pulmonary embolism. Thromb Haemost. 2008;100:943-8.
19. Sam A, Sanchez D, Gomez V, Wagner C, Kopecna D, Zamarro C, et al. The shock index and the simplified PESI for identification of low-risk patients with acute pulmonary embolism. Eur Respir J. 2011;37:762-6.
20. Le Gal G, Righini M, Sanchez O, Roy PM, Baba-Ahmed M, Perrier A, et al. A positive compression ultrasonography of the lower limb veins is highly predictive of pulmonary embolism on computed tomography in suspected patients. Thromb Haemost. 2006;95:963-6.
21. Righini M, Roy PM, Meyer G, Verschuren F, Aujesky D, Le Gal G. The Simplified Pulmonary Embolism Severity Index (PESI): validation of a clinical prognostic model for pulmonary embolism. J Thromb Haemost. 2011;9:2115-7.
22. Smulders YM. Pathophysiology and treatment of haemodynamic instability in acute pulmonary embolism: the pivotal role of pulmonary vasoconstriction. Cardiovasc Res. 2000;48:23-33.
23. Begieneman MP, van de Goot FR, van der Bilt IA, Vonk Noordegraaf A, Spreeuwenberg MD, Paulus WJ, et al. Pulmonary embolism causes endomyocarditis in the human heart. Heart. 2008;94:450-6.
24. Lankeit M, Jiménez D, Kostrubiec M, Dellas C, Hasenfuss G, Pruszczyk P, et al. Predictive value of the high-sensitivity troponin T assay and the simplified Pulmonary Embolism Severity Index in hemodynamically stable patients with acute pulmonary embolism: a prospective validation study. Circulation. 2011;124:2716-24.
25. Burrowes KS, Clark AR, Tawhai MH. Blood flow redistribution and ventilation-perfusion mismatch during embolic pulmonary arterial occlusion. Pulm Circ. 2011;1:365-76.
26. Konstantinides S, Geibel A, Heusel G, Heinrich F, Kasper W. Heparin plus alteplase compared with heparin alone in patients with submassive pulmonary embolism. N Engl J Med. 2002;347:1143-50.
27. Pollack CV, Schreiber D, Goldhaber SZ, Slattery D, Fanikos J, O'Neil BJ, et al. Clinical characteristics, management, and outcomes of patients diagnosed with acute pulmonary

embolism in the emergency department: initial report of EMPEROR (Multicenter Emergency Medicine Pulmonary Embolism in the Real World Registry). J Am Coll Cardiol. 2011;57:700-6.
28. Miniati M, Prediletto R, Formichi B, Marini C, Di Ricco G, Tonelli L, et al. Accuracy of clinical assessment in the diagnosis of pulmonary embolism. Am J Respir Crit Care Med. 1999;159:864-71.
29. Prandoni P, Lensing AW, Prins MH, Ciammaichella M, Perlati M, Mumoli N, et al. Prevalence of pulmonary embolism among patients hospitalized for syncope. N Engl J Med. 2016;375:1524-31.
30. Elliott CG, Goldhaber SZ, Visani L, DeRosa M. Chest radiographs in acute pulmonary embolism. Results from the International Cooperative Pulmonary Embolism Registry. Chest. 2000;118:33-8.
31. Shopp JD, Stewart LK, Emmett TW, Kline JA. Findings from 12-lead electrocardiography that predict circulatory shock from pulmonary embolism: systematic review and meta-analysis. Acad Emerg Med. 2015;22:1127-37.
32. Ceriani E, Combescure C, Le gal G, Nendaz M, Perneger T, Bounameaux H, et al. Clinical prediction rules for pulmonary embolism: a systematic review and meta-analysis. J Thromb Haemost. 2010;8:957-70.
33. Kline JA, Mitchell AM, Kabrhel C, Richman PB, Courtney DM. Clinical criteria to prevent unnecessary diagnostic testing in emergency department patients with suspected pulmonary embolism. J Thromb Haemost. 2004;2:1247-55.
34. Carpenter CR, Keim SM, Seupaul RA, Pines JM, Best Evidence in Emergency Medicine Investigator Group. Differentiating low-risk and no-risk PE patients: the PERC score. J Emerg Med. 2009;36:317-22.
35. Raja AS, Greenberg JO, Qaseem A, Denberg TD, Fitterman N, Schuur JD, et al. Evaluation of patients with suspected acute pulmonary embolism: best practice advice from the Clinical Guidelines Committee of the American College of Physicians. Ann Intern Med. 2015;163:701-11.
36. Geersing GJ, Erkens PM, Lucassen WA, Buller HR, Cate HT, Hoes AW, et al. Safe exclusion of pulmonary embolism using the Wells rule and qualitative D-dimer testing in primary care: prospective cohort study. BMJ. 2012;345:e6564.
37. Konstantinides SV, Meyer G, Becattini C, Bueno H, Geersing GJ, Harjola VP, et al. 2019 ESC guidelines for the diagnosis and management of acute pulmonary embolism developed in collaboration with the European Respiratory Society (ERS): the Task Force for the diagnosis and management of acute pulmonary embolism of the European Society of Cardiology (ESC). Eur Heart J. 2020;41(4):543-603.
38. Meyer G, Roy PM, Sors H, Sanchez O. Laboratory tests in the diagnosis of pulmonary embolism. Respiration. 2003;70:125-32.
39. Sista AK, Kuo WT, Mark S, David CM. Stratification, imaging, and management of acute massive and submassive pulmonary embolism. Radiology. 2017;284:5-24.
40. Paczyńska M, Sobieraj P, Burzyński Ł, Kostrubiec M, Wiśniewska M, Bienias P, et al. Tricuspid annulus plane systolic excursion (TAPSE) has superior predictive value compared to right ventricular to left ventricular ratio in normotensive patients with acute pulmonary embolism. Arch Med Sci. 2016;12:1008-14.
41. Bova C, Greco F, Misuraca G, Serafini O, Crocco F, Greco A, et al. Diagnostic utility of echocardiography in patients with suspected pulmonary embolism. Am J Emerg Med. 2003;21:180-3.
42. Kurnicka K, Lichodziejewska B, Goliszek S, Dzikowska-Diduch O, Zdonczyk O, Kozlowska M, et al. Echocardiographic pattern of acute pulmonary embolism: analysis of 511 consecutive patients. J Am Soc Echocardiogr. 2016;29:907-13.
43. Stein PD, Fowler SE, Goodman LR, Gottschalk A, Hales CA, Hull RD, et al. Multidetector computed tomography for acute pulmonary embolism. N Engl J Med. 2006;354:2317-27.
44. Patel S, Kazerooni EA, Cascade PN. Pulmonary embolism: optimization of small pulmonary artery visualization at multi-detector row CT. Radiology. 2003;227:455-60.
45. Qanadli SD, El Hajjam M, Vieillard-Baron A, Joseph T, Mesurolle B, Oliva VL, et al. New CT index to quantify arterial obstruction in pulmonary embolism. Am J Roentgenol. 2001;176:1415-20.
46. Righini M, Van Es J, Den Exter PL, Roy PM, Verschuren F, Ghuysen A, et al. Age-adjusted D-dimer cutoff levels to rule out pulmonary embolism. JAMA. 2014;311:1117-24.
47. Chan WS, Lee A, Spencer FA, Crowther M, Rodger M, Ramsay T, et al. Predicting deep venous thrombosis in pregnancy: out in "LEFt" field? Ann Intern Med. 2009;151:85-92.
48. Righini M, Jobic C, Boehlen F, Broussaud J, Becker F, Jaffrelot M, et al. Predicting deep venous thrombosis in pregnancy: external validation of the LEFT clinical prediction rule. Haematologica. 2013;98:545-8.
49. Simcox LE, Ormesher L, Tower C, Greer IA. Pulmonary thromboembolism in pregnancy: diagnosis and management. Breathe (Sheff). 2015;11:282-9.
50. Hunt BJ, Parmar K, Horspool K, Shephard N, Nelson-Piercy C, Goodacre S. The DiPEP (Diagnosis of PE in Pregnancy) biomarker study: an observational cohort study augmented with additional cases to determine the diagnostic utility of biomarkers for suspected venous thromboembolism during pregnancy and puerperium. Br J Haematol. 2018;180:694-704.
51. Jimenez D, Lobo JL, Fernandez-Golfin C, Portillo AK, Nieto R, Lankeit M, et al. Effectiveness of prognosticating pulmonary embolism using the ESC algorithm and the Bova score. Thromb Haemost. 2016;115:827-34.
52. Hobohm L, Hellenkamp K, Hasenfuss G, Munzel T, Konstantinides S, Lankeit M. Comparison of risk assessment strategies for not-high-risk pulmonary embolism. Eur Respir J. 2016;47:1170-8.
53. Dellas C, Tschepe M, Seeber V, Zwiener I, Kuhnert K, Schafer K, et al. A novel H-FABP assay and a fast prognostic score for risk assessment of normotensive pulmonary embolism. Thromb Haemost. 2014;111:996-1003.
54. Bova C, Sanchez O, Prandoni P, Lankeit M, Konstantinides S, Vanni S, et al. Identification of intermediate-risk patients with acute symptomatic pulmonary embolism. Eur Respir J. 2014;44:694-703.

55. Green EM, Givertz MM. Management of acute right ventricular failure in the intensive care unit. Curr Heart Fail Rep. 2012;9:228-35.
56. Mercat A, Diehl JL, Meyer G, Teboul JL, Sors H. Hemodynamic effects of fluid loading in acute massive pulmonary embolism. Crit Care Med. 1999;27:540-4.
57. Ternacle J, Gallet R, Mekontso-Dessap A, Meyer G, Maitre B, Bensaid A, et al. Diuretics in normotensive patients with acute pulmonary embolism and right ventricular dilatation. Circ J. 2013;77:2612-8.
58. Ventetuolo CE, Klinger JR. Management of acute right ventricular failure in the intensive care unit. Ann Am Thorac Soc. 2014;11:811-22.
59. Boulain T, Lanotte R, Legras A, Perrotin D. Efficacy of epinephrine therapy in shock complicating pulmonary embolism. Chest. 1993;104:300-2.
60. Ghignone M, Girling L, Prewitt RM. Volume expansion versus norepinephrine in treatment of a low cardiac output complicating an acute increase in right ventricular afterload in dogs. Anesthesiology. 1984;60:132-5.
61. Summerfield DT, Desai H, Levitov A, Grooms DA, Marik PE. Inhaled nitric oxide as salvage therapy in massive pulmonary embolism: a case series. Respir Care. 2012;57:444-8.
62. Meyer G, Vieillard-Baron A, Planquette B. Recent advances in the management of pulmonary embolism: focus on the critically ill patients. Ann Intensive Care. 2016;6:19.
63. Cossette B, Pelletier ME, Carrier N, Turgeon M, Leclair C, Charron P, et al. Evaluation of bleeding risk in patients exposed to therapeutic unfractionated or low-molecular-weight heparin: a cohort study in the context of a quality improvement initiative. Ann Pharmacother. 2010;44:994-1002.
64. Meyer G. Effective diagnosis and treatment of pulmonary embolism: improving patient outcomes. Arch Cardiovasc Dis. 2014;107:406-14.
65. Linnemann B, Scholz U, Rott H, Halimeh S, Zotz R, Gerhardt A, et al. Treatment of pregnancy-associated venous thromboembolism—position paper from the Working Group in Women's Health of the Society of Thrombosis and Haemostasis (GTH). Vasa. 2016;45:103-18.
66. Wan S, Quinlan DJ, Agnelli G, Eikelboom JW. Thrombolysis compared with heparin for the initial treatment of pulmonary embolism. Circulation. 2004;110:744-9.
67. Fesmire FM, Brown MD, Espinosa JA, Shih RD, Silvers SM, Wolf SJ, et al. Critical issues in the evaluation and management of adult patients presenting to the emergency department with suspected pulmonary embolism. Ann Emerg Med. 2011;57:628-52.e75.
68. Kearon C, Akl EA, Comerota AJ, Prandoni P, Bounameaux H, Goldhaber SZ, et al. Antithrombotic therapy for VTE disease: Antithrombotic Therapy and Prevention of Thrombosis, 9th ed: American College of Chest Physicians Evidence-Based Clinical Practice Guidelines. Chest. 2012;141(2 suppl):e419S-96S.
69. Jaff MR, McMurtry MS, Archer SL, Cushman M, Goldenberg N, Goldhaber SZ, et al. Management of massive and submassive pulmonary embolism, iliofemoral deep vein thrombosis, and chronic thromboembolic pulmonary hypertension. Circulation. 2011;123:1788-830.
70. Goldhaber SZ. PEITHO long-term outcomes study: data disrupt dogma. J Am Coll Cardiol. 2017;69:1545-8.
71. Konstantinides SV, Vicaut E, Danays T, Becattini C, Bertoletti L, Beyer-Westendorf J, et al. Impact of thrombolytic therapy on the long-term outcome of intermediate-risk pulmonary embolism. J Am Coll Cardiol. 2017;69:1536-44.
72. Meyer G, Vicaut E, Danays T, Agnelli G, Becattini C, Beyer-Westendorf J, et al. Fibrinolysis for patients with intermediate-risk pulmonary embolism. N Engl J Med. 2014;370:1402-11.
73. Perrott J, Henneberry RJ, Zed PJ. Thrombolytics for cardiac arrest: case report and systematic review of controlled trials. Ann Pharmacother. 2010;44:2007-13.
74. Truhlář A, Deakin CD, Soar J, Khalifa GE, Alfonzo A, Bierens JJ, et al. European Resuscitation Council Guidelines for Resuscitation 2015: Section 4. Cardiac arrest in special circumstances. Resuscitation. 2015;95:148-201.
75. Lavonas EJ, Drennan IR, Gabrielli A, Heffner AC, Hoyte CO, Orkin AM, et al. Part 10: special circumstances of resuscitation: 2015 American Heart Association guidelines update for cardiopulmonary resuscitation and emergency cardiovascular care. Circulation. 2015;132:S501-18.
76. Bottiger BW, Arntz HR, Chamberlain DA, Bluhmki E, Belmans A, Danays T, et al. Thrombolysis during resuscitation for out-of-hospital cardiac arrest. N Engl J Med. 2008;359:2651-62.
77. Sharifi M, Bay C, Skrocki L, Rahimi F, Mehdipour M, "MOPETT" Investigators. Moderate pulmonary embolism treated with thrombolysis (from the "MOPETT" trial). Am J Cardiol. 2013;111:273-7.
78. Kline JA, Nordenholz KE, Courtney DM, Kabrhel C, Jones AE, Rondina MT, et al. Treatment of submassive pulmonary embolism with tenecteplase or placebo: cardiopulmonary outcomes at 3 months: multicenter double-blind, placebo-controlled randomized trial. J Thromb Haemost. 2014;12:459-68.
79. Sharifi RD. The urokinase-pulmonary embolism trial. JAMA. 1974;227:1168-9.
80. Urokinase-streptokinase embolism trial. Phase 2 results. A cooperative study. JAMA. 1974;229:1606-13.
81. Tebbe U, Graf A, Kamke W, Zahn R, Forycki F, Kratzsch G, et al. Hemodynamic effects of double bolus reteplase versus alteplase infusion in massive pulmonary embolism. Am Heart J. 1999;138:39-44.
82. Becattini C, Agnelli G, Salvi A, Grifoni S, Pancaldi LG, Enea I, et al. Bolus tenecteplase for right ventricle dysfunction in hemodynamically stable patients with pulmonary embolism. Thromb Res. 2010;125:e82-6.
83. Kuo WT, Sista AK, Faintuch S, Dariushnia SR, Baerlocher MO, Lookstein RA, et al. Society of Interventional Radiology Position statement on catheter-directed therapy for acute pulmonary embolism. J Vasc Interv Radiol. 2018;29:293-7.
84. Kucher N, Boekstegers P, Muller OJ, Kupatt C, Beyer-Westendorf J, Heitzer T, et al. Randomized, controlled trial of ultrasound-assisted catheter-directed thrombolysis for acute intermediate-risk pulmonary embolism. Circulation. 2014;129:479-86.
85. Piazza G, Hohlfelder B, Jaff MR, Ouriel K, Engelhardt TC, Sterling KM, et al. A prospective, single-arm, multicenter

trial of ultrasound-facilitated, catheter-directed, low-dose fibrinolysis for acute massive and submassive pulmonary embolism. JACC Cardiovasc Interv. 2015;8:1382-92.

86. Kuo WT, Banerjee A, Kim PS, DeMarco FJ, Levy JR, Facchini FR, et al. Pulmonary Embolism Response to Fragmentation, Embolectomy, and Catheter Thrombolysis (PERFECT). Chest. 2015;148:667-73.

87. Iaccarino A, Frati G, Schirone L, Saade W, Iovine E, D'Abramo M, et al. Surgical embolectomy for acute massive pulmonary embolism: state of the art. J Thorac Dis. 2018;10:5154-61.

88. Lee T, Itagaki S, Chiang YP, Egorova NN, Adams DH, Chikwe J. Survival and recurrence after acute pulmonary embolism treated with pulmonary embolectomy or thrombolysis in New York State, 1999 to 2013. J Thorac Cardiovasc Surg. 2018;155:1084-90.e12.

89. Maj G, Melisurgo G, De Bonis M, Pappalardo F. ECLS management in pulmonary embolism with cardiac arrest: which strategy is better? Resuscitation. 2014;85:e175-6.

90. Agnelli G, Buller HR, Cohen A, Curto M, Gallus AS, Johnson M, et al. Apixaban for extended treatment of venous thromboembolism. N Engl J Med. 2013;368:699-70.

91. Weitz JI, Lensing AWA, Prins MH, Bauersachs R, Beyer-Westendorf J, Bounameaux H, et al. Rivaroxaban or aspirin for extended treatment of venous thromboembolism. N Engl J Med. 2017;376:1211-22.

92. Meyer G, Marjanovic Z, Valcke J, Lorcerie B, Gruel Y, Solal-Celigny P, et al. Comparison of low-molecular-weight heparin and warfarin for the secondary prevention of venous thromboembolism in patients with cancer: a randomized controlled study. Arch Intern Med. 2002;162:1729-35.

93. Louzada ML, Carrier M, Lazo-Langner A, Dao V, Kovacs MJ, Ramsay TO, et al. Development of a clinical prediction rule for risk stratification of recurrent venous thromboembolism in patients with cancer-associated venous thromboembolism. Circulation. 2012;126:448-54.

Acute Respiratory Distress Syndrome

Jigeeshu Vashisth Divatia, Kushal Rajeev Kalvit

CASE STUDY

A 28-year-old male is brought to the casualty with complaints of high-grade fever, upper respiratory tract infections (URTI), dry cough, and loose stools of 1-week duration. Over the past 2 days, he is progressively worsening and now has respiratory distress. On examination, he is tachycardic [heart rate (HR) of 96 beats/min], normotensive [blood pressure (BP) 116/80 mm Hg], and tachypneic [respiratory rate (RR) 35 breaths/min]. His saturation of peripheral oxygen (SpO_2) is 80% on room air, which falls to 70% on minimal exertion. Bilateral coarse crepitations are present. Chest X-ray shows bilateral consolidation, more on the right side. A throat swab sent 2 days back for H1N1 has come positive today.

Q1. What is the likely diagnosis? What should be the initial workup?

The patient is a young male with a history of high-grade fever and lung infiltrates with impaired oxygenation. The most likely diagnosis is pneumonia with acute hypoxemic (type I) respiratory failure (AHRF). The pathophysiologic mechanisms that account for the hypoxemia observed are a low ventilation/perfusion (V/Q) ratio and shunt. These two mechanisms lead to widening of the alveolar–arterial partial pressure of oxygen (PO_2) gradient (normal <15 mm Hg) while breathing room air. The difference between the two mechanisms is the response of the patient on breathing 100% oxygen. Hypoxemia predominantly due to low V/Q responds to oxygen supplementation, whereas hypoxemia due to shunt does not respond well to oxygen supplementation. The common causes of hypoxemic respiratory failure include the following:

- Pneumonia
- Chronic obstructive pulmonary disease (COPD)
- Pulmonary edema
- Pulmonary fibrosis
- Asthma
- Pneumothorax
- Pulmonary embolism
- Pulmonary arterial hypertension
- Pneumoconiosis
- Granulomatous lung diseases
- Cyanotic congenital heart disease
- Bronchiectasis
- Acute respiratory distress syndrome (ARDS)
- Fat embolism syndrome
- Kyphoscoliosis
- Obesity

Initial workup

Acute hypoxemic respiratory failure may be associated with a variety of clinical manifestations, including tachypnea and dyspnea. However, these are nonspecific, and respiratory failure may be present without dramatic signs or symptoms. Therefore, the analysis of arterial blood gas is extremely important in patients in whom AHRF is suspected. Chest radiography is essential. Electrocardiography (ECG) should be performed to evaluate the possibility of a cardiovascular cause of respiratory failure. ECG may also detect dysrhythmias resulting from hypoxemia or acidosis. Arterial blood gas analysis should be performed to confirm the diagnosis and to assess the severity of respiratory failure and guide management. The presence of anemia on a complete blood count in these patients will contribute to tissue hypoxia, whereas polycythemia may indicate chronic hypoxemic respiratory failure. Leukocytosis or leukopenia points to an infectious etiology. Evaluation of renal and hepatic function may be helpful in the evaluation and management of a patient in respiratory failure and to assess the presence of any multiorgan dysfunction. Abnormalities in electrolytes such as potassium, magnesium, and phosphorus may aggravate respiratory failure due to muscle weakness and also can affect functions of other organ systems such as cardiovascular and gastrointestinal systems.

Q2. What is ARDS?

Acute respiratory distress syndrome is a life-threatening condition requiring intensive care unit (ICU) admission and ventilatory support. It is defined by the presence of noncardiogenic pulmonary edema and hypoxemia due to direct or indirect injury to the lung parenchyma. It is a common endpoint of various direct and indirect insults. ARDS was first described by Ashbaugh and Petty in 1967. It was first described as adult respiratory distress syndrome to distinguish it from the neonatal respiratory distress syndrome, but after the recognition of ARDS in pediatric patients, the nomenclature has been changed to ARDS.[1]

Q3. What is the incidence and etiology of ARDS?

The incidence of ARDS varies in different studies due to variations in definitions and association with a lengthy list of causes and comorbidities. The National Institute of Health in 1977 had described an incidence of 75 per 100,000 population.[2] The *L*arge observational study to *UN*derstand the *G*lobal impact of *S*evere *A*cute respiratory *F*ailur*E* (LUNG SAFE) study found that ARDS was present in >10% of ICU patients, and the incidence was >20% in patients requiring invasive mechanical ventilation. The hospital mortality was around 40%.[3]

Acute respiratory distress syndrome is always associated with a risk factor; the risk increases with multiple risk factors. These factors can injure the lung directly or indirectly; accordingly, the risk factors are categorized as direct or indirect **(Table 1)**. This categorization is amply justified by the differences in pathogenesis, physiologic difference, and differing outcomes.[4]

Pneumonia and nonpulmonary sepsis are the most common causes of ARDS and are associated with the worst outcomes, while trauma-related ARDS has a significantly lower mortality.[4-6] COVID-19 infection and EVALI (e-cigarette or vaping product-use associated lung injury) are the newer causes of ARDS worldwide.[7]

TABLE 1: Risk factors associated with acute respiratory distress syndrome (ARDS).[4]

Factors causing direct lung injury	Factors causing indirect lung injury
• Pneumonia	• Sepsis
• COVID-19	• Multisystem trauma
• EVALI	• TRALI
• Aspiration	• Acute pancreatitis
• Lung contusion	• Drug overdose
• Inhalational injury	• Cardiopulmonary bypass
• Reperfusion injury	• Tropical infections (malaria, leptospirosis, scrub typhus)
• Near drowning	
• Fat embolism	

(EVALI: e-cigarette or vaping product-use associated lung injury; TRALI: transfusion-related acute lung injury)

Q4. What is the pathogenesis of ARDS? What are the pathophysiologic consequences of ARDS?

Pathogenesis

Acute respiratory distress syndrome is a condition initiated or triggered by injury to the alveolar epithelium and/or capillary endothelium. While alveolar epithelial injury is the initial insult in the conditions associated with direct lung injury, capillary endothelial injury is the initial trigger in the conditions associated with indirect lung injury. Ultimately, both mechanisms play a role in ARDS; hence, both events can be identified on histopathology at the time of diagnosis.[8] Alveolar epithelial cells are of two types: flat type I and cuboidal type II. Type I cells are most abundant (90% of epithelial cells) and are prone to damage. Type II cells are responsible for the production of surfactant, proliferation, production of type I cells, and transport of ions, and they are less prone to damage.[9] Loss of type II cells leads to the loss of usual transport and removal of fluid across the membrane.

There are three phases of ARDS identified on histopathology:[10,11]

1. Exudative phase occurs due to the injury to alveolar epithelium and capillary endothelium.
2. Proliferative phase starts 7–14 days after the initial insult and leads to repair of damaged epithelium/endothelium, restoration of barrier function, and proliferation of fibroblasts.
3. Fibrotic phase occurs in some patients as chronic inflammation sets in, leading to fibrosis of alveoli.

The most prominent feature in ARDS is the widespread loss of alveolar epithelial type I cells due to sloughing and apoptosis. One of the well-known markers for epithelial injury, the receptor of advanced glycosylation end-product (RAGE), is highly expressed on alveolar epithelial cells type I. Endothelial injury is also widespread. It causes increased permeability leading to leakage of plasma in the interstitial space and airspaces. Therefore, the alveolar fluid in ARDS is rich in protein, in contrast to the alveolar fluid in cardiogenic-pulmonary edema, which has low-protein content. Injury to endothelium also causes the release of inflammatory molecules, increased expression of cell surface adhesion molecules (e.g., selectin, intracellular adhesion molecule-1), and activation of procoagulant pathways by increased release of von Willebrand factor (vWF), especially in patients with sepsis and bacteremia. These, in turn, help in binding and transmigration of neutrophils across the endothelium.[12]

In addition, the other abnormalities contributing to pathogenesis of ARDS are as follows:

- Neutrophilic infiltration leading to inflammatory cascade
- Surfactant dysfunction

- Dysregulated intravascular and extravascular coagulation cascade.

Although neutrophils are not critical for the pathogenesis of ARDS, as evidenced by the incidence of ARDS in neutropenic patients, they play a crucial role in the initial inflammatory cascade. Neutrophils release a variety of proteases, e.g., elastase, collagenase, gelatinase A and gelatinase B, and reactive oxygen species, in addition to proinflammatory cytokines and chemokines. All these markers lead to a widespread inflammatory response, both pulmonary and extrapulmonary. Proinflammatory cytokine surge and further recruitment of neutrophils by resident macrophages also add to the inflammatory response.[12-14]

Surfactant dysfunction is the combined result of injury to type II epithelial cells, intra-alveolar flooding with proteinaceous fluids, and increased proteolysis. Both lipid and protein components of surfactant are abnormal. Surfactant dysfunction leads to abnormality in host defense and lung mechanics.[15-17]

Dysregulated intravascular and extravascular coagulation is mainly due to activated leukocytes and endothelial cells. Both increased procoagulant activity and impaired fibrinolysis have been described in ARDS. Tissue factor expression is increased on the surface of alveolar epithelium and resident macrophages, leading to increased procoagulant activity in the edema fluid. Elevated levels of plasminogen activator inhibitor-1 (PAI-1) and reduced levels of protein C have been implicated in the impaired fibrinolysis.[18]

Pathophysiologic consequences
The pathophysiologic consequences of ARDS include the following:
- Refractory hypoxemia and shunt
- Decreased lung compliance
- Pulmonary hypertension

Refractory hypoxemia and shunt: Physiological shunt increases in ARDS due to the following reasons:
- Flooding of the alveolar space with protein, exudates, and fluid
- Alveolar collapse due to increase in surface tension in the absence of surfactant
- Noncardiogenic pulmonary edema due to leaky alveolar–capillary membrane

All these lead to a mismatched V/Q as blood flowing through capillaries in the alveoli, which are collapsed, are not taking part in gas exchange. The inflammatory edema also leads to widened alveolar septum, leading to decreased diffusion across the alveolar–capillary membrane.[19-21]

Decreased compliance: Alveolar flooding and atelectasis along with alveolar–capillary membrane inflammation make the alveolar spaces very stiff, resulting in noncompliant lungs. In the late stages of ARDS, fibrosis also decreases the compliance of the lung.

Pulmonary hypertension and right ventricular (RV) failure: The development of pulmonary hypertension is a common occurrence in ARDS. It further worsens the hypoxemia by increasing dead-space ventilation and hypercarbia. Pulmonary hypertension develops due to hypoxic pulmonary vasoconstriction[22] and also due to local production of endothelin-1 and thromboxane A2. ARDS also causes remodeling of arterial, venous, and lymphatic circulation, leading to decrease in cross-section of the lumens due to the deposition of fibrin and collagen.[22,23] Formation of microthrombi and macrothrombi in pulmonary vessels is also common in ARDS. Microthrombi and macrothrombi have been demonstrated in 95% and 86% of autopsy specimens, respectively.[23] Pulmonary hypertension can lead to further hypoxia by right-to-left shunting across a patent foramen ovale and end-organ hypoperfusion due to RV failure leading to reduced cardiac output.[24]

Q5. What is the clinical definition of ARDS?

Clinical definition
Murray et al. proposed diagnostic criteria, which included hypoxemia [(partial pressure of oxygen in arterial blood (PaO_2)/fraction of inspired oxygen (FiO_2)], chest radiographic opacities (number of quadrants), positive end-expiratory pressure (PEEP) level, and low respiratory system compliance (C_{rs}). Murray further expanded their definition to describe the time course, which addressed prognostic and treatment implications of different phases and causes of ARDS.[25]

The American European Consensus Conference (AECC) on ARDS in 1994 considered four parameters to identify ARDS, namely timing of onset, oxygenation, absence of cardiac failure, and chest radiograph findings. ARDS was defined as impaired oxygenation of acute onset with a PaO_2/FiO_2 (PF) ratio < 200 and a pulmonary capillary wedge pressure < 18 mm Hg. Acute lung injury (ALI) with PF ratio < 300 was identified separately by AECC. ALI represented a broader spectrum of lung injury to include processes other than ARDS, which were associated with impaired gas exchange **(Table 2)**.[26]

*Berlin Definition 2012 **(Table 3)***
Meta-analysis of data from 4,188 patients, taken from four multicenter and three single-center datasets of ARDS patients, was used. All the four elements of AECC definition were updated. It also evaluated ancillary variables to update the definition and to increase the predictive validity in predicting clinical outcomes. It differs from AECC definition in each of the elements. It specifies the timing of onset within

TABLE 2: Differences between American European Consensus Conference (AECC) and Berlin definitions of acute respiratory distress syndrome (ARDS).[26,27]

Components	AECC definition	Berlin definition
Timing	Acute onset	Acute onset <1 week of inciting event
Chest imaging	Bilateral infiltrates on chest X-ray	Bilateral infiltrates on chest imaging not fully explained by effusion, lobar/lung collapse, or nodules
Origin of edema	No evidence of left atrial hypertension or PCWP <18 mm Hg	Respiratory failure not fully explained by cardiac failure or fluid overload
Oxygenation	• PaO_2/FiO_2 <300 is acute lung injury PaO_2/FiO_2 <200 is ARDS	• PaO_2/FiO_2 200–300 with PEEP or CPAP ≥ 5 cmH$_2$O: Mild ARDS • PaO_2/FiO_2 100–200 with PEEP or CPAP ≥ 5 cmH$_2$O: Moderate ARDS • PaO_2/FiO_2 < 100 with PEEP or CPAP ≥ 5 cmH$_2$O: Severe ARDS

(CPAP: continuous positive airway pressure; FiO$_2$: fraction of inspired oxygen; PaO$_2$: partial pressure of oxygen in arterial blood; PCWP: pulmonary capillary wedge pressure; PEEP: positive end-expiratory pressure)

TABLE 3: Berlin definition of acute respiratory distress syndrome (ARDS).[27,28]

Timing	Within 1 week of a known clinical insult or new or worsening respiratory symptoms
Chest radiograph	Bilateral opacities not fully explained by effusions, lobar/lung collapse, or nodules
Cause of edema	Respiratory failure not fully explained by cardiac failure or fluid overload. Need objective assessment (e.g., echocardiography) to exclude hydrostatic edema, if no risk factor present
Severity	Oxygenation criteria
Mild	200 mm Hg < PaO_2/FiO_2 ≤ 300 mm Hg with PEEP or CPAP ≥ 5 cmH$_2$O (formerly ALI by AECC criteria)
Moderate	100 mm Hg < PaO_2/FiO_2 ≤ 200 mm Hg with PEEP ≥ 5 cmH$_2$O (formerly ARDS by AECC criteria)
Severe	PaO_2/FiO_2 ≤ 100 mm Hg with PEEP ≥ 5 cmH$_2$O (formerly ARDS by AECC criteria)

(AECC: American European Consensus Conference; CPAP: continuous positive airway pressure; FiO$_2$: fraction of inspired oxygen; PaO$_2$: partial pressure of oxygen in arterial blood; PEEP: positive end-expiratory pressure)

7 days of a known insult.[27,28] To improve the interobserver agreement in the interpretation of chest radiographs consistent with ARDS, the Berlin definition further described the chest opacities in ARDS not be fully explained by effusions, lobar collapse, or nodules. In addition, 12 sample radiographs with interpretations as consistent, inconsistent, and equivocal for diagnosis of ARDS can be used.[28] The new definition has removed the term ALI and uses only ARDS. ARDS has been classified into three degrees of severity based on the PF ratio.[27] To meet the definition of PF ratio, the patient must be receiving ≥5 cmH$_2$O of continuous positive airway pressure (CPAP) or PEEP. In mild ARDS, this CPAP can be delivered through noninvasive ventilation (NIV):

1. *Mild (PaO_2/FiO_2: 201–300 mm Hg with PEEP or CPAP ≥ 5 cmH$_2$O)*
2. *Moderate (PaO_2/FiO_2: 101–200 mm Hg with PEEP ≥ 5 cmH$_2$O)*
3. *Severe (PaO_2/FiO_2: ≤100 mm Hg with PEEP ≥ 5 cmH$_2$O)*

For the calculation of the PF ratio, an arterial blood sample is needed. Recent studies have shown good correlation between SpO_2/FiO_2 ratio and PF ratio.[29] An SpO_2/FiO_2 ratio of 235 has been shown to correspond to a PF ratio of 200 and an SpO_2/FiO_2 ratio of 315 to a PF ratio of 300. One limitation of the SpO_2/FiO_2 ratio is that it is reliable only when SpO_2 is <98% because the oxyhemoglobin curve is flat above SpO_2 of 100%. The advantage with SpO_2 measurement is that it is noninvasive, can be done continuously, and is widely available in all setups.[30]

Q6. What are the modifications in the definition of ARDS?
The criteria for identifying ARDS in COVID-19 have not been modified. COVID-19 ARDS can be identified in any patient with COVID-19 infection who meets the Berlin ARDS criteria. In resource-limited settings, measurement of PaO$_2$ and application of PEEP via invasive ventilation is not always possible. Hence, a modified Kigali definition was proposed to identify ARDS in resource-limited settings. The three modifications in this definition were:[31]

1. Use of SpO_2/FiO_2 < 315 instead of PF ratio < 300
2. No PEEP requirement
3. Bilateral lung opacities identified by chest X-ray or lung ultrasound [no need of computed tomography (CT) scan]

A new global definition of ARDS has been proposed by a consensus statement in 2023, which is an expansion on the existing Berlin definition. The four points in this new definition are:[32]

1. High-frequency nasal oxygen (HFNO) > 30 L/min (intubation not required)
2. Hypoxemia defined as PF < 300 mm Hg or SF ratio < 315 with SpO_2 < 97%
3. Bilateral lung opacities identified by chest X-ray, CT, or lung ultrasound (any one of them)
4. PEEP, oxygen flow, or specific respiratory support devices are not required in case of resource-limited settings.

Q7. How will you differentiate ARDS from cardiogenic pulmonary edema (Table 4)?

The initial definition from AECC for ARDS required a pulmonary artery wedge pressure (PAWP) of <18 mm Hg without any clinical evidence of left atrial hypertension. This definition missed the diagnosis of ARDS in patients with left atrial hypertension or heart failure, whereas both can exist together. The Berlin definition allows for considering the presence of both hydrostatic and nonhydrostatic pulmonary edema provided the respiratory failure cannot be explained by heart failure alone. Even clinical vignettes were added in the supplementary article.

TABLE 4: Clinical differences between acute respiratory distress syndrome (ARDS) and cardiogenic pulmonary edema (CPE).[32-36]

Clinical parameter	ARDS	CPE
History	Variable	History of heart disease
Signs of cardiac failure	Usually absent	Commonly present
X-ray	Opacities are more or less uniformly distributed. Opacification persists for days to weeks (retrospective)	Opacities are prominent in perihilar areas. Opacification clears rapidly within hours with treatment (retrospective)
Ultrasound findings		
Pleural line	May be reduced, thickened, or appear coarse	Normal
Lung sliding	May be absent	Present
Lung pulse during ventilation	Can be seen	Not seen
B-lines-alveolar interstitial syndrome (AIS)	AIS with air bronchograms and spared areas	Homogeneous AIS with no spared areas
Consolidation	Shred sign or tissue-like sign	Not seen
Pleural effusion	Uncommon and exudative	Common and large transudative
Echocardiography	No new change in LV function	New or worsening LV function
IVC diameter	Usually normal and collapsing with respiration	Usually dilated and noncollapsible
PVPI using transpulmonary thermodilution technique	>3	<2

(IVC: inferior vena cava; LV: left ventricle; PVPI: pulmonary vascular pressure index)

The use of bedside echocardiography to rule out cardiogenic pulmonary edema has been encouraged if no identifiable precipitating factor for ARDS could be identified.[26] Till date, no laboratory study has been reliably able to differentiate between cardiogenic pulmonary edema and ARDS. B-type natriuretic peptide (BNP) levels at the time of admission could not differentiate between cardiogenic and noncardiogenic edema, and they also did not correlate with the measurements found on invasive hemodynamic monitoring.[30] Even N-terminal proBNP levels do not correlate with PAWP.[31]

Recently, lung ultrasound has been extensively used in the bedside assessment of critically ill patients in the ICU **(Figs. 1A to D)**.[32,33] In ARDS, a nonhomogeneous B-pattern and pleural line abnormality (shred sign) are usually found.[32] Bilateral B-pattern can be present in both cardiogenic and noncardiogenic pulmonary edema.[33-37]

Q8. How will you manage this patient in ICU?

Treatment

The treatment of ARDS is respiratory support and identification and treatment of the predisposing cause. With substantial improvement in supportive therapies, there has been a gradual decline in mortality attributable to ARDS over the last few decades. The most crucial step in treating ARDS is the identification of the predisposing factor and prompt therapy for it; for example, in sepsis-associated ARDS, early resuscitation, appropriate antibiotic, and early source control have shown good outcomes.[38]

The supportive therapy for ARDS mainly focuses on providing adequate gas exchange with lung-protective ventilation and minimizing ventilator-induced lung injury (VILI). The strategies to reach this objective can be pharmacologic, nonpharmacologic, or a combination of both **(Table 5)**.

Noninvasive ventilation/high-flow nasal cannula (HFNC): Noninvasive ventilation can reduce intrapulmonary shunt and the work of breathing, thus improving oxygenation. The advantages of NIV include avoiding deep sedation, allowing spontaneous breaths, minimal risk of nosocomial pneumonia, improved hemodynamics, and better V/Q matching. In a meta-analysis of 13 heterogeneous studies of NIV in ALI/ARDS (*n* = 540), there was a 50% NIV failure rate.[39]

Appropriate selection of patients for NIV is of paramount importance. NIV seems to be a reasonable choice in the subset of ARDS patients with an $PaO_2/FiO_2 > 150$ due to a lower failure rate.[40] On the other hand, patients with de novo acute respiratory failure (ARF) (without a previous cardiac or respiratory disease) have almost two times more chances of NIV failure compared to the patients with a previous

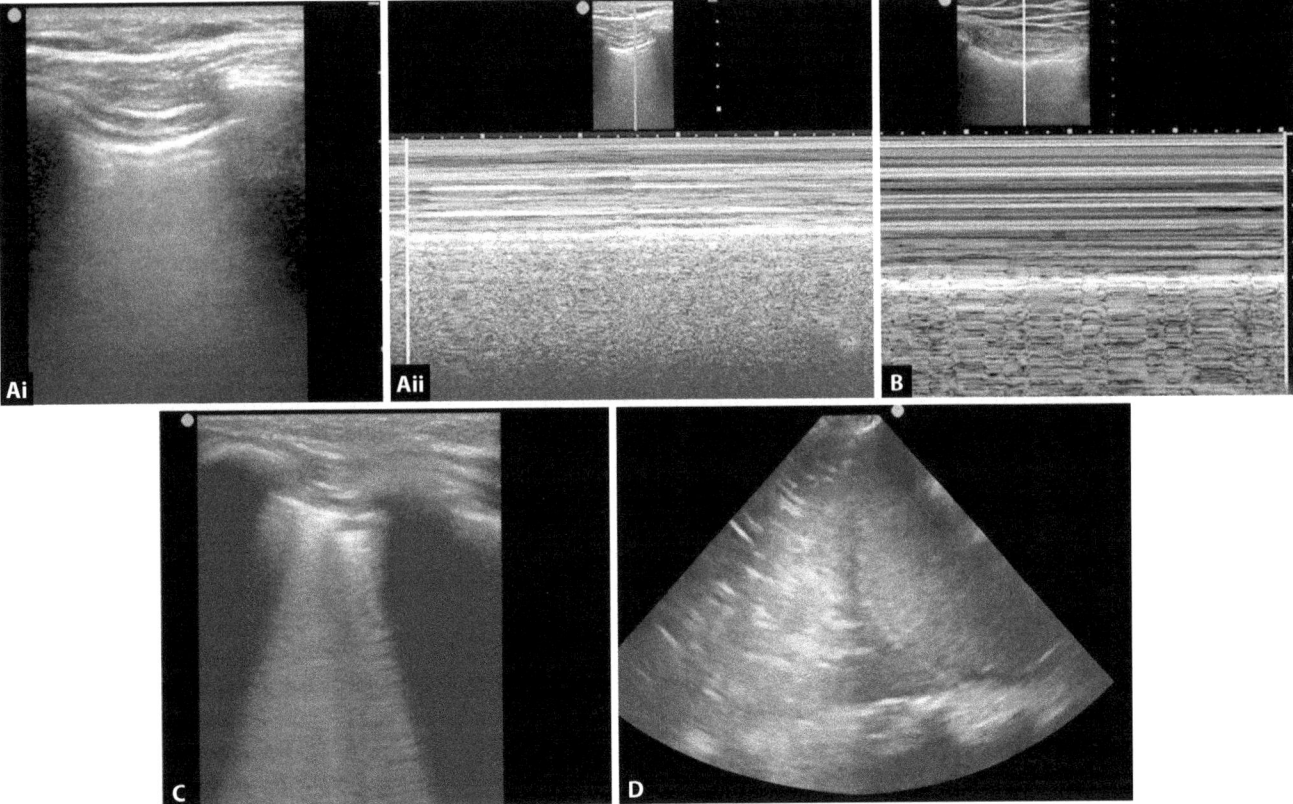

Figs. 1A to D: Possible findings at ultrasonographic lung examination. (A) Normal aeration with normal sliding, (Ai) B mode with A-lines pattern and (Aii) M mode showing seashore sign; (B) M mode showing lung pulse indicating lack of ventilation; (C) B lines indicating alveolar-interstitial syndrome (AIS); (D) lung consolidation, hyperechoic area with air bronchogram.

TABLE 5: Supportive strategies for acute respiratory distress syndrome (ARDS).

Nonpharmacologic strategies	Pharmacologic strategies
• Mechanical ventilation • Noninvasive ventilation/high-flow nasal cannula (HFNC) • Invasive ventilation with low tidal volumes • Positive end-expiratory pressure (PEEP) application	• Muscle relaxation • Corticosteroids • Diuretics to achieve negative fluid balance in the absence of shock
Rescue therapies: • Recruitment maneuvers • Prone positioning • High-frequency oscillation (HFO) • Extracorporeal carbon dioxide removal (ECCO$_2$R) • Extracorporeal membrane oxygenation (ECMO)	*Rescue therapy:* Inhaled vasodilators

cardiac or respiratory disease.[41] Other predictors of failure of NIV include higher heart rate, lower PF ratio, lower bicarbonate, high sepsis-related organ failure assessment (SOFA) score, and worsening of lung infiltrate 24 hours after admission. The likelihood of NIV failure is two to three times more in hypoxemic respiratory failure than in cardiogenic pulmonary edema or acute exacerbation of COPD. Higher hospital mortality is observed in patients with AHRF who fail NIV.[42]

A possible consequent risk of delaying tracheal intubation in patients managed with NIV also has a worse outcome. With the given amount of evidence, NIV should be avoided in de novo ARF and patients with severe ARDS. In other patients, NIV can be given with close monitoring for the signs of NIV failure. HFNC can deliver warmed and humidified high oxygen flow through the nose, which improves patient comfort.[43] It improves oxygenation, carbon dioxide (CO_2) clearance, and end-expiratory lung volume and thus decreases work of breathing. In the FLORALI trial, Frat et al. compared the efficacy of HFNC, NIV, and oxygen through a standard facemask in patients with AHRF without hypercapnia. They looked at the proportion of patients intubated at 28 days, all-cause mortality at 90 days, and ventilator-free days at 28 days. This trial also showed a high rate of failure with NIV with an intubation rate of 50%. Though the difference in intubation rate was not statistically significant in the three groups, the number of ventilator-free days was significantly higher in the HFNC group. On post hoc analysis, the intubation rate was significantly lower in the HFNC group and in the group of patients with the PF ratio <200. All-cause mortality was also lower in the HFNC group. Overall subjective patient comfort was much higher in the HFNC group.[44]

Invasive mechanical ventilation: Hypoxemic respiratory failure is the hallmark of ARDS. The alveolar spaces are flooded with proteinaceous exudative inflammatory fluid, leading to impaired oxygenation and a stiff lung with low lung compliance, which leads to increased work of breathing. Almost all patients with ARDS need some respiratory support, and a significant proportion of them need endotracheal intubation and invasive mechanical ventilation. There has been substantial evidence through clinical and experimental studies that mechanical ventilation leads to functional and structural alteration in the lung.[45] Mechanical ventilation perpetuates the lung injury in ARDS and contributes to the morbidity and mortality associated with ARDS.[46-48] Webb and Tierney in 1970 showed that high peak inspiratory pressure (PIP) produced severe damage in the lungs of rats, which was attenuated by the use of PEEP. Gattinoni[52] first described the concept of the "baby lung."[49] The ARDS lung was considered a homogeneous lung in radiographs, but it appeared inhomogeneous in CT scans with most of the densities present in the dependent parts of the lungs. The lungs are comprised of normally aerated, poorly aerated, nonaerated, and overinflated tissues. Effectively, the lung is divided into three zones: (1) A nonrecruitable zone, in the bases; (2) an injured but recruitable midzone, and (3) a spared though potentially overdistended zone in the apices. On quantitative estimation from the CT images, the volume of the normally aerated lungs in adult patients of severe ARDS was equivalent to the normally aerated lung of a healthy boy of 5-6 years age, supporting the concept of baby lung. The shunt fraction, degree of hypoxemia, and pulmonary hypertension relate to the nonaerated tissue of the lungs. Respiratory compliance correlates well with the remaining normally aerated lung tissue. Thus, compliance truly measures the volume of baby lung. In other words, we can say that the ARDS lung is not stiff but small. The modern mechanical ventilation strategy focuses mainly on minimizing VILI and near normalization of blood gases. It involves protective lung ventilation and keeping the lung open with the appropriate use of PEEP.

Lung-protective ventilation: Historically, a tidal volume of 12-15 mL/kg was routinely used for mechanical ventilation, but now it is well established that a low tidal volume, plateau-pressure limited ventilation has shown reduced mortality after the NIH ARDS Network published their first multicenter randomized controlled trial (RCT) in 2000.[50] Mortality in the traditional tidal volume group was 39.8% and 31% in the lower tidal volume [6 mL/kg predicted body weight (PBW) and plateau pressure < 30 cmH$_2$O] group ($p = 0.007$).

Permissive hypercapnia: In order to prevent VILI, the target tidal volume was decreased in the algorithm provided by the ARDS Net (**Box 1**). This, in turn, led to CO$_2$ retention and hypercapnic acidosis (HCA). In view of the proven mortality benefit with protective lung ventilation, this CO$_2$ rise is accepted as long as there is no harm with this respiratory acidosis. This practice is known as permissive hypercapnia.[51] The limits for PCO$_2$ and pH in permissive hypercapnia are not yet clear, but in the data from clinical trials on permissive hypercapnia, PCO$_2$ levels of 60-70 mm Hg and arterial pH of 7.20-7.25 have been found safe.[52-55]

Positive end-expiratory pressure: Positive end-expiratory pressure and/or recruitment maneuvers (RM) have been universally used to improve oxygenation in ARDS patients since the first description of ARDS. Over the last 50 years, the use of PEEP has shifted more toward minimizing lung injury than improving hypoxemia. The mechanisms explaining the beneficial effects of PEEP in ARDS lungs are as follows:

- Alveolar recruitment leading to increased functional residual capacity (FRC), leading to an improvement in —V/Q match.
- Stabilization of recruited lung and prevention of atelectrauma by avoiding cyclical alveolar collapse by splinting open alveoli
- Extravascular lung water redistribution

Even with all the evidences gained over the years about the beneficial effects of PEEP, one of the most debatable issues is to select the ideal or optimal PEEP. If PEEP is too low, recruitment will not be enough to improve hypoxemia, and if PEEP is too much, it will overstretch the normal baby lung leading to VILI and increased dead space.

Positive end-expiratory pressure titration: Setting the right PEEP is important as it not only helps in recruitment and oxygenation but also prevents VILI. An optimal PEEP is one that will help in recruitment, prevent cycles of recruitment and decruitment, and prevent alveolar overdistention. No single method has been optimized to set the right PEEP. Multiple methods have been used and proposed for setting optimal PEEP.

Oxygenation: In all ARDS Network studies, a combination of PEEP and FiO$_2$ was set to achieve and maintain a target SpO$_2$ (>88%). The tables proposed for the ARDS Network trial were based on expert opinion and not on robust evidence. At the same time, these tables did not consider individual lung mechanics. These tables were easy to use and had a face validity, as they were routinely used

> **BOX 1:** Ventilatory management of acute respiratory distress syndrome (ARDS) (ARDS Net protocol).[50]
>
> *Calculate predicted body weight (PBW):*
> - Males: PBW (kg) = 50 + 2.3 [(height in inches) – 60] or 50 + 0.91 [(height in cm) – 152.4]
> - Females: IBW (kg) = 45.5 + 2.3 [(height in inches) – 60] or 45.5 + 0.91 [(height in cm) – 152.4]
>
> Ventilator mode
> Volume assist/control until weaning
>
> *Tidal volume (V_t):*
> - Initial V_t: 6 mL/kg PBW
> - Measure inspiratory plateau pressure (P_{plat}, 0.5 seconds inspiratory pause) every 4 hours and after each change in PEEP or V_t
> - If P_{plat} >30 cmH$_2$O, decrease V_t to 5 or to 4 mL/kg
> - If P_{plat} <25 cmH$_2$O and V_t <6 mL/kg PBW
>
> *Respiratory rate (RR)*
> - With initial change in V_t, adjust RR to maintain minute ventilation
> - Make subsequent adjustments to RR to maintain pH 7.30–7.45, but do not exceed RR = 35/min and do not increase the set rate if PaCO$_2$ <25 mm Hg
>
> I:E ratio
> Acceptable range, 1:1–1:3 (no inverse ratio)
>
> FiO$_2$, PEEP, and arterial oxygenation
> Maintain PaO$_2$ = 55–80 mm Hg or SpO$_2$ = 88–95% using the following PEEP/FiO$_2$ combinations:
>
> | FiO$_2$ | 0.3 | 0.4 | 0.5 | 0.5 | 0.6 | 0.7 | 0.8 | 0.9 | 1 |
> |---|---|---|---|---|---|---|---|---|---|
> | PEEP | 5 | 5 | 8 | 8 | 10 | 12 | 14 | 16 | 18 | 18–24 |
>
> *Acidosis management:*
> - If pH < 7.30, increase RR until pH ≥ 730 or RR = 35/min
> - If pH remains <7.30 with RR = 35, consider bicarbonate infusion
> - If pH < 7.15, V_t may be increased (P_{plat} may exceed 30 cmH$_2$O)
>
> *Alkalosis management:*
> If pH > 7.45 and patient not triggering ventilator, decrease set RR but not below 6/min
>
> *Fluid management:*
> - Once patients are out of shock, adopt a conservative fluid management strategy
> - Use diuretics or fluids to target a central venous pressure (CVP) of <4 mm Hg or a pulmonary artery occlusion pressure (PAOP) of <8 mm Hg
>
> *Liberation from mechanical ventilation:*
> - Daily interruption of sedation
> - Daily screen for spontaneous breathing trial (SBT)
> - SBT when all of the following criteria are present:
>   - FiO$_2$ < 0.40 and PEEP < 8 cmH$_2$O
>   - Not receiving neuromuscular blocking agents
>   - Patient is awake and following commands
>   - Systolic arterial pressure > 90 mm Hg without vasopressor support
>   - Tracheal secretions are minimal, and the patient has a good cough and gag reflex
>
> *Spontaneous breathing trial:*
> - Place patient on 5 cmH$_2$O PEEP with 5 cmH$_2$O pressure support ventilation or T-piece
> - Monitor HR, RR, and oxygen saturation for 30–90 minutes
> - Extubate if there are no signs of distress (tachycardia, tachypnea, agitation, hypoxia, diaphoresis)
>
> (FiO$_2$: fraction of inspired oxygen; HR: heart rate; I:E: inspiratory to expiratory; IBW: ideal body weight; PaCO$_2$: partial pressure of carbon dioxide in arterial blood; PaO$_2$: partial pressure of oxygen in arterial blood; PEEP: positive end-expiratory pressure; SpO$_2$: saturation of peripheral oxygen)

in all the trials by the ARDS Network. It is largely believed that higher PEEP should be limited to patients with high recruitability to extract maximal benefit and to avoid lung injury. Chiumello et al.[56] concluded that simple PEEP selection methods, such as Lung Open Ventilation Strategy study table, correlated recruitability better than the complex PEEP selection methods based on lung mechanics, such as ExPress (progressively increasing PEEP until the airway plateau pressure of 28–30 cm), stress index < 1 (discussed below), and esophageal pressure (PEEP set equal to the absolute value of esophageal pressure), as judged by whole-lung CT scans in static conditions at 5 and 45 cmH$_2$O.

Pressure–volume loop

Pressure–volume (PV) loop is the graphical representation of the relationship between pressure and volume as the lung inflates and deflates (**Fig. 2**). The lower inflection point (LIP) mainly represents the point where alveolar recruitment starts. The rapid rise after the LIP represents alveolar recruitment. PEEP above the LIP increases the compliance of the lung by recruitment. Upper inflection point (UIP) is the pressure above which the compliance decreases, and here the lungs start to get overdistended. The rapid rise in pressure at the beginning of inspiration after the LIP indicates alveolar recruitment. This pressure is high as reinflation of collapsed alveolus needs higher pressure than distending an inflated one. The part of the loop which is linear from LIP to UIP represents the ideal pressure at which the alveoli are open and continue to distend gradually with the rise in pressure with increasing compliance. This is known as the curve of optimal compliance.

Amato et al.[57] popularized the concept of setting ideal PEEP based on the PV curve and identification of the LIP and UIP. They recommended to set PEEP at a level 2 cmH$_2$O more than the LIP. A number of issues are faced while using this method to set the ideal or optimal PEEP:

- Deep sedation (and often paralysis) is required to get a correct PV curve.
- In a mechanically ventilated patient, a quasi-static PV loop maneuver is required with a low flow rate (<10 L/min) to minimize the effects of airway resistance on the peak pressure and bring it closer to the plateau pressure.
- It is often difficult to identify the LIP and UIP.
- Esophageal manometry is required to calculate the actual lung compliance instead of respiratory system compliance.

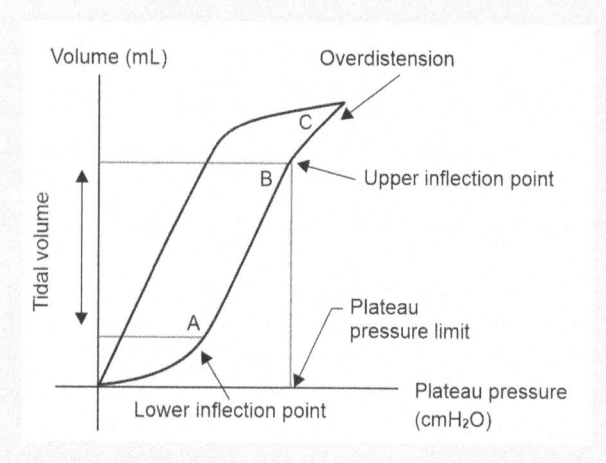

Fig. 2: Pressure–volume loop showing inflection points.

The inflation limb may not be indicative of recruitment; rather, it can be due to some other mechanics, e.g., inflation of an edematous lung.

Driving pressure: Driving pressure (ΔP) is the ratio of tidal volume to the static compliance of the respiratory system.

ΔP = tidal volume (V_t)/respiratory system compliance (C_{rs})

Clinically, driving pressure is the difference between alveolar plateau pressure and PEEP, i.e.,

$$\Delta P = P_{plat} - PEEP$$
$$P_{plat} - PEEP = V_t/C_{rs}$$
$$C_{rs} = V_t/P_{plat} - PEEP$$

Both PEEP and tidal volume are independent variables and can be altered by the physician, but plateau pressure and compliance are dependent variables, so any change in the independent variable affects the dependent variable.

When increasing the tidal volume or PEEP, if there is recruitment, then driving pressure will decrease and compliance increases, but if there is overdistension, then worsening of compliance and increase in driving pressure occur. Driving pressure and compliance are interrelated. Driving pressure may be defined better as the amount of cyclical alveolar deformation imposed on ventilating lung units.

When we measure compliance (C_{rs}), we are actually measuring the compliance of the thorax as a whole, and the lungs are just a part of it. Hence, if we need to know the distending pressure of the lungs alone, we need to measure transpulmonary pressure (alveolar-pleural pressure/esophageal pressure), which is clinically not feasible.

Ventilator-induced lung injury is due to lung stress and strain, which is proportional to the pressure applied to the lung. As lung stress and strain are difficult to measure in clinical practice, airway driving pressure can be used to predict lung injury. The higher the driving pressure, the greater the lung injury.[55]

Recently, Amato et al.[59] showed in their multilevel mediation analysis of 3,562 ARDS patients from nine previous RCTs that ΔP is a better predictor of ARDS outcome.[56] The independent variables associated with improved outcome were driving pressure, PaO$_2$/FiO$_2$ ratio at entry, pH at entry, and risk of death (APACHE, SAPS). The authors did multiple resampling, considering subgroups of patients with matched mean levels for one variable but different mean levels for another ranking variable, and found that increased driving pressure was associated with increased mortality.

Thus, driving pressure is an independent predictor of survival in patients with ARDS, and the reduction in tidal volume or increase in PEEP was found beneficial only if associated with a decrease in driving pressure (ΔP).

Low driving pressure is associated with improved survival, but achieving a lower driving pressure may be a challenge. In patients with ARDS with good recruitable lung after applying RM and appropriate PEEP, the functional lung size increases, and transpulmonary pressure gets evenly distributed, leading to better compliance and lower driving pressure.

Stress index: Another easy bedside surrogate method to know the change in compliance is the stress index **(Fig. 3)**.[57] It is noted from the terminal part of the pressure–time curve of volume-controlled breath with constant flow in a paralyzed patient. When the terminal part of the pressure–time curve is concave downward, it represents good compliance (stress index < 1); when it is concave upward, it represents poor compliance (stress index > 1) whereas a flat shape represents normal compliance (stress index = 1). To know the real stress on the lung, we need to measure the transpulmonary stress index, and it is clinically challenging. Transpulmonary stress index can be substituted by the airway pressure stress index since there is good correlation between them.[58,59] Airway stress index is a simple bedside tool to track respiratory compliance to ventilator adjustments and is hence used to predict lung injury during ventilation.[60] Both tidal volume and PEEP can be titrated to the stress index to limit lung injury.[61] Stress index reflects the respiratory compliance, which in turn has an impact on driving pressure ($C_{rs} = V_t/P_{plat} - PEEP$), so a low stress index will have a low driving pressure and vice versa. Hence, both stress index and driving pressure can be used as indicators of lung stress. Driving pressure has shown to have a close correlation with transpulmonary driving pressure and reflects lung stress.[62] Driving pressure is easy to measure, more objective, and easier to keep a trend as compared to the stress index.

Transpulmonary pressure: The measured airway pressure is not always a reliable estimate of lung stress. Conditions that increase the chest wall elastance (kyphoscoliosis, chest wall edema, obesity) can elevate airway pressure without an increase in lung stress. Hence, the measurement of transpulmonary pressure (P_L) has been advocated as the true marker of global lung stress. P_L is calculated as the difference between plateau pressure and pleural pressure. Pleural pressure is estimated with the help of an esophageal balloon catheter as it cannot be measured directly. PEEP should be set to keep the end-inspiratory P_L < 15–20 cmH$_2$O and the difference between end-inspiratory P_L and end-expiratory P_L (ΔP_L) between 10 and 15 cmH$_2$O. The EP-Vent study demonstrated that esophageal pressure-guided PEEP titration resulted in better oxygenation as compared to the ARDS Net protocol.[63] However, the EP-Vent2 trial did not demonstrate any significant difference in the survival or ventilator-free days when PEEP titration was done by esophageal pressure or the high FiO$_2$-PEEP table.[64] Transpulmonary pressure method is not yet popular owing to the expertise required for esophageal balloon catheter insertion and interpretation.

Q9. What is VILI? What are the major considerations during invasive mechanical ventilation?

To understand the principles of invasive ventilation and VILI, it is important to understand the evolution of concepts of respiratory mechanics of ARDS and the heterogeneous nature of lungs in ARDS. CT revealed the nonhomogeneous nature of lungs, with the densities concentrated primarily in the most dependent regions.[52] The amount of normally aerated tissue, measured at end-expiration, was around 200–500 g in severe ARDS, i.e., roughly equivalent to the normally aerated tissue of a 5–6-year-old healthy boy. This finding gave rise to the concept of "baby lung."[52] The total compliance of the lungs actually corresponds with the size of this baby lung. Hence, high tidal volume ventilation in ARDS patients can cause overdistention of the normally aerated baby lung, leading to lung injury. This can be prevented by using low tidal volumes while maintaining adequate oxygenation and accepting high PCO$_2$, i.e., permissive hypercapnia. There is no clear cutoff for accepting PCO$_2$, but PCO$_2$ levels of 60–70 and pH levels of 7.2–7.25 have been found to be safe in the literature.[65] During positive pressure ventilation, the ventilator applies a force to the lung structure, which develops an internal tension equal and opposite to the applied pressure. This tension is called "stress." This stress is responsible for elongation of the lung fibers from their resting position, which is called "strain." A rough equivalent of the stress in the whole lung is the distending pressure or transpulmonary pressure (airway pressure minus the pleural pressure), while the strain is the change in the size of the lung from its resting position at end expiration.[52] VILI is

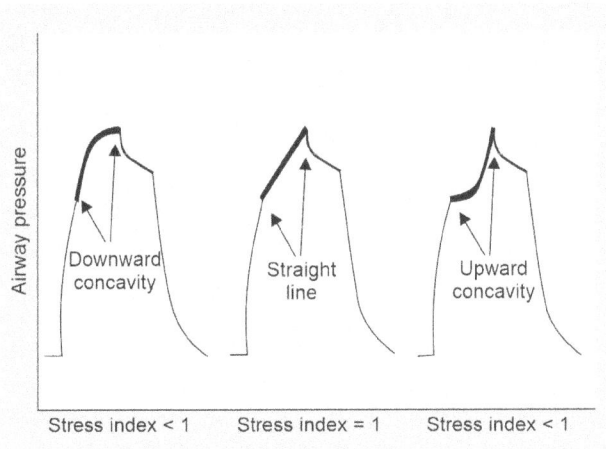

Fig. 3: Pressure time scalar waveforms showing stress index.
Courtesy: Kulkarni and Divatia (2009).[60]

excessive mechanical strain or stress applied to lung globally or regionally, causing lung injury.

Classically, *barotrauma* (pressure-mediated lung injury) and *volutrauma* (overdistension-mediated lung injury) have been described as mechanisms of VILI.

Atelectrauma and shear stress injury: Cyclical opening and closing of atelectatic but recruitable lung units during tidal ventilation contribute to lung injury called atelectrauma. Collapse of one lung unit causes deformation of adjacent units because the interalveolar septum stretches inward toward the collapsed unit. As a result, the adjacent air-filled alveolus undergoes additional shear strain as it inflates nonuniformly. Therefore, repeated opening and closing of atelectatic lung units during mechanical ventilation cause significant shear stress at their junctions with aerated lung units.[66] This results in damage to the capillary endothelium and the alveolar membrane. This is termed cyclical shear stress injury.

Biotrauma: Alveolar overdistension along with the repeated collapse and reopening of the alveoli can trigger a cascade of proinflammatory cytokines that induce both a pulmonary and systemic cytokine response, aggravating lung injury and causing systemic multiorgan dysfunction.[66]

Low tidal ventilation reduces the overdistension-related lung injury. Addition of PEEP can reduce VILI by increasing the resting end-expiratory lung volume in the recruitable lung. Hence, it avoids atelectrauma by preventing its cyclical collapse. However, in a poorly recruitable lung, PEEP may overdistend the normally aerated lung, increasing its strain. Studies have investigated the effect of high PEEP versus low PEEP but did not find significant mortality benefit suggesting that high PEEP is not beneficial in all patients.[67,68]

Mechanical power (MP) and VILI: Conceptually, VILI is caused by the delivery of a critical amount of mechanical energy to the lung.[69] The energy delivered to the lung during positive pressure ventilation causes structural deformation sufficient to activate mechanotransduction-related inflammation or create micro-wounding and to break molecular bonds of the fibers composing the extracellular matrix. The energy delivered may be so great as to cause stress-at-rupture (e.g., pneumothorax). When it is below the stress-at-rupture threshold, if delivered for a sufficient time, it results in VILI (termed *ergotrauma*). Thus, energy and time define MP. A simplified equation for determination of MP during volume-controlled ventilation is as follows:

$$MP = 0.098 \times RR \times V_t \times [PIP - 1/2(P_{plat} - PEEP)]$$

Other supportive measures
Sedation: It is usually mandatory in ARDS patients receiving lung-protective ventilation. Deep sedation is preferred in the initial stages to improve synchrony, to prevent VILI, especially when neuromuscular blockade is warranted. Secondary analysis of a large ICU database has shown that benzodiazepines, as compared to propofol, were associated with a higher number of days of ventilatory support, longer duration of ICU stay, and higher mortality.[70] Lighter levels of sedation are targeted once there is no requirement of muscle paralysis. Pain and sedation scores should be frequently assessed using validated scales.[71] In conclusion, sedation should be adequate and deep enough in the early stages of ARDS, especially when patients are receiving neuromuscular blockade. Analgesia and lighter sedation or no sedation are preferred when the clinician starts preparing for weaning from mechanical ventilation.

Fluid management: Pulmonary edema is the hallmark of ARDS; hence, logically keeping the patient "dry" may help in oxygenation and outcome. At the same time, the presence of circulatory shock warrants adequate fluid resuscitation to maintain the peripheral perfusion in the initial stages. In hemodynamically stable ARDS patients (FACTT trial), the conservative strategy of fluid management improved lung function and shortened the duration of mechanical ventilation and intensive care without increasing nonpulmonary organ failure, without any change in mortality.[72]

Nutrition: As in any other ICU patient, the management of ARDS patients also includes nutrition. The enteral route of nutrition is safer and better than the parenteral route.[73] No individual dietary component or composition has yet been proven to be of particular benefit over others in ARDS. The goal of nutritional support is the provision of sufficient nutrients along with correction and prevention of deficiency of micro- or macronutrients.[74] Various combinations of omega-3 fatty acids, ribonucleotides, glutamine, and arginine have been investigated in ARDS for immunomodulation. There was a beneficial effect on the infection rate, but there was no mortality benefit.[75] Even one large study of omega-3 fatty acids and antioxidants was terminated early in view of excess mortality in patients receiving omega-3 fatty acids.[76] One study found that a high-fat, low-carbohydrate diet reduced the duration of mechanical ventilation in patients with respiratory failure. The authors suggested that the reason for the beneficial effect was a decrease in the respiratory quotient with a decrease in CO_2 production, though the most common reason for high respiratory quotient remains to be overfeeding.[77] A study of clinical outcomes in 1,000 ARDS patients randomized to full calorie versus trophic (10 cc/h) enteral feeds did not show any difference in mortality or other clinical outcomes.[78] Overall, there is still no compelling evidence to support the use of anything other than standard (enteral) nutritional support, with avoidance of overfeeding.

Q10. What is the role of steroids in ARDS?

The anti-inflammatory actions of corticosteroids have made these drugs the most studied. Alveolar fibrosis in ARDS and the antifibrotic properties of steroids have been investigated.

Steroids in early ARDS: Earlier studies investigated the use of high-dose methylprednisolone in early ARDS. Bernard et al. in 1987 used methylprednisolone (4 doses of 30 mg/kg) and found no improvement in oxygenation, lung compliance, or severity of ARDS at 45 days, as compared with the placebo group.[79] Similar results were seen when high-dose steroids were used in septic shock patients.[80] Further trials used a lower dose of steroids. In the 2002 trial by Annane,[84,85] which investigated low-dose steroids in septic shock, a retrospective subgroup analysis of ARDS patients showed a reduction in mortality in those patients who had received 7 days of low-dose corticosteroids and mineralocorticoids.[81,82] Meduri[86] published the results of a double-blind, placebo-controlled trial, in which patients of early severe ARDS were randomized to receive methylprednisolone infusion (1 mg/kg/day) versus placebo for 28 days.[83] They observed downregulation of systemic inflammation, significant improvement in both pulmonary and extrapulmonary organ dysfunction, and reduction in the duration of mechanical ventilation and ICU length of stay with methylprednisolone. On long-term follow-up of 12 months, they found no difference in mortality between the groups. A higher incidence of septic shock patients in the placebo group may have contributed to this.

Steroids in late ARDS: The effectiveness of steroids in the late fibroproliferative phase of ARDS became an area of interest for researchers after the initial trials showed a lack of favorable outcomes in the early stages of ARDS. Meduri[87] et al. reported a case series of nine patients with ARDS and fibrotic changes on open lung biopsy.[84] The use of 2–3 mg/kg/day of methylprednisolone resulted in improvement in lung injury scores, chest X-ray appearance, and oxygenation in all patients. A larger case series of 25 patients was published by the same author in 1994 using similar doses of methylprednisolone followed by a tapering dose over 6 weeks, resulting in a marked improvement in most indices of lung function.[85]

The ARDS Clinical Trials Network conducted a multicenter trial of steroids in late persistent ARDS. About 180 ARDS patients were recruited 7–28 days after the diagnosis and randomly assigned to receive either methylprednisolone or placebo. The steroids were tapered over a 3-week period unless the patient remained ventilated at 21 days when the steroids were tapered over 4 days. There was no mortality benefit at day 60 and day 180. There was increased 60- and 180-day mortality in patients who were started on steroids at least 14 days after diagnosis. Methylprednisolone increased ventilator-free days and shock-free days, with improvement in oxygenation and respiratory system compliance. As compared with placebo, methylprednisolone did not increase the rate of infectious complications but was associated with a higher rate of neuromuscular weakness. Thus, they concluded against the routine use of steroids in ARDS and also warned about the increased rate of death in ARDS if steroids were started after 14 days of diagnosis of ARDS.[86]

The use of steroids in ARDS still remains controversial. Both meta-analysis and cohort studies reported a trend toward improved outcome with steroids. No excess adverse events were found. Marked heterogeneity was seen in the included studies.[87]

A 2019 Cochrane systematic review on corticosteroids in ARDS concluded with low-certainty evidence that corticosteroids might improve the number of ventilator-free days up to day 28 in ARDS; however, the review was unable to draw firm conclusions about mortality or other outcomes.[88] In patients with ARF requiring mechanical ventilation due to SARS-CoV-2, the RECOVERY trial[89] reported that 6 mg dexamethasone given daily for 10 days increased survival in COVID-19 patients receiving oxygen or mechanical ventilation. Thus, the use of dexamethasone has become the standard of care in COVID-19 patients receiving oxygen or mechanical ventilation. Villar et al. conducted a randomized clinical trial (DEXA-ARDS) comparing dexamethasone to standard care for patients with moderate-to-severe ARDS. Patients in the dexamethasone group had 4.8 more ventilator-free days compared with untreated patients and a 15% absolute risk reduction in 60-day mortality. However, there were methodological issues with this trial, including lack of complete masking and high use of corticosteroids before enrollment.[90]

Timing of steroid dosing: Evidence suggests that fibrosis starts at a very early stage of ARDS. Inflammatory cytokines have been documented in bronchoalveolar lavage fluid and plasma of ARDS patients from the outset of their disease. Experimental studies and animal studies suggest that earlier use of steroids is more likely to prevent progression of ARDS.[91] The timing of steroid differed significantly in two major studies. The ARDS Net study recruited patients at least 7 days into the course of their disease, whereas Meduri's group recruited patients within 3 days of diagnosis. One interpretation of these trials is that steroids may only be effective if given early in lung injury, before the inflammatory process has caused irreversible damage to the alveoli.[92,93]

Steroid dose: Very little data is available on the relationship between steroid dose and response in critically sick patients. It will be immature to say that a "one-dose-fits-all-strategy" will be successful because of:[94]

- Extremely complex and multifaceted nature of inflammatory response

- Wide variance in metabolism and tissue distribution among individuals
- Uncertainty about the targets of steroids—whether local or systemic

Q11. What are the rescue therapies for refractory hypoxemia?

Rescue therapies (Table 6)

Rescue measures or rescue therapies are required in the patients who are profoundly hypoxemic with maximum ventilatory support. Initially, these patients are managed with deep sedation and neuromuscular blockade to prevent asynchrony and improve recruitment.

Rescue therapies have been used in patients with persistent hypoxemia in spite of deep sedation and neuromuscular blockade; however, the benefits of many of these therapies are yet to be proven.

Neuromuscular blockade: This is the first step before using any rescue therapy. Neuromuscular blocking agents (NMBA) used in the initial stage of severe ARDS (defined as PF ratio <150) have been shown to reduce mortality. In the ACURYSYS trial,[95] the effect of neuromuscular blockade for 48 hours started within 48 hours of diagnosis of severe ARDS has shown to improve outcome. Crude 28- and 90-day mortality were significantly lower in the group receiving cisatracurium; the hazard ratio for death at 90 days in the cisatracurium group was 0.68. The cisatracurium group had more ventilator-free days without an increase in muscle weakness. The explanation for the improved outcome in the group with neuromuscular blockade is not clear. Neuromuscular blockade leads to the abolition of spontaneous efforts. There was improved control of inspiratory volume, preventing volutrauma and reduction in transpulmonary pressure, which reduced the incidence of barotrauma. In terms of lung mechanics, improved synchrony led to better recruitment, reduced atelectrauma, improved compliance, and oxygenation. All these led to less pulmonary and systemic inflammation, producing a better outcome.[96] However, NMBA use has its own side effects, the most prominent of which is ICU-acquired weakness. The recent ROSE trial was a larger trial that showed no significant difference in survival with the use of continuous infusion of NMBA in severe ARDS.[97] Hence, the use of NMBA infusion should be used only in selected cases of severe ARDS to improve patient–ventilator synchrony.

Recruitment maneuver: Lung-protective ventilation with low tidal volume limits injury due to overdistension. PEEP is applied to avoid atelectrauma by splinting open alveoli and preventing cyclical alveolar collapse. In hypoxemic ARDS, RM is applied to reopen the recruitable lung. RMs are used to recruit collapsed but potentially recruitable alveoli.[98] RM is followed by constant application of higher (than before) PEEP to keep the lungs open to increase end-expiratory lung volume. This will help the patient by preventing cyclical collapse.[99] Moreover, recruitment may reduce VILI caused by overdistension of healthy alveoli. However, RMs may directly overdistend aerated lung units and could, paradoxically, lead to increased VILI.[100-102] Several methods of recruitment have been employed in clinical and experimental settings with varying results.

Sustained inflation: The most common approach is to set the ventilator on CPAP mode and increase the pressure to 30–40 cmH_2O for 30–40 seconds. Severe hemodynamic compromise may happen during this maneuver and requires proper hemodynamic monitoring. This can even be done with pressure-controlled ventilation.[103] The effects of RM were variable in the patients with ARDS and had higher adverse effects (hypotension and desaturation occurred in

TABLE 6: Interventions with increasing severity of acute respiratory distress syndrome (ARDS).

Intervention	Mild ARDS PaO_2/FiO_2 > 200 and <300	Moderate ARDS PaO_2/FiO_2 >100 and <200	Severe ARDS PaO_2/FiO_2 <100
Tidal volume	Low tidal volume		
Ventilation	Noninvasive ventilation or invasive ventilation	Invasive ventilation	Invasive ventilation
PEEP	Low–moderate	Low–moderate	High
Neuromuscular blockade		If PaO_2/FiO_2 < 150	Yes
Prone position		If PaO_2/FiO_2 < 150	Yes
$ECCO_2R$		May be used	May be used
HFOV			May be used
ECMO			Yes

($ECCO_2R$: extracorporeal carbon dioxide removal; ECMO: extracorporeal membrane oxygenation; FiO_2: fraction of inspired oxygen; HFOV: high-frequency oscillatory ventilation; PaO_2: partial pressure of oxygen in arterial blood; PEEP: positive end-expiratory pressure)

22% of patients receiving RMs, while serious complication like increased air leak through chest tube occurred in <5% patients).[104-106] Due to the uncertainty of benefits with RM and the potential for complications with repeated RM, it is unjustified to use scheduled RM.

Stepwise RM or decremental PEEP method (open lung approach): In this approach, both plateau pressure and PEEP are gradually increased with the driving pressure kept constant (e.g., 15 cmH$_2$O). After the recruitment, the PEEP is kept high (e.g., 20–25 cmH$_2$O). PEEP is then gradually decreased in 2-cm decrement, and the compliance is measured at each step to get the best compliance.[107] Some have used arterial oxygenation or even dead space to identify the optimal PEEP while decreasing the PEEP.[108,109] After identifying the PEEP at which the best compliance or oxygenation is not maintained, the RM is applied again. After this second recruitment, PEEP is set 2 cm above the PEEP level identified with the best compliance. Marini[102] suggested that the stepwise approach is much better than the sustained inflation, as it is better tolerated from a hemodynamic point of view **(Figs. 4A and B)**. One alternative way for recruitment is to keep the patient in PCV with the inspiratory pressure fixed and gradually increasing the PEEP.

Recruitment maneuver in prone position: Prone position helps in facilitation of recruitment. Kacmarek[109] showed that oxygenation was better with RM in prone position than in supine position; also a lesser amount of PEEP was needed in prone position to maintain the same PF ratio.[111] Lim et al.[110] also showed in canine lung injury models that prone position increased the effect of low PEEP recruitments; at the same time, the hemodynamic impairment due to high PEEP was decreased in prone position.[112] Similarly, Cakar et al.[111] found that RMs with lower PEEP were more effective in prone position.[113]

Prone positioning: As in the case of the application of PEEP, the indications and applications of prone ventilation have changed over time. Prone positioning was first utilized in mid-1970s.[114] The proposed mechanisms by which prone ventilation helps in improving oxygenation are as follows:[115,116]

- Recruitment and improved ventilation of the previously dependent dorsal lung via regional changes in chest wall

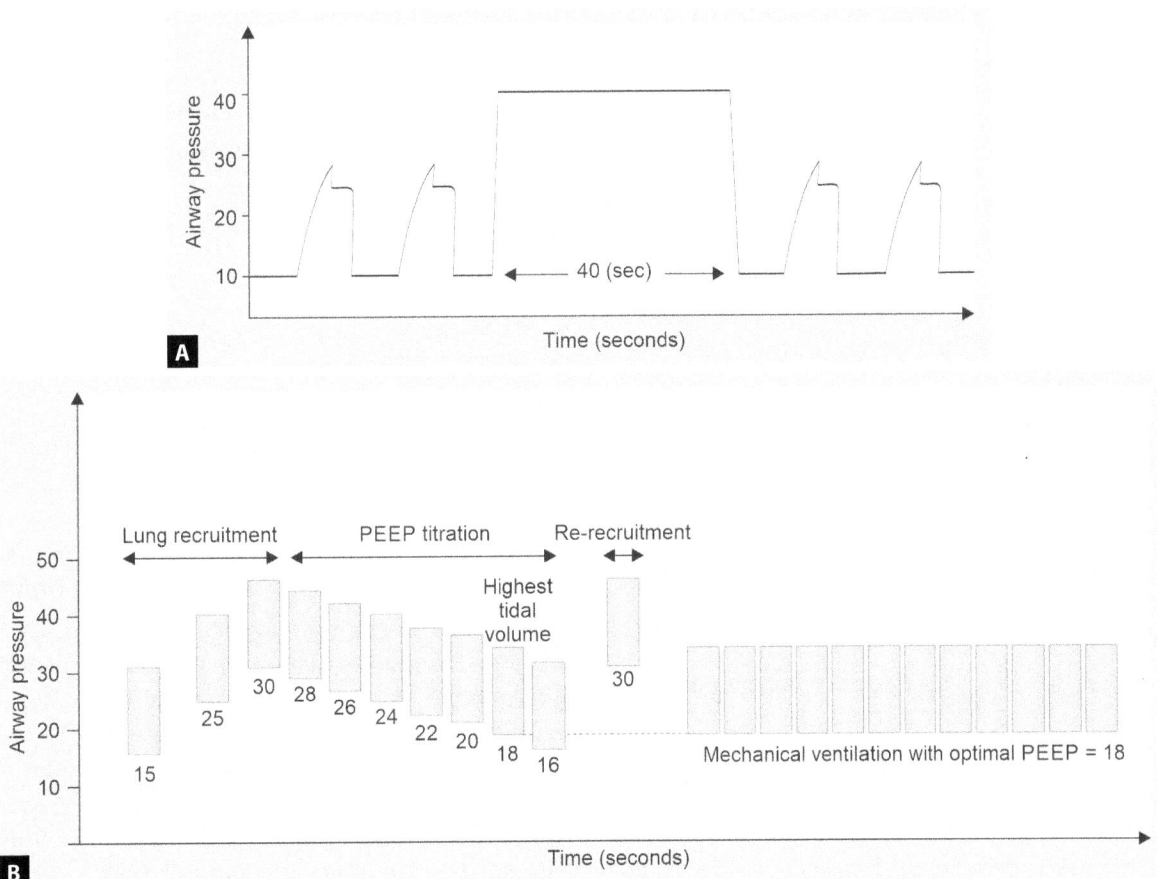

Figs. 4A and B: Pressure–time curve with recruitment maneuvers: (A) Sustained inflation with CPAP of 40 cmH$_2$O for 40 seconds; (B) Stepwise recruitment using decremental PEEP, keeping driving pressure constant to obtain optimal PEEP. (PEEP: positive end-expiratory pressure)

mechanics and reduced lung compression by the heart and mediastinum
- Gravitationally distributed better perfusion toward the better-ventilated previously ventral lung
- Better ventilation–perfusion matching with better clearance of CO_2
- More homogeneous ventilation and reduced chances of VILI

TABLE 7: Contraindications to prone positioning.	
Absolute	Relative
Unstable spinal fractures	• Open abdominal wound • Unmonitored raised intracranial pressure • Pregnancy • Severe hemodynamic instability • Severe facial trauma or facial surgery in last 15 days

Indications for prone position: The beneficial effect of prone positioning is not only the improvement in oxygenation but also the prevention of VILI with reduction in transpulmonary pressure and more homogeneous distribution of stress and strain throughout the lungs.[117,118] Accordingly, it should be applied at the early stage as first-line therapy. Despite the physiological advantages with prone ventilation, earlier trials did not show any mortality benefit, though these trials were not done with the ideal body weight (IBW) driven tidal volumes. The Proning Severe ARDS Patients (PROSEVA) study group showed significant reduction in mortality with prone ventilation.[117] They had given prone position in patients with PF ratio < 150 for 16 consecutive hours and ventilated with protective lung ventilation strategy. There was significant reduction in 28- and 90-day mortality. After these trials, a meta-analysis of the combined data of these studies found that there was a significant benefit of prone ventilation in patients ventilated with tidal volume > 8 mL/kg of IBW.[118]

Timing and duration for prone ventilation: Prone ventilation should be started in hypoxemic ARDS as soon as possible. In initial trials, proning sessions were of 7–8 hours, which was later increased to >12 hours.[119,120] In the PROSEVA trial, proning was given as 17-hour sessions and was used for 4 days on average. In PSII trial, it was further increased to 18 hours and 8 days.

Risk management/safety: Given the high rates of complications [e.g., dislocation of endotracheal tube (ETT), pressure sores, etc.], experts have concluded that prone positioning should be limited to patients with severe hypoxemia and undertaken only in high expertise centers with experience in safe technique.[121]

Contraindications: Absolute contraindication is an unstable spine fracture. Other relative contraindications are enumerated in **Table 7**. Acute abdomen is not a contraindication for prone position ventilation.

High-frequency oscillatory ventilation (HFOV)
High-frequency oscillatory ventilation has also been used to improve oxygenation by increasing mean airway pressure to promote alveolar recruitment. At the same time, small tidal volumes avoid the risk of overdistention. HFOV has been successfully used in neonates and pediatric patients since 1983. Studies have shown higher survival rates for patients in premature infants with ARDS. There was a resurgence of interest in HFOV for adults after a low tidal volume strategy was shown to be effective. HFOV delivers tidal volumes of 1–3 mL/kg at very high rates, usually between 100 and 600/min. HFOV use has failed to demonstrate improvement in outcomes in adults.[122]

Initial settings and management of a patient on HFOV (Table 8): Bias flow is the continuous flow of gas responsible for replenishing oxygen and removing CO_2 from the patient circuit, and it is started at 20 L/min. A large number of patients will need to be paralyzed at this flow rate. The need for neuromuscular block (NMB) may be eliminated by increasing the bias flow rate, but CO_2 retention is a potential concern. Bias flow is set between 25 and 40 L/min.

Inspiratory time is usually set at 33%.

Mean airway pressure (mPaw) is set at 25–34 cmH_2O or at 3–5 cm above the patient's previous conventional ventilator mPaw.

Frequency (f): Initial frequency should be based on the most recent arterial blood gas:
- pH < 7.10 = 4 Hz
- pH 7.10–7.19 = 5 Hz
- pH 7.20–7.35 = 6 Hz
- pH > 7.35 = 7 Hz

FiO_2: Initially set at 1.0, it is gradually reduced as per improvement in oxygenation.

Tidal volume (V_t) depends on the oscillatory pressure amplitude (ΔP) and frequency. Lowering the frequency allows more time for gas exchange, leading to larger V_t.[124,125]

Mechanisms of gas exchange in HFOV: During HFOV, the alveolar minute ventilation increases exponentially with tidal volume, but unlike conventional ventilation, alveolar ventilation decreases with increase in frequency and vice versa. Increase in frequency decreases the delivered tidal volume by dampening the pressure delivery, thus decreasing alveolar ventilation, giving rise to CO_2 retention. The mechanism of gas exchange at such a very low tidal volume involves several phenomena, which are given in the following text.[126-128]

TABLE 8: Initial and ongoing assessment of the patient on high-frequency oscillatory ventilation (HFOV).[123]	
ABG	• 30 minutes postinitiation • Frequency based on clinical status • Within an hour of any major change in setting
CXR	• Within an hour postinitiation • Daily • Whenever lung hyperinflation or collapse is suspected
CWF	Check for degree of vibration noted and symmetry *Changes in CWF:* • Increases with improvement in compliance • Decreases with worsening of compliance • Noted only on one side of the chest, if tube gets migrated to one lung or in the presence of unilateral pneumothorax
Auscultation	• Breath sounds cannot be heard • Listen for changes in intensity of the piston sound
Heart and GI sounds	• Stop the piston temporarily • Lung inflation and oxygenation will be maintained
Vital signs	HR, BP, MAP, and urine output hourly
Perfusion	Monitor adequate perfusion status by monitoring capillary refill time, skin turgor and color, urine output changes, base excess
Secretions	*Secretions are suspected if there are:* • Rapid rise in $PaCO_2$ • Decrease in oxygenation • Decrease in CWF • Suctioning should be done whenever needed to minimize de-recruitment

(ABG: arterial blood gas; BP: blood pressure; CWF: chest wiggle factor; CXR: chest X-ray; GI: gastrointestinal; HR: heart rate; MAP: mean arterial pressure; $PaCO_2$: partial pressure of carbon dioxide in arterial blood)

Bulk flow: Bulk flow or bulk convention is the most important mechanism in HFOV. It also helps in gas exchange in areas with low regional dead space volumes, such as in proximal gas exchange units. The importance of bulk flow has been shown in anesthetized canine models where partial pressure of carbon dioxide in arterial blood ($PaCO_2$) rose significantly once the volume delivered per oscillation was decreased to lower than the volume of rebreathing circuit. Even in clinical practice, the volume delivered per oscillation changes much more than expected, depending on the changes in the applied frequency.[129]

Convective gas exchange: The spatial distribution of inspiratory gas flow and expiratory gas flow is different in HFOV. As a result, convection in opposing currents happens in the same airway, giving rise to convective gas exchange, which is more pronounced at the bifurcation of airways.[130]

Pendelluft means "swinging air." It describes the movement of gas within the lung because of dynamic pressure gradients between lung units through differences in the timing of inflation and deflation. Regional differences in inertance and compliance of the peripheral airways and lung units—and hence differences in local respiratory time constants—result in differences in the timing of inflation and deflation at a steady state during HFOV. Lung units that are inflating even as others are deflating may receive gas from the deflating lung units. This inter-regional airflow increases gas mixing and enhances gas exchange.[131]

Cardiac contractions also enhance gas mixing and contribute to gas exchange during HFOV. The strong contractions of the heart act as a percussive force for gas mixing. Indeed, during apneic ventilation, cardiac oscillations may account for over 50% of oxygen uptake and nearly 40% of CO_2 clearance.[132]

Evidence against the use of HFOV: The OSCILLATE trial, an international study from the Canadian Critical Care Trials Group, compared HFOV in early, moderate-to-severe ARDS (PaO_2/FiO_2 ratio ≤ 200 mm Hg) with conventional protective ventilation.[133] The study was terminated early following interim analysis as they found that in-hospital mortality was higher in the HFOV group, which was quite significant. Patients who received HFOV were more likely to be treated with neuromuscular blockade and vasopressors and received higher doses of sedatives compared with controls. The OSCAR study was conducted simultaneously in the United Kingdom and involved a similar population of patients.[134] The investigators reported a higher 30-day mortality rate with HFOV compared to the conventional group. There did not appear to be any differences between the groups in terms of vasopressor support or fluid administration. It is unclear why the HFOV trials failed. The relatively high mean airway pressures may have been associated with increased regional overdistension and VILI.

Alternatively, increased intrathoracic pressures may have resulted in hypotension, RV dysfunction, fluid overload, hypoperfusion, and multiple organ dysfunction syndrome (MODS).

In conclusion, on the basis of current evidence, HFOV should not be used as a primary mechanical ventilation mode in ARDS, and its use as rescue therapy should be reserved until proven strategies have been exhausted.

Extracorporeal membrane oxygenation
Extracorporeal membrane oxygenation (ECMO) removes blood from the body, oxygenates it, removes CO_2, and returns it back to the body. This comprises a mechanical system and can be used to support failing lung or heart or both. In case of failing lung (as in ARDS), blood is withdrawn from a central

vein into the extracorporeal circuit through a mechanical pump and then passed through an oxygenator, where blood passes along one side of a membrane, which provides the interface for diffusion of gases. The oxygenated blood is (after proper warming or cooling) returned to another central vein. This is known as venovenous ECMO (VV-ECMO). In patients with cardiac dysfunction or cardiopulmonary dysfunction, blood is collected through a central vein and returned to a central artery, and thus both oxygenation and support to systemic circulation are maintained. This is known as venoarterial ECMO (VA-ECMO).[135]

Indications and contraindications for ECMO in ARDS: [136,137]

Indications:

- Severe hypoxemia [e.g., PF ratio < 80, despite the application of high levels of PEEP (15–20 cmH_2O)] for at least 6 hours in patients with potentially reversible respiratory failure
- Uncompensated hypercapnia with acidemia (pH < 7.15) despite the best possible ventilator settings
- Very severe ARDS defined as any one of the three criteria:
  - PF ratio ~ 50 mm Hg for >3 hours
  - PF ratio < 80 mm Hg for >6 hours
  - Arterial blood pH < 7.25 with a partial pressure of arterial CO_2 of at least 60 mm Hg for >6 hours

Contraindications for ECMO in ARDS:

Absolute: Any condition that precludes the use of anticoagulation therapy.

Relative: High-pressure ventilation (end-inspiratory plateau pressure > 30 cmH_2O) for >7 days

- High FiO_2 requirements (>0.8) for >7 days
- Limited vascular access
- Any condition or organ dysfunction that would limit the likelihood of overall benefit from ECMO, such as severe, irreversible brain injury or untreatable metastatic cancer

Evidence for the utility of ECMO in ARDS: Older studies with the technology of ECMO did not find a significant difference in survival with extracorporeal CO_2 removal.[138,139] Peek et al. (CESAR trial) studied the outcome of referral to an ECMO center in patients with severe, potentially reversible respiratory failure as judged by Murray score > 3.0 or pH < 7.20. The ECMO patients had a significantly better chance of survival without severe disability.[140] A recent study (EOLIA trial 2018) of early initiation of ECMO in severe ARDS (PF ratio < 50 mm Hg for >3 hours; or <80 mm Hg for >6 hours; or an arterial blood pH < 7.25) was designed to demonstrate an absolute mortality reduction of 20% and relative risk reduction of 33%. It was terminated prematurely after 75% recruitment. There was a statistically nonsignificant reduction in mortality (46 vs. 35%).[141] This amounts to a clinically important 24% relative reduction in mortality and could have been demonstrated in an adequately powered trial. Further, the results of this trial should not undermine role of ECMO as rescue therapy.

Extracorporeal carbon dioxide removal ($ECCO_2R$)

This technique uses a venovenous or arteriovenous extracorporeal device at low blood flow rates primarily to remove CO_2. This technique could allow clinicians to use ultraprotective lung ventilation, low tidal volumes, lower P_{plat}, and lower driving pressure while avoiding the adverse effects due to hypercapnia and respiratory acidosis.[142] However, in the recently concluded REST trial, this strategy did not significantly reduce 90-day mortality.[143]

Airway pressure release ventilation in ARDS

Airway pressure release ventilation (APRV): This allows patients to breathe spontaneously while receiving high airway pressure with an intermittent pressure release. The high pressure is used for alveolar recruitment. By promoting spontaneous breathing, it might improve alveolar recruitment to the dorsal caudal regions of the lungs. Although arterial oxygenation might be better with APRV, evidence is lacking to support improved outcomes. Given that the transalveolar distending pressures are probably high during spontaneous breathing with APRV, the potential for lung injury is of concern.[144]

Airway pressure release ventilation is a mode of ventilation, which is based on the open lung approach and provides partial ventilatory support. This mode provides both safety and comfort, safety in terms of low chances of VILI and hemodynamic compromise while providing adequate ventilatory support without dangerously high pressures in the lung and comfort in terms of unrestricted spontaneous breathing with greater patient–ventilator synchrony. APRV had been historically viewed as CPAP at two alternate pressure levels, and accordingly, the mandatory breath is known as "P_{high}" and the duration of mandatory breath is called "T_{high}." In a similar manner, the expiratory pressure and time (release time) are known as "P_{low}" and "T_{low}," respectively.[145]

In a small study of 24 patients with ARDS, V/Q distribution was better with APRV with spontaneous breathing compared to pressure support ventilation (PSV).[146] Zhou et al. compared APRV and low tidal volume lung-protective ventilation (LTV) in patients with ARDS. They observed that patients ventilated in the APRV mode had a significantly higher ventilator-free day and a shorter ICU stay. APRV also led to better oxygenation, respiratory system compliance, and lower plateau pressures. Although the mortality in the APRV group was numerically lower, it could not reach statistical significance. The settings used in this study were a P_{high} equal to the plateau pressure and a P_{low} equal to 5 cmH$_2$O, and a T_{low} adjusted to terminate the peak expiratory flow to >50%.[147] A meta-analysis of seven RCTs showed that APRV, in comparison with LTV, could reduce the duration of ventilation, ICU length of stay, and hospital mortality. Hence, APRV remains a promising tool that can be used either as a rescue therapy or as the primary mode of ventilation.[148]

Q12. What are the endotypes of ARDS?
Acute respiratory distress syndrome shows great heterogeneity in its clinical presentation, pathogenesis, severity, and response to treatment. It is difficult to predict which patients would survive or worsen based on clinical criteria alone. Therefore, the association of genetic variants with ARDS risk and the genetic susceptibility of ARDS has been suggested. Calfee et al., based on the data from ARMA and ALVEOLI trials, identified two broad endotypes of ARDS, namely hyperinflammatory and hypoinflammatory. The hyperinflammatory group is characterized by increased levels of proinflammatory cytokines, lower serum bicarbonate, and high vasopressor requirements, while the opposite was true in case of the hypoinflammatory subgroup. These were identified by latent class analysis, a statistical method to identify certain groups in a heterogeneous population.[149] Interestingly, these groups have different responses to different treatment modalities. While the hyperinflammatory group responds well to higher PEEP and a liberal fluid strategy, the hypoinflammatory group responds poorly or may even experience higher mortality with the same therapies.[150] This biological heterogeneity could partly explain the failure of many pharmacological therapies in treating ARDS. Hence, the identification of biological endotypes and targeted therapies can be a way forward.

Q13. What are the biomarkers of ARDS?
Owing to the heterogeneous presentation and natural course, identifying biomarkers has become the need of the hour to diagnose ARDS early, better risk stratification, better prognostication, and tailoring the therapy accordingly. Studies have identified several biomarkers released in the process of lung injury as follows:[151]
- *Epithelial:* Soluble receptor for advanced glycation end-products (sRAGE), Krebs von den Lungen-6 (KL-6), surfactant protein-D (SP-D), and keratinocyte growth factor (KGF)
- *Endothelial:* Angiopoietin-2, vWF, and VEGF
- *Inflammatory:* Proinflammatory factors [interleukin (IL)-1, IL-6, IL-18, tumor necrosis factor (TNF)-α] and anti-inflammatory factors (IL-10, IL-1RA)
- *Coagulation:* PAI-1

Many of these markers correlate with ARDS mortality and need further studies to identify cutoff levels and targeted therapies. Moreover, metabolomic studies are ongoing to identify certain metabolic products that may help in risk stratification or prediction of organ injury in ARDS. Of the thousands of metabolic markers, only octane has been validated and is the only breath biomarker of ARDS. Acetaldehyde and 3-methylheptane are under investigation for earlier identification of ARDS.[152] Urinary levels of hydrogen peroxide correlate with increased mortality, while urinary nitric oxide (NO) levels are associated with improved survival.[153,154]

Q14. What are the therapies under investigation for ARDS?
Many pharmacological therapies have been tried in clinical trials to treat ARDS. These therapies include statins, omega-3 fatty acids, β-agonists, keratinocyte growth factor, mesenchymal stem cells and multipotent progenitor cells, nebulized heparin, dilmapimod (MAPK inhibitor), solnatide (inhaled peptide), surfactants, inhaled NO, sivelestat (neutrophil elastase inhibitor), *N*-acetylcysteine, interferon-β-1a, vitamin D, and aspirin. Many of these molecules have shown promising results in the preliminary studies and are under investigation in RCTs. Unfortunately, none of these studies have shown a mortality benefit in ARDS. Therefore, currently, they are not recommended in the treatment of ARDS.[155]

Conclusion
ARDS is a common disease associated with significant morbidity and mortality. It has become especially relevant in today's era due to a worldwide pandemic of SARS-CoV-2. Treatment of ARDS mainly involves treating the primary cause and providing protective lung ventilation to ensure adequate oxygenation while preventing further lung injury. Although huge progress has been made in understanding the disease and improving clinical outcomes through decades of research, further research directed toward the prevention and novel treatment modalities should be our future goal.

REFERENCES
1. Ashbaugh DG, Bigelow DB, Petty TL, Levine BE. Acute respiratory distress in adults. Lancet. 1967;2:319-23.
2. Murray JF, Division of Lung Diseases, National Heart, Lung, and Blood Institute. Mechanisms of acute respiratory failure. Am Rev Respir Dis. 1977;115:1071-8.
3. Bellani G, Laffey JG, Pham T, Fan E, Brochard L, Esteban A, et al. Epidemiology, patterns of care, and mortality for patients with acute respiratory distress syndrome in intensive care units in 50 countries. JAMA. 2016;315:788-800.
4. Rubenfeld GD, Caldwell E, Peabody E, Weaver J, Martin DP, Neff M, et al. Incidence and outcomes of acute lung injury. N Engl J Med. 2005;353:1685-93.

5. Zilberberg MD, Epstein SK. Acute lung injury in the medical ICU: comorbid conditions, age, etiology, and hospital outcome. Am J Respir Crit Care Med. 1998;157:1159-64.
6. Calfee CS, Eisner MD, Ware LB, Thompson BT, Parsons PE, Wheeler AP, et al. Trauma-associated lung injury differs clinically and biologically from acute lung injury due to other clinical disorders. Crit Care Med. 2007;35:2243-50.
7. Meyer NJ, Gattinoni L, Calfee CS. Acute respiratory distress syndrome. Lancet. 2021;398(10300):622-37.
8. Tomashefski JF. Pulmonary pathology of acute respiratory distress syndrome. Clin Chest Med. 2000;21:435-66.
9. Lee KS, Choi YH, Kim YS, Baik SH, Oh YJ, Sheen SS, et al. Evaluation of bronchoalveolar lavage fluid from ARDS patients with regard to apoptosis. Respir Med. 2008;102:464-9.
10. Thille AW, Esteban A, Fernandez-Segoviano P, Rodriguez JM, Aramburu JA, Vargas-Errazuriz P, et al. Chronology of histological lesions in acute respiratory distress syndrome with diffuse alveolar damage: a prospective cohort study of clinical autopsies. Lancet Respir Med. 2013;1:395-401.
11. Bachofen M, Weibel ER. Structural alterations of lung parenchyma in the adult respiratory distress syndrome. Clin Chest Med. 1982;3:35-56.
12. Lee WL, Downey GP. Neutrophil activation and acute lung injury. Curr Opin Crit Care. 2001;7:1-7.
13. Janz DR, Ware LB. Biomarkers of ALI/ARDS: pathogenesis, discovery, and relevance to clinical trials. Sem Respir Crit Care Med. 2013;34:537-48.
14. Calfee CS, Budev MM, Matthay MA, Church G, Brady S, Uchida T, et al. Plasma receptor for advanced glycation end-products predicts duration of ICU stay and mechanical ventilation in patients after lung transplantation. J Heart Lung Transplant. 2007;26:675-80.
15. Cheng IW, Ware LB, Greene KE, Nuckton TJ, Eisner MD, Matthay MA. Prognostic value of surfactant proteins A and D in patients with acute lung injury. Crit Care Med. 2003;31:20-7.
16. Greene KE, Wright JR, Steinberg KP, Ruzinski JT, Caldwell E, Wong WB, et al. Serial changes in surfactant-associated proteins in lung and serum before and after onset of ARDS. Am J Respir Crit Care Med. 1999;160:1843-50.
17. Gunther A, Ruppert C, Schmidt R, Markart P, Grimminger F, Walmrath D, et al. Surfactant alteration and replacement in acute respiratory distress syndrome. Respir Res. 2001;2:353-64.
18. Bastarache JA, Fremont RD, Kropski JA, Bossert FR, Ware LB. Procoagulant alveolar microparticles in the lungs of patients with acute respiratory distress syndrome. Am J Physiol Lung Cell Mol Physiol. 2009;297:L1035-41.
19. Albert RK. The role of ventilation-induced surfactant dysfunction and atelectasis in causing acute respiratory distress syndrome. Am J Respir Crit Care Med. 2012;185:702-8.
20. Suratt BT, Parsons PE. Mechanisms of acute lung injury/acute respiratory distress syndrome. Clin Chest Med. 2006;27:579-89.
21. Cressoni M, Caironi P, Polli F, Carlesso E, Chiumello D, Cadringher P, et al. Anatomical and functional intrapulmonary shunt in acute respiratory distress syndrome. Crit Care Med. 2008;36:669-75.
22. Moloney ED, Evans TW. Pathophysiology and pharmacological treatment of pulmonary hypertension in acute respiratory distress syndrome. Eur Respir J. 2003;21:720-7.
23. Cornet AD, Hofstra JJ, Swart EL, Girbes AR, Juffermans NP. Sildenafil attenuates pulmonary arterial pressure but does not improve oxygenation during ARDS. Intensive Care Med. 2010;36:758-64.
24. Mekontso Dessap A, Boissier F, Leon R, Carreira S, Campo FR, Lemaire F, et al. Prevalence and prognosis of shunting across patent foramen ovale during acute respiratory distress syndrome. Crit Care Med. 2010;38:1786-92.
25. Murray JF, Matthay MA, Luce JM, Flick MR. An expanded definition of the adult respiratory distress syndrome. Am Rev Respir Dis. 1988;138:720-3.
26. Bernard GR, Artigas A, Brigham KL, Carlet J, Falke K, Hudson L, et al. The American-European Consensus Conference on ARDS. Definitions, mechanisms, relevant outcomes, and clinical trial coordination. Am J Respir Crit Care Med. 1994;149:818-24.
27. Ranieri VM, Rubenfeld GD, Thompson BT, Ferguson ND, Caldwell E, Fan E, et al. Acute respiratory distress syndrome: the Berlin definition. JAMA. 2012;307:2526-33.
28. Ferguson ND, Fan E, Camporota L, Antonelli M, Anzueto A, Beale R, et al. The Berlin definition of ARDS: an expanded rationale, justification, and supplementary material. Intensive Care Med. 2012;38:1573-82.
29. Rice TW, Wheeler AP, Bernard GR, Hayden DL, Schoenfeld DA, Ware LB. Comparison of the SpO_2/FiO_2 ratio and the PaO_2/FiO_2 ratio in patients with acute lung injury or acute respiratory distress syndrome. Chest. 2007;132:410-7.
30. Chen W, Janz DR, Shaver CM, Bernard GR, Bastarache JA, Ware LB. Clinical characteristics and outcomes are similar in ARDS diagnosed by SpO_2/FiO_2 ratio compared with PaO_2/FiO_2 ratio. Chest. 2015;148:1477-83.
31. Riviello ED, Buregeya E, Twagirumugabe T. Diagnosing acute respiratory distress syndrome in resource limited settings: the Kigali modification of the Berlin definition. Curr Opin Crit Care. 2017;23(1):18-23.
32. Matthay MA, Arabi Y, Arroliga AC, Bernard GR, Bersten AD, Brochard LJ, et al. A new global definition of acute respiratory distress syndrome. Am J Respir Crit Care Med. 2023;207:A6229.
33. Levitt JE, Vinayak AG, Gehlbach BK, Pohlman A, Van Cleve W, Hall JB, et al. Diagnostic utility of B-type natriuretic peptide in critically ill patients with pulmonary edema: a prospective cohort study. Crit Care. 2008;12:R3.
34. Determann RM, Royakkers AA, Schaefers J, de Boer AM, Binnekade JM, van Straalen JP, et al. Serum levels of N-terminal proB-type natriuretic peptide in mechanically ventilated critically ill patients–relation to tidal volume size and development of acute respiratory distress syndrome. BMC Pulm Med. 2013;13:42.
35. Lichtenstein DA. Ultrasound in the management of thoracic disease. Crit. Care Med. 2007;35:250-61.
36. Volpicelli G, Elbarbary M, Blaivas M, Lichtenstein DA, Mathis G, Kirkpatrick AW, et al. International evidence-based recommendations for point-of-care lung ultrasound. Intensive Care Med. 2012;38:577-91.

37. Copetti R, Soldati G, Copetti P. Chest sonography: a useful tool to differentiate acute cardiogenic pulmonary edema from acute respiratory distress syndrome. Cardiovasc Ultrasound. 2008;6:16-26.
38. Bouhemad B, Liu ZH, Arbelot C, Zhang M, Ferarri F, Le-Guen M, et al. Ultrasound assessment of antibiotic-induced pulmonary reaeration in ventilator-associated pneumonia. Crit Care Med. 2010;38:84-92.
39. Peris A, Zagli G, Barbani F, Tutino L, Biondi S, di Valvasone S, et al. The value of lung ultrasound monitoring in H1N1 acute respiratory distress syndrome. Anesthesia. 2010;65:294-97.
40. Tagami T, Ong MEH. Extravascular lung water measurements in acute respiratory distress syndrome: why, how, and when? Curr Opin Crit Care. 2018;24:209-15.
41. Rhodes A, Evans LE, Alhazzani W, Levy MM, Antonelli M, Ferrer R, et al. Surviving Sepsis Campaign: international guidelines for management of sepsis and septic shock: 2016. Crit Care Med. 2017;45:486-552.
42. Agarwal R, Aggarwal AN, Gupta D. Role of noninvasive ventilation in acute lung injury/acute respiratory distress syndrome: a proportion meta-analysis. Respir Care. 2010;55:1653-60.
43. Thille AW, Contou D, Fragnoli C, Córdoba-Izquierdo A, Boissier F, Brun-Buisson C, et al. Non-invasive ventilation for acute hypoxemic respiratory failure: intubation rate and risk factors. Crit Care. 2013;17(6):R269.
44. Carrillo A, Gonzalez-Diaz G, Ferrer M, Martinez-Quintana ME, Lopez-Martinez A, Llamas N, et al. Non-invasive ventilation in community-acquired pneumonia and severe acute respiratory failure. Intensive Care Med. 2012;38:458-66.
45. Schettino G, Altobelli N, Kacmarek RM. Noninvasive positive-pressure ventilation in acute respiratory failure outside clinical trials: experience at the Massachusetts General Hospital. Crit Care Med. 2008;36:441-7.
46. Lee JH, Rehder KJ, Williford L, Cheifetz IM, Turner DA. Use of high flow nasal cannula in critically ill infants, children, and adults: a critical review of the literature. Intensive Care Med. 2013;39:247-57.
47. Frat JP, Thille AW, Mercat A, Girault C, Ragot S, Perbet S, et al. High flow oxygen through nasal cannula in acute hypoxemic respiratory failure. N Engl J Med. 2015;372:2185-96.
48. Dos Santos CC, Slutsky AS. Invited review: mechanisms of ventilator-induced lung injury: a perspective. J Appl Physiol. 2000;89:1645-55.
49. Ranieri VM, Suter PM, Tortorella C, De Tullio R, Dayer JM, Brienza A, et al. Effect of mechanical ventilation on inflammatory mediators in patients with acute respiratory distress syndrome: a randomized controlled trial. JAMA. 1999;282:54-61.
50. Ranieri VM, Giunta F, Suter PM, Slutsky AS. Mechanical ventilation as a mediator of multisystem organ failure in acute respiratory distress syndrome. JAMA. 2000;284:43-4.
51. Parsons PE, Eisner MD, Thompson BT, Matthay MA, Ancukiewicz M, Bernard GR, et al. Lower tidal volume ventilation and plasma cytokine markers of inflammation in patients with acute lung injury. Crit Care Med. 2005;33:1-6.
52. Gattinoni L, Pesenti A. The concept of "baby lung". Intensive Care Med. 2005;31(6):776-84.
53. Brower RG, Matthay MA, Morris A, Schoenfeld D, Thompson BT, Wheeler A. Ventilation with lower tidal volumes as compared with traditional tidal volumes for acute lung injury and the acute respiratory distress syndrome. N Engl J Med. 2000;342:1301-8.
54. Laffey JG, O'Croinin D, McLoughlin P, Kavanagh BP. Permissive hypercapnia—role in protective lung ventilatory strategies. Intensive Care Med. 2004;30:347-56.
55. Hickling KG, Walsh J, Henderson S, Jackson R. Low mortality rate in adult respiratory distress syndrome using low-volume, pressure-limited ventilation with permissive hypercapnia: a prospective study. Crit Care Med. 1994;22:1568-78.
56. Chiumello D, Cressoni M, Carlesso E, Caspani ML, Marino A, Gallazzi E, et al. Bedside selection of positive end-expiratory pressure in mild, moderate, and severe acute respiratory distress syndrome. Crit Care Med. 2014;42:252-64.
57. Amato MB, Barbas CS, Medeiros DM, Magaldi RB, Schettino GP, Lorenzi-Filho G, et al. Effect of a protective-ventilation strategy on mortality in the acute respiratory distress syndrome. N Engl J Med. 1998;338:347-54.
58. Davide C, Eleonora C, Matteo B, Massimo C. Airway driving pressure and lung stress in ARDS patients. Crit Care. 2016;20:276.
59. Amato MBP, Meade MO, Slutsky AS, Brochard L, Costa ELV, Schoenfeld DA, et al. Driving pressure and survival in the acute respiratory distress syndrome. N Engl J Med. 2015;372:747-55.
60. Kulkarni AP, Divatia JV. Ventilator-induced lung injury. In: Nayar V, Peter JV, Kishen R, Srinivas S (Eds). Critical Care Update. New Delhi: Jaypee Brothers Medical Publishers; 2009. pp. 48-58.
61. Pan C, Chen L, Zhang Y-H, Liu W, Urbino R, Ranieri VM, et al. Physiological correlation of airway pressure and transpulmonary pressure stress index on respiratory mechanics in acute respiratory failure. Chinese Med J. 2016;129:1652-7.
62. Chiumello D, Carlesso E, Mietto C, Protti M, Berto V, Marino A, et al. Stress index: is the airway pressure a good surrogate of the transpulmonary pressure? C23. Mechanical ventilation: from start to finish. Am J Respir Crit Care Med. 2010;181:A4076.
63. Talmor D, Sarge T, Malhotra A, O'Donnell CR, Ritz R, Lisbon A, et al. Mechanical ventilation guided by esophageal pressure in acute lung injury. N Engl J Med. 2008;359(20):2095-104.
64. Beitler JR, Sarge T, Banner-Goodspeed VM, Gong MN, Cook D, Novack V, et al. Effect of titrating positive end-expiratory pressure (PEEP) with an esophageal pressure-guided strategy vs an empirical high PEEP-FiO$_2$ strategy on death and days free from mechanical ventilation among patients with acute respiratory distress syndrome: a randomized clinical trial. JAMA. 2019;321(9):846-57.
65. Hickling KG, Henderson SJ, Jackson R. Low mortality associated with low volume pressure limited ventilation with permissive hypercapnia in severe adult respiratory distress syndrome. Intensive Care Med. 1990;16(6):372-77.
66. Beitler JR, Malhotra A, Thompson BT. Ventilator-induced lung injury. Clin Chest Med. 2016;37(4):633-46.

67. Brower RG, Lanken PN, Macintyre N, Matthay MA, Morris A, Ancukiewicz M, et al. Higher versus lower positive end-expiratory pressures in patients with the acute respiratory distress syndrome. N Engl J Med. 2004;351(4):327-36.

68. Meade MO, Cook DJ, Guyatt GH. Ventilation strategy using low tidal volumes, recruitment maneuvers, and high positive end-expiratory pressure for acute lung injury and acute respiratory distress syndrome: a randomized controlled trial. JAMA. 2008;299:637-45.

69. Vasques F, Duscio E, Cipulli F, Romitti F, Quintel M, Gattinoni L. Determinants and prevention of ventilator-induced lung injury. Crit Care Clin. 2018;34(3):343-56.

70. Terragni P, Filippini C, Slutsky A, Birocco A, Tenaglia T, Grasso S, et al. Accuracy of plateau pressure and stress index to identify injurious ventilation in patients with acute respiratory distress syndrome. Anesthesiology. 2013;119:880-9.

71. Ferrando C, Suárez-Sipmann F, Gutierrez A, Tusman G, Carbonell J, García M, et al. Adjusting tidal volume to stress index in an open lung condition optimizes ventilation and prevents overdistension in an experimental model of lung injury and reduced chest wall compliance. Crit Care. 2015;19:9.

72. Miñana A, Ferrando C, Arocas B, Gutiérrez A, Soro M, Belda J. Matching tidal volume to stress index in an open lung condition optimizes ventilation and prevents VILI in an experimental model of lung injury and intra-abdominal hypertension: 5AP1-3. Eur J Anesthesiol. 2014;31:76-7.

73. Lonardo NW, Mone MC, Nirula R, Kimball EJ, Ludwig K, Zhou X, et al. Propofol is associated with favorable outcomes compared with benzodiazepines in ventilated intensive care unit patients. Am J Resp Crit Care Med. 2014;189:1383-94.

74. Barr J, Fraser GL, Puntillo K, Ely EW, Gelinas C, Dasta JF, et al. Clinical practice guidelines for the management of pain, agitation, and delirium in adult patients in the intensive care unit. Crit Care Med. 2013;41:263-306.

75. Wiedemann HP, Wheeler AP, Bernard GR, Thompson BT, Hayden D, deBoisblanc B, et al. Comparison of two fluid-management strategies in acute lung injury. N Engl J Med. 2006;354:2564-75.

76. Heyland DK, Cook DJ, Guyatt GH. Enteral nutrition in the critically ill patients: a critical review of the evidence. Intensive Care Med. 1993;19:435-42.

77. Cerra FB, Benitez MR, Blackburn GL, Irwin RS, Jeejeebhoy K, Katz DP, et al. Applied nutrition in ICU patients: a consensus statement of the American College of Chest Physicians. Chest. 1997;111:769-78.

78. Heys SD, Walker LG, Smith I, Eremin O. Enteral nutritional supplementation with key nutrients in patients with critical illness and cancer: a meta-analysis of randomized controlled clinical trials. Ann Surg. 1999;229:467-77.

79. Rice TW, Wheeler AP, Thompson BT, deBoisblanc BP, Steingrub J, Rock P, et al. Enteral omega-3 fatty acid, gamma-linolenic acid, and antioxidant supplementation in acute lung injury. JAMA. 2011;306:1574-81.

80. Al-Saady NM, Blackmore CM, Bennett ED. High fat, low carbohydrate, enteral feeding lowers $PaCO_2$ and reduces the period of ventilation in artificially ventilated patients. Intensive Care Med. 1989;15:290-5.

81. Rice TW, Wheeler AP, Thompson BT, Steingrub J, Hite RD, Moss M, et al. Initial trophic vs full enteral feeding in patients with acute lung injury: the EDEN randomized trial. JAMA. 2012;307:795-803.

82. Bernard GR, Luce JM, Sprung CL, Rinaldo JE, Tate RM, Sibbald WJ, et al. High-dose corticosteroids in patients with the adult respiratory distress syndrome. N Engl J Med. 1987;317:1565-70.

83. Sprung CL, Caralis PV, Marcial EH, Pierce M, Gelbard MA, Long WM, et al. The effects of high-dose corticosteroids in patients with septic shock. A prospective, controlled study. N Engl J Med. 1984;311:1137-43.

84. Annane D, Sebille V, Charpentier C, Bollaert PE, François B, Korach JM, et al. Effect of treatment with low doses of hydrocortisone and fludrocortisone on mortality in patients with septic shock. JAMA. 2002;288:862-71.

85. Annane D, Sebille V, Bellissant E. Effect of low doses of corticosteroids in septic shock patients with or without early acute respiratory distress syndrome. Crit Care Med. 2006;34:22-30.

86. Meduri GU, Golden E, Freire AX, Taylor E, Zaman M, Carson SJ, et al. Methylprednisolone infusion in early severe ARDS: results of a randomized controlled trial. Chest. 2007;131:954-63.

87. Meduri GU, Belenchia JM, Estes RJ, Wunderink RG, el Torky M, Leeper Jr KV. Fibroproliferative phase of ARDS. Clinical findings and effects of corticosteroids. Chest. 1991;100:943-52.

88. Lewis SR, Pritchard MW, Thomas CM, Smith AF. Pharmacological agents for adults with acute respiratory distress syndrome. Cochrane Database Syst Rev. 2019;7(7):CD004477.

89. Horby P, Lim WS, Emberson JR, Mafham M, Bell JL, Linsell L, et al. Dexamethasone in hospitalized patients with COVID-19. N Engl J Med. 2021;384(8):693-704.

90. Villar J, Ferrando C, Martínez D. Dexamethasone treatment for the acute respiratory distress syndrome: a multicentre, randomised controlled trial. Lancet Respir Med. 2020;8:267-76.

91. Meduri GU, Chinn AJ, Leeper KV, Wunderink RG, Tolley E, Winer-Muram HT, et al. Corticosteroid rescue treatment of progressive fibroproliferation in late ARDS. Patterns of response and predictors of outcome. Chest. 1994;105:1516-27.

92. Steinberg KP, Hudson LD, Goodman RB, Hough CL, Lanken PN, Hyzy R, et al. Efficacy and safety of corticosteroids for persistent acute respiratory distress syndrome. N Engl J Med. 2006;354:1671-84.

93. Tang BM, Craig JC, Eslick GD, Seppelt I, McLean AS. Use of corticosteroids in acute lung injury and acute respiratory distress syndrome: a systematic review and meta-analysis. Crit Care Med. 2009;37(5):1594-603.

94. Headley AS, Tolley E, Meduri GU. Infections and the inflammatory response in acute respiratory distress syndrome. Chest. 1997;111:1306-21.

95. Papazian L, Forel JM, Gacouin M, Penot-Ragon C, Perrin G, Loundou A, et al. Neuromuscular blockers in early acute respiratory distress syndrome. N Engl J Med. 2010;363:1107-16.

96. Forel JM, Roch A, Marin V, Michelet P, Demory D, Blache JL, et al. Neuromuscular blocking agents decrease inflammatory

response in patients presenting with acute respiratory distress syndrome. Crit Care Med. 2006;34:2749-57.
97. National Heart, Lung, and Blood Institute PETAL Clinical Trials Network, Moss M, Huang DT, Brower RG, Ferguson ND, Ginde AA, et al. Early neuromuscular blockade in the acute respiratory distress syndrome. N Engl J Med. 2019;380(21):1997-2008.
98. Lapinsky SE, Mehta S. Bench-to-bedside review: recruitment and recruiting maneuvers. Crit Care. 2005;9:60-5.
99. Trembley LN, Slutsky AS. Ventilator-induced lung injury: from the bench to the bedside. Intensive Care Med. 2006;32:24-33.
100. Dreyfuss D, Saumon G. Ventilator-induced lung injury: lessons from experimental studies. Am J Respir Crit Care Med. 1998;157:294-323.
101. Hess DR, Bigatello LM. Lung recruitment: the role of recruitment maneuvers. Respir Care. 2002;47(3):308-17.
102. Brower RG, Morris A, MacIntyre N, Matthay MA, Hayden D, Thompson T, et al. Effects of recruitment maneuvers in patients with acute lung injury and acute respiratory distress syndrome ventilated with high positive end-expiratory pressure. Crit Care Med. 2003;31(11):2592-7.
103. Meade MO, Cook DJ, Griffith LE, Hand LE, Lapinsky SE, Stewart TE, et al. A study of the physiologic responses to a lung recruitment maneuver in acute lung injury and acute respiratory distress syndrome. Respir Care. 2008;53(11):1441-9.
104. Fan E, Checkley W, Stewart TE, Muscedere J, Lesur O, Granton JT, et al. Complications from recruitment maneuvers in patients with acute lung injury: secondary analysis from the lung open ventilation study. Respir Care. 2012;57(11):1842-9.
105. Kacmarek RM, Villar J. Management of refractory hypoxemia in ARDS. Minerva Anesthesiol. 2013;79(10):1173-9.
106. Toth I, Leiner T, Mikor A, Szakmany T, Bogar L, Molnar Z. Hemodynamic and respiratory changes during lung recruitment and descending optimal positive end-expiratory pressure titration in patients with acute respiratory distress syndrome. Crit Care Med. 2007;35(3):787-93.
107. Fengmei G, Jin C, Songqiao L, Congshan Y, Yi Y. Dead space fraction changes during PEEP titration following lung recruitment in patients with ARDS. Respir Care. 2012;57(10):1578-85.
108. Richard JC, Lyazidi A, Akoumianaki E, Mortaza S, Cordioli RL, Lefebvre JC, et al. Potentially harmful effects of inspiratory synchronization during pressure preset ventilation. Intensive Care Med. 2013;39(11):2003-10.
109. Kacmarek RM. Strategies to optimize alveolar recruitment. Curr Opin Crit Care. 2001;7:15-20.
110. Lim CM, Koh Y, Chin JY, Lee JS, Lee SD, Kim WS, et al. Respiratory and hemodynamic effects of the prone position at two different levels of PEEP in a canine acute lung injury model. Eur Respir J. 1999;13:163-8.
111. Cakar N, der Kloot TV, Youngblood M, Adams A, Nahum A. Oxygenation response to a recruitment manoeuvre during supine and prone positions in an oleic acid induced lung injury model. Am J Respir Crit Care Med. 2000;161:1949-56.
112. O'Gara B, Fan E, Talmor DS. Controversies in the management of severe ARDS: optimal ventilator management and use of rescue therapies. Semin Respir Crit Care Med. 2015;36:823-34.
113. Guerin C, Baboi L, Richard JC. Mechanisms of the effects of prone positioning in acute respiratory distress syndrome. Intensive Care Med. 2014;40:1634-42.
114. Cornejo RA, Diaz JC, Tobar EA, Bruhn AR, Ramos CA, Gonzalez RA, et al. Effects of prone positioning on lung protection in patients with acute respiratory distress syndrome. Am J Respir Crit Care Med. 2013;188:440-8.
115. Gattinoni L, Tognoni G, Pesenti A, Taccone P, Mascheroni D, Labarta V, et al. Effect of prone positioning on the survival of patients with acute respiratory failure. N Engl J Med. 2001;345:568-73.
116. Mancebo J, Fernandez R, Blanch L, Rialp G, Gordo F, Ferrer M, et al. A multicenter trial of prolonged prone ventilation in severe acute respiratory distress syndrome. Am J Respir Crit Care Med. 2006;173:1233-9.
117. Guerin C, Reignier J, Richard JC, Beuret P, Gacouin A, Boulain T, et al. Prone positioning in severe acute respiratory distress syndrome. N Engl J Med. 2013;368:2159-68.
118. Beitler JR, Shaefi S, Montesi SB, Devlin A, Loring SH, Talmor D, et al. Prone positioning reduces mortality from acute respiratory distress syndrome in the low tidal volume era: a meta-analysis. Intensive Care Med. 2014;40:332-41.
119. Mentzelopoulos SD, Roussos C, Zakynthinos SG. Prone position reduces lung stress and strain in severe acute respiratory distress syndrome. Eur Respir J. 2005;25:534-44.
120. Taccone P, Pesenti A, Latini R, Polli F, Vagginelli F, Mietto C, et al. Prone positioning in patients with moderate and severe acute respiratory distress syndrome: a randomized controlled trial. JAMA. 2009;302:1977-84.
121. Sud S, Friedrich JO, Adhikari NK, Taccone P, Mancebo J, Polli F, et al. Effect of prone positioning during mechanical ventilation on mortality among patients with acute respiratory distress syndrome: a systematic review and meta-analysis. CMAJ. 2014;186:E381-90.
122. Kessel I, Waisman D, Barnet-Grinnes O, Ben Ari TZ, Rotschild A, et al. Benefits of high frequency oscillatory ventilation for premature infants. Isr Med Assoc J. 2010;12:144-9.
123. Derdak S, Mehata S, Stewart TE, Smith T, Rogers M, Buchman TG, et al. High-frequency oscillatory ventilation for ARDS in adults: a randomized controlled trial. Am J Respir Crit Care Med. 2002;166:801-8.
124. Ritacca FV, Stewart TE. High frequency oscillatory ventilation in adults: a review of the literature and practical applications. Crit Care. 2003;7:385-90.
125. Fessler HE, Derdak S, Ferguson ND, Hager DN, Kacmarek RM, Thompson BT, et al. A protocol for high-frequency oscillatory ventilation in adults: results from a roundtable discussion. Crit Care Med. 2007;35(7):1649-54.
126. Slutsky AS, Drazen JM. Ventilation with small tidal volumes. N Engl J Med. 2002;347:630-1.
127. Pillow JJ. High-frequency oscillatory ventilation: mechanisms of gas exchange and lung mechanics. Crit Care Med. 2005;33:S135-41.
128. Rossing TH, Slutsky AS, Lehr JL, Drinker PA, Kamm R, Drazen JM. Tidal volume and frequency dependence of carbon dioxide elimination by high-frequency ventilation. N Engl J Med. 1981;305:1375-9.

129. Hager DN, Fessler HE, Kaczka DW, Shanholtz CB, Fuld MK, Simon BA, et al. Tidal volume delivery during high frequency oscillatory ventilation in adults with acute respiratory distress syndrome. Crit Care Med. 2007;35:1522-9.
130. Scherer PW, Haselton FR. Convective exchange in oscillatory flow through bronchial-tree models. J Appl Physiol. 1982;53:1023-33.
131. Greenblatt EE, Butler JP, Venegas JG, Winkler T. Pendelluft in the bronchial tree. J Appl Physiol. 2014;117:979-88.
132. Cybulsky IJ, Abel JG, Menon AS, Salerno TA, Lichtenstein SV, Slutsky AS. Contribution of cardiogenic oscillations to gas exchange in constant-flow ventilation. J Appl Physiol (1985). 1987;63:564-70.
133. Ferguson ND, Cook DJ, Guyatt GH, Mehta S, Hand L, Austin P, et al. High-frequency oscillation in early acute respiratory distress syndrome. N Engl J Med. 2013;368:795-805.
134. Young D, Lamb SE, Shah S, MacKenzie I, Tunnicliffe W, Lall R, et al. High-frequency oscillation for acute respiratory distress syndrome. N Engl J Med. 2013;368:806-13.
135. Gattinoni L, Carlesso E, Langer T. Clinical review: extracorporeal membrane oxygenation. Crit Care. 2011;15:243.
136. Hemmila MR, Rowe SA, Boules TN, Miskulin J, McGillicuddy JW, Schuerer DJ, et al. Extracorporeal life support for severe acute respiratory distress syndrome in adults. Ann Surg. 2004;240:595-607.
137. Patroniti N, Zangrillo A, Pappalardo F, Peris A, Cianchi G, Braschi A, et al. The Italian ECMO network experience during the 2009 influenza A (H1N1) pandemic: preparation for severe respiratory emergency outbreaks. Intensive Care Med. 2011;37:1447-57.
138. Zapol WM, Snider MT, Hill JD, Fallat RJ, Bartlett RH, Edmunds LH, et al. Extracorporeal membrane oxygenation in severe acute respiratory failure: a randomized prospective study. JAMA. 1979;242:2193-6.
139. Morris AH, Wallace CJ, Menlove RL, Clemmer TP, Orme Jr JF, Weaver LK, et al. Randomized clinical trial of pressure-controlled inverse ratio ventilation and extracorporeal CO_2 removal for adult respiratory distress syndrome. Am J Respir Crit Care Med. 1994;149:295-305.
140. Peek GJ, Mugford M, Tiruvoipati R, Wilson A, Allen E, Thalanany MM, et al. Efficacy and economic assessment of conventional ventilatory support versus extracorporeal membrane oxygenation for severe adult respiratory failure (CESAR): a multicenter randomized controlled trial. Lancet. 2009;374:1351-63.
141. Combes A, Hajage D, Capellier G, Demoule A, Lavoué S, Guervilly C, et al. Extracorporeal membrane oxygenation for severe acute respiratory distress syndrome. N Engl J Med. 2018;378:1965-75.
142. Morelli A, Del Sorbo L, Pesenti A, Ranieri VM, Fan E. Extracorporeal carbon dioxide removal ($ECCO_2R$) in patients with acute respiratory failure. Intensive Care Med. 2017;43(4):519-30.
143. McNamee JJ, Gillies MA, Barrett NA, Perkins GD, Tunnicliffe W, Young D, et al. Effect of lower tidal volume ventilation facilitated by extracorporeal carbon dioxide removal vs standard care ventilation on 90-day mortality in patients with acute hypoxemic respiratory failure: the REST randomized clinical trial. JAMA. 2021;326(11):1013-23.
144. Varpula T, Valta P, Niemi R, Takkunen O, Hynynen M, Pettilä VV. Airway pressure release ventilation as a primary ventilatory mode in acute respiratory distress syndrome. Acta Anaesthesiol Scand. 2004;48(6):722-31.
145. Porhomayon J, El-Solh AA, Nader ND. Applications of airway pressure release ventilation. Lung. 2010;188:87-96.
146. González M, Arroliga AC, Frutos-Vivar F, Raymondos K, Esteban A, Putensen C, et al. Airway pressure release ventilation versus assist-control ventilation: a comparative propensity score and international cohort study. Intensive Care Med. 2010;36(5):817-27.
147. Zhou Y, Jin X, Lv Y, Wang P, Yang Y, Liang G, et al. Early application of airway pressure release ventilation may reduce the duration of mechanical ventilation in acute respiratory distress syndrome. Intensive Care Med. 2017;43(11):1648-59.
148. Zhong X, Wu Q, Yang H, Dong W, Wang B, Zhang Z, et al. Airway pressure release ventilation versus low tidal volume ventilation for patients with acute respiratory distress syndrome/acute lung injury: a meta-analysis of randomized clinical trials. Ann Transl Med. 2020;8(24):1641.
149. Calfee CS, Delucchi K, Parsons PE, Thompson BT, Ware LB, Matthay MA, et al. Subphenotypes in acute respiratory distress syndrome: latent class analysis of data from two randomised controlled trials. Lancet Respir Med. 2014;2(8):611-20.
150. Famous KR, Delucchi K, Ware LB, Kangelaris KN, Liu KD, Thompson BT, et al. Acute respiratory distress syndrome subphenotypes respond differently to randomized fluid management strategy. Am J Respir Crit Care Med. 2017;195(3):331-8. Erratum in: Am J Respir Crit Care Med. 2018;198(12):1590. Erratum in: Am J Respir Crit Care Med. 2019;200(5):649.
151. Spadaro S, Park M, Turrini C, Tunstall T, Thwaites R, Mauri T, et al. Biomarkers for acute respiratory distress syndrome and prospects for personalised medicine. J Inflamm. 2019;16:1.
152. Bos LDJ. Diagnosis of acute respiratory distress syndrome by exhaled breath analysis. Ann Transl Med. 2018;6(2):33.
153. Mathru M, Rooney MW, Dries DJ, Hirsch LJ, Barnes L, Tobin MJ. Urine hydrogen peroxide during adult respiratory distress syndrome in patients with and without sepsis. Chest. 1994;105(1):232-6.
154. McClintock DE, Ware LB, Eisner MD, Wickersham N, Thompson BT, Matthay MA, et al. Higher urine nitric oxide is associated with improved outcomes in patients with acute lung injury. Am J Respir Crit Care Med. 2007;175(3):256-62.
155. Battaglini D, Fazzini B, Silva PL, Cruz FF, Ball L, Robba C, et al. Challenges in ARDS definition, management, and identification of effective personalized therapies. J Clin Med. 2023;12(4):1381.

Approach to Tropical Infections in the ICU

Ashit Hegde

CASE STUDIES

Case 1

A 45-year-old female is admitted with fever, altered sensorium, hypotension, and thrombocytopenia in the month of August.

Q1. What is the differential diagnosis?
This patient could be suffering from any of the tropical infections, viz:
- Severe malaria
- Severe dengue
- Severe leptospirosis
- Severe rickettsial infection
- Severe typhoid (rare nowadays)

Of course, she could be suffering from any severe community-acquired bacterial infection as well.

Q2. Are there any clinical or laboratory features that help in the differential diagnosis of a tropical infection?
- *Leptospirosis:* Patients usually present in crops (usually 12–15 days after an episode of flooding in the area).
- Hemoptysis, conjunctival suffusion, and muscle pain suggest leptospirosis.
- Right hypochondriac pain is common in severe dengue.
- A narrow pulse pressure is indicative of dengue.
- *Hemoglobin (Hb):* A significant anemia is more likely in severe malaria, a raised hematocrit is characteristic of severe dengue.
- *White blood cell (WBC):* Increased in leptospirosis and scrub typhus, decreased in dengue. In malaria, the WBC count may be normal, decreased, or raised.
- *Platelets:* All of the tropical infections can cause thrombocytopenia. Platelet counts below 40,000 are usually seen in malaria and dengue.
- Jaundice is unusual in dengue unless the patient has severe hepatic damage.
- *Transaminases:* The transaminases are usually modestly raised in the tropical infections and serum glutamic-oxaloacetic transaminase (SGOT) is higher than the serum glutamic-pyruvic transaminase (SGPT). Very high levels may be seen in dengue.
- *Raised creatine phosphokinase (CPK):* This suggests leptospirosis especially if the CPK level is higher than the SGOT and SGPT levels.
- Renal dysfunction at onset is a feature of malaria and leptospirosis. In leptospirosis, the renal failure is usually nonoliguric and hypokalemic.

Case continued: The patient was treated with intravenous (IV) fluids and ceftriaxone and doxycycline (pending investigation).

Preliminary investigations:

Hb 8.5 g%, WBC: 3600/cmm (N51, L39, M8, E2), platelet count: 25000/cmm

SGOT: 280 IU/L, SGPT 206 IU/L, bilirubin 3.5 mg% (D2)

Blood urea nitrogen (BUN): 18 mg%, creatinine 1.0 mg%, Na 130 mEq/L, K 4.1 mEq/L

Q3. What would be the best test to confirm or rule out malaria in this case?[1]
Laboratory diagnosis of malaria Light microscopy of Giemsa-stained blood smears is the accepted standard. Thick smears are used to estimate the parasite density and the response to treatment. However, the parasite density may be underestimated in *Plasmodium falciparum* sometimes because of sequestration of the parasites in the microcirculation.

Thin smears are used to determine the species. Thin-smear examination can provide additional information, such as the presence of intraleukocytic pigment which is a poor prognostic sign.

Rapid diagnostic tests in malaria are quite useful in the diagnosis of severe malaria. These tests are based on the detection of histidine-rich protein 2 (HRP-2) (*P. falciparum*) or pan-specific or species-specific *Plasmodium* lactate dehydrogenase (pLDH) or pan-specific aldolase. These tests remain positive for up to 28 days and cannot be used to monitor response to treatment. The sensitivity of these tests decreases with low parasite density [unlikely in intensive care unit (ICU) patients].

Peripheral smear examination (if done properly) is more sensitive than the rapid diagnostic test. Unfortunately, there is a shortage of technicians who have the time and skill to properly examine the peripheral smear. It is therefore recommended that both the tests—peripheral smear examination and rapid diagnostic tests are performed in a suspected case of severe malaria.

Q4. The patient's peripheral smear reveals trophozoites of *P. falciparum*. The infestation rate is 3%. The rapid diagnostic test is also positive for *P. falciparum*. Is this a case of severe *falciparum* malaria?[2]

According to the World Health Organization (WHO), severe *falciparum* malaria is diagnosed in patients with any of the following:

Clinical features:
- Impaired consciousness
- Multiple convulsions—more than two episodes in day
- Respiratory distress (acidotic breathing)
- Systolic blood pressure <70 mm Hg in adults
- Clinical jaundice plus evidence of other vital organ dysfunction
- Hemoglobinuria
- Spontaneous bleeding
- Pulmonary edema (radiological)

Laboratory tests:
- Severe anemia
- Hypoglycemia
- Acidosis
- Renal impairment
- Hyperlactatemia
- *Hyperparasitemia*
- In some patients with severe malaria, the infestation rate may be misleadingly low because most of the parasites are sequestered in the peripheral circulation. *Organ dysfunction is therefore an important determinant of severity.*

Q5. What is the pathophysiology of severe *falciparum* malaria?[3]

Infected cells form knobs on red blood cell (RBC) surfaces. These knobs express an adhesive protein called PFEMP (*P. falciparum* erythrocyte membrane protein).

PFEMP mediates attachment of the infected RBCs to receptors on capillary and venular endothelium. The infected RBCs also adhere to other uninfected cells. Organ dysfunction is due to sequestration and obstruction to blood flow, endothelial dysfunction, and local inflammation.

Q6. How would you treat this patient?[4,5]

Artesunate 2.4 mg/kg body weight IV or intramuscular (IM) given on admission (time = 0), then at 12 hours and 24 hours, then once a day is the recommended treatment.

The reconstituted solution should be given stat because it is not very stable.

Artemether: 3.2 mg/kg IM is an alternative but its absorption is erratic.

When the patient's condition improves, oral artemisinin-based combination therapy should be prescribed.

Q7. Is there any role for combining artemisinin with quinine in patients with severe malaria?

There is no role for combining artemisinin with quinine. The combination only increases potential toxicity without any greater efficacy.

Q8. Are there any additional aspects in the management of patients with severe *falciparum* malaria?[6]

Fluid therapy: Fluids should be carefully administered to patients with severe malaria because these patients are vulnerable to both underhydration (and risk of renal impairment) and overhydration (and risk of pulmonary and cerebral edema). In general, liberal fluid administration should be avoided unless there is clearly a history of fluid loss.

Concomitant use of antibiotics: Severe malaria can often be complicated by secondary bacterial infections. The intensivist should consider administering antibiotics (after obtaining blood cultures) to patients with shock, respiratory distress, renal dysfunction, or altered sensorium.

Exchange transfusion: There is no evidence supporting its efficacy in severe malaria. The procedure is very labor-intensive and consumes a large volume of blood and is not without significant risk. There is no role for routine exchange transfusion.

Q9. How do you manage acute respiratory distress syndrome (ARDS) in malaria?[7]

Fluids should be administered cautiously to patients with severe malaria because they are at high risk of developing pulmonary edema/ARDS.

Acute respiratory distress syndrome is probably caused by an immune response to the infected RBCs which are sequestered in the pulmonary circulation. An immune response to the *Plasmodium* antigen even after the parasitemia has been cleared can also occur. ARDS may therefore occur as a late complication even in patients in whom the parasite load has decreased. Management of ARDS in *falciparum* malaria is no different from the management of routine ARDS. ARDS in *falciparum* malaria usually tends to be short-lived and patients with *falciparum* malaria and ARDS can often be successfully managed with a closely supervised trial of noninvasive ventilation (NIV).

Q10. How do you manage acute kidney injury (AKI) in patients with severe malaria?[8]

Acute kidney injury may occur due to a variety of factors—infected erythrocytes causing mechanical obstruction, oxidative tubular damage, immune-mediated glomerular damage, and alterations in the renal microcirculation. The prognosis of AKI in malaria is usually good. Most patients need only conservative management with special attention to fluid balance.

Q11. Is any modification of the dose of antimalarial drugs needed in patients with renal profile?

Artemisinin derivatives does not need adjustment. In the rare instances, when the patient is receiving quinine instead of artemisinin, the dose should be reduced by one-third after 48 hours.

Q12. What other complications can develop in patients with severe malaria?

These patients may develop convulsions, hypoglycemia, severe anemia, and splenic rupture.

Q13. What about the prevention/management of these other complications?[5-7]

Only supportive care is indicated for a majority of these complications.

There is no role for prophylactic anticonvulsants in patients with cerebral malaria. Hypoglycemia was more common when quinine was the drug of choice for treatment of severe *falciparum* malaria. Pregnant patients are also at risk of developing hypoglycemia and blood sugar levels should be monitored in these patients. Splenic rupture is an occasional complication (more common with *vivax* malaria). Conservative treatment and close monitoring is the preferred option. Splenectomy is reserved as a last resort.

Delayed-onset anemia might develop 2–3 weeks after IV artesunate treatment in nonimmune patients.

Q14. Is there any other drug that you would prescribe once the patient recovers?

A single dose of primaquine 45 mg [without testing for glucose-6-phosphate dehydrogenase (G6PD)] is recommended as a gametocidal agent to prevent transmission of malaria in the community.

Q15. What if the patient was a young pregnant female with severe malaria? Would the management be any different?[9]

Hypoglycemia and pulmonary edema are more common in pregnant patients and patients need careful monitoring.

Parenteral artesunate is still the treatment of choice in all trimesters.

Q16. What if this patient had severe *vivax* malaria instead of *falciparum* malaria?[10]

Vivax malaria can also be associated with multiple organ dysfunction much like *falciparum* malaria. It is not yet very clear why *vivax* malaria has changed its character and has become more virulent of late.

The treatment of severe *Plasmodium vivax* malaria is the same as that of *P. falciparum*. The patients should also be prescribed primaquine after testing for G6PD enzyme activity to prevent a relapse.

Case 2

A 36-year-old male is transferred to the ICU from the floors in view of severe abdominal pain, vomiting, and dyspnea. He had fever, body ache, and headache for 6 days and was admitted to hospital 3 days prior.

On examination: In respiratory distress, extremities cold, pulse 106/min, blood pressure (BP) 86/76 mm Hg. Air entry is reduced bilaterally. Peripheral oxygen saturation (SpO_2) 90% on 4L/min of nasal O_2.

Investigations done on floor:
- *Hb 17 g% WBC 2,500/cmm (N50, L38 M9, E3), platelets 24,000/cmm*
- *BUN 14 mg%, serum creatinine 0.9 mg%, Na 134 mEq/L, K 4.1 mEq/L*
- *SGOT: 176 IU/L, SGPT: 132 IU/L, bilirubin 1.0 mg%, alkaline phosphatase 88 IU/L*
- *Smear for malaria negative; rapid malarial test negative*
- *NS1: negative, immunoglobulin M (IgM) anti-dengue: negative, IgG anti-dengue: positive*
- *X-ray chest: Bilateral infiltrates, bilateral effusions*

Q1. What is the diagnosis and why?

The patient probably has severe dengue with shock. He has an undifferentiated fever, leukopenia, and severe thrombocytopenia; his IgG anti-dengue level is positive, suggesting that he is suffering from dengue.

He has hypotension, a narrow pulse pressure, and an increased hematocrit and evidence of a bilateral pleural effusion suggesting that he is in hypovolemic shock due to a capillary leak caused by severe dengue.

Q2. Why is the IgM anti-dengue negative but IgG anti-dengue positive in this patient?[11]

This patient is probably suffering from secondary dengue (the second attack) which generally tends to be more severe.

After the first attack of dengue the viremia lasts for 5–6 days during which time the NS1 antigen remains positive. The IgM antibodies begin to rise from around day 3–4 and peak at around day 6, the IgG antibodies begin to rise after day 6 and peak around day 9.

Primary dengue confers transient immunity against all the four serotypes of dengue but lifelong immunity only against the particular serotype that caused the infection. An individual can therefore develop only one attack of dengue during a season but can develop dengue up to four times in a lifetime.

If the patient gets a second attack of dengue, the antibodies from the previous attack are now non-neutralizing antibodies and are no longer protective, but they bind to the virus and allow the virus easier entry into the mononuclear phagocytes where they replicate more easily and stimulate a much greater immune response than the primary infection. This phenomenon is termed antibody-dependent enhancement (ADE). In secondary dengue therefore, the duration of viremia is shorter because the antigen–antibody complexes formed by the enhanced immune response clear the virus faster. NS1 levels therefore may become negative earlier than in primary infection. The IgG anti-dengue levels begin to rise much earlier in secondary dengue even before the IgM levels rise. Depending on whether it is primary or secondary dengue and depending on which day the tests are done, the results of testing will vary. In a suspected case of dengue, it is therefore important to test for NS1 antigen, IgM anti-dengue, and IgG anti-dengue in order not to miss the diagnosis.

Q3. What is the pathophysiology of severe dengue?[11,12]

The enhancing antibodies allow greater replication of virus and a more pronounced immune response. The antigen–antibody complexes activate complement which is deposited on various tissues, the blood vessel and platelets. Activated T cells release a host of cytokines as well. As a result, there is increased vascular permeability and a coagulopathy leading to a capillary leak with intravascular volume depletion and hemoconcentration along with bleeding manifestations.

Q4. How is the severity of dengue classified?[13]

Dengue is classified as:
- Dengue without warning signs
- Dengue with warning signs
- Severe dengue

Dengue with warning signs
The warning signs are:
- Abdominal pain or tenderness
- Persistent vomiting
- Clinical fluid accumulation
- Mucosal bleed
- Lethargy, restlessness
- Liver enlargement >2 cm
- Increase in hematocrit with rapid decrease in platelet count.

Patients with any of these warning signs need to be admitted and closely observed.

Severe dengue is diagnosed when the patient has either severe plasma leakage, severe hemorrhage, or severe organ involvement. Plasma leakage classified as severe when it causes either shock (dengue shock syndrome) or fluid accumulation with respiratory distress.

Any severe bleeding as evaluated by clinician qualifies as severe hemorrhage.

Severe organ involvement is indicated by:
- *Liver:* Aspartate aminotransferase (AST) or alanine aminotransferase (ALT) ≥1,000 IU/L
- *Central nervous system (CNS):* Impaired consciousness
- Severe involvement of the heart or other organs

Patients with severe dengue need to be admitted to the ICU.

Patients with dengue and certain comorbidities also need to be admitted and monitored closely. These comorbidities include extremities of age, diabetes, hypertension, pregnancy, coronary artery disease, immunocompromised patients, and patients on steroids or anticoagulants.

Q5. How would you manage this patient who has been transferred to the ICU with hypotension?[13-15]

The most common cause of death in dengue shock patients is hypovolemic state caused by plasma leakage and/or bleeding with inadequate or delayed fluid and/or blood resuscitation.

This patient needs aggressive fluid resuscitation to begin with—about 10 mL/kg/h.

The patient needs to be re-evaluated frequently. If at the end of 1 hour the patient has improved as evidenced by an increase in the systolic BP and a decrease in the pulse pressure, an improvement in pulse rate, warmer extremities, decrease in hematocrit, etc., the rate of fluid infusion may be gradually decreased with frequent monitoring of vital signs and hematocrit.

If after 1 hour the patient has not shown improvement, the hematocrit should be checked. If the hematocrit has increased or remained unchanged. Another fluid bolus of 10 mL/kg/h may be tried and the patient needs to be re-evaluated again after 1 hour. Infusion of albumin may be considered in patients who do not improve and have a persistently high hematocrit.

Patients who do not show any improvement but have a drop in their hematocrit should be examined for bleeding and will need transfusions.

Q6. What are the other causes of refractory hypotension in patients with severe dengue?

In patients who remain hypotensive in spite of adequate resuscitation, cardiac dysfunction due to myocarditis, intra-abdominal hypertension, secondary bacterial infections, and secondary hemophagocytic lymphohistiocytosis (HLH) should be considered. Severe acidosis, hypoglycemia, and hypocalcemia may also contribute to hypotension.

Q7. When would you consider stopping the IV fluids?

Fluid resuscitation may be stopped when:
- The hematocrit is stable and there is no bleeding.
- The systolic blood pressure has risen and pulse pressure has increased.
- Urine output >0.5 mL/kg/h
- There is clinical evidence of improved organ perfusion.

Q8. Day 7 of the illness: The patient feels better, pulse rate is 76/min, BP 130/82 mm Hg, Hb has decreased to 13 g% (from 17), platelet count has increased to 32,000/cmm. How would you manage the patient now?

Once the capillary leak stops, there is a gradual reabsorption of the fluid.

The hematocrit stabilizes or may be lower due to the dilutional effect of reabsorbed fluid.

During this recovery phase, continuing fluid therapy may cause pulmonary edema. The patient may be administered diuretics cautiously during this phase.

Q9. What is the role of prophylactic platelet transfusions in dengue?[16]

There is no role for prophylactic platelet transfusions in dengue. A study demonstrated that there was no correlation between bleeding manifestations and the platelet count and that there were more side effects in patients who were given prophylactic platelet transfusions.

Q10. What is the expanded dengue syndrome?[17]

Dengue can sometimes present with several atypical features affecting a variety of organs. These manifestations are referred to as the expanded dengue syndrome. The patient may have neurologic manifestations such as Guillain–Barré syndrome, cortical venous thrombosis, encephalitis, and hypokalemic periodic paralysis. Cardiac manifestations include myocarditis, tachy- and bradyarrhythmias, pericarditis, etc. Patients may have rhabdomyolysis and myoglobinuric renal failure, hemolytic uremic syndrome, and IgA nephropathy. They may also develop immune thrombocytopenic purpura (ITP) and secondary HLH.

Q11. When would you suspect secondary HLH in patients with severe dengue?[18]

In rapidly deteriorating patients with severe dengue who have persistent fever, cytopenia, and markedly elevated ferritin and liver enzyme levels, secondary HLH should be considered.

Secondary HLH should also be suspected in patients in whom the fever and cytopenia persist beyond a week.

Case 3

A 45-year-old manual laborer is admitted with a history of fever for 3 days. He also gives history of hemoptysis and breathlessness for 1 day. The city had been flooded because of intense rains 13 days prior admission.

On examination:
The patient is drowsy, tachypneic, and has pulse 102/min and BP 98/60 mm Hg. He is icteric, and conjunctival suffusion is present; he has severe pain over the thighs and calves. His SpO_2 on room air is 82%.

Q1. What is the most likely diagnosis?

The patient has conjunctival suffusion and icterus, he has severe muscle pain. He probably has alveolar hemorrhage (hemoptysis, dyspnea, hypoxia). He is drowsy. The patient is most probably suffering from severe leptospirosis.

Q2. What are the investigations you would order in this patient?

A complete blood count (CBC), renal profile, liver profile, CPK, X-ray chest, 2D echocardiogram (ECHO), polymerase chain reaction (PCR) for *Leptospira* (or a tropical fever panel), and a test for IgM anti-*Leptospira* antibodies need to be ordered.

Q3. What would you expect to find in these investigations?[19]

- *Complete blood count:* The patient may have a mild anemia, there will usually be a neutrophilic leukocytosis (or at least a left shift), the platelet counts will be moderately reduced.
- *Liver profile:* The SGOT and SGPT levels will be moderately high with SGOT levels being greater than SGPT (SGOT rises much more because muscle and heart are also involved). Bilirubin levels will be significantly high.
- *Renal profile:* The BUN and creatinine will be raised. The potassium levels will tend be normal or low in spite of kidney injury because the disease affects tubular function.[20]
- *CPK* levels will be raised because of muscle injury.
- *X-ray chest* will reveal bilateral infiltrates probably due to alveolar hemorrhage.

- *2D ECHO* may reveal evidence of decreased myocardial function due to myocarditis. Myocardial involvement is often underdiagnosed in leptospirosis.
- *PCR* is a sensitive and specific technique which can detect the presence of DNA in the very early stage of the disease, but may become negative when the leptospiremic phase ends.
- *An enzyme-linked immunosorbent assay (ELISA) to detect IgM antibodies against Leptospira* may help in the diagnosis of leptospirosis. However, very early on in the infection, it may fail to detect the presence of antibodies. PCR together with IgM ELISA can be used to confirm the diagnosis, early on in the acute stage of the infection.[21,22]

Q4. What is the pathophysiology of severe leptospirosis?[19]
Water (especially during episodes of flooding) contaminated by the urine of infected rats is the most common source of infection. The organisms gain entry through cuts in the skin. The twisting motion of periplasmic flagella allows leptospires to then enter the host bloodstream in a few minutes.

Human toll-like receptor 4 (TLR-4) is unable to recognize leptospiral lipopolysaccharide (LPS). This allows leptospires to hide themselves from the host innate immune response, providing them enough time to cause damage before they get detected.

This leptospiremic phase is followed by an immune phase which classically begins 7–10 days after the onset of symptoms. Often the two phases merge. As leptospires bind to host cells, cytokines [interleukin 6 (IL-6), IL-10, and tumor necrosis factor alpha (TNF-α)] and antimicrobial peptides (AMPs) are released to limit the invasive damages caused by the bacteria. Phagocytic cells engulf these organisms. However, leptospires are capable of replicating and surviving in phagolysosomes.

In vain, the host immune system continuously releases excessive amounts of cytokines, producing a destructive response instead of a beneficial one.

Q5. How will you manage this patient?[19,23]
Treatment: In patients with severe leptospirosis, treatment with crystalline penicillin or ceftriaxone is recommended. Doxycycline/tigecycline may be used in patients allergic to the beta-lactams. Paradoxical worsening may occur in patients treated with beta-lactam antibiotics due to a Jarisch–Herxheimer-like reaction.

Organ dysfunction and hypotension are treated with standard supportive care.

Nonoliguric patients with renal dysfunction may need careful fluid replacement and potassium supplementation. Oliguria and hyperkalemia are poor prognostic indicators and early dialysis may be considered in such patients.

A closely supervised trial of NIV/high-flow nasal cannula (HFNC) may be tried first in patients with ARDS/alveolar hemorrhage. If the patient needs intubation and mechanical ventilation, the principles of management are the same as for any other ARDS.

There are anecdotal reports of high-dose steroids being used for alveolar hemorrhage especially early in the course of the disease and for brief periods. However, there are also reports of an increased incidence of nosocomial infections in patients who receive high-dose steroids. More evidence is needed before steroids are routinely recommended for the treatment of pulmonary leptospirosis.

A few centers have reported the use of desmopressin for alveolar hemorrhage. Plasma exchange and ECMO have been tried in severely ill patients. More evidence is needed before these procedures can be routinely recommended.

Case 4

A 35-year-old male is admitted to ICU with fever, altered sensorium, hypotension, and hypoxia. He gives a history of fever for 1 week prior to admission. There is no focal neurologic deficit, no neck stiffness; he needs vasopressors and supplemental oxygen.

Q1. What is the differential diagnosis?
This is most likely to be a severe tropical infection. It might also be due to severe bacterial sepsis. It is unlikely to be a primary CNS infection because several other systems are also affected.

Q2. Is there any important clinical finding that should be looked for in any patient with a suspected severe tropical infection?
Such patients should be closely examined for an eschar which is an area of necrotic skin. In females, it is commonly present in the chest and abdomen and in males it is present in the axilla, groin, and genitalia. Unusual sites of eschar are in the cheek, ear lobe, and dorsum of the feet. If an eschar is seen in a patient with an undifferentiated fever, it is very likely that this patient has scrub typhus.[24]

Case continued: This patient had an eschar on his scrotum.

Q3. What investigations would you ask for in this patient and what would you expect to find on investigation?[25]
- *Complete blood count:* There might be a mild anemia, neutrophilic leukocytosis, and moderate thrombocytopenia.
- There might be evidence of disseminated intravascular coagulation (DIC) in severe cases.
- Liver functions and renal functions might be deranged.
- X-ray chest might reveal bilateral infiltrates consistent with ARDS.

- The tests that might be used to diagnose scrub typhus in our country are:
- The Weil Felix test is most commonly used to diagnose scrub typhus in India. Though it is a cheap and easily available test, it is not very sensitive.
- IgM antibodies to scrub are more specific and sensitive. The cutoff values are not clearly defined however, and might depend upon the prevalence of scrub typhus in the community. A lateral flow assay to detect antibodies to scrub is now available.
- PCR for scrub typhus is very sensitive and specific. However, it is not widely available. It may be falsely negative in patients who have received antibiotics.
- A PCR from the eschar might be even more sensitive.

The eschar must be carefully looked for and empiric treatment for *Rickettsia* must be initiated in every patient who presents to the ICU with a severe undifferentiated illness.

Q4. What is the pathophysiology of severe scrub typhus?[25,26]

This is a disease which occurs when an infected chigger (*the larval stage of trombiculid mites*) bites an individual and inoculates *Orientia tsutsugamushi* which are intracellular coccobacilli having an affinity for the capillary endothelium.

Disseminated vasculitis with perivasculitis is the hallmark of scrub typhus, and involvement of the *brain and lungs* are the most important factors in any fatal outcome.

Q5. Which organs are commonly involved in severe scrub typhus?

Patients may present with liver failure, renal failure, DIC, and shock. ARDS and an encephalitis-like syndrome are also being increasingly reported in our country.

Q6. How would you manage this patient?[25,26]

Organs that have been affected need the standard methods of organ support.

Doxycycline or azithromycin are the recommended antibiotics for the treatment of scrub typhus. A recent paper from India[27,28] suggests that a combination of doxycycline and azithromycin might result in better outcomes in patients with severe scrub typhus than either drug alone. Other drugs that have been used are chloramphenicol and *rifampicin*.

REFERENCES

1. World Health Organization. Universal Access to Malaria Diagnostic Testing: An Operational Manual. Geneva: World Health Organization; 2011.
2. World Health Organization. World Health Organization Guidelines For Malaria. Geneva: World Health Organization; 2022.
3. Pasvol G. Management of severe malaria: interventions and controversies. Infect Dis Clin North Am. 2005;19(1):211-40.
4. World Health Organization. WHO Guidelines for Malaria. Geneva: World Health Organization; 2023.
5. Dondorp A, Nosten F, Stepniewska K, Day N, White N; South East Asian Quinine Artesunate Malaria Trial (SEAQUAMAT) group. Artesunate versus quinine for treatment of severe falciparum malaria: a randomised trial. Lancet. 2005;366(9487):717-25.
6. Cheng MP, Yansouni CP. Management of severe malaria in the intensive care unit. Crit Care Clin. 2013;29(4):865-85.
7. Plewes K, Leopold SJ, Kingston HWF, Dondorp AM. Malaria: What's New in the Management of Malaria? Infect Dis Clin North Am. 2019;33(1):39-60.
8. Silva GBD Junior, Pinto JR, Barros EJG, Farias GMN, Daher EF. Kidney involvement in malaria: an update. Rev Inst Med Trop Sao Paulo. 2017;59:e53.
9. Rogerson SJ, Hviid L, Duffy PE, Leke RF, Taylor DW. Malaria in pregnancy: pathogenesis and immunity. Lancet Infect Dis. 2007;7(2):105-17.
10. Rahimi BA, Thakkinstian A, White NJ, Sirivichayakul C, Dondorp AM, Chokejindachai W. Severe vivax malaria: a systematic review and meta-analysis of clinical studies since 1900. Malar J. 2014;13:481.
11. Muller DA, Depelsenaire AC, Young PR. Clinical and Laboratory Diagnosis of Dengue Virus Infection. J Infect Dis. 2017;215(suppl_2):S89-95.
12. Oishi K, Saito M, Mapua CA, Natividad FF. Dengue illness: clinical features and pathogenesis. J Infect Chemother. 2007;13(3):125-33.
13. World Health Organization. Dengue Guidelines for Diagnosis, Treatment, Prevention and Control. Geneva: SEAMEO Regional Tropical Medicine and Public Health Network; 2009.
14. World Health Organization. Handbook for Clinical Management of Dengue. Geneva: World Health Organization; 2012.
15. Lee TH, Lee LK, Lye DC, Leo YS. Current management of severe dengue infection. Expert Rev Anti Infect Ther. 2017;15(1):67-78.
16. Lye DC, Archuleta S, Syed-Omar SF, Low JG, Oh HM, Wei Y, et al. Prophylactic platelet transfusion plus supportive care versus supportive care alone in adults with dengue and thrombocytopenia: a multicentre, open-label, randomised, superiority trial. Lancet. 2017;389(10079):1611-8.
17. World Health Organization. Comprehensive Guidelines for Prevention and Control of Dengue and Dengue Haemorrhagic Fever. New Delhi: WHO, SEARO; revised and expanded edition. 2011.
18. Giang HTN, Banno K, Minh LHN, Trinh LT, Loc LT, Eltobgy A, et al. Dengue hemophagocytic syndrome: A systematic review and meta-analysis on epidemiology, clinical signs, outcomes, and risk factors. Rev Med Virol. 2018;28(6):e2005.
19. Haake DA, Levett PN. Leptospirosis in humans. Curr Top Microbiol Immunol. 2015;387:65-97.
20. Seguro AC, Lomar AV, Rocha AS. Acute renal failure of leptospirosis: nonoliguric and hypokalemic forms. Nephron. 1990;55(2):146-51.
21. Cumberland P, Everard CO, Levett PN. Assessment of the efficacy of an IgM-elisa and microscopic agglutination test

21. (MAT) in the diagnosis of acute leptospirosis. Am J Trop Med Hyg. 1999;61(5):731-4.
22. Brown PD, Gravekamp C, Carrington DG, van de Kemp H, Hartskeerl RA, Edwards CN, et al. Evaluation of the polymerase chain reaction for early diagnosis of leptospirosis. J Med Microbiol. 1995;43(2):110-4.
23. Jiménez JIS, Marroquin JLH, Richards GA, Amin P. Leptospirosis: Report from the task force on tropical diseases by the World Federation of Societies of Intensive and Critical Care Medicine. J Crit Care. 2018;43:361-5.
24. Raina SK. Eschar in scrub typhus: A valuable clue to the diagnosis. J Postgrad Med. 2013;59(4):342-3.
25. Kore VB, Mahajan SM. Recent Threat of Scrub Typhus in India: A Narrative Review. Cureus. 2022;14(10):e30092.
26. Peter JV, Sudarsan TI, Prakash JA, Varghese GM. Severe scrub typhus infection: Clinical features, diagnostic challenges and management. World J Crit Care Med. 2015;4(3):244-50.
27. Varghese GM, Dayanand D, Gunasekaran K, Kundu D, Wyawahare M, Sharma N, et al; INTREST Trial Investigators. Intravenous Doxycycline, Azithromycin, or Both for Severe Scrub Typhus. N Engl J Med. 2023;388(9):792-803.
28. Walker DH, Blanton LS. Progress in Treating a Neglected Tropical Disease. N Engl J Med. 2023;388(9):843-4.

CHAPTER 9

Sepsis and Septic Shock

Divya Pal, Deepak Govil

CASE STUDY

A 63-year-old male patient, a known diabetic and chronic alcoholic, was brought to the casualty by relatives with complaints of fever, altered sensorium, and loose stools of 3 days' duration. On examination, the patient was drowsy, tachycardic (heart rate 130/min) with a thready pulse, hypotensive [blood pressure (BP) 86/40 mm Hg], and tachypneic (respiratory rate of 30/min). His abdomen was distended and tense. A standing chest X-ray showed gas under the diaphragm. A computed tomography (CT) abdomen showed pneumoperitoneum and free fluid in the peritoneal cavity, suggesting peritonitis. The arterial blood gas (ABG) revealed pH 7.10, partial pressure of oxygen (PO_2) 67 mm Hg on FiO_2 0.4, partial pressure of carbon dioxide (PCO_2) 36 mm Hg, and HCO_3 15 mmol/L, and the electrolytes were Na 126 mmol/L and Cl 88 mmol/L. The random blood sugar was 168 mg/dL.

Q1. From the history and examination, what is your diagnosis?

The working diagnosis at present is perforation peritonitis and septic shock with metabolic acidosis.

Sepsis is defined as a life-threatening organ dysfunction caused by dysregulated host response to infection. Septic shock is a subset of sepsis in which underlying circulatory and cellular or metabolic abnormalities are profound enough to substantially increase mortality. Patients with septic shock can be identified with a clinical construct of sepsis with persisting hypotension requiring vasopressors to maintain a mean arterial pressure (MAP) of 65 mm Hg and having a serum lactate level >2 mmol/L (18 mg/dL) despite adequate volume resuscitation.[1]

Q2. How will you resuscitate and manage the patient?

Sepsis and septic shock are a medical emergency. Resuscitation, treatment, and diagnostic workup should commence immediately and simultaneously. The surviving

BOX 1: One-hour surviving sepsis care bundle.

- Measure lactate level. Remeasure if initial lactate is >2 mmol/L
- Obtain blood cultures prior to administration of antibiotics
- Administer broad-spectrum antibiotics
- Rapidly administer 30 mL/kg crystalloid for hypotension or lactate ≥4 mmol/L
- Apply vasopressors, if the patient is hypotensive during or after fluid resuscitation to maintain mean arterial pressure (MAP) ≥65 mm Hg

sepsis campaign (SSC) guidelines 2018 have combined the 3- and 6-hour bundle into a single 1-hour bundle, which includes five essential steps of initial management **(Box 1)**.[2]

The latest SSC guidelines 2021 have *suggested* administration of at least 30 mL/kg of intravenous (IV) crystalloid fluid within the first 3 hours of resuscitation in patients with sepsis-induced hypoperfusion or septic shock (downgraded from previous). They have also suggested to use dynamic measures over the static ones and to use serum lactates, capillary refill time as adjuncts to assess perfusion and guide fluid resuscitation. Use of balance salt solution over normal saline has been suggested. In patients who have received large volumes of crystalloids, they suggest using albumin. The recommendation is against the use of starches and gelatin for resuscitation.[3]

Q3. Discuss the role of biomarkers in patients with sepsis.

Numerous biomarkers for sepsis have been evaluated, and there are many more under clinical development.[4-6] Despite the multiple advances, till date, no biomarker has been found to be reliable to answer the question—whether the patient has sepsis or not. Different biomarkers identified in sepsis can be categorized as follows: (1) The systemic manifestations based, that is, host response biomarkers—C-reactive protein (CRP) and procalcitonin (PCT); (2) microbiology based, that is, pathogen specific; and (3) based on organ dysfunction. This is known as "the three-vector approach to sepsis."[7]

Host response biomarkers: Serum PCT is the only biomarker that is widely used in clinical practice. It is a precursor of the hormone calcitonin and is not detected in healthy individuals. The level of PCT increases in response to any proinflammatory stimulus with peak values correlating with the intensity of stimulus. False-positive results have been associated with severe trauma, circulatory shock, pancreatitis, burns, and major surgery.[8] Localized infections such as mediastinitis and empyema can show spuriously low PCT levels. False-negative results have also been found in patients when the sample is tested too early in infection.[9] The presence of neutropenia, immunosuppression, renal failure, or dialysis can also affect the levels of PCT.[7] Albeit a recent meta-analysis[10] showed a mean sensitivity of 0.77 [95% confidence interval (CI) 0.72–0.81] and specificity of 0.79 (95% CI 0.74–0.84) to differentiate sepsis from other causes of inflammatory response, no cutoff value could be derived because of the heterogeneity of the studies in the final analysis. In patients with suspected respiratory tract infection, cutoffs between 0.1 and 0.5 ng/mL have been calculated.[11] Despite the current limitations, multiple studies have used PCT to start and stop antibiotics. The Procalcitonin to Reduce Antibiotic Treatments in Acutely ill patients (PRORATA) trial[12] included an initial PCT to help assess whether to start antibiotics in addition to subsequent daily PCT levels to help decide when to stop antibiotics. The PCT group had significantly more antibiotics-free days (14.3 vs. 11.6 days) and an overall 23% relative reduction in days of antibiotic exposure (mean 10.3 vs. 13.3 days) when a cutoff value of <0.5 μg/L or a decrease of ≥80% from the baseline was used to stop antibiotics. In Stop Antibiotics on Procalcitonin guidance Study (SAPS),[13] the PCT group had significantly less days of antibiotic exposure (5 vs. 7 days) and also had lower mortality at 28 days (20 vs. 25% in control group, $p = 0.0122$) and at 1 year (36 vs. 43%, $p = 0.0188$), when a similar algorithm-based antibiotic approach was used. A suggested algorithm for discontinuation of antibiotics is described in **Flowchart 1**.

Procalcitonin-based antibiotic regimes have been successfully used in patients with suspected respiratory tract infections. In the Procalcitonin-guided Antibiotic Therapy and Hospitalization in Patients with Lower Respiratory Tract Infections (ProHOSP) study,[14] the PCT group had a significantly lower mean duration of antibiotics (5.7 vs. 8.7 days), with no difference in adverse events [including death, intensive care unit (ICU) admission and recurrent infection]. The authors proposed an algorithm-based approach for management of patients with suspected respiratory tract infections **(Flowchart 2)**. If the serum biomarkers levels remain elevated on day 3 or day 4 of antibiotic therapy, then the clinician should think of treatment failure or alternative diagnosis and approach to treatment.

The SSC guidelines 2021 *suggest* against the use of PCT plus clinical evaluation for decision regarding when to initiate antimicrobials, as compared to clinical evaluation alone. They *suggest* using PCT and clinical evaluation to decide when to discontinue antimicrobials over clinical evaluation alone, in adults who were diagnosed with sepsis or septic shock and have adequate source control.[3]

As per the American Thoracic Society and Infectious Diseases Society of America (*ATS/IDSA*) 2019 guidelines for diagnosis and treatment of adults with CAP, empiric antibiotic therapy should be initiated in adults with clinically suspected and radiographically confirmed CAP, regardless of the initial serum PCT level (strong recommendation).[15] Even though previously in some studies, it was suggested that PCT levels of ≤0.1 mg/L had a higher probability of having viral infection, while levels ≥0.25 mg/L had a higher probability of bacterial pneumonia, in a recent multicenter study in patients admitted with CAP, the authors concluded that no particular threshold of PCT could differentiate between the pneumonia of viral or bacterial etiology. But higher levels of PCT were associated with the likelihood of bacterial etiology and more so the typical bacteria.[16]

The other biomarker that has been recently approved by US Food and Drug Administration (FDA) is SeptiCyte LAB. It consists of four ribonucleic acid (RNA) biomarkers (CEACAM 4, LAMP1, PLA2G7, and PLAC8). The overall area under the curve (AUC) in validation cohorts was 0.88[17] in differentiating between inflammatory responses due to infectious and noninfectious origins.

Reevaluation of the clinical status and measurement of serum PCT levels are mandatory after 6–24 hours in all persistently sick and hospitalized patients in whom antibiotics are withheld. The PCT algorithm can be overruled by prespecified criteria, for example, in patients with immediately life-threatening disease. In all patients with a very high PCT value on admission

Flowchart 1: Procalcitonin-based algorithm for sepsis.

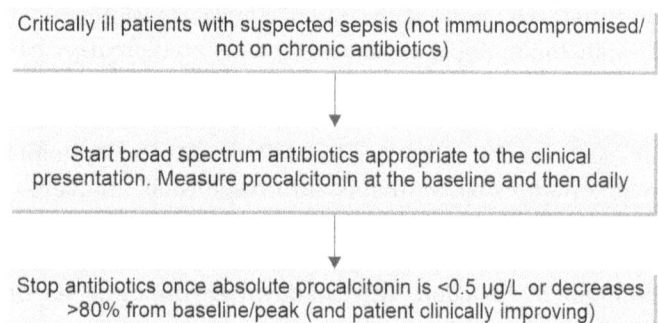

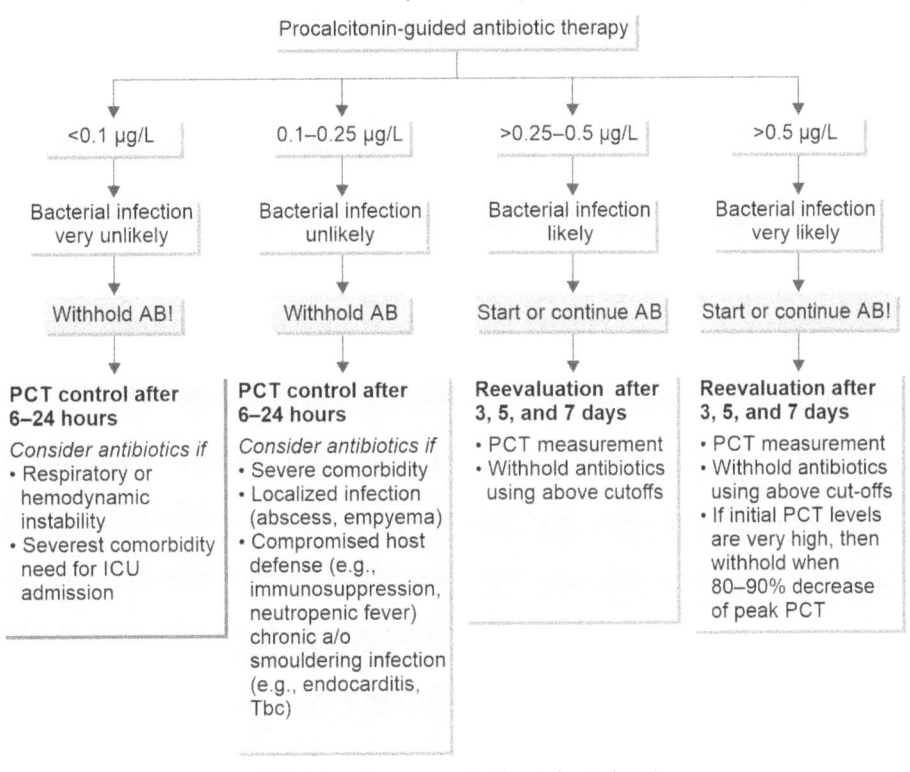

Flowchart 2: Antibiotic stewardship based on procalcitonin (PCT) cutoff ranges.

(ICU: intensive care unit; Tbc: tuberculosis)
Source: Reproduced from Schuetz et al.[14]

(e.g., >10 µg/L), discontinuation of antibiotics is encouraged if levels decreased below 80-90% of the initial value. In patients discharged and, thus, likely uncomplicated resolution of the infection or in patients transferred to an institution not taking part in this trial, the recommended total duration of antibiotic therapy was based on the last PCT level and was as follows: >1 µg/L 7 days, 0.5-0.99 µg/L 5 days, 0.25-0.49 µg/L 3 days, <0.25 µg/L stop antibiotic, <0.1 µg/L stop antibiotic.[14]

C-reactive protein is an acute-phase reactant made in liver, whose levels start to rise 4-6 hours after any inflammatory insult and peak in 36-50 hours. Unlike PCT, its levels are not affected by immunosuppression, renal failure, or dialysis. Rather than absolute CRP value, the CRP ratio from day 0 to subsequent days has been found to be of more relevance. But there is no strong evidence to suggest use of CRP to guide initiation or discontinuation of antimicrobial therapy.[7]

Pathogen-specific biomarkers: These could either be based on the detection of nucleic acid of the microorganism or antigen based, but the latter are more commonly used in practice in critically ill patients.

Fungal antigen-based tests include serum (1,3)-β-D-glucan (BDG), serum or BAL (bronchoalveolar lavage) galactomannan (GM), and serum or CSF (cerebrospinal fluid) cryptococcal antigen test.

Serum 1,3-BDG has high sensitivity (~0.81) and low specificity (~0.60) for invasive candidiasis, turns positive 24-72 hours earlier than blood culture, and has a high negative predictive value (NPV) >95% at low prevalence. Taking two consequent samples, combining it with other biomarkers, and increasing the cutoff value can help increase its specificity and positive predictive value. It is more sensitive for detection of *Pneumocystis jirovecii* pneumonia in human immunodeficiency virus (HIV) patients compared to non-HIV patients and has a higher NPV ≥95% in non-HIV and low/intermediate disease likelihood subset of patients. Interruption of empirical antifungal therapy guided by serum BDG has been found to be safe and linked with a shorter course of antifungal therapy in critically ill patients with suspected invasive candidiasis.[18] Serum 1,3BDG assay has been approved by the FDA as an adjunct to cultures for the diagnosis of invasive fungal infections.[19]

Galactomannan antigen can be used for diagnosis of invasive pulmonary aspergillosis. Increasing the cutoff (ODI ≥1) is associated with higher sensitivity and specificity in both serum and BAL. Serum GM can be falsely positive in certain conditions such as intestinal mucositis or use of β-lactams. BAL GM is of more use in making the diagnosis in nonneutropenic critically ill patients compared to serum GM.

Cryptococcal antigen test is highly sensitive (~0.99) and specific (≥0.95) in both serum and CSF for diagnosis of cryptococcal meningitis and can detect all the cryptococcal serotypes. A negative serum cryptococcal antigen test can rule out cryptococcal meningitis in HIV patients with neurological symptoms.[7]

Diagnosis of *Clostridium difficile* infection (CDI) can be made based on a two-step algorithm with a positive glutamate dehydrogenase (GDH) followed by positive free toxins A/B in the stool sample. These tests have low positive predictive value (PPV) and high NPV at low prevalence, so either of them should not be used alone for diagnosis.[7]

Other pathogen-specific biomarkers that are used include the influenza A/B antigen test on nasal swab, SARS-CoV-2 (severe acute respiratory syndrome coronavirus 2) antigen test on nasal swab or other respiratory samples, Streptococcus urinary antigen test, and Legionella urinary antigen test for CAP. (Some other biomarkers are summarized in **Table 1**.)[20]

In view of persistent hypotension and acidosis, the patient was intubated and ventilated with a tidal volume (TV) of 6 mL/kg of ideal body weight (IBW). MAP was 56 mm Hg in spite of fluid boluses. The PCT levels were found to be 152 ng/mL. Antibiotics were initiated. A surgical consult was obtained, and it was decided to perform an emergency laparotomy. Laparotomy revealed a perforated sigmoid mass with gross fecal contamination and peritonitis.

Q4. What is the MAP target for the patient?
Target MAP for this patient is at least 65 mm Hg. A higher MAP target of 80–85 mm Hg has not been found to reduce mortality, but it is associated with an increased incidence of arrhythmias. In patients with chronic hypertension, a higher MAP has been associated with reduced need for renal replacement therapy (RRT) without beneficial outcomes in terms of mortality.[21] A recent pilot study demonstrated a reduced mortality in elderly patients (age >75 years) with a lower MAP target (13 vs. 60%, p = 0.03).[22] SSC 2021 recommends an initial target MAP of 65 mm Hg over higher MAP targets.[3]

Back in the ICU, the patient continued to be oliguric and metabolic acidosis worsened. Vasopressor requirement was increasing, and his (PaO_2/FiO_2) ratio dropped. Two-dimensional (2D) echo revealed global left ventricular (LV) dysfunction and ejection fraction (LVEF) of 45%. RRT was contemplated and was discussed with the relatives. Blood culture showed heavy growth of Escherichia coli. The patient gradually improved after three sessions of continuous renal replacement therapy (CRRT), and his urine output (UOP) has improved to 30 mL/h. His oxygenation has improved, and he is drowsy but obeying commands. Sedation has been stopped, and he is being contemplated for weaning.

Q5. What is the current perspective on early goal-directed therapy (EGDT) in patients with septic shock?
Rivers[23] and his team showed that early aggressive goal-directed resuscitation of a patient with septic shock improved outcomes in terms of mortality (30.5 vs. 46.5%, p = 0.009). The protocol used also found its way in subsequent surviving sepsis guidelines. Subsequently, three large trials, Australasian Resuscitation in Sepsis Evaluation (ARISE),[24] Protocolised Management in Sepsis (ProMISe),[25] and Protocolized Care for Early Septic Shock (ProCESS)[26] did not show any outcome benefit when compared to standard protocol-based treatment. After these trials, the SSC withdrew the recommendation for EGDT. The targets suggested by Rivers are not found to be harmful and can still be used in resource-limited settings.

Q6. What is the role of venous oxygen saturation (SvO_2), central venous oxygen saturation ($ScvO_2$), and pCO_2 gap in sepsis?
Mixed SvO_2 is a useful parameter in assessing the balance between oxygen demand and supply. SvO_2 is typically decreased in patients with low-flow states due to high oxygen extraction, but it is normal or high in those with distributive shock. $ScvO_2$, which is measured in the superior vena cava, reflects the oxygen saturation of the venous blood from the upper half of the body. Under normal circumstances, $ScvO_2$ is slightly less than SvO_2, but in critically ill patients, it is often greater because of increased oxygen extraction in hepatosplanchnic and coronary circulation but not in cerebral circulation as the blood flow and O_2 extraction there remain constant.

Measuring SvO_2 requires a pulmonary artery catheter, which is associated with many complications, and thus $ScvO_2$ is used as a surrogate for SvO_2 and this has been validated in various studies.[27,28] EGDT by Rivers included $ScvO_2$ as a resuscitation target and showed a significant reduction in mortality, which could not be replicated in subsequent trials. When compared with lactates as a resuscitation goal, $ScvO_2$-targeted therapy has been found to have a trend toward increased mortality.[29]

The major drawback of $ScvO_2$ and SvO_2 measurements in sepsis is that of heterogeneity in microcirculation. In septic shock, tissues which are close to the perfused capillaries consume normal amounts of oxygen and those far from the perfused capillaries remain hypoxic. Also, due to microcirculatory disturbances and mitochondrial dysfunction, oxygen extraction capabilities of the tissues are affected with varying degrees.[30,31] This heterogeneity results

TABLE 1: Role of different biomarkers in sepsis.[20]

Biomarker	Function
Acute-phase proteins	
CRP, hsCRP	• Response to infection and other inflammatory stimuli • Predictive for increased 28-day mortality in patients with sepsis • Hyperinflammatory phenotype
Complement	Prognosis of disease severity
PTX-3	• Discrimination of sepsis and septic shock, prediction of septic shock • Diagnosis of sepsis and septic shock during the first week in the ICU
Cytokines and chemokines	
IL-10	Hypoinflammatory phenotype, mortality prognosis at 30 days and 6 months
TNF-α, IL-1, IL-6	IL-6 all-cause mortality prognosis at 30 days and 6 months, IL-1 and IL-6 acute phase of sepsis. It was increased in the hyperinflammatory phenotype
DAMPs	
Calprotectin	• PCT to distinguish between patients with sepsis and patients without sepsis in the ICU • Predictive for 30-day mortality
HMGB-1	Worst prognosis and higher 28-day mortality
Endothelial cells and BBB markers	
Ang-1	It stabilizes the endothelium and inhibits vascular leakage by constitutively activating the Tie-2 receptor
Ang-2	It can disrupt microvascular integrity by blocking the Tie-2 receptor, which results in vascular leakage. Individuals with septic shock had higher levels of Ang-2 than those with sepsis
OCLN	Increase related to sepsis severity and positive correlation with SOFA scores. The absence of OCLN in the cerebral microvascular endothelium was related to more severe disease and intense inflammatory response
PAI-1	Sepsis severity prognosis, predictor of mortality, an increase may indicate DIC
sICAM-1, sVCAM-1	Sepsis severity prognosis, prognosis of 90-day mortality in patients with sepsis and septic shock in the ICU
E-selectin	Sepsis severity prognosis, increase related to SOFA and APACHE-II, predicts mortality
Gut permeability markers	
Citrulline	The decrease may indicate early acute bowel dysfunction
I-FABP	Indicates early intestinal damage in patients with sepsis and septic shock, risk of septic shock
D-lactic acid	Indicates early intestinal damage in patients with sepsis and septic shock
Noncoding RNAs—lnc-MALAT1, lnc-MEG3	
miRNA—miR-125a, miR-125b	
Membrane receptors, cell proteins, and metabolites	
CD64	Prognosis of disease severity, 28-day mortality predictor
NSE	• Diagnosis of sepsis-associated encephalopathy • 30-day mortality risk • Neuronal injury marker in sepsis
TREM-1	Sepsis indicator, predictive of septic shock
Peptide precursor of the hormone and hormone	
PCT	Diagnosis of sepsis
NT-proBNP	In the acute phase of sepsis, it indicates a risk of long-term impairment of physical function and muscle strength, predict mortality risk
Neutrophil, cells, and related biomarkers	
Lactate	Predictive of mortality
MPO	• Increase in patients with DIC, indicates organ dysfunction • Mortality predictor at 28 and 90 days

Contd...

Contd...

Biomarker	Function
Resistin	Sepsis indicator, risk of septic shock, 28-day mortality predictor
Lipoproteins	
LDL-C	Protective effect against sepsis, the decrease can cause a risk of sepsis and admission to the ICU
HDL	Low levels: Mortality prognosis and adverse clinical outcomes

(Ang-1: angiopoietin-1; Ang-2: angiopoietin-2; APACHE-II: acute physiology and chronic health evaluation II; ARDS: acute respiratory distress syndrome; BBB: blood–brain barrier; CD: cluster of differentiation; CRP: C-reactive protein; DAMPs: damage-associated molecular patterns; DIC: disseminated intravascular coagulation; HDL: high density lipoprotein; HMGB1: high mobility group box 1; hsCRP: high sensitivity C-reactive protein; I-FABP: intestinal fatty acid binding protein; ICU: intensive care unit; IL: interleukin; LDL: low-density lipoprotein; lnc-MALAT1: long non-coding metastasis-associated lung adenocarcinoma transcript 1; lnc-MEG3: long non-coding RNA maternally expressed gene 3; miR-125a: micro RNA-125a; miR-125b: micro RNA-125b; MPO: myeloperoxidase; NSE: neuron-specific enolase; NT-proBNP: N-terminal pro-brain natriuretic peptide; OCLN: occludin; PAI-1: plasminogen activator inhibitor 1; PCT: procalcitonin; PTX-3: pentraxin-3; RNA: ribonucleic acid; S100B: calcium-binding protein B; sFlt-1: soluble fms-like tyrosine kinase 1; sICAM-1: soluble intercellular adhesion molecule 1; SIRS: systemic inflammatory response syndrome; SOFA: sequential organ failure assessment; sVCAM-1: soluble vascular cell adhesion molecule 1; T-chol: total cholesterol; TNF-α: tumor necrosis factor alpha; TREM-1: triggering receptor expressed on myeloid cells-1)

in a normal or high $ScvO_2$ despite tissue hypoxia,[32] and a high normal $ScvO_2$ cannot differentiate if the oxygen delivery is adequate or excess.

Despite the drawbacks, $ScvO_2$ can still be used as a part of resuscitation bundle, especially in patients with septic shock with low $ScvO_2$ values, who are at the highest risk of death.[33]

A relatively newer strategy involving $ScvO_2$ and venous-arterial carbon dioxide (CO_2) gap was proposed. In septic shock, oxygen supply may be adapted to the oxygen extraction capabilities of the tissues, and oxygen diffusion is also affected because of shunt or reduced perfusion. The total cardiac output may not be adequate to wash out the CO_2 produced during tissue metabolism, and tissue CO_2 will increase. Since CO_2 is at least 20 times more soluble than oxygen, it can easily diffuse from the hypoperfused tissues and enter venous circulation, thereby unmasking cellular hypoxia.[34] Many clinical studies have shown an inverse correlation between cardiac index and venous arterial CO_2 gap $[P(v-a)CO_2]$. Patients with a gap of >6 mm Hg have been found to have significantly lower cardiac output.[35,36] Normalization of an increased CO_2 gap has been shown to correlate with improvement in tissue perfusion. Vallée et al., have suggested a CO_2 gap of 6 mm Hg as an additional marker to identify inadequate resuscitation after achieving a target $ScvO_2$ of 70%.[37] A simplified $ScvO_2$ and pCO_2-based resuscitation algorithm is described in **Flowchart 3**.

An increase in blood lactate levels reflects abnormal cellular function. In patients with sepsis and septic shock, an increase in lactates is primarily because of anaerobic metabolism secondary to a low flow state. Increased glycolysis and inhibition of pyruvate dehydrogenase also contribute to high lactate levels in septic shock. Both single, abnormal lactate values and the duration of lactates above 2 mmol/L have been associated with multiorgan failure and mortality.[38] In a multicenter, randomized noninferiority trial, a 6-hour resuscitation targeting a 10% reduction in lactates was found to be noninferior to $ScvO_2$-based resuscitation, though a trend toward lower mortality was seen in the lactate group.[22] In patients with sepsis and hypotension with baseline lactate levels of >3 mmol/L, a 20% decrease every 2 hours of resuscitation has been associated with reduced mortality (33.9 vs. 43.5%) with an adjusted hazard ratio (HR) of 0.61. Patients in the lactate group also had lower organ failure scores, reduced days on mechanical ventilation, and lesser days in ICU.[29]

Q7. How and when do you use vasopressors in septic shock? Which vasopressor would you prefer?

Sepsis and septic shock are a state of vasoplegia. Catecholamine infusion remains the first line of therapy for vasoplegic state, albeit differences exist among the choice of drug and timing of initiation of therapy. Dopamine, norepinephrine, epinephrine, phenylephrine, vasopressin, terlipressin, and angiotensin 2 are the few vasopressors that have been used in septic shock.

Dopamine has a dose-dependent effect on α-1, β-1 adrenergic and dopaminergic-1 receptors. It causes an increase in peripheral vascular tone, increased inotropic and chronotropic effects with higher dosages. Though stimulation of dopaminergic receptors has shown to maintain splanchnic and renal perfusion, it can also suppress the hypothalamic–pituitary axis, causing harmful immunological effects. Dopamine was routinely used as a first-line therapy in patients with septic shock. In a multivariate analysis, age, cancer, medical admissions, higher mean sequential organ failure assessment (SOFA) score, higher mean fluid balance, and dopamine administration were independent risk factors for ICU mortality in patients with shock.[39] In a large multicenter trial comparing the use of dopamine and norepinephrine as a first-line vasopressor in patients with

Flowchart 3: Central venous oxygen saturation (ScvO$_2$) and partial pressure of carbon dioxide (pCO$_2$) based resuscitation.

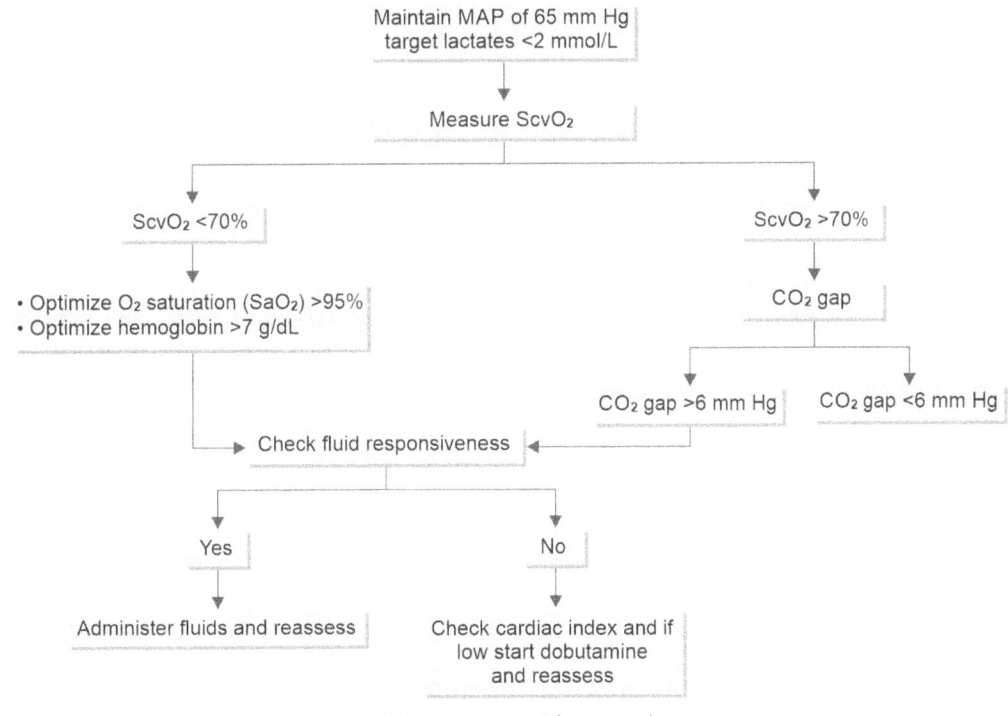

(MAP: mean arterial pressure)

septic shock, De Backer et al.,[40] showed that there was no difference in mortality in both groups (52.5% in the dopamine group and 48.5% in the norepinephrine group; odds ratio with dopamine, 1.17; 95% CI, 0.97–1.42; p = 0.10), albeit use of dopamine was associated with a higher incidence of arrhythmias and higher incidence of 28-day mortality in a subgroup of patients with cardiogenic shock. The higher risk of arrhythmias associated with dopamine precludes its use in septic shock.

SSC guidelines 2021 strongly *recommend* use of norepinephrine as the vasopressor of choice over others in septic shock because of its predominant peripheral vasoconstrictor property.[3] A meta-analysis comparing norepinephrine with dopamine showed that use of norepinephrine was associated with reduced mortality [risk ratio (RR) 0.89; 95% CI, 0.81–0.98], resulting in absolute risk reduction of 11%, and dopamine use resulted in an increased incidence of arrhythmias.[41] The same meta-analysis did not show any difference between norepinephrine and epinephrine (RR 0.96, 95% CI, 0.77–1.21, I^2 = 0%, n = 4) in terms of mortality. Epinephrine has been associated with increased lactate production due to stimulation of β-2-adrenergic receptors in skeletal muscles and therefore can preclude the use of lactate as a target resuscitation parameter.[3]

Vasopressin levels have been found to be inappropriately low in septic shock due to reduced baroreceptor-mediated release and depletion of secretory stores of neurohypophysis.[42] In a large randomized controlled trial [Vasopressin and Septic Shock Trial (VASST)], low-dose vasopressin (0.03 U/min) in addition to norepinephrine did not result in any improvement in mortality at 28 days (35.4 and 39.3%, respectively; p = 0.26; 95% CI for absolute risk reduction in the vasopressin group, −2.9 to 10.7%) and 90 days (43.9 and 49.6%, respectively; p = 0.11; 95% CI for absolute risk reduction, −1.3 to 12.8%), or organ functions.[43] There was a trend toward better survival in a subgroup of patients with low-dose norepinephrine (<15 µg) without any adverse effects. The VANISH trial[44] showed a reduced need for RRT in patients treated with vasopressin, but there was no difference in the incidence of renal failure-free days or mortality. Since no clear benefit has been shown in clinical trials with addition of epinephrine or vasopressin to norepinephrine, norepinephrine still remains the vasopressor of choice in vasodilatory shock. SSC 2021 suggests adding vasopressin instead of escalating the dose of norepinephrine in adults with septic shock where the MAP levels are inadequate on norepinephrine (usually when the norepinephrine dose ranges between 0.25 and 0.5 µg/kg/min) (weak recommendation).[3]

For adults with septic shock and inadequate MAP levels despite norepinephrine and vasopressin, SSC 2021 suggests adding epinephrine (weak recommendation). The suggestion by SSC 2021 is against the use of terlipressin for adults with septic shock because of no difference in mortality but an increased incidence of adverse consequences (digital ischemia, mesenteric ischemia, diarrhea) related to its use compared to norepinephrine in their meta-analysis.[3]

The United States FDA approved the use of angiotensin II for septic shock in 2017. The presence of hypovolemia and renal hypoperfusion in septic shock activates the renin–angiotensin–aldosterone system (RAAS), sympathetic nervous system, and hypothalamic–pituitary–adrenal axis, leading to excessive release of renin and angiotensin II. The angiotensin II, an octapeptide, has strong vasopressor activity and thereby increases BP. It also helps in maintaining glomerular filtration by preferentially constricting the efferent arteriole and increasing intraglomerular pressure. In a double blinded, randomized controlled trial, addition of angiotensin II to conventional high-dose vasopressors (0.2 μg/kg/min of norepinephrine or equivalent), resulted in achievement of MAP target in higher number of patients in the intervention group [114 of 163 patients, 69.9% vs. 37 of 158 patients, 23.4%, odds ratio (OR), 7.95; 95% CI, 4.76–13.3; $p <0.001$], better cardiovascular SOFA scores, and a trend toward improved mortality.[45] Because of the limited availability of a good-quality evidence and experience in sepsis, the SSC panel considered that angiotensin II should not be used as a first-line agent and that it may have a role as an adjunctive vasopressor therapy.[3]

Early administration of vasopressors not only reduces the amount of fluid administered in the first 24 hours but also increases the MAP and organ perfusion. In a retrospective analysis of 213 patients of septic shock, an increase in mortality by 5.3% was observed with every hour delay in administration of norepinephrine during the first 6 hours of resuscitation.[46] In a multicenter retrospective analysis of 6,514 patients, delay in administration of vasopressors was associated with a higher risk of mortality (adjusted OR 1.02/h, 95% CI 1.01–1.03, $p <0.001$).[47] The 1-hour bundle of SSC recommends use of vasopressors if the patient is hypotensive during or after fluid resuscitation to maintain MAP ≥65 mm Hg.

This patient had developed a global LV dysfunction with a drop of LVEF to 45%, which subsequently improved after 3 days.

Q8. Discuss septic cardiomyopathy (SCM) and the role of inotropes in septic shock.

Septic cardiomyopathy is a transient cardiac dysfunction due to sepsis resulting in impaired cardiac contractility. There is formal definition, but experts agree that it is an acute and reversible (usually within 7–10 days) uni- or biventricular systolic and/or diastolic cardiac dysfunction with decreased ejection fraction, which is not due to coronary disease. There is LV dilatation with normal or low filling pressure perhaps due to an increase in the LV compliance and increase in LV end-diastolic volume, and regional wall dysfunction is absent. The patients with SCM tend to be either hypokinetic or normokinetic, unlike those without SCM who tend to be hyperkinetic. It is different from Takotsubo cardiomyopathy (which can also be precipitated by sepsis), wherein the contractile function of the mid- to apical segments of the left ventricle is depressed, and there is hyperkinesis of basal walls causing apical ballooning.[48,49] The pathophysiology of SCM has been briefed in **Flowchart 4**.

Echocardiography remains the mainstay modality for diagnosis of SCM. Biomarkers such as cardiac troponin (cTn) and brain natriuretic peptide (BNP) correlate with illness severity and mortality in sepsis but are not diagnostic of SCM. Vieillard-Baron found that patients with a hyperkinetic profile (i.e., small LV, supranormal ejection fraction, tachycardia, high cardiac index), reflecting a persistent vasoplegic state, had a higher mortality rate (~100%) compared to patients who developed SCM with a hypo- or normokinetic profile.[50] Therapeutic interventions for SCM include fluid expansion to restore central blood volume and simultaneously avoid overload, inotropes, and vasopressors, particularly norepinephrine in the relevant subset.[48-50] Other adjunctive

Flowchart 4: Mechanisms of sepsis-induced cardiomyopathy. Endotoxins cause depressed cardiac contractility, which is mediated by enhanced nitric oxide (NO) production. Tumor necrosis factor and interleukin-1β also contribute to NO overproduction. NO is believed to act in the heart by decreasing myofibril response to calcium, inducing mitochondrial dysfunction, and downregulating β-adrenergic receptors. These reactions lead to sepsis-induced cardiomyopathy. Methylene blue, an inhibitor of the NO pathway, counteracts the myocardial depression. Histones occur inside the nucleus and can be released into circulation because of extensive inflammation and cellular death during sepsis. Since cardiac dysfunction can be ameliorated by antihistone antibodies in a septic mouse model, histones may be implicated in the pathophysiology of sepsis-induced cardiomyopathy.

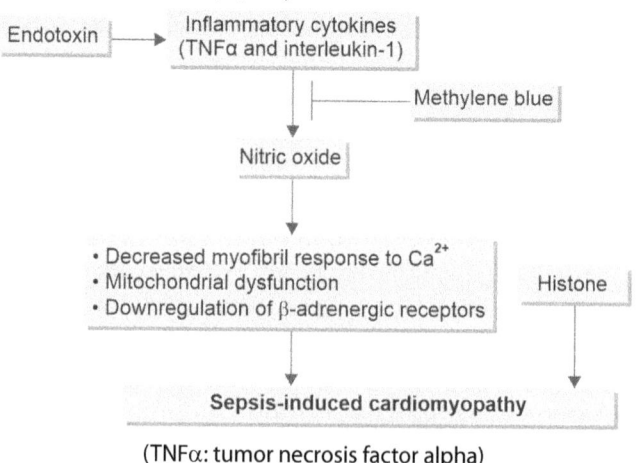

(TNFα: tumor necrosis factor alpha)
Source: Sato and Nasu (2015).[49]

treatment options include methylene blue (with no proven outcome benefit) and mechanical support in the form of intra-aortic balloon pump or venoarterial extracorporeal membrane oxygenation in select patients with refractory sepsis-induced cardiogenic shock, keeping in mind the high invasiveness and associated risk of complications.

SSC 2021 guidelines suggest either adding dobutamine to norepinephrine or using epinephrine alone in adults with septic shock and cardiac dysfunction with persistent hypoperfusion (persistent shock, lactic acidosis, and oliguria) despite adequate volume status and arterial BP.[3] Dobutamine helps by increasing LV ejection fraction and cardiac index, but it can increase myocardial demand, vasodilation may worsen hemodynamics, and its use may not be associated with improved outcomes.[48,49]

Levosimendan, an inodilator, is a calcium-sensitizing drug. The SSC 2021 panel has issued a weak recommendation against its use based on lack of benefit, safety profile, cost, and its limited availability.

Q9. What is the role of early source control in sepsis?

Every patient with sepsis and a potential amenable source of infection should be dealt with at the earliest. In a large observational study of 154 patients with gastrointestinal perforation, time to initiation of surgery was an independent predictor of mortality in multiple logistic regression analyses (OR, 0.29; 95% CI, 0.16–0.47; p <0.0001).[51] The survival rate fell as surgery initiation was delayed and was 0% for times >6 hours. Thus, all source control measures should be undertaken as early as possible, and prolonged medical management and resuscitative efforts without adequate source control might not be fruitful.

Prompt removal of intravascular access devices that are a possible source of sepsis or septic shock is recommended by SSC 2021 after other vascular access has been established.

Q10. Discuss sepsis-associated acute kidney injury (SA-AKI) and role of sodium bicarbonate in septic shock with metabolic acidosis.

It is not infrequent to see AKI in patients with sepsis. In fact, sepsis is responsible for 45–70% cases of AKI in critically ill patents. The presence of SA-AKI has been found to be having a poorer prognosis compared to either of the two entities separately. The 28th Acute Disease and Quality Initiative (ADQI) consensus statement defined SA-AKI as the occurrence of AKI within 7 days of sepsis onset [AKI diagnosed according to Kidney Disease Improving Global Outcome (KDIGO) criteria and sepsis as defined by the Sepsis-3 criteria].[52] AKI within 48 hours of sepsis diagnosis is referred to as early SA-AKI and that between 48 hours and 7days is referred to as late SA-AKI. The pathophysiology of SA-AKI has been summarized in **Flowchart 5**.

The 28th ADQI consensus suggests using validated functional, stress, and damage-related biomarkers in addition to KDIGO criteria to diagnose SA-AKI. It also suggests using selected functional and stress- or injury-related biomarkers for clinical assessment to identify and discriminate patients with sepsis at risk of transient or persistent SA-AKI (**Table 2**).[52,53]

Management of SA-AKI: Hemodynamic management should be done as recommended by SSC 2021 guidelines. Dynamic measures of fluid responsiveness should preferably be used to assess the need for fluid administration. It is recommended by the 28th ADQI consensus to perform daily and cumulative fluid balance monitoring and depending upon the severity and progression, strict UOP and renal function monitoring should be done. The choice of fluid should be guided by the acid–base and electrolyte imbalances, and the balanced salt solutions and normal saline should be used for resuscitation accordingly. The recent BaSICS and PLUS trials and meta-analysis found no clinical benefit of balanced solutions over the use of 0.9% saline solutions.[54,55] The recommendation is against the use of starch, gelatin, and dextran; however, albumin and bicarbonate can be used on a per-patient basis.

Severe metabolic acidosis causes myocardial dysfunction, peripheral vasodilation, and impaired response to catecholamines, leading to further hemodynamic instability. Treatment of the underlying disease process is the cornerstone for the management of metabolic acidosis. Administration of bicarbonate can increase the extracellular acidemia but might worsen intracellular acidosis by increasing the production of CO_2, thus resulting in fluid overload and ionized hypocalcemia. The impact of alkali administration on reducing vasopressor requirements, improving hemodynamics, and overall outcomes is not known. A recent analysis from a large database of patients with metabolic acidosis showed that the use of sodium bicarbonate did not improve mortality in the overall population (HR 1.07, 95% CI 0.95–1.19; p = 0.264), but a trend toward better outcomes was noted in patients with stage 2, stage 3 acute kidney injury, and in patients with severe metabolic acidosis (pH <7.2).[56] Large, prospective trials are needed to settle the debate on the use of sodium bicarbonate in sepsis with metabolic acidosis. SSC 2021 suggests that sodium bicarbonate therapy can be used for adults with septic shock and severe metabolic acidemia (pH ≤7.2) and acute kidney injury [Acute Kidney Injury Network (AKIN) score 2 or 3].[3]

Depending upon the hemodynamic status of the patients, vasopressors, inotropes, and diuretics can be used, norepinephrine being the vasopressor of choice; however, in certain subtypes of SA-AKI, others such as vasopressin

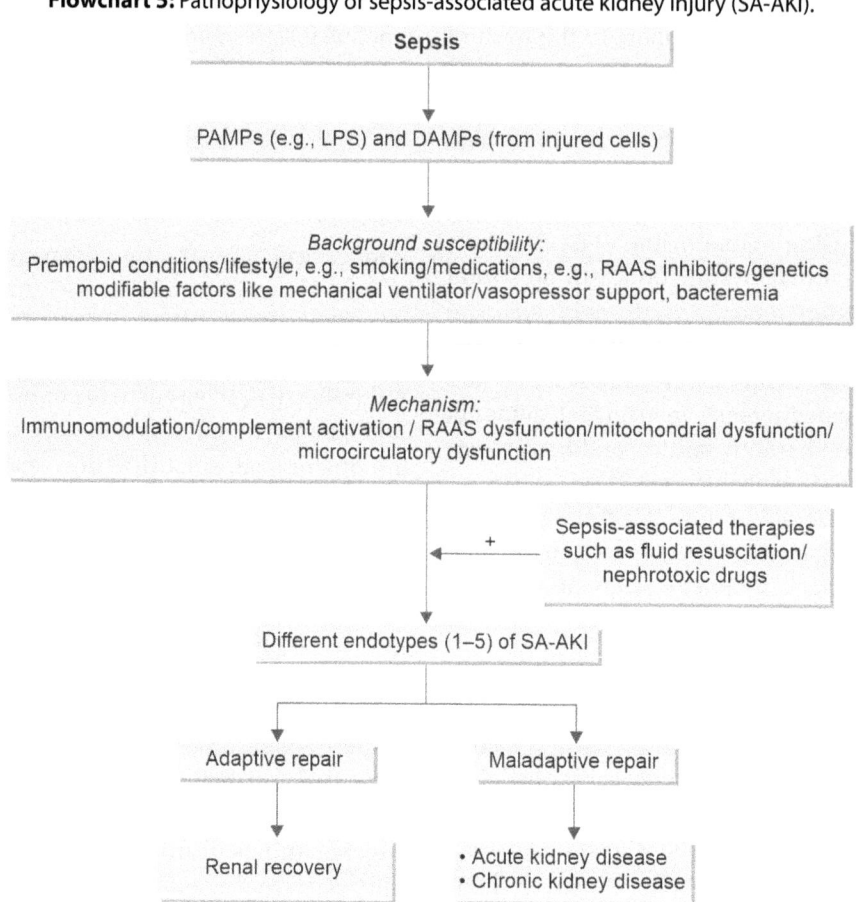

Flowchart 5: Pathophysiology of sepsis-associated acute kidney injury (SA-AKI).

(DAMP: damage-associated molecular pattern; LPS: lipopolysaccharide; PAMP: pathogen-associated molecular pattern; RAAS: renin–angiotensin–aldosterone system)

or angiotensin II may be preferred. In patients with fluid overload, it is recommended to use diuretics. Initiation of RRT in SA-AKI should be done as in AKI due to other causes, and extracorporeal blood purification techniques to remove pathogens, toxins, inflammatory mediators, and immunomodulatory support may be considered.[52]

Q11. What is the role of steroids in sepsis and septic shock?

Sepsis is associated with intense inflammatory activity. Both pro- and anti-inflammatory mediators are produced in response to pathogen invasion. Proinflammatory cytokines have been shown to inhibit adrenocorticotropic hormone (ACTH) secretion, suppress intracellular glucocorticoid function, and also cause peripheral steroid resistance, leading to adrenal failure.[57] Corticosteroid deficiency can cause vasopressor-refractory shock and precipitate organ failure. The major role played by steroids in inflammation and high incidence of corticosteroid insufficiency in septic shock leads to the use of steroids in sepsis, especially septic shock.

In the Hydrocortisone for Prevention of Septic Shock (HYPRESS) trial,[58] use of continuous infusion of hydrocortisone (200 mg) for 5 days followed by tapering dose till day 11 did not prevent the development of shock at 14 days. There was also no difference in other patient outcomes, but the treatment group had a higher incidence of infection and weaning failure. Due to lack of evidence, steroids are not recommended in patients with sepsis without shock.

In a Cochrane review of 33 randomized trials, use of corticosteroids was associated with reduced 28-day mortality (RR 0.87, 95% CI, 0.76–1.00; $p = 0.05$, random-effects model).[59] The quality of evidence was very low due to heterogeneity, inconsistency among trials, and imprecision. Use of steroids was associated with better shock reversal, better organ function scores, and reduced stay in intensive care, without any serious adverse effects such as gastrointestinal bleeding, superinfection, or neuromuscular weakness. Use of steroids was associated with an increased risk of metabolic derangements such as hypernatremia and hyperglycemia. A subsequent meta-analysis did not show any mortality benefit with any dose of corticosteroids in septic shock.[60] No specific steroid (hydrocortisone, dexamethasone, methylprednisolone) has been found to

TABLE 2: Biomarkers associated with acute kidney injury (AKI).[52,53]

Type of biomarker	Biomarker subclass	Parameters	Comments and utility
Functional	• Glomerular function/filtration biochemical biomarker	• Serum creatinine	• Most commonly used biomarker. Used to define AKI
		• Serum or urine cystatin C	• FDA approved
		• Plasma proenkephalin (penKID)	• Not FDA approved
	• Nephron function global assessment biomarker	• Urine output	
	• Nephron capacity	• Frusemide stress test 2-hour urine output • Renal reserve testing	• Validated for prediction of worsening AKI in critically ill patients
Damage biomarkers	• Nephron injury global assessment	• Urine microscopy	• Can detect injury along the entire nephron (from glomerulus to tubules). Urine microscopy scores are there but still not validated
		• Dipstick albuminuria	• Point of care, cheap, as an initial screening tool for kidney disease
	• Renal tubular injury biochemical biomarker	• Urinary/serum NGAL	• Rises in sepsis and inflammation. Peaks 4–6 hours after renal tubular injury
		• Urinary KIM-1 • Soluble Fas	• FDA approved. Increase 12–24 hours after tubular injury, peaking at 2–3 days
AKI stress biomarkers	Biochemical biomarker	Urine TIMP2*IGFBP7	FDA approved. It is supposed to predict the risk of developing stage 2–3 AKI within 12 hours of assessment
Others		• FeNa	• Differentiates prerenal AKI from renal tubular injury
		• Renal resistive index	• On doppler ultrasound, to monitor vascular and renal parenchymal disease
		• Infrarenal venous flow	• On doppler ultrasound, to assess renal congestion

(FDA: Food and Drug Administration; FeNa: fractional excretion of sodium; KIM-1: kidney injury molecule-1; NGAL: neutrophil gelatinase-associated lipocalin)

be superior to other in patients with septic shock in terms of mortality, though shock reversal was better with boluses or infusion of hydrocortisone.[61] The recent guidelines for management of corticosteroid insufficiency in critical illness have recommended low dose and short duration of hydrocortisone (<400 mg/day for 3 days) in septic shock with a low quality of evidence.[62]

The recently published ADRENAL trial did not show any mortality benefit with use of hydrocortisone at 90 days (27.9% in the hydrocortisone group vs. 28.8% in the placebo group, OR 0.95; 95% CI; 0.82–1.10; $p = 0.50$).[63] In a multicenter trial, addition of fludrocortisone 50 µg once a day with hydrocortisone 50 mg every 6 hours, in patients with high-dose vasopressors, was associated with significant reduction of mortality at 90 days (43.0 vs. 49.1%, relative risk of 0.88 at 95% CI)[64] without serious adverse effects.

The SSC guidelines 2021 suggest using intravenous hydrocortisone 200 mg/day for adults with septic shock and an ongoing requirement for vasopressor therapy (to be started when the dose of norepinephrine or epinephrine is ≥0.25 µg/kg/min and at least 4 hours after initiation).[3]

Q12. Discuss the role of adjuvant therapies such as ulinastatin, CytoSorb®, and polymyxin hemoperfusion in the management of patients with septic shock.

Polymyxin B and CytoSorb® hemoadsorption: Extracorporeal blood purification techniques have been used based on the concept that removal of inflammatory cytokines, endotoxins, or both will modulate the host immune response and provide better outcomes in sepsis and septic shock.

Hemoadsorption or hemoperfusion techniques place the blood in direct contact with sorbents which attracts solutes by various chemical mechanisms such as hydrophobic interaction, ionic bonding, van der Waals interaction, and hydrogen bonding. Polymyxin B-derived immobilized fibers, with high molecular weight adsorption potential, have been used for endotoxin removal. The Early Use of Polymyxin B Hemoperfusion in Abdominal Sepsis

(EUPHAS) multicenter trial,[65] conducted in 10 Italian ICUs, in patients in septic shock after emergency laparotomy for intra-abdominal sepsis, showed a significant reduction in mortality (32 vs. 53%, $p = 0.03$) with two treatment sessions of polymyxin hemoadsorption. But the benefit has not been replicated in subsequent studies. In a multicenter trial in French ICUs, use of two sessions of polymyxin hemoperfusion after abdominal emergency surgery for peritonitis did not show any improvement in organ function scores, with a trend toward increased mortality [27.7 vs. 19.5% ($n = 113$), $p = 0.14$ (OR 1.5872, 95% CI 0.8583–2.935] in the intervention group, though nonsignificant.[66] In a recent meta-analysis of six trials (857 patients), use of polymyxin B hemoperfusion did not show any mortality benefit (the pooled RR was 1.03, 95% CI 0.78–1.36; $n = 797$) in patients with sepsis and septic shock. There was no difference in organ dysfunction scores over 24–72 hours after the intervention (standardized mean difference –0.26; 95% CI –0.64 to 0.12, $n = 797$), though the heterogeneity between the trials was high ($I^2 = 78\%$).[67] In the recently concluded EUPHRATES multicenter trial, use of polymyxin hemoadsorption did not show any improvement in mortality [37.7% (84 of 223) in the polymyxin group vs. 34.5% (78 of 226)] in the sham group [risk difference (RD), 3.2%; 95% CI, –5.7% to 12.0%; relative risk (RR), 1.09; 95% CI, 0.85–1.39; $p = .49$]. There was no improvement in mortality in patients with multiorgan failure [44.5% (65 of 146)] in the polymyxin B hemoperfusion group and [43.9% (65 of 148)] in the sham group (RD, 0.6%; 95% CI, –10.8% to 11.9%; RR, 1.01; 95% CI, 0.78–1.31; $p = .92$).[68]

CytoSorb® is a cartridge made of biocompatible polystyrene divinyl benzene copolymer beads, which adsorbs cytokines. In experimental studies, CytoSorb® use has been associated with significant reduction posttreatment cytokine levels, especially interleukin-6 (IL-6), IL-10, and tumor necrosis factor-α (TNF-α). Its use has been associated with improved survival in experimental animals. In a case series of 26 critically ill patients with septic shock, use of CytoSorb® was associated with better hemodynamic stability (reduction in vasopressor dosage by 67%) and reduction in blood lactate levels by 26.4%.[69] Early administration of CytoSorb® was associated with better outcomes. In a randomized controlled trial of patients with septic shock, treatment with CytoSorb for 6 hours a day for 7 consecutive days did not result in reduction of plasma IL-6 levels post treatment. The treatment arm had significantly higher mortality (44.7 vs. 26%, $p = 0.039$).[70]

Due to conflicting and insufficient evidence, SSC 2021 guidelines suggest against using polymyxin B hemoperfusion and have made no recommendation on the use of other blood purification techniques for adults with sepsis or septic shock.[3]

Ulinastatin: Ulinastatin, a serine protease inhibitor, is secreted by degradation of inter-α-trypsin inhibitors by neutrophil elastase. By inhibiting serine proteases, ulinastatin blunts the rise of proinflammatory cytokines and also inhibits secretion of proinflammatory cytokines such as IL-6 and IL-8. It also downregulates thromboxane B2 production and modulates TNF-α mediated hypotension, thereby appearing to play a role in the prevention of organ failure.

Though early use of ulinastatin has been associated with good outcomes in patients with severe acute pancreatitis, severe burns, and postcardiopulmonary bypass surgery, the data in sepsis and septic shock are not convincing. In a randomized controlled trial, use of ulinastatin (200,000 IU units twice daily for 5 days) within 48 hours of onset of shock was associated with lower organ failures, more ventilator-free days, without any improvement in mortality [10.2% (6/59 deaths) with ulinastatin vs. 20.6% (13/63 deaths) in the placebo group; $p = 0.11$].[71] Immunomodulation using combination of ulinastatin and thymosin α1 has been shown to reduce organ failure and improve outcomes in few small trials.[72]

Q13. Discuss sepsis-associated encephalopathy (SAE).
Sepsis-associated encephalopathy is a multifactorial syndrome, characterized as diffuse cerebral dysfunction induced by the dysregulated host response to the infection without clinical or laboratory evidence of direct brain infection or other types of encephalopathy.[73] The important feature of SAE is a generalized cerebral dysfunction with absence of any focal neurological deficit. Presence of sepsis, particularly extracranial infection, and an impaired mental state (especially awareness and cognition) are a prerequisite to make a diagnosis of SAE.[73]

Uncontrolled neuroinflammation and ischemic injury are the two main mechanisms involved in the development of brain injury. Inflammatory mediators, disruption of blood–brain barrier (BBB), alterations in neurotransmitters, mitochondrial dysfunction, and schema are among the different factors involved. In the pathogenesis, however, the specific mechanism of SAE development is not known[74] **(Flowchart 6)**. SAE acts as a vicious cycle of immunosuppression **(Fig. 1)**. Understanding the pathophysiology will help to define a strategy to interfere with the brain injury and identify a potential target to reverse the immunosuppression. The treatment mainly comprises management of sepsis and any potential neurotoxic factors. Other nonpharmacological interventions include early mobilization, sedation discontinuation, etc.

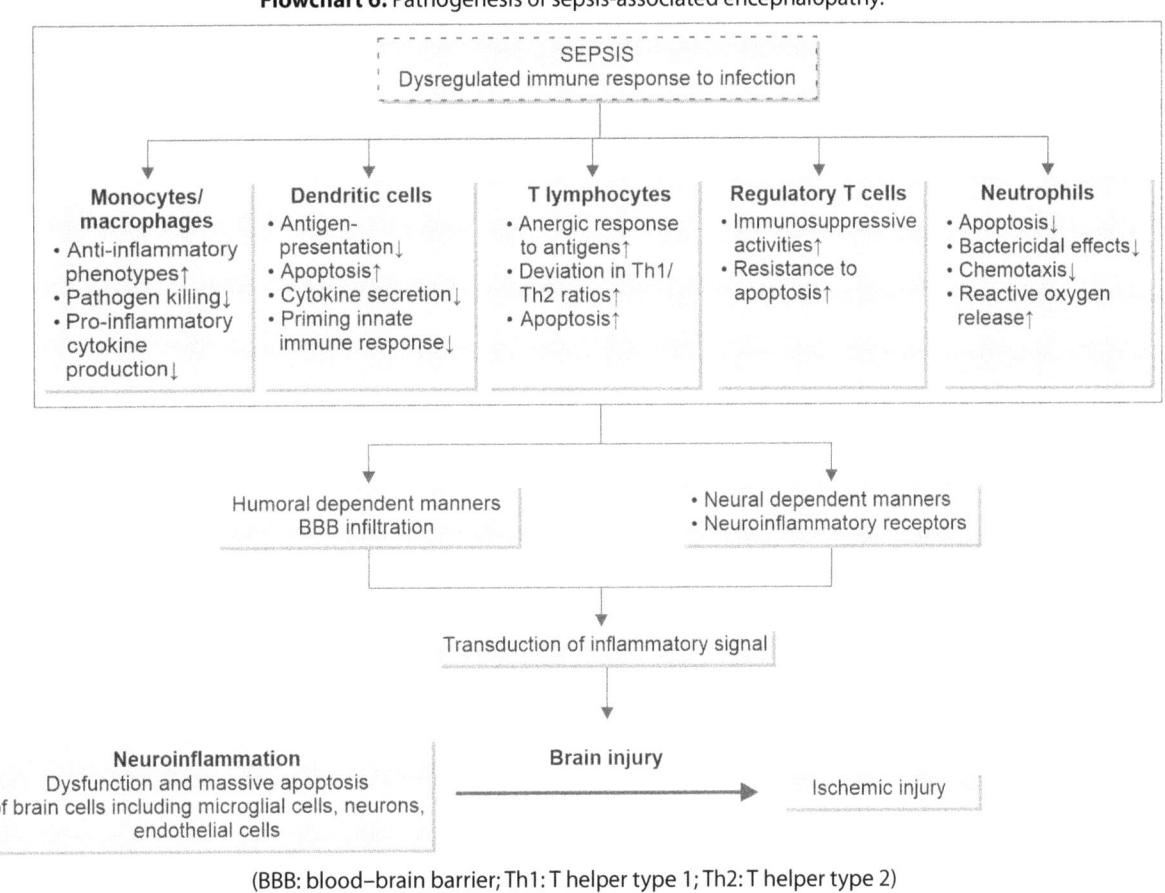

Flowchart 6: Pathogenesis of sepsis-associated encephalopathy.

(BBB: blood–brain barrier; Th1: T helper type 1; Th2: T helper type 2)
Source: Ren et al. (2020).[74]

Q14. On the second day of his ICU admission, this patient had a platelet count of $100 \times 10^9/L$ and prothrombin time-international normalized ratio (PT-INR) of 1.6. What do you attribute this to? What is sepsis-induced coagulopathy (SIC) and how is it different from disseminated intravascular coagulation (DIC)?

On the basis of the clinical history and the SIC criteria, this patient has SIC.

Coagulopathy in patients with sepsis is a dynamic phenomenon beginning with coagulation disorder, which may progress to SIC and further to overt DIC, which is the decompensated coagulation disorder[75] **(Flowchart 7)**.

The International Society on Thrombosis and Haemostasis (ISTH) scientific standardization subcommittee defined DIC in 2001 as "an acquired syndrome characterized by intravascular activation of coagulation with loss of localization arising from different causes that can originate from and cause damage to the microvasculature, which if sufficiently severe, can produce organ dysfunction." The laboratory criteria for diagnosis of DIC have been discussed and compared with the SIC criteria given by ISTH SSC and the Japanese Association for Acute Medicine (JAAM) DIC criteria in **Table 3**. The JAAM DIC criteria, however, need revision as they include systemic inflammatory response syndrome (SIRS) as one of the parameters which has been removed from the Sepsis-3.0 definition. Various DIC criteria were compared by Wang et al., and they did not find any difference in the AUC for these diagnostic criteria. The SIC criteria are the simplest among all, and it has been found in studies that most overt DIC patients were previously diagnosed with SIC criteria. The idea behind the SIC criteria is to timely diagnose DIC and initiate anticoagulant therapy. In a retrospective study, patients with SIC based on SIC criteria have been found to be good candidates for heparin therapy. The limitation of SIC criteria is that it can misdiagnose other conditions that mimic SIC. The differential diagnosis of SIC includes thrombotic thrombocytopenic purpura (TTP), atypical hemolytic uremic syndrome (aHUS), heparin-induced thrombocytopenia (HIT), hemophagocytic syndrome, and antiphospholipid antibody syndrome. The treatment of sepsis-associated DIC includes management of underlying disease, optimizing tissue perfusion, and a possible role of anticoagulant therapy in high disease severity patients. Heparin is the most commonly used anticoagulant

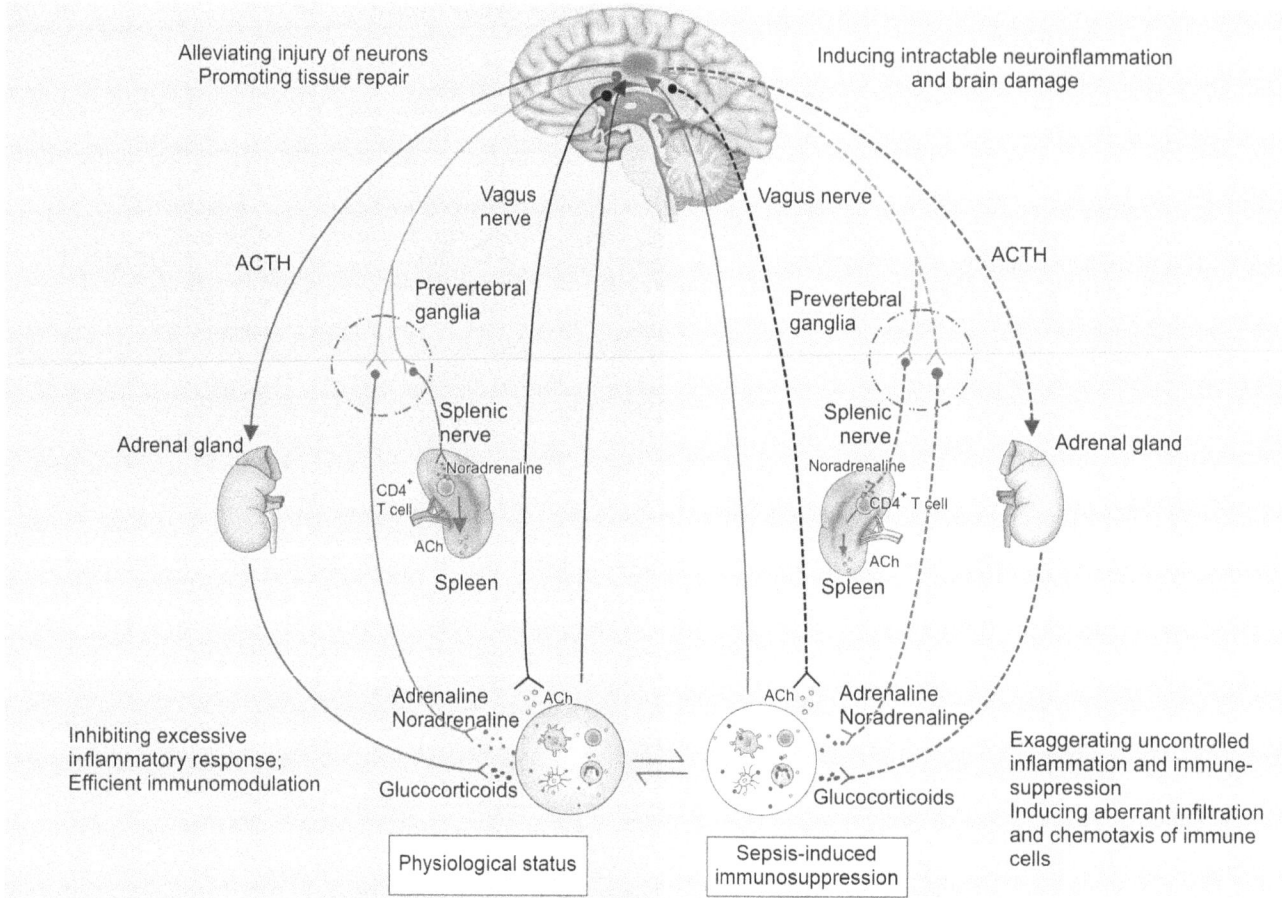

Fig. 1: Sepsis-associated encephalopathy (SAE): A vicious cycle of sepsis-induced immunosuppression. In the physiological condition, the brain – hypothalamic–pituitary–adrenal (HPA) axis, sympathetic and parasympathetic nervous system, maintain homeostasis, inhibiting excessive inflammation and enabling efficient immunomodulation. Appropriate infiltration of immune cells into the central nervous system is beneficial for functional integrity and viability of neurons. However, sepsis-induced immunosuppression leads to intractable neuroinflammation, resulting in serious cognitive impairment. (ACh: acetylcholine; ACTH: adrenocorticotropic hormone)
Source: Ren et al. (2020).[74]

among all in patients with SIC. Use of recombinant thrombomodulin and antithrombin has been recommended by the Japanese sepsis guidelines.[75,76] However, there is no robust/international evidence to support their efficacy, and SSC 2021 guidelines do not support their use for SIC. Further studies are needed regarding therapeutic agents in SIC to improve the outcomes.

Q15. What is symmetric peripheral gangrene (SPG)?
Tissue necrosis that involves the distal extremities bilaterally is known as SPG. It is not a very frequent phenomenon but can be seen in critically ill patients. When there is predominantly a nonacral necrosis, it is termed purpura fulminans (PF). Circulatory shock, DIC, and profound natural anticoagulant depletion are the key features that have been observed in these patients.[77] **(Table 4)**. Knight et al., defined SPG as symmetrical distal ischemic damage in two or more sites in the absence of major vascular occlusive disease.[78]

The treatment options for prevention of SPG/procoagulant-anticoagulant misbalance include administration of unfractionated heparin (FDA approved for DIC; associated with risk of fatal bleeding in severe DIC), low molecular weight heparin for thromboprophylaxis, antithrombin III and protein C concentrates (but availability of concentrates and measurements is a limiting factor), plasma infusion or exchange. However, none of these therapies have been proven to be efficacious in SPG.[77]

Q16. What are multidrug resistant (MDR), extensively drug resistant (XDR), and pan drug resistant (PDR) organisms? What is their significance? How does the infection with each of these organisms affect the ICU outcomes?
Multidrug resistance is defined as resistance or nonsusceptibility to at least one agent in three or more antimicrobial categories. XDR is defined as resistance

or nonsusceptibility to at least one agent in all but two or lesser antimicrobial categories (i.e., bacterial isolates remain susceptible to only one or two categories). PDR is defined as resistance or nonsusceptibility to all agents in all antimicrobial categories (i.e., no agents tested as susceptible for that organism). Intrinsic resistance of organisms (*Providencia* for aminoglycosides, Proteus for tigecycline and polymyxins, *Citrobacter* for aminopenicillins and cefazolin) for a specific class of antimicrobial should be taken in consideration before identifying a particular organism as MDR or XDR.[79]

The World Health Organization, in its global report on surveillance of antimicrobial resistance, reported an extremely high risk of fluoroquinolone and third-generation cephalosporin resistance *E. coli* and *Klebsiella* (>50%), with certain countries reporting alarming rates (>50%) of carbapenem resistance. Inappropriate use of antimicrobials is the most common risk factor for acquired antimicrobial resistance. Mechanical ventilation, length of stay in ICU and hospital, the severity of illness, recent surgery, and invasive procedures are other factors that contribute to antimicrobial resistance.[80]

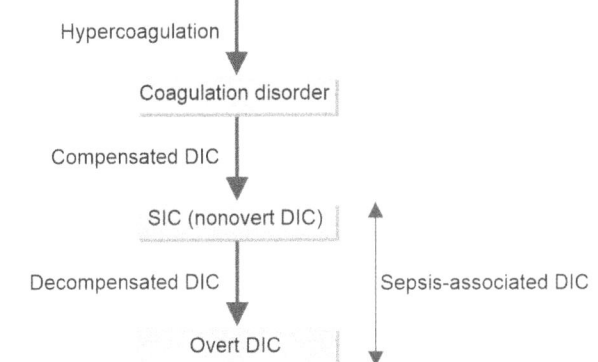

Flowchart 7: Initiation and advancement of coagulation disorder in sepsis.

(DIC: disseminated intravascular coagulation; SIC: sepsis-induced coagulopathy)
Source: Iba et al. (2023).[75]

TABLE 4: Symmetric peripheral gangrene (SPG) in critical illness—characteristics.

DIC state	As in circulatory shock, mainly the cardiogenic and/or septic shock
Natural anticoagulant depletion	Consumptive coagulopathy (DIC), shock liver, chronic liver disease, colloid transfusion causing hemodilution. Implicated anticoagulants include protein C activity <20%, protein S, antithrombin activity <40%
Localizing features	Distal extremities, because of the reduced blood flow. Begins 2–5 days after the onset of shock liver
Pathophysiology	Microthrombi formation

(DIC: disseminated intravascular coagulation)

TABLE 3: Comparison of overt disseminated intravascular coagulation (DIC) versus sepsis-induced coagulopathy (SIC) scoring systems.[75,76]

Parameter	Points	ISTH overt DIC	SIC	JAAM-DIC
Platelet count (×10⁹/L)	3	–	–	<80 or ≥50% decrease within 24 hours
	2	<50	<100	–
	1	50–100	100–150	80–120 or ≥30% decrease within 24 hours
FDP or D-dimer	3	Strong increase	–	≥25 µg/mL
	2	Moderate increase	–	–
	1	–	–	10–25 µg/mL
PT-INR	2	≥6 seconds	>1.4 (PT-INR)	–
	1	3–6 seconds	1.2–1.4	≥1.2 (PT ratio)
Fibrinogen (g/L)	1	<1	–	–
Total SOFA score	2	–	≥2	–
	1	–	1	–
Total score		≥5 (overt DIC)	≥4 (SIC)	≥4 (JAAM-DIC)

Note: Total SOFA includes respiratory, cardiovascular, hepatic and renal SOFA.

(FDP: fibrin degradation product; ISTH: International Society on Thrombosis and Haemostasis; JAAM: Japanese Association for Acute Medicine; PT-INR: prothrombin time-international normalized ratio; SOFA: sequential organ failure assessment)

In a prospective observational study of patients with ICU-acquired pneumonia, infection with MDR organisms was associated with significantly higher mortality (OR 2.89; p <0.05; 95% CI) and longer stay in the ICU.[81]

Q17. What are ESBLs? What is their significance? Describe Ambler classification of β-lactamases. Differentiate between AmpC, ESBL, and New Delhi metallo-β-lactamase (NDM).

The ESBL stands for extended-spectrum β-lactamase.

Classification of β-lactamases: Ambler classification divides β-lactamases into four groups (A, B, C, and D) based upon their amino acid sequence. Classes A, C, and D belong to serine β-lactamases group and class B belongs to metallo-β-lactamases (MBLs), which require bivalent zinc ion for substrate hydrolysis. MBL have a broader substrate spectrum and can hydrolyze virtually all existing β-lactams except the monobactams. Based on the primary amino acid sequence, MBL are subdivided into three classes (B1, B2, and B3).[82]

Recently, Bush and Jacoby have proposed a functional classification of β-lactamases, based on selective resistance of different classes of β-lactam antibiotics.[83] Accordingly, β-lactamases are classified into three groups—group 1 (Ambler class C) cephalosporinases; group 2 (Ambler classes A and D) broad-spectrum, inhibitor-resistant, and extended-spectrum β-lactamases and serine carbapenemases; and group 3 MBLs.

Difference between ESBL, Amp C, and NDM-1: Extended-spectrum β-lactamase is an enzyme that hydrolyzes β-lactam ring of various antibiotics, rendering the bacteria resistant to the various classes of antibiotics. Various types of ESBL are explained in **Table 5**.[84] Infection caused by ESBL organisms are increasing both in the hospital environment and in the community. In the United States, the incidence of ESBL-producing strains of *E. coli* increased from 7.8% in 2010 to 18.3% in 2014, but this was as high as 27.7% for strains representing hospital-acquired infection in 2014, the majority of which produced CTX type.[85] A meta-analysis of 16 studies showed increased mortality in patients with ESBL bloodstream infections (relative risk, 1.85; p <0.001).[86] Strict infection control policies with restricted antibiotic policy should be in place to reduce the increasing burden of resistant organisms.

AmpC β-lactamases are important cephalosporinases (Ambler class C, Bush and Jacoby group 1) encoded by Enterobacteriaceae and few other organisms. The enzymes are located in bacterial periplasm. AmpC enzymes can hydrolyze many cephalosporins including cephamycins such as cefoxitin and cefotetan; oxyimino-cephalosporins such as ceftazidime, cefotaxime, and ceftriaxone; and monobactams such as aztreonam and most penicillins. Inhibition of murine biosynthesis of bacterial cell wall leads to a significant increase in induction of AmpC enzyme by a complex mechanism. Bacteria with AmpC β-lactamases can be successfully treated with carbapenems.[87]

New Delhi metallo-β-lactamase-1 is a carbapenemase (Ambler class B, Bush and Jacoby Group 3) that rapidly hydrolyzes the carbapenem antibiotics including meropenem and imipenem, apart from cephalosporins such as ceftazidime, cefotaxime, and cefpirome. In contrast, NDM-1 is susceptible to tigecycline and monobactam. The enzymes are plasmid coded, rendering them hazardous as they can easily be transferred to other microorganisms by horizontal gene transfer. Up to 17 different variants of NDM-1 have been isolated. Bacteria with NDM-1 can be treated with tigecycline and aztreonam.[88,89]

The latest IDSA 2023 guidelines on the treatment of antimicrobial resistant gram-negative infections are summarized in **Table 6**.[90]

Q18. What contact precautions will you observe in ICUs for patients with proven infections with MDR organisms?

All patients in ICU should ideally be screened for colonization with resistant organisms such as MRSA (methicillin-resistant *Staphylococcus aureus*), VRE

TABLE 5: Various examples of extended-spectrum β-lactamases (ESBLs).

Type	Substrate antibiotics	Susceptible antibiotics (not hydrolyzed) and inhibition
Temoneira (TEM)	• Penicillin • First generation of cephalosporin	Oxyimino-cephalosporins (ceftazidime, cefotaxime, ceftriaxone)
Sulfhydryl variable (SHV)	• Penicillin • Piperacillin • Tigecycline	Oxyimino-cephalosporins
Cefotaxime (CTX)	Stronger ability to hydrolyze cefotaxime	Can be inhibited by tazobactam
Oxacillin (OXA)	Oxacillin and cloxacillin	Cannot be inhibited by clavulanate

TABLE 6: Infectious Diseases Society of America (IDSA) multidrug resistance gram-negative bacteria (MDR-GNB) 2023 guidelines.[90]

Condition	Preferred line of treatment	Alternative agents	Additional information
Extended-spectrum β-lactamase-producing Enterobacterales (ESBL-E)			
Uncomplicated cystitis	Nitrofurantoin and trimethoprim–sulfamethoxazole (TMP–SMX)—safe and effective	• Carbapenems and the fluoroquinolones (ciprofloxacin or levofloxacin)—preserve for future, avoid toxicities • Single-dose aminoglycosides—no strong data • Single-dose oral fosfomycin—only against ESBL-E cystitis caused by *E. coli*	
Pyelonephritis and cUTI	TMP–SMX, ciprofloxacin, or levofloxacin—achieve adequate and sustained concentrations in the urine	• Ertapenem, meropenem, and imipenem–cilastatin: When resistance or toxicities prevent use of TMP–SMX or fluoroquinolones, or early in the treatment course if a patient is critically ill • Aminoglycosides	Fosfomycin and nitrofurantoin do not achieve adequate concentrations in the renal parenchyma and are *not* advised for pyelonephritis or cUTI
Infections outside of the urinary tract	• Carbapenems—meropenem, imipenem–cilastatin, or ertapenem • For patients who are critically ill and/or hypoalbuminemic, meropenem or imipenem–cilastatin is preferred. Ertapenem is highly protein bound. In above states, the free fraction of ertapenem increases, leading to a decrease in the serum half-life	• Consider transitioning to oral TMP–SMX, ciprofloxacin, or levofloxacin, if susceptible, and appropriate clinical response is achieved • Ceftazidime–avibactam, meropenem–vaborbactam, imipenem–cilastatin–relebactam, and cefiderocol: Reserved for infections caused by organisms exhibiting carbapenem resistance	• Avoid oral step-down to nitrofurantoin, fosfomycin, amoxicillin–clavulanate, doxycycline, or omadacycline for ESBL-E bloodstream infections • Piperacillin–tazobactam and cefepime are *not* to be given, even if susceptibility to piperacillin–tazobactam is demonstrated
AmpC β-lactamase-producing Enterobacterales (AmpC-E)			
• *Enterobacter cloacae* complex, *Klebsiella aerogenes*, and *Citrobacter freundii* are the most common Enterobacterales at moderate to high risk for clinically significant AmpC production • β-Lactam antibiotics have the potential for inducing *AmpC* genes. Aminopenicillins (i.e., amoxicillin, ampicillin), narrow-spectrum (i.e., first generation) cephalosporins, and cephamycins are potent *AmpC* inducers			
Uncomplicated cystitis	Nitrofurantoin or TMP–SMX	Aminoglycosides (for uncomplicated cystitis, pyelonephritis, and cUTI caused by AmpC-E)	• Ceftazidime–avibactam, meropenem–vaborbactam, imipenem–cilastatin–relebactam, and cefiderocol be preferentially reserved for treating infections caused by organisms exhibiting carbapenem resistance • Piperacillin–tazobactam/ceftolozane–tazobactam not to be used as a treatment option for AmpC-E infection
Invasive infections	TMP–SMX or fluoroquinolones		
Carbapenem-resistant Enterobacterales (CRE)			
Infection with Enterobacterales without carbapenemase production	If susceptible to meropenem and imipenem (i.e., MICs ≤1 µg/mL), but are not susceptible to ertapenem (i.e., MICs ≥1 µg/mL), the use of extended-infusion meropenem (or imipenem–cilastatin) is suggested		

Contd...

Contd...

Condition	Preferred line of treatment	Alternative agents	Additional information
Uncomplicated cystitis	Nitrofurantoin, TMP–SMX, ciprofloxacin, or levofloxacin	A single dose of an aminoglycoside, oral fosfomycin (for *E. coli* only), colistin, ceftazidime–avibactam, meropenem–vaborbactam, imipenem–cilastatin–relebactam, cefiderocol	Polymyxin B should not be used as treatment for uncomplicated CRE cystitis, due to its predominantly nonrenal clearance
Pyelonephritis and cUTI	• TMP–SMX, ciprofloxacin, or levofloxacin, if susceptible • Ceftazidime–avibactam, meropenem–vaborbactam, imipenem–cilastatin–relebactam, and cefiderocol	Aminoglycosides	
Infections outside of the urinary tract, when carbapenemase testing results are either not available or negative	• Ceftazidime–avibactam, meropenem–vaborbactam, and imipenem–cilastatin–relebactam • For a patient with CRE infection within previous 12 months, or a previous metallo-β-lactamase (MBL)-producing organisms, combination of ceftazidime–avibactam plus aztreonam, or cefiderocol as monotherapy should be preferred while AST results to newer β-lactam agents and carbapenemase testing are awaited	• Tigecycline or eravacycline (CRE infections not involving the bloodstream or urinary tract). Activity is independent of the presence or type of carbapenemase • Minocycline-use with caution	• Ceftazidime–avibactam has activity against most KPC- and OXA-48-like-producing CRE isolates • Meropenem–vaborbactam and imipenem–cilastatin–relebactam are active against CRE with KPC but not against OXA-48-like. None of these have activity against MBL. But CRE with KPC has been found to be the most common. So in the absence of carbapenemase testing, these are the suggested antibiotics • The panel advises against the use of extended-infusion carbapenems with or without the addition of a second agent for the treatment of CRE infections
Infections outside of the urinary tract caused by CRE with KPC production	Meropenem–vaborbactam, ceftazidime–avibactam, and imipenem–cilastatin–relebactam	Cefiderocol	
Infections outside of the urinary tract caused by CRE with NDM production	Ceftazidime–avibactam plus aztreonam or cefiderocol	• Tigecycline or eravacycline (CRE infections not involving the bloodstream or urinary tract). Activity is independent of the presence or type of carbapenemase • Minocycline—use with caution	
Infections outside of the urinary tract caused by CRE with OXA-48	Ceftazidime–avibactam	• Cefiderocol • Tigecycline or eravacycline (CRE infections not involving the bloodstream or urinary tract). Activity is independent of the presence or type of carbapenemase • Minocycline—use with caution	

Polymyxin B and colistin are not suggested for the treatment of infections caused by CRE. Combination antibiotic therapy (a β-lactam agent in combination with an aminoglycoside, fluoroquinolone, tetracycline, or polymyxin) is not suggested for the treatment of infections caused by CRE

Contd...

Contd...

Condition	Preferred line of treatment	Alternative agents	Additional information
Pseudomonas aeruginosa with difficult-to-treat resistance (DTR)			
Infections caused by MDR *P. aeruginosa*	• If susceptible to both traditional noncarbapenem β-lactam agents (i.e., piperacillin–tazobactam, ceftazidime, cefepime, aztreonam) and carbapenems, prefer the former • If not susceptible to carbapenems but susceptible to traditional β-lactams, the latter to be given as high-dose extended-infusion, and repeat AST is encouraged (a novel β-lactam agent may be an alternative)	For critically ill patients or those with poor source control with *P. aeruginosa* isolates resistant to carbapenems but susceptible to traditional β-lactams, the use of a novel β-lactam agent that tests susceptible is recommended	
Uncomplicated cystitis	Ceftolozane–tazobactam, ceftazidime–avibactam, imipenem–cilastatin–relebactam, and cefiderocol	• A single dose of tobramycin or amikacin • Colistin, but not polymyxin B, is an alternate consideration as it converts to its active form in the urinary tract	Oral fosfomycin *not* to be used (presence of the *fosA* gene, which is intrinsic to *P. aeruginosa*)
Pyelonephritis and cUTI	Ceftolozane–tazobactam, ceftazidime–avibactam, imipenem–cilastatin—relebactam, cefiderocol		
Infections outside of the urinary tract	Ceftolozane–tazobactam, ceftazidime–avibactam, and imipenem–cilastatin–relebactam	Cefiderocol	
DTR-*P. aeruginosa* with MBL production	Cefiderocol		

- Combination antibiotic therapy is not suggested for infections caused by DTR-*P. aeruginosa* if susceptibility to ceftolozane–tazobactam, ceftazidime–avibactam, imipenem–cilastatin–relebactam, or cefiderocol has been confirmed
- Use of nebulized antibiotics for the treatment of respiratory infections caused by DTR-*P. aeruginosa* is not suggested

Carbapenem-resistant Acinetobacter baumannii (CRAB)			
	• Combination therapy with at least two agents, at least until clinical improvement, even if a single agent demonstrates activity • High-dose ampicillin-sulbactam (total daily dose of 6–9 g of the sulbactam component) is suggested as a component of combination therapy for CRAB, regardless of whether susceptibility has been demonstrated • Possible options to combine with it include tetracycline derivatives (minocycline/tigecycline), polymyxin B, or cefiderocol		• Sulbactam is a competitive, irreversible β-lactamase inhibitor that, in high doses, saturates PBP1a/1b and PBP3 of *A. baumannii* isolates. • Cefiderocol to be used where intolerance or resistance to other agents prevents their use • The antibiotic sulbactam–durlobactam completed phase 3 clinical studies but is not currently FDA-approved • Nebulized antibiotics are not suggested for the treatment of respiratory infections caused by CRAB

Contd...

Contd...

Condition	Preferred line of treatment	Alternative agents	Additional information
Stenotrophomonas maltophilia			
Infections caused by *S. maltophilia*	Either of the two approaches: 1. The use of two of the following agents: TMP–SMX, minocycline/tigecycline, cefiderocol, or levofloxacin 2. Ceftazidime–avibactam plus aztreonam (when critical illness is evident or intolerance or inactivity of other agents is observed)		• Dose range of 8–12 mg/kg (trimethoprim component) of TMP–SMX • High-dose minocycline (200 mg IV/orally every 12 hours) favored over tigecycline (100 mg IV every 12 hours) • Tetracycline derivatives not suggested for *S. maltophilia* UTIs

(AST: antimicrobial susceptibility test; cUTI: complicated urinary tract infection; IV: intravenous; MICs: minimum inhibitory concentrations; UTIs: urinary tract infections)

TABLE 7: Contact precautions in an intensive care unit (ICU).

Organism	Indication for isolation		Duration
Methicillin-resistant *Staphylococcus aureus* (MRSA)	Antibiotic resistance	Positive screening swab [by culture or nucleic acid testing (NAT)] or evidence of active infection	• At least 1–3 negative swabs done at an interval of 1 week for patients not on MRSA antibiotics • Can be extended for patients with chronic wounds • Ideal duration for patients on antibiotics (for MRSA) is not known. The testing for patients on antibiotics should be done 72 hours after discontinuation of antibiotics, and the contact precautions should be extended till the sample tests negative
Vancomycin-resistant *Enterococci* (VRE)	Antibiotic resistance	Positive screening swab (by culture or NAT) or evidence of active infection	• At least 1–3 negative swabs done at an interval of 1 week for patients not on VRE antibiotics • Can be extended for immunocompromised patients, patients with broad-spectrum antibiotics, and ICUs with high VRE isolates • Ideal duration for patients on antibiotics (for VRE) is not known. The testing for patients on antibiotics should be done 72 hours after discontinuation of antibiotics, and the contact precautions should be extended till the sample tests negative
Extended-spectrum β-lactamase (ESBL)	Antibiotic resistance	Culture of ESBL-secreting organisms	Duration of index hospitalization
Carbapenem-resistant organisms (CRO)	Antibiotic resistance	Positive screening swab (by culture or NAT) or evidence of active infection	Indefinite contact precautions
Clostridium difficile	Prevention of transmission	Liquid stool positive for toxin	At least for 48 hours after resolution of diarrhea

(vancomycin-resistant *Enterococci*), and CRO (carbapenem-resistant organism). Standard contact precautions include isolation of the patient and wearing of cap, gown, and gloves before touching the patient or surroundings. The reason for isolation and duration is described in **Table 7**. The Society of Healthcare Epidemiology has proposed appropriate guidelines for the duration of isolation practices in acute care settings.[91]

Q19. What are the guidelines about infection control as per SSC 2021?

The guidelines recommend administering antimicrobials within 1 hour of recognition in adults with a high likelihood of sepsis or septic shock. For such patients only with a high risk of MRSA or fungal infection, empiric MRSA coverage or antifungal therapy, respectively, is recommended. They have made no recommendation regarding the use of antiviral agents. Daily assessment for de-escalation of antimicrobials is suggested.[3]

Q20. What care would you take while ventilating this patient? What other general care would you like to provide? Is Vitamin C administration recommended?

A low tidal volume ventilation strategy (6 mL/kg), with an upper limit goal for plateau pressures of 30 cmH$_2$O, is recommended by SSC 2021. The recommendation is against using incremental positive end expiratory pressure (PEEP) strategy. They recommend using prone ventilation trial of >12 hours in adults with sepsis-induced moderate–severe acute respiratory distress syndrome (ARDS).

Venous thromboembolism (VTE) prophylaxis: They recommend using pharmacologic VTE prophylaxis in absence of any contraindication, with a preference for low molecular weight heparin over unfractionated heparin.

A restrictive transfusion strategy is recommended.

Nutrition: Early initiation of enteral nutrition (within 72 hours), if possible, should be done. It is recommended to start insulin therapy if the glucose level is ≥180 mg/dL in patients with sepsis or septic shock.

They suggest against using intravenous vitamin C for patients with sepsis and septic shock.[3]

REFERENCES

1. Singer M, Deutschman CS, Seymour CW, Shankar-Hari M, Annane D, Bauer M, et al. The third international consensus definitions for sepsis and septic shock (Sepsis-3). JAMA. 2016;315(8):801-10.
2. Levy MM, Evans LE, Rhodes A. The surviving sepsis campaign bundle: 2018 update. Intensive Care Med. 2018;44(6):925-8.
3. Evans L, Rhodes A, Alhazzani W, Antonelli M, Coopersmith CM, French C, et al. Surviving sepsis campaign: international guidelines for management of sepsis and septic shock 2021. Intensive Care Med. 2021;47:1181-247.
4. Pierrakos C, Vincent JL. Sepsis biomarkers: a review. Crit Care. 2010;14(1):R15.
5. Bloos F, Reinhart K. Rapid diagnosis of sepsis. Virulence. 2014;5(1):154-60.
6. Reinhart K, Bauer M, Riedemann NC, Hartog CS. New approaches to sepsis: molecular diagnostics and biomarkers. Clin Microbiol Rev. 2012;25(4):609-34.
7. Povoa P, Coelho L, Dal-Pizzol F, Ferrer R, Huttner A, Morris AC, et al. How to use biomarkers of infection or sepsis at the bedside: guide to clinicians. Intensive Care Med. 2023;49:142-53.
8. Becker KL, Snider R, Nylen ES. Procalcitonin assay in systemic inflammation, infection, and sepsis: clinical utility and limitations. Crit Care Med. 2008;36(3):941-52.
9. Christ-Crain M, Muller B. Procalcitonin in bacterial infections—hype, hope, more or less? Swiss Med Wkly. 2005;135(31-32):451-60.
10. Wacker C, Prkno A, Brunkhorst FM, Schlattmann P. Procalcitonin as a diagnostic marker for sepsis: a systematic review and meta-analysis. Lancet Infect Dis. 2013;13(5):426-35.
11. Schuetz P, Chiappa V, Briel M, Greenwald JL. Procalcitonin algorithms for antibiotic therapy decisions: a systematic review of randomized controlled trials and recommendations for clinical algorithms. Arch Intern Med. 2011;171(15):1322-31.
12. Bouadma L, Luyt CE, Tubach F, Cracco C, Alvarez A, Schwebel C, et al. Use of procalcitonin to reduce patients' exposure to antibiotics in intensive care units (PRORATA trial): a multicentre randomised controlled trial. Lancet. 2010;375(9713):463-74.
13. De Jong E, Van Oers JA, Beishuizen A, Vos P, Vermeijden WJ, Hass LE, et al. Efficacy and safety of procalcitonin guidance in reducing the duration of antibiotic treatment in critically ill patients: a randomised, controlled, open-label trial. Lancet Infect Dis. 2016;16(7):819-27.
14. Schuetz P, Christ-Crain M, Wolbers M, Schild U, Thomann R, Falconnier C, et al. Procalcitonin guided antibiotic therapy and hospitalization in patients with lower respiratory tract infections: a prospective, multicenter, randomized controlled trial. BMC Health Serv Res. 2007;7:102.
15. Metlay JP, Waterer GW, Long AC, Anzueto A, Brozek J, Crothers K, et al. Diagnosis and treatment of adults with community-acquired pneumonia. An Official Clinical Practice Guideline of the American Thoracic Society and Infectious Diseases Society of America. Am J Respir Crit Care Med. 2019;200(7):e45-67.
16. Self WH, Balk RA, Grijalva CG, Williams DJ, Zhu Y, Anderson EJ, et al. Procalcitonin as a marker of etiology in adults hospitalized with community-acquired pneumonia. Clin Infect Dis. 2017;65(2):183-90.
17. McHugh L, Seldon TA, Brandon RA, Kirk JT, Rapisarda A, Sutherland AJ, et al. A molecular host response assay to discriminate between sepsis and infection-negative systemic inflammation in critically ill patients: discovery and validation in independent cohorts. PLoS Med. 2015;12(12):e1001916.
18. De Pascale G, Posteraro B, D'Arrigo S, Spinazzola G, Gaspari R, Bello G, et al. (1,3)-β-D-Glucan-based empirical antifungal interruption in suspected invasive candidiasis: a randomized trial. Crit Care. 2020;24:550.
19. Pappas PG, Kauffman CA, Andes DR, Clancy CJ, Marr KA, Ostrosky-Zeichner L, et al. Clinical practice guideline for the management of candidiasis: 2016 update by the Infectious Diseases Society of America. Clin Infect Dis. 2016;62:e1-50.
20. Barichello T, Generoso JS, Singer M, Dal-Pizzol F. Biomarkers for sepsis: more than just fever and leukocytosis—a narrative review. Crit Care. 2022;26:14.
21. Asfar P, Meziani F, Hamel JF, Grelon F, Megarbane B, Anguel N, et al. High versus low blood-pressure target in patients with septic shock. N Engl J Med. 2014;370(17):1583-93.
22. Lamontagne F, Meade MO, Hebert PC, Asfar P, Lauzier F, Seely AJE, et al. Higher versus lower blood pressure targets for vasopressor therapy in shock: a multicentre pilot randomized controlled trial. Intensive Care Med. 2016;42(4):542-50.
23. Rivers E, Nguyen B, Havstad S, Ressler J, Muzzin A, Knoblich B, et al. Early goal-directed therapy in the treatment of severe sepsis and septic shock. N Engl J Med. 2001;345(19):1368-77.

24. Peake SL, Delaney A, Bailey M, Bellomo R, Cameron PA, Cooper DJ, et al. Goal-directed resuscitation for patients with early septic shock. N Engl J Med. 2014;371(16):1496-506.
25. Mouncey PR, Osborn TM, Power GS, Harrison DA, Sadique MZ, Grieve RD, et al. Trial of early, goal-directed resuscitation for septic shock. N Engl J Med. 2015;372(14):1301-11.
26. Yealy DM, Kellum JA, Huang DT, Barnato AE, Weissfeld LA, Pike F, et al. A randomized trial of protocol-based care for early septic shock. N Engl J Med. 2014;370(18):1683-93.
27. Reinhart K, Rudolph T, Bredle DL, Hannemann L, Cain SM. Comparison of central-venous to mixed-venous oxygen saturation during changes in oxygen supply/demand. Chest. 1989;95(6):1216-21.
28. Reinhart K, Kuhn HJ, Hartog C, Bredle DL. Continuous central venous and pulmonary artery oxygen saturation monitoring in the critically ill. Intensive Care Med. 2004;30(8):1572-8.
29. Jones AE, Shapiro NI, Trzeciak S, Arnold RC, Claremont HA, Kline JA, et al. Lactate clearance vs central venous oxygen saturation as goals of early sepsis therapy: a randomized clinical trial. JAMA. 2010;303(8):739-46.
30. Ince C, Sinaasappel M. Microcirculatory oxygenation and shunting in sepsis and shock. Crit Care Med. 1999;27(7):1369-77.
31. Fink MP. Cytopathic hypoxia. Is oxygen use impaired in sepsis as a result of an acquired intrinsic derangement in cellular respiration? Crit Care Clin. 2002;18(1):165-75.
32. De Backer D, Ospina-Tascon G, Salgado D, Favory R, Creteur J, Vincent JL. Monitoring the microcirculation in the critically ill patient: current methods and future approaches. Intensive Care Med. 2010;36(11):1813-25.
33. Boulain T, Garot D, Vignon P, Lascarrou JB, Desachy A, Botoc V, et al. Prevalence of low central venous oxygen saturation in the first hours of intensive care unit admission and associated mortality in septic shock patients: a prospective multicentre study. Crit Care. 2014;18(6):609.
34. Mallat J, Lemyze M, Tronchon L, Vallet B, Thevenin D. Use of venous-to-arterial carbon dioxide tension difference to guide resuscitation therapy in septic shock. World J Crit Care Med. 2016;5(1):47-56.
35. Bakker J, Vincent JL, Gris P, Leon M, Coffernils M, Kahn RJ. Veno-arterial carbon dioxide gradient in human septic shock. Chest. 1992;101(2):509-15.
36. Mecher CE, Rackow EC, Astiz ME, Weil MH. Venous hypercarbia associated with severe sepsis and systemic hypoperfusion. Crit Care Med. 1990;18(6):585-9.
37. Vallée F, Vallet B, Mathe O, Parraguette J, Mari A, Silva S, et al. Central venous-to-arterial carbon dioxide difference: an additional target for goal-directed therapy in septic shock? Intensive Care Med. 2008;34(12):2218-25.
38. Jansen TC, van Bommel J, Woodward R, Mulder PG, Bakker J. Association between blood lactate levels, sequential organ failure assessment subscores, and 28-day mortality during early and late intensive care unit stay: a retrospective observational study. Crit Care Med. 2009;37(8):2369-74.
39. Sakr Y, Reinhart K, Vincent JL, Sprung CL, Moreno R, Ranieri VM, et al. Does dopamine administration in shock influence outcome? Results of the Sepsis Occurrence in Acutely Ill Patients (SOAP) Study. Crit Care Med. 2006;34:589-97.
40. De Backer D, Biston P, Devriendt J, Madl C, Chochrad D, Aldecoa C, et al. Comparison of dopamine and norepinephrine in the treatment of shock. N Engl J Med. 2010;362(9):779-89.
41. Avni T, Lador A, Lev S, Leibovici L, Paul M, Grossman A. Vasopressors for the treatment of septic shock: systematic review and meta-analysis. PLoS One. 2015;10(8):e0129305.
42. Landry DW, Levin HR, Gallant EM, Ashton Jr RC, Seo S, D'Alessandro D, et al. Vasopressin deficiency contributes to the vasodilation of septic shock. Circulation. 1997;95(5):1122-5.
43. Russell JA, Walley KR, Singer J, Gordon AC, Hebert PC, Cooper DJ, et al. Vasopressin versus norepinephrine infusion in patients with septic shock. N Engl J Med. 2008;358(9):877-87.
44. Gordon AC, Mason AJ, Thirunavukkarasu N, Perkins GD, Cecconi M, Cepkova M, et al. Effect of early vasopressin vs norepinephrine on kidney failure in patients with septic shock: the VANISH randomized clinical trial. JAMA. 2016;316(5):509-18.
45. Khanna A, English SW, Wang XS, Ham K, Tumlin J, Szerlip H, et al. Angiotensin II for the treatment of vasodilatory shock. N Engl J Med. 2017;377(5):419-30.
46. Bai X, Yu W, Ji W, Lin Z, Tan S, Duan K, et al. Early versus delayed administration of norepinephrine in patients with septic shock. Crit Care. 2014;18(5):532.
47. Beck V, Chateau D, Bryson GL, Pisipati A, Zanotti S, Parrillo JE, et al. Timing of vasopressor initiation and mortality in septic shock: a cohort study. Crit Care. 2014;18(3):R97.
48. L'Heureux M, Sternberg M, Brath L, Turlington J, Kashiouris MG. Sepsis-induced cardiomyopathy: a comprehensive review. Curr Cardiol Rep. 2020;22(5):35.
49. Sato R, Nasu M. A review of sepsis-induced cardiomyopathy. J Intensive Care. 2015;3:48.
50. Vieillard-Baron A. Septic cardiomyopathy. Ann Intensive Care. 2011;1:6.
51. Azuhata T, Kinoshita K, Kawano D, Komatsu T, Sakurai A, Chiba Y, et al. Time from admission to initiation of surgery for source control is a critical determinant of survival in patients with gastrointestinal perforation with associated septic shock. Crit Care. 2014;18(3):R87.
52. Zarbock A, Nadim MK, Pickkers P, Gomez H, Bell S, Joannidis M, et al. Sepsis-associated acute kidney injury: consensus report of the 28th Acute Disease Quality Initiative workgroup. Nat Rev Nephrol. 2023;19;401-17.
53. Poston JT, Koyner JL. Sepsis associated acute kidney injury. BMJ. 2019;364:k4891.
54. Zampieri FG, Machado FR, Biondi RS, Freitas FGR, Veiga VC, Figueiredo RC, et al. Effect of intravenous fluid treatment with a balanced solution vs 0.9% saline solution on mortality in critically ill patients: the BaSICS randomized clinical trial. JAMA. 2021;326(9):1-12.
55. Finfer S, Micallef S, Hammond N, Navarra L, Bellomo R, Billot L, et al. Balanced multielectrolyte solution versus saline in critically ill adults. N Engl J Med. 2022;386(9):815-26.

56. Zhang Z, Zhu C, Mo L, Hong Y. Effectiveness of sodium bicarbonate infusion on mortality in septic patients with metabolic acidosis. Intensive Care Med. 2018;44(11):1888-95.
57. Prigent H, Maxime V, Annane D. Clinical review: corticotherapy in sepsis. Crit Care. 2004;8(2):122-9.
58. Keh D, Trips E, Marx G, Wirtz SP, Abduljawwad E, Bercker S, et al. Effect of hydrocortisone on development of shock among patients with severe sepsis: the HYPRESS randomized clinical trial. JAMA. 2016;316(17):1775-85.
59. Annane D, Bellissant E, Bollaert PE, Briegel J, Keh D, Kupfer Y, et al. Corticosteroids for treating sepsis. Cochrane Database Syst Rev. 2015;(12):CD002243.
60. Volbeda M, Wetterslev J, Gluud C, Zijlstra JG, van der Horst IC, Keus F. Glucocorticosteroids for sepsis: systematic review with meta-analysis and trial sequential analysis. Intensive Care Med. 2015;41(7):1220-34.
61. Gibbison B, Lopez-Lopez JA, Higgins JP, Miller T, Angelini GD, Lightman SL, et al. Corticosteroids in septic shock: a systematic review and network meta-analysis. Crit Care. 2017;21(1):78.
62. Annane D, Pastores SM, Rochwerg B, Arlt W, Balk RA, Beishuizen A, et al. Guidelines for the diagnosis and management of critical illness-related corticosteroid insufficiency (CIRCI) in critically ill patients (Part I): Society of Critical Care Medicine (SCCM) and European Society of Intensive Care Medicine (ESICM) 2017. Intensive Care Med. 2017;43(12):1751-63.
63. Venkatesh B, Finfer S, Cohen J, Rajbhandari D, Arabi Y, Bellomo R, et al. Adjunctive glucocorticoid therapy in patients with septic shock. N Engl J Med. 2018;378(9):797-808.
64. Annane D, Renault A, Brun-Buisson C, Megarbane B, Quenot JP, Siami S, et al. Hydrocortisone plus fludrocortisone for adults with septic shock. N Engl J Med. 2018;378(9):809-18.
65. Cruz DN, Antonelli M, Fumagalli R, Foltran F, Brienza N, Donati A, et al. Early use of polymyxin B hemoperfusion in abdominal septic shock: the EUPHAS randomized controlled trial. JAMA. 2009;301(23):2445-52.
66. Payen DM, Guilhot J, Launey Y, Lukaszewicz AC, Kaaki M, Veber B, et al. Early use of polymyxin B hemoperfusion in patients with septic shock due to peritonitis: a multicenter randomized control trial. Intensive Care Med. 2015;41(6):975-84.
67. Fujii T, Ganeko R, Kataoka Y, Furukawa TA, Featherstone R, Doi K, et al. Polymyxin B-immobilized hemoperfusion and mortality in critically ill adult patients with sepsis/septic shock: a systematic review with meta-analysis and trial sequential analysis. Intensive Care Med. 2018;44(2):167-78.
68. Dellinger RP, Bagshaw SM, Antonelli M, Foster DM, Klein DJ, Marshall JC, et al. Effect of targeted polymyxin B hemoperfusion on 28-day mortality in patients with septic shock and elevated endotoxin level: the EUPHRATES randomized clinical trial. JAMA. 2018;320(14):1455-63.
69. Kogelmann K, Jarczak D, Scheller M, Drüner M. Hemoadsorption by CytoSorb in septic patients: a case series. Crit Care. 2017:21(1):74.
70. Schädler D, Pausch C, Heise D, Meier-Hellmann A, Brederlau J, Weiler N, et al. The effect of a novel extracorporeal cytokine hemoadsorption device on IL-6 elimination in septic patients: a randomized controlled trial. PLoS One. 2017;12(10):e0187015.
71. Karnad DR, Bhadade R, Verma PK, Moulick ND, Daga MK, Chafekar ND, et al. Intravenous administration of ulinastatin (human urinary trypsin inhibitor) in severe sepsis: a multicenter randomized controlled study. Intensive Care Med. 2014;40(6):830-8.
72. Huang SW, Guan XD, Chen J, Yang BO. Clinical study and long-term evaluation of immunomodulation therapy on trauma, severe sepsis and multiple organ dysfunction syndrome patients. Zhongguo Wei Zhong Bing Ji Jiu Yi Xue. 2006;18(11):653-6.
73. Chaudhary N, Duggal AK. Sepsis associated encephalopathy. Adv Med. 2014;2014:762320.
74. Ren C, Yao RQ, Zhang H, Feng YW, Yao YM. Sepsis-associated encephalopathy: a vicious cycle of immunosuppression. J Neuroinflammation. 2020;17:14.
75. Iba T, Helms J, Connors JM, Levy JH. The pathophysiology, diagnosis, and management of sepsis-associated disseminated intravascular coagulation. J Intensive Care. 2023;11:24.
76. Iba T, Levy JH. Sepsis-induced coagulopathy and disseminated intravascular coagulation. Anesthesiology. 2020;132:1238-45.
77. Warkentin TE, Ning S. Symmetrical peripheral gangrene in critical illness. Transfus Apher Sci. 2021;60:103094.
78. Knight Jr TT, Gordon SV, Canady J, Rush DS, Browder W. Symmetrical peripheral gangrene: a new presentation of an old disease. Am Surg. 2000;66:196-9.
79. Magiorakos AP, Srinivasan A, Carey RB, Carmeli Y, Falagas ME, Giske CG, et al. Multidrug resistant, extensively drug-resistant and pandrug-resistant bacteria: an international expert proposal for interim standard definitions for acquired resistance. Clin Microbiol Infect. 2012;18(3):268-81.
80. Souli M, Galani I, Giamarellou H. Emergence of extensively drug-resistant and pandrug-resistant gram-negative bacilli in Europe. Euro Surveill. 2008;13(47):19045.
81. Martin-Loeches I, Torres A, Rinaudo M, Terraneo S, de Rosa F, Ramirez P, et al. Resistance patterns and outcomes in intensive care unit (ICU)-acquired pneumonia. Validation of European Centre for Disease Prevention and Control (ECDC) and the Centers for Disease Control and Prevention (CDC) classification of multidrug resistant organisms. J Infect. 2015;70(3):213-22.
82. Palzkill T. Metallo-β-lactamase structure and function. Ann N Y Acad Sci. 2013;1277:91-104.
83. Bush K, Jacoby GA. Updated functional classification of β-lactamases. Antimicrob Agents Chemother. 2010;54(3):969-76.
84. Amelia A, Nugroho A, Harijanto PN. Diagnosis and management of infections caused by Enterobacteriaceae producing extended-spectrum b-lactamase. Acta Med Indones. 2016;48(2):156-66.
85. Lob SH, Nicolle LE, Hoban DJ, Kazmierczak KM, Badal RE, Sahm DF. Susceptibility patterns and ESBL rates of *Escherichia coli* from urinary tract infections in Canada and the United States, SMART 2010-2014. Diagn Microbiol Infect Dis. 2016;85(4):459-65.

86. Schwaber MJ, Carmeli Y. Mortality and delay in effective therapy associated with extended-spectrum beta-lactamase production in Enterobacteriaceae bacteraemia: a systematic review and meta-analysis. J Antimicrob Chemother. 2007;60(5):913-20.
87. Jacoby GA. AmpC β-lactamases. Clin Microbiol Rev. 2009;22(1):161-82.
88. Liang Z, Li L, Wang Y, Chen L, Kong X, Hong Y, et al. Molecular basis of NDM-1, a new antibiotic resistance determinant. PLoS One. 2011;6(8):e23606.
89. Khan AU, Maryam L, Zarrilli R. Structure, genetics and worldwide spread of New Delhi metallo-β-lactamase (NDM): a threat to public health. BMC Microbiol. 2017;17(1):101.
90. Tamma PD, Aitken SL, Bonomo RA, Mathers AJ, van Duin D, Clancy CJ. Infectious Diseases Society of America 2023 guidance on the treatment of antimicrobial resistant gram-negative infections. Clin Infect Dis. 2023;ciad428.
91. Banach DB, Bearman G, Barnden M, Hanrahan JA, Leekha S, Morgan DJ, et al. Duration of contact precautions for acute-care settings. Infect Control Hosp Epidemiol. 2018;39(2):127-44.

CHAPTER 10

Acute Coronary Syndrome

Kushal Rajeev Kalvit, Akshaya Ramaswami, Atul Prabhakar Kulkarni

CASE STUDY

*A 72-year-old male, a known case of diabetes mellitus, hypertension, and dyslipidemia, presented with acute-onset shortness of breath and left-sided chest pain of half hour duration. On examination, the peripheries were cold and clammy. His vitals were: Heart rate (HR) 116/min, blood pressure (BP) 86/60 mm Hg, and respiratory rate (RR) 28/min. Bilateral crackles were present all over the chest. His electrocardiogram (ECG) is shown in **Figure 1**.*

Q1. What are the clinical features of acute coronary syndrome (ACS)?

The most common symptom of ACS is typical ischemic chest pain, which is characterized by the following features:
- The pain is diffusely located over the entire chest, and typically the patient finds it difficult to localize the pain, which is usually characterized as a crushing or squeezing discomfort rather than as a pain sensation.
- It is generally provoked by activity or exertion and does not vary with respiration or change in position.
- It radiates to other parts of the body with radiation to both arms or one arm being highly suggestive of an ACS. Other areas where the pain radiates include the epigastrium, shoulders, neck and throat, back, lower jaw, and teeth.
- The duration of pain is generally longer than 10 minutes.

Other symptoms include:
- Shortness of breath, which may be associated with orthopnea
- Nausea, vomiting
- Diaphoresis
- Dizziness or light-headedness
- Fatigue

One-third of patients presenting with ACS have atypical presentation (angina equivalents), i.e., they present without chest pain. They may present with nausea, vomiting, shortness of breath, epigastric pain, syncope, or even cardiac arrest. These presentations are more common in diabetics, elderly, females, psychiatry patients, etc. Atypical presentations of ACS often cause a delay in diagnosis, and this leads to an increase in hospital mortality.

Q2. What is the Fourth Universal Definition of acute myocardial infarction (AMI)?

Acute myocardial injury is defined as the elevation of cardiac troponin values with at least one value above the 99th

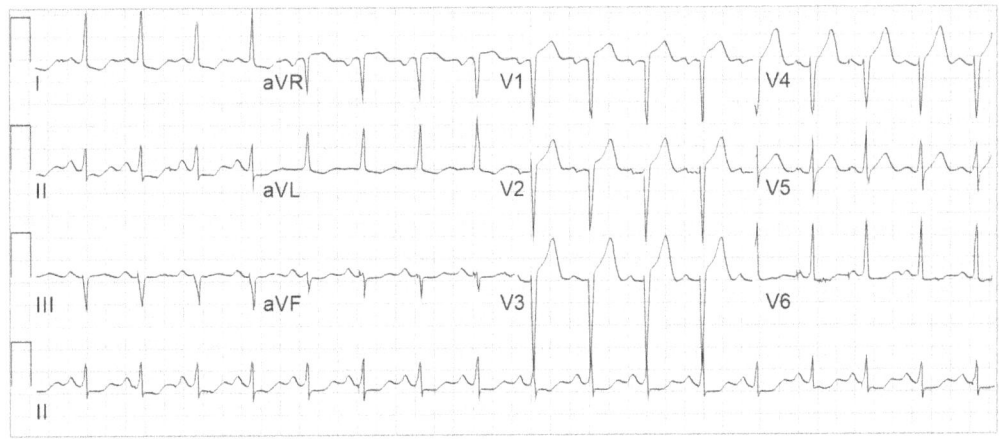

Fig. 1: Electrocardiogram (ECG) at the time of admission.

percentile of the upper reference limit (URL). It is considered as acute if there is a rise/fall in the cardiac troponin values.

Acute myocardial infarction is defined as acute myocardial injury in the presence of clinical evidence of acute myocardial ischemia. This clinical evidence may be any one of the following:
- Symptoms of myocardial ischemia
- New ischemic ECG changes
- Development of pathologic Q waves
- Imaging evidence of new loss of viable myocardium or new regional wall motion abnormality (RWMA)
- Identification of a thrombus on coronary angiography or autopsy.[1]

Q3. What are the types of AMI?

Type 1: Spontaneous thrombotic myocardial infarction (MI) due to atherosclerotic plaque rupture, fissuring, ulceration, erosion, or dissection.

Type 2: MI due to a mismatch between myocardial oxygen supply and demand triggered by processes other than coronary artery thrombosis such as hypertensive emergency or arrhythmias.

Type 3: Cardiac death in a clinical setting (symptoms and/or ECG changes) suggestive of MI without any definite biochemical evidence of myocardial injury (elevated troponins).

Type 4a: Percutaneous coronary intervention (PCI) procedure-related MI (within 48 hours of the index procedure associated with a rise in cardiac troponin more than times the 99th percentile of URL in patients with normal troponins at baseline; if baseline troponin elevated, then the variation should be >20%).

Type 4b: Stent thrombosis-related MI.

Type 4c: Stent restenosis-related MI.

Type 5: Coronary artery bypass graft (CABG)-related MI (within 48 hours of the index procedure associated with a rise in cardiac troponin more than 10 times the 99th percentile of URL in patients with normal troponins at baseline; if baseline troponin elevated, then the variation should be >20%).

Q4. What are the features in ECG suggestive of ACS?

ST-elevation myocardial infarction (STEMI) is characterized by new or presumed new ST elevation at the J point in two or more anatomically contiguous leads defined as ≥0.1 mV (1 mm) in all leads other than V2-3, where the cutoffs are as follows:
- ≥0.2 mV (2 mm) in males ≥40 years
- ≥0.25 mV (2.5 mm) in males <40 years
- ≥0.15 mV (1.5 mm) in females

Findings suggestive of non-ST-elevation myocardial infarction (NSTEMI) on ECG include:
- New or presumed new horizontal or down-sloping ST depressions ≥0.05 mV (0.5 mm) in two or more anatomically contiguous leads.
- T-wave inversion ≥0.1 mV (1 mm) in two or more anatomically contiguous leads with prominent R wave or R/S ratio >1.

There are certain ECG changes which are considered STEMI equivalents, i.e., while they do not fit the ECG definition of a STEMI, they indicate critical MI and should be managed with emergent reperfusion therapy. These changes include:
- *De Winter's T waves:* Upsloping ST depression >1 mm at J point with tall prominent symmetric upright T waves in two or more leads from V2 to V6—suggestive of left anterior descending (LAD) occlusion.
- ST depression >0.5 mm and a positive terminal T wave in V1–V3—suggestive of posterior wall MI.
- ST elevation in aVR/V1 with diffuse ST depression >1 mm (in at least 8 leads)—suggestive of triple vessel disease or left main coronary artery disease occlusion.
- Deep T-wave inversions in precordial leads V1–V4 with minimal or no ST elevation known as the Wellens pattern—suggestive of high-grade stenosis in LAD.

The presence of a presumed new left bundle branch block (LBBB) does not predict MI per se. At the same time, patients with suspicion of myocardial ischemia and LBBB should be treated as STEMI *regardless* of whether the LBBB was previously known. Criteria such as the modified Sgarbossa criteria or the Barcelona criteria may be applied to assist in the diagnosis. Similar urgent attention should be given to suspected acute myocardial ischemia and right bundle branch block (RBBB) on ECG.[2,3]

Q5. How can the area of infarct be localized with the help of ECG?

Localization of ischemia and thereby determination of the suspect culprit artery can be done broadly by determining the ECG leads showing the ischemic changes **(Table 1)**.

TABLE 1: Localization of ischemia and determination of suspect culprit artery.

Anatomic location of infarct	Leads showing ischemic changes	Leads showing reciprocal changes
Anterior wall	V1–V6	
Anteroseptal	V1–V4	V7–V9 (posterior leads)
Apical/lateral	V4–V6 and I, AvI	II, III, aVF
Inferior wall	II, III, aVF	V4–V6, I, aVL
Right ventricular	Right precordial leads (V4R, V5R, V6R)	
Posterior	V7–V9	V1–V3

Q6. What are the causes of ST-segment elevation and elevated cardiac troponins other than ACS?

ST-segment elevation:
- Acute pericarditis
- Early repolarization pattern
- Left ventricular hypertrophy (LVH)
- LBBB (V1–V3)
- Myocarditis
- Myocardial trauma/tumor
- Stress cardiomyopathy

Elevated cardiac troponins:
- Tachy- or bradyarrhythmias
- PCI or cardiac surgery
- Coronary artery spasm
- Coronary artery vasculitis
- Severe hypertension
- Aortic dissection
- Severe hypoxia/hypoperfusion
- Sepsis
- Renal failure
- Pulmonary embolism
- Stroke/subarachnoid hemorrhage (SAH)
- Major burns
- Electrocution
- Cardiotoxic drugs/toxins
- Acute heart failure of any cause [stress cardiomyopathy, myocarditis, peripartum cardiomyopathy (PPCM)].[4]

Q7. What is the initial management of ACS?

Any patient with suspected ACS requires a 12-lead ECG within 10 minutes of presentation. If the initial ECG is nondiagnostic and the clinical suspicion remains high, ECG may have to be repeated every 20–30 minutes. Based on the presence or absence of significant ST elevation, ACS may be classified into STEMI and non-ST-elevation acute coronary syndrome (NSTE-ACS) (NSTEMI and unstable angina), respectively. NSTEMI and unstable angina are differentiated based on the presence of elevated cardiac troponins with elevation present in NSTEMI.

Cardiac troponin levels should be sent in all patients with suspected ACS. If the initial troponin level is normal but the clinical suspicion is high, a repeat troponin level should be sent after 3–6 hours.

Two-dimensional (2D) echocardiography should be performed at the bedside to look for new-onset RWMAs and for the mechanical complications of MI as well such as rupture of the chordae tendinae, ventricular free wall, or the interventricular septum.

The initial assessment and emergency interventions for a patient with ACS include the following:
- Stabilize airway, breathing, and circulation.
- Continuous cardiac monitoring is to be instituted and supplemental oxygen is to be used as required to maintain oxygen saturation (SpO_2) >90%.
- An oral loading dose of aspirin, a $P2Y_{12}$ receptor blocker, and a statin are to be administered in all patients with ACS.
- *Pain relief:*
  - Sublingual nitroglycerin (NTG) 0.4 mg can be given (up to 3 tablets at 5-minute intervals).
  - Intravenous (IV) NTG can be considered in cases refractory to sublingual NTG.
- Selection of a reperfusion strategy
- If the patient has no signs of heart failure, is hemodynamically stable, and has no history of reactive airway disease, oral beta-blockers should be started (metoprolol 25–50 mg OD).
- Atrial and ventricular arrhythmias are to be managed as per advanced cardiac life support (ACLS) protocol.
- Heart failure is to be managed using positive pressure ventilation, afterload-reducing agent (such as NTG), and diuretics depending on the clinical profile.

Q8. Discuss the choice of reperfusion strategy in patients with STEMI and NSTEMI.

All patients with STEMI presenting within 12 hours of symptom onset need to undergo reperfusion therapy in the form of either fibrinolysis or primary PCI. Primary PCI is the preferred therapy over fibrinolysis in STEMI based on the results of multiple randomized controlled trials (RCTs) (AIR PAMI, STOPAMI-1, STOPAMI-2, DANAMI-2). If the patient has presented to a PCI-capable center, the time to PCI should be within 60 minutes of STEMI diagnosis. If the patient has presented to a non-PCI center, then the patient should be transferred to a PCI-capable center only if the PCI can be done within 120 minutes of STEMI diagnosis. In primary PCI, the radial approach is the preferred one and a drug-eluting stent is chosen over a bare metal stent. Stenting only of the infarct-related artery (IRA) is to be done in the index procedure while the remaining atherosclerotic arteries can be stented before hospital discharge in a separate procedure. However, complete revascularization of all stenosed/thrombosed arteries can be done in case of cardiogenic shock or resuscitation after cardiac arrest.

If this timeline cannot be followed, fibrinolysis should be chosen as the reperfusion therapy. Fibrinolysis should be done within 10 minutes of STEMI diagnosis. The success of fibrinolysis is ascertained by a repeat ECG after 60–90 minutes and >50% reduction in ST-elevation.

Fibrinolysis is considered as "failed" in the presence of ongoing or recurrent chest pain, hemodynamic instability, electrical instability, or cardiac arrest. Such cases need a "rescue PCI" strategy. All cases of STEMI with successful fibrinolysis should be shifted to a PCI-capable center in 2–24 hours for angiography.

If STEMI patients present 12–48 hours after symptom onset, primary PCI should be done in the presence of hemodynamic instability or arrhythmias. Primary PCI may also be considered if the patient is hemodynamically stable. There is no role of PCI if the patient has presented after 48 hours of symptom onset.

Patients with NSTEMI need to be risk stratified before deciding the urgency of angiography. Patients with hemodynamic instability, electrical instability, cardiogenic shock, acute heart failure, mechanical complications, and refractory chest pain despite medical therapy are deemed to be at "very high risk" and need invasive angiography within 2 hours. Patients resuscitated after cardiac arrest but without ST-segment elevation and patients with a GRACE score >140 are deemed to be at "high risk" and need invasive angiography within 24 hours. There is no role of fibrinolysis in patients with NSTEMI.[5,6]

Q9. Which are the fibrinolytic agents for patients with STEMI?

Approved fibrinolytic agents are as follows:
- Streptokinase 1.5 million units over 30–60 minutes.
- Reteplase 10 U over 2 minutes and repeat 10 U at 30 minutes.
- Alteplase 15 mg bolus over 1–2 minutes, then 0.75 mg/kg over 30 minutes, then 0.5 mg/kg over 60 minutes.
- Tenecteplase bolus over 5–10 seconds; weight-based dosing (30 mg for <60 kg and 35 mg for 60–69 kg).

Fibrin-specific third-generation agents such as reteplase and tenecteplase are preferred over the other agents. The absolute contraindications which need to be ruled out prior to initiation of fibrinolysis are as follows:
- History of intracranial hemorrhage, intracranial primary or metastatic malignancy, cerebral vascular malformation.
- History of ischemic stroke in the last 3 months (except in the last 3 hours).
- Symptoms/signs of aortic dissection.
- Significant head or facial trauma in the last 3 months.
- Active bleeding (except menses).

Q10. Discuss the principles of antiplatelet therapy in STEMI and NSTEMI.

Platelet adhesion and aggregation are the two events that need to be targeted in thrombotic occlusion of coronary arteries. All patients with STEMI or NSTEMI need to be treated with dual antiplatelet therapy (DAPT), which consists of aspirin and another $P2Y_{12}$ receptor blocker. DAPT needs to be given at least for 12 months and may be extended up to 36 months.

Aspirin is given as a 300 mg loading dose orally in the form of nonenteric coated tablets that need to be crushed/chewed to achieve blood levels quickly. The maintenance dose is 75 mg OD for all patients. In cases where aspirin cannot be given orally such as postesophagectomy or postgastrectomy perioperative MI, IV aspirin can be given as a 250 mg loading dose followed by 100 mg OD as a maintenance dose.

The choice of $P2Y_{12}$ receptor blocker in STEMI depends on whether revascularization is planned and if fibrinolytic agents are going to be administered.

- If primary PCI is planned, either ticagrelor or prasugrel is the preferred drug. Both drugs are preferred over clopidogrel based on the TRITON TIMI 38 and PLATO trials on patients with STEMI and NSTEMI undergoing primary PCI. The PRAGUE-18 and ISAR REACT 5 trials compared ticagrelor and prasugrel head-to-head. The PRAGUE-18 study was stopped early and showed no significant difference between the two. Although the ISAR REACT 5 study showed an increased risk of adverse events with ticagrelor use, the trial had its own limitations including open-label design, modest sample size, and no difference in the STEMI subgroup. Ticagrelor is administered as a 180 mg loading dose followed by 90 mg BD as a maintenance dose. Prasugrel is administered as a 60 mg loading dose followed by 10 mg OD as a maintenance dose. A previous history of ischemic stroke/transient ischemic attack (TIA) is an absolute contraindication for prasugrel therapy while age >75 years and weight <60 kg are relative contraindications.
- If a fibrinolytic agent is being administered, clopidogrel is preferred over ticagrelor or prasugrel. Clopidogrel is administered as a loading dose of 300 mg orally followed by 75 mg OD as the maintenance dose. There is no need to routinely switch from clopidogrel to other $P2Y_{12}$ blockers even if PCI is done after fibrinolysis. Switching to another $P2Y_{12}$ receptor blocker may be done if the PCI is performed >24 hours after fibrinolysis and if the angiography reveals high-risk features.
- If neither fibrinolysis nor PCI is performed, ticagrelor is to be given at the same dose as for primary PCI.
- For the uncommon patient where oral drugs cannot be given, IV cangrelor can be given as the $P2Y_{12}$ receptor blocker at a dose of 30 µg/kg bolus followed by 4 µg/kg/min to be continued till the PCI procedure is complete.

In case of NSTEMI, the $P2Y_{12}$ receptor blocker has to be given in the same doses as discussed above. If an invasive strategy is chosen, prasugrel is preferred over ticagrelor and needs to be given after the angiography is done. Routine pretreatment with $P2Y_{12}$ blockers of patients planned for PCI is not recommended unless the coronary anatomy is known. There is no role of routine administration of glycoprotein (GP) IIb/IIIa inhibitors such as tirofiban, eptifibatide, or abciximab in patients with STEMI/NSTEMI. GP IIb/IIIa inhibitors may be given in the event of intraprocedural bailout due to no-reflow phenomenon, large thrombus burden, or coronary artery dissection.

Q11. Discuss the principles of anticoagulant therapy in STEMI and NSTEMI.

Anticoagulants are required in all cases of STEMI and NSTEMI to prevent clot extension and clot reformation. The commonly used anticoagulants are unfractionated heparin (UFH), low-molecular-weight heparin (LMWH), fondaparinux, and bivalirudin. The choice of anticoagulant depends on the revascularization strategy.

- For patients with primary PCI, UFH infusion is started before the procedure with a loading dose of 70–100 U/kg and a target activated clotting time (ACT) >250 seconds. The infusion is continued throughout the procedure and is stopped after a successful PCI. UFH is preferred over enoxaparin due to easier titratability. If enoxaparin is chosen as the initial anticoagulant, the loading dose is given as 30 mg IV along with 1 mg/kg subcutaneously (s/c) BD (first s/c dose to be given with IV dose).
- For patients with primary fibrinolysis, UFH infusion is preferred if the patient is planned for immediate angiography after fibrinolysis (pharmacoinvasive strategy). It should continue till the PCI is complete. If angiography is not planned, then either enoxaparin or fondaparinux is preferred. Anticoagulation should continue for either 8 days or until discharge, whichever comes first.

Q12. Which are the other medical therapies in ACS?

- Sublingual NTG is administered at a dose of 0.4 mg every 5 minutes for three doses for ongoing chest pain. Nitrates act by dilatation of coronary arteries to improve perfusion, venodilation to reduce preload, and arterial dilation to some extent with a reduction in afterload. It should not be administered if the systolic blood pressure (SBP) is <90 mm Hg, HR is <50/min, or there is right ventricular (RV) infarction, concomitant hypertrophic obstructive cardiomyopathy (HOCM) or aortic stenosis, or intake of phosphodiesterase inhibitors in the last 24 hours. If the chest pain is not relieved after three sublingual doses, NTG IV infusion may be required. It is usually started at 5–10 μg/min and uptitrated every 5 minutes till a maximum dose of 400 μg/min. Nitrates rapidly develop tolerance within 24 hours and are to be administered only for relief of symptoms.
- Patients with ACS who do not have hypotension, bradycardia, or heart block typically receive oral beta-blockers as a part of the initial therapy. Cardioselective drugs such as metoprolol or atenolol are preferred with a target HR of 55–70/min and SBP of >90 mm Hg.
- Routine use of morphine is not recommended.
- Oxygen therapy should not be routinely administered if the SpO_2 is >94%. The AVOID trial showed that patients treated with oxygen even if the SpO_2 >94% had a larger myocardial scar at follow-up.
- Statins are typically prescribed to all patients with ACS to lower the low-density lipoprotein-cholesterol (LDL-C) and for their pleiotropic effects. Atorvastatin 80 mg OD or rosuvastatin 10–20 mg OD are the preferred agents.

REFERENCES

1. Thygesen K, Alpert JS, Jaffe AS, Chaitman BR, Bax JJ, Morrow DA, et al. Fourth Universal Definition of Myocardial Infarction (2018). J Am Coll Cardiol. 2018;72(18):2231-64.
2. Macfarlane PW. New ECG criteria for acute myocardial infarction in patients with left bundle branch block. J Am Heart Assoc. 2020;9(14):e017119.
3. Miranda DF, Lobo AS, Walsh B, Sandoval Y, Smith SW. New insights into the use of the 12-lead electrocardiogram for diagnosing acute myocardial infarction in the emergency department. Can J Cardiol. 2018;34(2):132-45.
4. Park KC, Gaze DC, Collinson PO, Marber MS. Cardiac troponins: from myocardial infarction to chronic disease. Cardiovasc Res. 2017;113(14):1708-18.
5. Collet JP, Thiele H, Barbato E, Barthélémy O, Bauersachs J, Bhatt DL, et al. 2020 ESC Guidelines for the management of acute coronary syndromes in patients presenting without persistent ST-segment elevation. Eur Heart J. 2021;42(14): 1289-367.
6. Ibanez B, James S, Agewall S, Antunes MJ, Bucciarelli-Ducci C, Bueno H, et al. 2017 ESC Guidelines for the management of acute myocardial infarction in patients presenting with ST-segment elevation: the Task Force for the management of acute myocardial infarction in patients presenting with ST-segment elevation of the European Society of Cardiology (ESC). Eur Heart J. 2018;39(2):119-77.

Eclampsia and Cerebral Venous Thrombosis

Dilip R Karnad

CASE STUDY

A 24-year-old primiparous woman with normal antenatal history was shifted to intensive care unit (ICU) following sudden-onset convulsions at 36 weeks of gestation. Her past medical history was uneventful. On arrival to ICU, she was conscious, oriented, following commands, and did not have any focal neurological deficits. She was hemodynamically stable [heart rate (HR) 100 beats/min, blood pressure (BP) 170/110 mm Hg] and her systemic examination was unremarkable. Her laboratories revealed: hemoglobin (Hb): 11 g/dL, platelets: 150×10^9/L, and white blood cell count: 12.5×10^9/L. Her other investigations were serum urea: 46 mg/dL, uric acid: 6 mg/dL, and creatinine: 1.50 mg/dL. The liver function tests (LFTs) were: bilirubin: 1.8 mg/dL, alanine aminotransferase (ALT): 350 IU/L, and aspartate aminotransferase (AST): 240 IU/L. Her coagulation profile was prothrombin time (PT): 13 seconds, international normalized ratio (INR): 1.1, and activated partial thromboplastin time (APTT) was 45 seconds.

Q1. What is the most likely diagnosis? List the differential diagnosis.

In a parturient presenting with new-onset seizures in third trimester, associated with hypertension along with features of organ dysfunction in the form of raised serum creatinine and liver enzymes, the most likely diagnosis is eclampsia.

The differential diagnoses for parturient presenting with new-onset seizures are given below:
- *Unique*: Eclampsia
- Concurrent causes such as metabolic hypocalcemia, hyponatremia, hypoglycemia, toxins like alcohol or drug withdrawal, infections like meningitis, encephalitis, cerebral malaria, head trauma, hemorrhage, and ischemia.
- *Exacerbated by the pregnant state*: Cerebral venous thrombosis (CVT), thrombotic thrombocytopenic purpura (TTP), hemolytic uremic syndrome (HUS).
- *Incidental*: Brain tumors, aneurysm

The history, physical examination, blood investigations, and neuroimaging provide clues to diagnosis.

New-onset seizures <20 weeks of pregnancy are unlikely to be due to eclampsia. Structural disease, metabolic disorder, or molar pregnancy should be suspected and confirmed with relevant investigations.[1]

If the seizures are associated with fever, vomiting, features of raised intracranial pressure (ICP) like altered sensorium, projectile vomiting, infectious causes like meningitis or encephalitis should be considered. Cerebrospinal fluid (CSF) analysis and neuroimaging help in confirmation.

Usually eclampsia is not associated with persistent neurological deficits and therefore suggests some anatomic defect. Causes of sudden development of neurologic symptoms include stroke, tumors, and abscess.[2] Seizures occurring >20 weeks without high BP recordings or organ dysfunction and without neurological deficits point toward metabolic causes, toxins, and infections. Antecedent trauma followed by seizures should be evaluated with imaging and treated accordingly.

In parturient presenting with seizure and thrombocytopenia, the most common differentials other than eclampsia are hemolysis, elevated liver enzymes, low platelet count (HELLP) syndrome and TTP/HUS. Usually following delivery eclampsia and HELLP improve, however delivery does not alter course of HUS and TTP.

Q2. What is the American College of Obstetricians and Gynecologists (ACOG) classification of hypertensive disorders of pregnancy?

The ACOG classified hypertensive disorders of pregnancy into:[3]
- Pre-eclampsia–eclampsia
  - Pre-eclampsia without severe features
  - Pre-eclampsia with severe features
  - Eclampsia
- Chronic hypertension

- Pre-eclampsia superimposed upon chronic/preexisting hypertension
- Gestational hypertension

Pre-eclampsia is a hypertensive disease in a pregnant lady with multisystem involvement characterized by new-onset hypertension, i.e., BP greater than 140/90 mm Hg on two occasions at least 4 hours apart that develops after 20 weeks of gestation along with either proteinuria (>300 mg/day) or presence of severe systemic involvement. When proteinuria is absent, pre-eclampsia can be defined as new-onset hypertension (BP >140/90 mm Hg 4 hours apart) along with the new onset of either renal insufficiency, thrombocytopenia, pulmonary edema, impaired liver function, cerebral disturbance, or visual disturbance.

Pre-eclampsia with severe features refers to women who present with high BP (>160/110 mm Hg) or features suggestive of organ dysfunction **(Table 1)**.

Eclampsia: It is the convulsive manifestation of pre-eclampsia characterized by occurrence of new-onset, generalized, tonic–clonic seizures. It is one of the clinical manifestations at the severe end of the pre-eclampsia spectrum.

Chronic hypertension: It is defined as hypertension that is present prepregnancy or is detected on at least two occasions before the 20th week of gestation or that persists longer than 12 weeks postpartum.

Pre-eclampsia superimposed upon chronic/preexisting hypertension: Superimposed pre-eclampsia is defined by the new onset of proteinuria, significant end-organ dysfunction, or both after 20 weeks of gestation in a woman with chronic/preexisting hypertension.

Gestational hypertension refers to new onset hypertension, i.e., BP >140/90 mm Hg on two occasions at least 4 hours apart that develops after 20 weeks of gestation without proteinuria or other symptoms/signs suggestive of pre-eclampsia-related end-organ dysfunction.

Q3. How will you manage the patient?
Principles of management of this patient include:
- Management of airway, breathing to prevent hypoxia during, and postseizures
- Control of BP
- Drugs for prevention of seizures (eclampsia) in a patient with pre-eclampsia
- Treatment of seizures
- Prevention of recurrence of seizures
- Delivery of fetus

Management of airway and breathing: This patient is conscious, oriented, and stable, and hence requires only observation. Supplemental oxygen and assessment for need of intubation and ventilation should be considered in patients with altered level of consciousness. Further episodes of seizure warrant care to prevent trauma during seizure.

Control of BP: The ACOG recommends use of antihypertensive medications in women with pre-eclampsia with severe features like BP >160/110 mm Hg or features of organ dysfunction.

Several drugs have been tried for treatment of acute severe hypertension in pregnancy-induced hypertension (PIH). A Cochrane review of 35 trials (3,573 patients) found no significant difference in terms of BP control or mortality between hydralazine, labetalol, and nifedipine. Choice of antihypertensive (hydralazine, labetalol, or nifedipine) can be based on clinician's experience and the women's preferences. Treatment with diazoxide was found to result in severe hypotension and hence it is not recommended. Treatment with nimodipine, magnesium sulfate, and ketanserin was found to be inferior due to persistent hypertension. Although nimodipine and magnesium sulfate are indicated for women who require an anticonvulsant for prevention or treatment of eclampsia, their role in pre-eclampsia is limited due to poor BP control.[4]

Prevention of seizures (eclampsia) in a patient with pre-eclampsia: Magnesium sulfate is the drug of choice for the prevention of seizure. Several drugs such as diazepam, midazolam, phenytoin, and lytic cocktail (chlorpromazine,

TABLE 1: Pre-eclampsia with severe features.[3]

Criteria based on blood pressure only	Criteria based on blood pressure and end-organ dysfunction
Blood pressure ≥160 mm Hg or diastolic blood pressure ≥110 mm Hg on two occasions at least 4 hours apart after 20 weeks of pregnancy while patient is on bed rest	Systolic blood pressure ≥140 mm Hg or diastolic blood pressure ≥90 mm Hg (with or without proteinuria) after 20 weeks of pregnancy along with one or more of the following signs and symptoms of significant end-organ dysfunction: • Thrombocytopenia—platelets <100,000/mm^3 • Severe, persistent epigastric or right upper quadrant pain unresponsive to medication and not accounted for by an alternative diagnosis or serum transaminase concentration more than or equal to two times upper limit of normal or both • Progressive renal insufficiency (serum creatinine >1.1 mg/dL or doubling of serum creatinine from baseline in the absence of other renal disease) • Pulmonary edema • New-onset cerebral or visual disturbance

promethazine, and pethidine) have been used in the past for prevention of recurrence of seizures. Magnesium Sulfate for Prevention of Eclampsia (MAGPIE) was a multicenter, multinational trial done at 175 hospitals in 33 nations with 10,141 patients comparing magnesium sulfate versus placebo for prevention of seizures (eclampsia) in patients with pre-eclampsia. Patients in treatment arm received standard intramuscular (IM) or intravenous (IV) regimen magnesium sulfate (vide infra). Women who received magnesium sulfate had significantly lower risk of eclampsia as compared to placebo [(0.8 vs. 1.9%), relative risk 0.42 (0.29–0.60)] and statistically nonsignificant reduction in maternal mortality [(0.2 vs. 0.4%), relative risk 0.55 (0.26-1.14)] without any significant increase in adverse effects to mother or baby.[5] Based on this trial, magnesium sulfate is used as first-line therapy for prevention of seizures.

Treatment of seizures: Patients who present with sudden onset of seizure in hospital are initially managed with benzodiazepines like diazepam IV bolus of 5-10 mg or lorazepam slow IV bolus of 2-4 mg.[6]

Prevention of recurrence of seizures: Magnesium sulfate is used to prevent recurrence. Systemic reviews which compared magnesium sulfate with lytic cocktail, diazepam, and phenytoin demonstrated reduction in both maternal mortality and recurrence of seizures with magnesium sulfate without any increase in maternal or fetal morbidity. Hence, magnesium sulfate is the drug of choice for prevention of recurrence of seizures.[7,8]

Anticonvulsant mechanism of action of magnesium sulfate: It is yet unclear how magnesium sulfate acts as anticonvulsant in prevention of eclamptic seizures. Possible underlying anticonvulsant mechanisms of action of magnesium sulfate in eclampsia are likely to be multifactorial, being vasodilation, N-methyl-D-aspartate (NMDA) receptor antagonism, calcium receptor antagonism, central anticonvulsant, and protection of the blood–brain barrier (BBB) to decrease cerebral edema formation.[9]

Magnesium regimens: Magnesium sulfate regimen approved for the management of eclampsia is IV Zuspan and IM Pritchard regimen. The IV regimen consists of an IV loading dose of 4 g followed by maintenance IV infusion at the rate of 1 g/h.[10] The IM regimen consists of initial IV bolus of 4 g IV and 10 g IM [(5 g in each buttock)] followed by 5 g every 4 hourly IM.[11]

Monitoring of patient on magnesium regimens (Table 2): Patients on magnesium sulfate should be monitored for features suggestive of hypermagnesemia like absence of deep tendon reflexes and urine output <100 mL/4 h.[12]

Delivery of fetus: Delivery of fetus helps in reversing the pathophysiology of PIH and should be done promptly after

TABLE 2: Clinical signs of rising plasma magnesium level.[12]

Clinical signs	Plasma level of magnesium	
	(mmol/L)	(mg/dL)
Normal	0.7–1	1.7–2.4
Therapeutic	1.8–3.0	4.4–7.3
Loss of deep tendon reflexes	3.5–5	8.5–12
Respiratory paralysis	5–6.5	12–15.8
Cardiac arrhythmias	>7.5	>18.2
Cardiac arrest	>12.5	30.4

Note: Conversion factor for magnesium 2.43 mg/dL = 1 mmol/L

stabilizing the mother ensuring fetal viability. Preferred route of delivery is cesarean section (CS), however, vaginal delivery may be attempted in carefully selected cases.[13]

A third-trimester parturient with new-onset seizures, high BP, and organ dysfunction due to raised creatinine and liver enzymes makes diagnosis of eclampsia obvious. The patient does not require further investigations or neuroimaging at this stage.

However, further workup in the form of CSF study, toxicology screening, neuroimaging, and electroencephalography (EEG) is warranted in patients who develop persistent neurological deficits, intractable seizures, and prolonged loss of consciousness.

Q4. How will you manage the patient if she continues to have seizures?

If patients on magnesium prophylaxis continue to have seizures, additional boluses of IV magnesium sulfate 2-4 g over 5-10 minutes can be given while monitoring for features of magnesium toxicity (e.g., loss of patellar reflex, respirations <12 per minute and urine output <100 mL/4 h). If patient continues to have seizures, she should be treated in line of status epilepticus similar to a nonpregnant patient. Benzodiazepines like lorazepam (2-4 mg), other antiepileptics like phenytoin (15-20 mg/kg IV with a repeat dose of 10 mg/kg in 20 minutes), or levetiracetam (500 mg IV followed by 500 mg IV or orally every 12 hours) can be given.[1] In patients with recurrent seizures in spite of prophylaxis, intubation and paralysis may be warranted in order to maintain oxygenation. Persistent or recurrent seizures in spite of adequate prophylaxis warrant evaluation for intracranial lesions or stroke.

Q5. What will be the management for persistent hypertension?

As discussed above, the definitive management of pre-eclampsia is delivery of the fetus. Delivery helps in reversing pathophysiology of PIH and minimizes the risk of development of serious maternal and fetal complications.

The ACOG recommends immediate delivery in parturient beyond 34 weeks with maternal or fetal complication in those having pre-eclampsia with severe features after maternal stabilization. However, in parturients who are at minimal risk for adverse maternal or fetal outcomes and period of gestation <34 weeks, expectant management can be done in centers with good maternal and neonatal intensive care facilities. In parturients <34 weeks, administration of corticosteroids for fetal lung maturity is recommended as it has been found to reduce incidence of respiratory distress syndrome, neonatal death, and intraventricular hemorrhage. Either two 12-mg doses of betamethasone can be given intramuscularly 24 hours apart or four doses of 6 mg dexamethasone can be administered intramuscularly every 12 hours. If such parturient develops organ dysfunction or risks of adverse maternal or fetal outcomes, immediate delivery after maternal stabilization is recommended and there is no role for expectant management.[2]

Q6. What are the various causes of altered LFT in pregnancy? How do you differentiate between them?

The differential diagnosis of raised LFT in a parturient are HELLP syndrome, acute fatty liver of pregnancy (AFLP), HUS, TTP, systemic lupus erythematosus (SLE), hepatitis, antiphospholipid antibody (APLA) syndrome, cholecystitis, pancreatitis, etc. **(Table 3)**.

HELLP syndrome: HELLP is a syndrome which is characterized by hemolysis, elevated liver enzymes, and a low platelet count.

Diagnosis of HELLP requires all three components to be present, and if only one or two elements of the triad are present then it is called partial or incomplete HELLP syndrome.

The incidence of HELLP is <1% if all pregnancies are considered, however, it is more common in women with severe pre-eclampsia where the incidence can go up to 10-20%. Patients generally present with nausea, vomiting, and pain in the right upper abdominal quadrant or epigastrium. Few patients complain of headache or visual disturbance.[14]

Criteria to diagnose HELLP (Tennessee classification): Presence of all the following characteristics is required for diagnosis of "complete HELLP syndrome".

- Microangiopathic hemolytic anemia with characteristic schistocytes (also called helmet cells) on blood smear; other signs suggestive of hemolysis include burr cells, increased lactate dehydrogenase (LDH), and decreased haptoglobin due to destruction of red cells and total bilirubin ≥1.2 mg/dL.
- Platelet count ≤100,000 cells/mm^3
- Serum AST more than two times upper limit of normal (usually >70 IU/L).

The Mississippi Triple-class system classifies the disorder based on the nadir platelet count anytime during the disease **(Table 4)**.

AFLP: The clinical presentation of AFLP varies and may include nausea, vomiting, and abdominal pain usually in the region of epigastrium or right upper quadrant, anorexia, confusion, and irritability along with cholestatic liver abnormalities. HELLP and AFLP share several clinical features and hence it may be difficult to distinguish between them. Hypertension and proteinuria are generally absent in AFLP. Thrombocytopenia is associated with HELLP whereas deranged coagulation is seen with AFLP. AFLP can rapidly progress to fulminant hepatic failure and may require liver transplant.[15]

TABLE 3: Clinical, hematological, and biochemical profile of differential diagnosis of altered liver function test (LFT)*.[14-19]

	HELLP	AFLP	TTP/HUS	SLE	Hepatitis
Onset	>20 weeks	Third trimester	Second or third trimester	Anytime	Anytime
Hemolytic anemia	+++	+	+++	+	–
Thrombocytopenia	+++	+/–	+++	+	+
Coagulation abnormalities	+/–	+++	+/–	+/–	++
Deranged liver enzymes	+++	+++	++	+/–	+++
Raised bilirubin	+	+	+/–	+	+/++
Renal abnormalities	+/–	++	+++ (more in HUS)	++	–/=
Neurologic features like altered sensorium, irritability, and seizures	+/–	++	+++ (more in TTP)	+	–

*Actual clinical presentation in individual patient may vary.
(AFLP: acute fatty liver of pregnancy; HELLP: hemolysis, elevated liver enzymes, low platelet count; HUS: hemolytic uremic syndrome; SLE: systemic lupus erythematosus; TTP: thrombotic thrombocytopenic purpura)

TABLE 4: HELLP syndrome classification based on Mississippi Triple-class system.[14]

Class	Platelet count	AST or ALT	LDH
Class 1	<50,000/mm³	>70 IU/L	>600 IU/L
Class 2	50,000–10,000/mm³	>70 IU/L	>600 IU/L
Class 3	100,000–150,000/mm³	>40 IU/L	>600 IU/L

(ALT: alanine aminotransferase; AST: aspartate aminotransferase; LDH: lactate dehydrogenase)

Immune thrombocytopenic purpura (ITP) is an immune-mediated disorder characterized by thrombocytopenia which usually manifests as bleeding disorder which may present as purpura and petechiae. The incidence and severity of ITP in pregnant women is same as nonpregnant women. Pregnancy does not increase the incidence of ITP nor does it exacerbate existing disease. Maternal and fetal mortality is very low even though platelet counts may be very low.[16]

Thrombotic microangiopathy: HUS and TTP are thrombotic angiopathies with pathophysiological characteristics similar to HELLP syndrome which includes endothelial injury, platelet-aggregating microthrombi, thrombocytopenia, and anemia.[17]

Thrombotic thrombocytopenic purpura can present before 20 weeks of gestation whereas HELLP presents after 20 weeks. TTP/HUS is usually associated with isolated thrombocytopenia, however, HELLP may be associated with coagulopathy (prolongation of PT/APTT) and in severe cases disseminated intravascular coagulation (DIC). TTP is characterized by pentad of fever, microangiopathic hemolytic anemia, mental status changes, renal failure, and thrombocytopenia, though all features need not be present for diagnosis. HUS usually causes renal failure and may present in the postpartum period.[18]

Systemic lupus erythematosus is an autoimmune disorder which affects multiple organs. It is known for SLE to flare during pregnancy; however most of these flares are mild-to-moderate.[19] SLE flare may present with clinical picture (including thrombocytopenia) difficult to distinguish from pre-eclampsia/HELLP syndrome. The underlying mechanism of thrombocytopenia in SLE is increased peripheral platelet destruction induced by antiplatelet antibodies and/or circulating immune complexes. APLAs (lupus anticoagulant and/or anticardiolipin antibodies) may be present in 30–40% of the cases.[16] Possibility of an undiagnosed SLE, although not very common, should be kept in mind in case of a suspected case of PIH.

Hepatitis may present with features of abdominal pain, vomiting, nausea, weight loss. Patients will have acute presentation and will have elevated liver enzymes. Hepatitis E-associated thrombocytopenia is also common.[16]

Q7. How will you manage a patient with HELLP syndrome?

The HELLP syndrome carries increased risk of eclampsia, acute renal failure, DIC, abruptio placentae, pulmonary edema, severe ascites, acute respiratory distress syndrome (ARDS), sepsis and shock as well as increased risk of maternal death. Once patient is diagnosed as HELLP, initial management consists of stabilization of mother, assessment of fetus, and decision of delivery.[20]

Delivery management options for a patient with HELLP can be divided into these main categories:

- *Immediate delivery:* This is indicated in pregnancy >34 weeks or earlier if patient has features of organ dysfunctions such as renal failure, DIC, suspected abruptio placentae, liver infarction or hemorrhage, and nonreassuring fetal status.
- Delivery after maternal stabilization is indicated in women with period of gestation before fetal viability, i.e., 23–24 weeks.
- *Expectant management:* In parturients with HELLP syndrome, with gestational age >23 weeks and before 34 weeks, delivery can be delayed for 24–48 hours for a course of steroids for fetal lung maturity.[2,20]

Role of steroids: Benefits of corticosteroid administration on neonatal lung maturation in <34 weeks of pregnancy are well accepted. However, there is lack of definitive evidence regarding maternal benefits of steroids administration in HELLP syndrome. Initial observational studies and small randomized trials which compared corticosteroids with placebo found improvement in clinical parameters such as BP and urine output as well as biochemical parameters such as platelet counts, LDH, and AST.[21,22] However, subsequent large, well-designed randomized clinical trials which evaluated the use of dexamethasone failed to show improvement in maternal outcome as well as biochemical parameters in patients with HELLP syndrome.[23,24] A Cochrane review of corticosteroids with placebo/no treatment/other drugs or comparing various corticosteroid regimens in women with HELLP syndrome found no difference between groups in rates of maternal death or severe maternal morbidity, or perinatal/infant death and concluded there was no clear evidence of benefit on substantive clinical outcomes. However, those receiving steroids showed significantly greater improvement in platelet counts.[25] The ACOG recommends use of corticosteroids for fetal lung maturity in parturients <34 weeks of pregnancy and also suggests a possible benefit of corticosteroids in improving maternal platelet count.[2]

Q8. There was loss of baseline variability of fetal HR. A decision for emergency CS was taken and patient was shifted to operation theatre (OT) for CS. What are the clinically significant complications that should be anticipated?

Airway changes occur during pregnancy such as capillary engorgement and edema of the upper airway. This tends to increase the risk of bleeding during manipulation of the upper airway, in addition to an increased risk of difficult ventilation and intubation of trachea. In parturient with pre-eclampsia, these airway changes are exaggerated, hence increasing the risk. Suctioning and placement of devices should be done gently to prevent bleeding. Pregnant patients are predisposed to regurgitation, aspiration, and development of aspiration pneumonitis also called as Mendelson's syndrome. The gravid uterus moves stomach and pylorus cephalad and increases intragastric pressure. The lower esophageal tone is reduced due to relaxation by progesterone. The placenta secretes gastrin which reduces gastric pH. Gastric emptying is delayed during labor. Due to all these reasons, all parturients in labor are considered to be full stomach with an increased risk for aspiration.[26]

Thrombocytopenia is commonly seen in patients with pre-eclampsia. Both quantitative and qualitative functions are affected. Problems with platelet activation, increased consumption, and decreased lifespan of platelets are noticed in pre-eclampsia. When the platelet count reduces to <1 lakh, the risk of bleeding is considerably increased which further increases when levels drop to <50,000/mm^3. Platelet transfusion is considered if platelet count is <50,000/mm^3 and patient is taken up for CS.[27] Neuraxial anesthesia is generally avoided in patients with thrombocytopenia due to increased risk of development of spinal–epidural hematoma due to engorgement of epidural veins seen in pregnancy. General consensus is to avoid neuraxial puncture in patients with platelet count <75,000/mm^3, however ideal threshold and effect of transfusion pre-puncture have not been studied prospectively in a large population.

Hemodynamic alterations: Depending on mode of anesthesia, patients are at increased risk of hypertension or hypotension during surgery. During general anesthesia, laryngoscopy and surgical stimulation can cause urges in BP whereas induction can itself cause hypotension as these patients are intravascularly volume-deficient.

High incidence of failed ventilation and intubation makes this modality unpopular. Neuraxial anesthesia is generally safe and recommended in pre-eclampsia. The two major concerns with the use of neuraxial techniques are—(1) the potential for a large drop in BP due to the combination of depleted intravascular volume and sympathetic blockade, and (2) epidural–spinal hematoma in women with severe thrombocytopenia. Incidence of hypotension postspinal blockade in pre-eclamptic woman is found to be lesser than normal pregnant woman. In view of risk of epidural–spinal hematoma in women with severe thrombocytopenia (<75,000/mm^3), neuraxial anesthesia is generally avoided below this threshold.[28]

Magnesium sulfate has several interactions with anesthetic agents. It prolongs the duration of action of non-depolarizing muscle relaxants; hence, previously discontinuation of magnesium sulfate in operating room was practiced. However, this may lead to reduction in the threshold of seizure and increases the risk of eclampsia. Discontinuation of magnesium sulfate does not prevent interaction of anesthetic agents, it in fact may increase risk of intraoperative and postoperative seizures. Hence, the ACOG recommends continued intraoperative administration of parenteral magnesium sulfate during delivery.

These patients are at increased risk of eclampsia, renal failure, postpartum hemorrhage (PPH), pulmonary edema, acute renal failure, DIC, ARDS, coagulopathy, hepatic rupture, sepsis, and shock. Hence, these patients should be carefully monitored in postpartum period for 24–48 hours.

Q9. What intraoperative monitoring is required in these patients?

Routine monitoring such as electrocardiography (ECG), oxygen saturation, BP, and temperature should be done. The underlying mechanism of hypertension in patients with pre-eclampsia is increased systemic vascular resistance with decrease in circulating plasma volume. If these patients develop hypotension or decreased urine output, fluid boluses need to be given. Invasive hemodynamic monitoring may be considered in case of persistence of hemodynamic instability or oliguria despite fluid boluses. Traditionally, central venous catheter is used for measurement of central venous pressure (CVP). A single value of CVP is rarely useful and should not be used for interpretation of fluid status; instead trends of changes from baseline on administration of bolus should be used. Possibility of higher pulmonary capillary wedge pressure (PCWP) at lower CVP value in this unique population should be kept in mind. Even though there is an increased risk of pulmonary edema due to increases in hydrostatic pressure in pulmonary bed, this does not warrant placement of pulmonary artery catheter for measurement of PCWP. Central venous catheter can be inserted in patients requiring vasoactive medications to maintain BP or for administration of medications in case of difficult venous access due to edema or multiple previous attempts at difficult peripheral vein cannulation.

Invasive arterial line is avoided unless patient is having high BP requiring IV infusions of antihypertensives. It allows for continuous measurement of BP as well as frequent sampling for arterial blood gas (ABG).[29]

In mechanically ventilated patients, pulse pressure variation (PPV) or stroke volume variation (SVV) can be used to assess volume status, however, these have not been validated in pregnancy. Echocardiographic measures like inferior vena cava (IVC) variability with respiration are inaccurate in spontaneously breathing patient and useful in only mechanical ventilated patients. Other measurements using echocardiography such as left ventricular end diastolic area (LVEDA) maybe used as measure of preload.

Intravenous access: Wide-bore cannula should be secured as these patients are at risk of PPH and may require resuscitation. These patients are usually edematous and may have had multiple punctures for blood collection and cannulation. Hence, venous access may be difficult. If central venous cannulation is planned, platelet count and coagulation parameters should be checked. Ultrasound-guided venous access is preferred due to higher incidence of coagulation disorders and inability to give Trendelenburg position due to increased abdominal girth. It may be prudent to transfuse platelets to raise level above $50,000/mm^3$ prior to insertion of ultrasound-guided central venous catheter.

Q10. What are your management priorities within the first postoperative 24 hours?

General postpartum care: Patients with pre-eclampsia/eclampsia/HELLP should be monitored for recurrence of seizures, maternal complications such as DIC, PPH, pulmonary edema, subcapsular hepatic hematoma, and retinal detachment and shock. Hence, these patients should be monitored for 48–72 hours. Routine vital signs should be monitored. If patients are on magnesium, signs suggestive of toxicity should be looked for. Seizures are common postpartum, hence, patient should be closely monitored. Investigations such as complete blood count, renal function test, LFT, and coagulation profile should be repeated daily for a few days.

Postoperative pain control: These patients are at a higher risk for respiratory depression especially if they are receiving both magnesium and opioids. Titrated doses of opioids should be given with monitoring of respiratory rate and oxygen saturation with pulse oximetry. Antidotes like naloxone and calcium may need to be used in case toxicity is seen.

Hypertension or pre-eclampsia: Postpartum development of hypertension or pre-eclampsia could be due to persistence of severe hypertension or exacerbation of hypertension in women with gestational hypertension, pre-eclampsia, or chronic hypertension or could be new onset presentation itself. Antihypertensives are recommended if BP is persistently above 150/100 mm Hg. Magnesium sulfate is recommended if the patient develops new-onset hypertension with features suggestive of severe pre-eclampsia.

She is shifted to the recovery room and recovered uneventfully from anesthesia. After 6 hours, she complains of severe headache. She had one episode of vomiting and one more episode of seizure. Post seizure, she noticed weakness in the right side of body.

Q11. What is the differential diagnosis?

Headache, vomiting, seizure, and hemiparesis in postpartum period indicates structural lesion. Structural lesions which may present in the postpartum period are ischemic stroke, hemorrhage, undetected intracranial neoplasms, and CVT. Hemorrhage could be due to rupture of an aneurysm, arteriovenous (AV) malformation, or due to coagulopathy secondary to HELLP. Ischemic stroke could be due to arterial occlusions, pre-eclampsia/eclampsia, intracranial/extracranial atherothrombosis, or cardioembolism from valvular heart disease.[30,31] CVT is more common in pregnant patients due to hypercoagulability and venous stasis and may present as stroke.

Neuroimaging is an important initial investigation. Noncontrast CT helps to differentiate acute causes of stroke and helps to rule out hemorrhage. It can also diagnose brain edema and raised ICP. Contrast CT would help in identification of tumor, abscess, and meningitis. Magnetic resonance imaging (MRI) with diffusion-weighted images has a high sensitivity for detection of regions of early infarcts. In patients with high suspicion of CVT, CT or MRI venogram can be used.

Cerebral venous thrombosis: As pregnancy is a hypercoagulable state. These patients are at increased risk of venous thromboembolism (VTE) as well as intracranial venous thrombosis. During pregnancy, coagulation system adapts to hemostatic challenge of delivery by increasing procoagulants concentration and inhibiting anticoagulants.[32]

Pregnancy and puerperium account for about 20% of all CVT cases.[32] CVT usually presents in third trimester or during puerperium.[33] Reported risk of CVT in pregnancy is about 8.9/100,000 deliveries.[33] A higher incidence of 4.5/1,000 has been previously reported. CS and infections are independent risk factors for obstetric CVT and the patients undergoing CS have three times more incidence of CVT.[34-36] Normal pregnancy is a state of compensated hypercoagulable state with increase in coagulation factors such as fibrinogen, II, VII, VIII, IX, X, XII and von Willebrand factor along with reduction of protein S and tissue plasminogen activator.[36] These changes are complicated by volume depletion which may happen at the time of delivery. Other possible risk factors implicated in the development of CVT are dehydration, traumatic instrumental delivery, and increased homocysteine concentration. However, association between these factors and CVT have not been clear.[37]

Onset can be acute, subacute, or chronic. CVT patients present with features of raised ICT and focal neurological deficit due to venous ischemia/infarction/hemorrhage or a combination of both. Uncommonly, they can present with cavernous sinus syndrome, subarachnoid hemorrhage, and multiple cranial nerve palsies.

Most patients of CVT may present with headache. It can be diffuse or localized. It can present as an isolated feature or associated with other features of raised ICP. Location of headache can be variable and has no relation to the location of thrombus. Some patients may present with severe headache—migraine type or cluster headache or thunderclap headache of subarachnoid hemorrhage.[37]

Seizures can be generalized or focal. Patients with CVT present with seizures more commonly than other cerebrovascular diseases. Severe cases of CVT can present with features of encephalopathy such as alteration in consciousness, apathy, and cognitive dysfunction.

Due to venous ischemia, infarction, and hemorrhage in CVT, patients can present with focal neurological deficits such as hemiplegia, hemiparesis, monoparesis, aphasia as well as sensory symptoms. Patients may also present with altered mental status and confusion. Alteration of mental status is usually mild to moderate.

Investigations for CVT: Investigations such as complete blood count, coagulation parameters like PT and APTT, and biochemistry are done in CVT to look for contributory factors like hypercoagulable state, any infection, and inflammation. The D-dimer measurement has been evaluated in CVT and found that it is a sensitive tool for diagnosis of CVT however, specificity is low.

Computed tomography (CT) of head is imaging of choice to rule out other differential diagnosis like stroke or hemorrhage. CT signs of CVT are divided into direct and indirect signs. Direct signs include dense triangle sign, cord sign, and delta or "empty triangle sign". Dense triangle sign is presence of a fresh thrombus seen in posterior part of sagittal sinus in noncontrast CT. Cord sign is visualization of hyperdense, thrombosed cortical veins whereas delta or empty triangle sign is a visualization of nonfilling of confluence of sinus on contrast-enhanced CT. Indirect signs of CVT on head CT are more frequent and include intense contrast enhancement of falx and tentorium, dilated transcerebral veins, small ventricles, and parenchymal abnormalities. Ischemic lesion which cross arterial boundaries is suggestive of CVT.[38] Advantages of CT are that it is quick, easily available, provides good visualization of venous sinuses, and it is useful in patients with implants and pacemaker. However, CT is not very sensitive and is positive in only 30% of cases of CVT. Other disadvantages are exposure to ionizing radiation and risk of contrast reactions.[37]

Magnetic resonance imaging is more sensitive than CT for the diagnosis of CVT. MRI detects thrombosis, edema, hemorrhage, infarction, and other consequences of CVT. MRI findings depend on the interval between time of imaging and onset of thrombus formation. On T2-weighted images, venous thrombus is hypointense in the first week and hyperintense on T1 and T2 images in the second week. After the first month, thrombosed sinuses may exhibit a variable pattern which includes even an isointense signal. Parenchymal brain lesions, secondary to venous occlusion, (cerebral edema, or venous infarction), appear as hypointense or isointense on T1-weighted MRI and hyperintense on T2-weighted MRI.[37]

Magnetic resonance venography (MR venography, angiography) has advantage of avoiding contrast by using noncontrast methods like time-of-flight (TOF) technique. It can detect absence of flow in cerebral venous sinuses, however, the interpretation can be confounded by normal anatomic variants such as sinus hypoplasia and asymmetric flow.[39] Contrast-enhanced MR venography can provide better visualization of cerebral venous channels, and gradient echo or susceptibility-weighted sequences will show normal signal in a hypoplastic sinus and abnormally low signal in the presence of thrombus.[40]

Computed tomographic venography helps in the demonstration of filling defects, sinus wall enhancement, and increased collateral venous drainage. Head CT may be normal in initial stages. CT venography has been found to be equivalent to MR venography or intra-arterial imaging. It is useful in settings where MR is not possible.[41]

Cerebral angiography, in the current scenario, is done when there is clinical suspicion for CVT but CT venography or MR venography is inconclusive.

Venous infarction in CVT: Presence of a venous infarct in neuroimaging should raise suspicion of CVT. CVT is associated with a high venous pressure leading to vasogenic edema in the white matter. Venous infarction is frequently associated with hemorrhage; however presence of hemorrhage does not seem to be a contraindication to anticoagulation.[37]

Management of CVT: Anticoagulation is the treatment of choice for CVT. It helps to prevent thrombus growth as well as induce recanalization. Unfractionated heparin (UFH) as well as low-molecular-weight heparin (LMWH) have be used for treatment of CVT. Patients treated with LMWH are less likely to develop new intracranial hemorrhage, have lower hospital mortality, and have a better functional prognosis after 6 months compared with UFH. Hence, LMWH is the preferred choice.[42-44] Guidelines for treatment of deep venous thrombosis (DVT), pulmonary embolus in pregnancy, and the puerperium recommend LMWH over UFH due to lack of teratogenic effects. For CVT, which is a disease of third trimester and puerperium, guidelines suggest use of LMWH over UFH.[36] UFH is preferred when a surgical intervention is a likely possibility as it can be easily reversed.

Thrombolytic therapy may be indicated if patient continues to deteriorate clinically despite therapeutic anticoagulation. Intravascular treatment options available are direct catheter thrombolysis or direct mechanical thrombectomy with or without thrombolysis. Though endovascular treatment for CVT are increasing these days, their benefits have not been evaluated in randomized controlled trials and are only supported by case reports and case series.[45-48]

Pathophysiology of cerebral edema associated with CVT is a combination of vasogenic and cytotoxic edema. Even though theoretically steroids may have a role in CVT by decreasing vasogenic edema, studies did not show any benefit of steroids and in fact steroids were found to be associated with higher incidence of death or disability in patients without parenchymal lesions on neuroimaging.[49] Surgical thrombectomy is usually not done but may be considered if despite maximal medical therapy patient deteriorates neurologically. If progressive edema leads to cerebral hernia, decompressive craniectomy may be required.

REFERENCES

1. Guntupalli K, Hall N, Karnad D, Bandi V, Belfort M. Critical Illness in Pregnancy. Chest. 2015;148:1093-104.
2. Wright WL. Neurologic complications in critically ill pregnant patients. Handb Clin Neurol. 2017;141:657-74.
3. Hypertension in pregnancy. Report of the American College of Obstetricians and Gynecologists' Task Force on Hypertension in Pregnancy. Obstet Gynecol. 2013;122:1122-31.
4. Duley L, Meher S, Jones L. Drugs for treatment of very high blood pressure during pregnancy. Cochrane Database Syst Rev. 2013;(7):CD001449.
5. Altman D, Carroli G, Duley L, Farrell B, Moodley J, Neilson J, et al. Do women with pre-eclampsia, and their babies, benefit from magnesium sulphate? The Magpie Trial: a randomised placebo-controlled trial. Lancet. 2002;359:1877-90.
6. Munro PT. Management of eclampsia in the accident and emergency department. J Accid Emerg Med. 2000;17:7-11.
7. Duley L, Gulmezoglu AM, Chou D. Magnesium sulphate versus lytic cocktail for eclampsia. Cochrane Database Syst Rev. 2010;(9):CD002960.
8. Duley L, Henderson-Smart D. Magnesium sulphate versus diazepam for eclampsia. Cochrane Database Syst Rev. 2003;(4):CD000127.
9. Euser AG, Cipolla MJ. Magnesium sulfate for the treatment of eclampsia: a brief review. Stroke. 2009;40:1169-75.
10. Abbade JF, Costa RA, Martins AM, Borges VT, Rudge MV, Peraçoli JC. Zuspan's scheme versus an alternative magnesium sulfate scheme: Randomized clinical trial of magnesium serum concentrations. Hypertens Pregnancy. 2010;29:82-92.
11. Seth S, Nagrath A, Singh DK. Comparison of low dose, single loading dose, and standard Pritchard regimen of magnesium sulfate in antepartum eclampsia. Anatol J Obstet Gynecol. 2010;1:1-4.
12. Lu J, Nightingale CH. Magnesium sulfate in eclampsia and pre-eclampsia. Clin Pharmacokinet. 2000;38:305-14.
13. Townsend R, O'Brien P, Khalil A. Current best practice in the management of hypertensive disorders in pregnancy. Integr Blood Press Control. 2016;9:79-94.
14. Haram K, Svendsen E, Abildgaard U. The HELLP syndrome: Clinical issues and management. A Review. BMC Pregnancy Childbirth. 2009;9:8.
15. Minakami H, Morikawa M, Yamada T, Yamada T, Akaishi R, Nishida R. Differentiation of acute fatty liver of pregnancy from syndrome of hemolysis, elevated liver enzymes and low platelet counts. J Obstet Gynaecol Res. 2014;40:641-9.
16. Stavrou E, McCrae KR. Immune thrombocytopenia in pregnancy. Hematol Oncol Clin North Am. 2009;23:1299-316.
17. Franchini M. Thrombotic microangiopathies: an update. Hematology. 2006;11:139-46.
18. Mayer SA, Aledort LM: Thrombotic microangiopathy: differential diagnosis, pathophysiology and therapeutic strategies. Mt Sinai J Med. 2005;72:166-75.
19. Petri M, Howard D, Repke J. Frequency of lupus flare in pregnancy. The Hopkins Lupus Pregnancy Center experience. Arthritis Rheum.1991;34:1538-45.
20. Sibai BM. Diagnosis, controversies, and management of the syndrome of hemolysis, elevated liver enzymes, and low platelet count. Obstet Gynecol. 2004;103:981-91.
21. Magann EF, Bass D, Chauhan SP, Sullivan DL, Martin RW, Martin JN Jr. Antepartum corticosteroids: disease stabilization in patients with the syndrome of hemolysis, elevated liver enzymes, and low platelets (HELLP). Am J Obstet Gynecol. 1994;171:1148-53.
22. Vigil-De Gracia P, García-Cáceres E. Dexamethasone in the post-partum treatment of HELLP syndrome. Int J Gynaecol Obstet. 1997;59:217-21.
23. Fonseca JE, Méndez F, Cataño C, Arias F. Dexamethasone treatment does not improve the outcome of women with HELLP syndrome: a double-blind, placebo-controlled, randomized clinical trial. Am J Obstet Gynecol. 2005;193:1591-8.
24. Katz L, de Amorim MM, Figueiroa JN, Pinto e Silva JL. Postpartum dexamethasone for women with hemolysis, elevated liver enzymes, and low platelets (HELLP) syndrome: a double-blind, placebo-controlled, randomized clinical trial. Am J Obstet Gynecol. 2008;198:283.e1-8.

25. Woudstra DM, Chandra S, Hofmeyr GJ, Dowswell T. Corticosteroids for HELLP (hemolysis, elevated liver enzymes, low platelets) syndrome in pregnancy. Cochrane Database Syst Rev. 2010;(9):CD008148.
26. Flood P, Rollins MD. Anesthesia for Obstetrics. In: Miller RD (Ed). Miller's Anesthesia, 8th edition. Philadelphia: Elsevier; 2015. pp. 2328-58.
27. Estcourt LJ, Malouf R, Hopewell S, Doree C, Veen JV. Use of platelet transfusions prior to lumbar punctures or epidural anaesthesia for the prevention of complications in people with thrombocytopenia. Cochrane Database Syst Rev. 2018;4:CD011980.
28. Wallace DH, Leveno KJ, Cunningham FG, Giesecke AH, Shearer VE, Sidawi JE. Randomized comparison of general and regional anesthesia for cesarean delivery in pregnancies complicated by severe preeclampsia. Obstet Gynecol. 1995;86:193-9.
29. Anthony J, Schoeman L. Fluid management in pre-eclampsia. Obstet Med. 2013;6:100-4.
30. Feske SK. Stroke in pregnancy. Semin Neurol. 2007;27:442-52.
31. Grear KE, Bushnell CD. Stroke and pregnancy: clinical presentation, evaluation, treatment and epidemiology. Clin Obstet Gynecol. 2013;56:350-9.
32. Khealani BA, Mapari UU, Sikandar R. Obstetric cerebral venous thrombosis. J Pak Med Assoc. 2006;56:490-3.
33. Lanska DJ, Kryscio RJ. Stroke and intracranial venous thrombosis during pregnancy and puerperium. Neurology. 1998;51:1622-28.
34. Bansal BC, Gupta RR, Prakash C. Stroke during pregnancy and puerperium in young females below the age of 40 years as a result of cerebral venous/venous sinus thrombosis. Jpn Heart J. 1980;21:171-83.
35. Lanska DJ, Kryscio RJ. Risk Factors for peripartum and postpartum stroke and intracranial venous thrombosis. Stroke. 2000;31:1274-82.
36. Marwah S, Mohindra R. Diagnosis and management of obstetric cerebral venous thrombosis: a stringent challenge. Int J Reprod Contracept Obstet Gynecol. 2016;5:4095-8.
37. Saposnik G, Barinagarrementeria F, Brown RD Jr, Bushnell CD, Cucchiara B, Cushman M, et al; American Heart Association Stroke Council and the Council on Epidemiology and Prevention. Diagnosis and management of cerebral venous thrombosis: a statement for healthcare professionals from the American Heart Association/American Stroke Association. Stroke. 2011;42:1158-92.
38. Dash D, Prasad K, Joseph L. Cerebral venous thrombosis: An Indian perspective. Neurol India. 2015;63:318-28.
39. Ivancevic MK, Geerts L, Weadock WJ, Chenevert TL. Technical principles of MR angiography methods. Magn Reson Imaging Clin N Am. 2009;17:1-11.
40. Ferro JM, Canhão P, Stam J, Bousser MG, Barinagarrementeria F; ISCVT Investigators. Prognosis of cerebral vein and dural sinus thrombosis: results of the International Study on Cerebral Vein and Dural Sinus Thrombosis (ISCVT). Stroke. 2004;35:664-70.
41. Majoie CB, van Straten M, Venema HW, den Heeten GJ. Multisection CT venography of the dural sinuses and cerebral veins by using matched mask bone elimination. AJNR Am J Neuroradiol. 2004;25:787-91.
42. Misra UK, Kalita J, Chandra S, Kumar B, Bansal V. Low molecular weight heparin versus unfractionated heparin in cerebral venous sinus thrombosis: a randomized controlled trial. Eur. J. Neurol. 2012;19:1030-6.
43. Coutinho JM, Ferro JM, Canhão P, Barinagarrementeria F, Bousser MG, Stam J; ISCVT Investigators. Unfractionated or low-molecular weight heparin for the treatment of cerebral venous thrombosis. Stroke. 2010;41:2575-80.
44. Bates SM, Greer IA, Pabinger I, Sofaer S, Hirsh J. Venous thromboembolism, thrombophilia, antithrombotic therapy, and pregnancy: American College of Chest Physicians Evidence-Based Clinical Practice Guidelines (8th Edition). Chest. 2008;133:844S-86S.
45. Horowitz M, Purdy P, Unwin H, Carstens G 3rd, Greenlee R, Hise J, et al. Treatment of dural sinus thrombosis using selective catheterization and urokinase. Ann Neurol. 1995;38:58-67.
46. Frey JL, Muro GJ, McDougall CG, Dean BL, Jahnke HK. Cerebral venous thrombosis: combined intrathrombus rtPA and intravenous heparin. Stroke. 1999;30:489-94.
47. Canhão P, Falcão F, Ferro JM. Thrombolytics for cerebral sinus thrombosis: A systematic review. Cerebrovasc Dis. 2003;15:159-66.
48. Stam J, Majoie CB, van Delden OM, van Lienden KP, Reekers JA. Endovascular thrombectomy and thrombolysis for severe cerebral sinus thrombosis: A prospective study. Stroke. 2008;39:1487-90.
49. Canhão P, Cortesão A, Cabral M, Ferro JM, Stam J, Bousser MG, et al. Are steroids useful to treat cerebral venous thrombosis? Stroke. 2008;39:105-10.

CHAPTER 12

Subarachnoid Hemorrhage

Suresh Ramasubban, Rupak Banerjee

CASE STUDY

A 74-year-old female, hypertensive on irregular treatment is brought to the hospital with history of severe headache, vomiting, and loss of consciousness. On examination, she has a Glasgow Coma Scale (GCS) of 3 (E1M1V1). Her heart rate is 46 beats/min, she is in sinus rhythm. Her blood pressure (BP) is 210/140 mm Hg. Her right-side pupil is dilated and fixed while the left side pupil is not reacting to light, but normal in size. A computed tomography (CT) scan of head shows diffuse subarachnoid hemorrhage (SAH) and a neurosurgeon is called into examine the patient.

Q1. How will you initially examine the patient? What are the scores available to prognosticate the patient? Discuss in brief the pathophysiology of raised intracranial pressure (ICP) and intracranial compliance.

This 74-year-old lady is presenting with history of headache, nausea, vomiting, and loss of consciousness. She is presenting with impaired responsiveness, an acute life-threatening emergency that requires prompt intervention so as to preserve both life and brain function. Coma is defined as the state of unarousable unresponsiveness and the patient in this vignette has presented in such a state. Alertness is maintained by the ascending reticular activating system, which is a network of neurons originating in the upper pons and mid brain and is projected to the diencephalon and from there to the cerebral cortex. Alteration in a person's alertness is a result of lesions either in the brainstem or bilateral cerebral hemispheres.

The patient's coma can be due to a variety of medical and neurologic disease, and the list of potential diseases causing coma is extremely large. To evaluate patients with impaired consciousness we need to have a brief history, general examination, and a pertinent neurological examination.

History: Patients presenting with coma often are not in a situation to give a history. Therefore, history from relatives, friends, and witnesses should be taken, and a few pertinent questions need to be asked to them.

- Time course of loss of consciousness—abrupt, gradual, and fluctuating
- Any focal signs or symptoms which preceded the loss of consciousness
- Any previous neurological episodes
- Any recent medical illness
- Medication history.

General examination: A comatose patient should have a quick general examination, and this should not be ignored as the examination can reveal clues to the etiology of coma. General examination should focus on vital signs, especially BP and temperature, as both hypothermia and hyperthermia may be present in comatose patients. The bedside vital signs act as an important addendum to the neurological examination as it helps in assessing the autonomic nervous system. The primary purpose is to evaluate for the Cushing's triad, which consists of hypertension, decreased heart rate, and irregular respiration.

Neurological examination: An urgent neurological examination is required and is directed to find out whether the coma is structural or metabolic. Neurological examination should focus on:
- Level of consciousness
- Motor response
- Brainstem response.

Level of consciousness: This can be described by using various terms such as stupor, obtundation, and somnolence. However, it is useful to describe patient's "spontaneous behavior" and "response to stimulation" to assess his level of consciousness. Arousability should be assessed by noise that is speaking in the ear of the patient and by somatosensory stimulation. The response to arousability is manifested in the form of vocalization, movement of the limbs, and eye opening. The GCS[1] is a commonly used scale to assess consciousness level by the hierarchy of responses **(Table 1)**. GCS helps in assessing the depth of impaired consciousness;

TABLE 1: Glasgow coma scale.

Behavior	Response	Score
Eye opening response	Spontaneously	4
	To speech	3
	To pain	2
	No response	1
Best verbal response	Oriented to time, place, and person	5
	Confused	4
	Inappropriate words	3
	Incomprehensible sounds	2
	No response	1
Best motor response	Obeys commands	6
	Localizes pain	5
	Flexion withdrawal to pain	4
	Abnormal flexion (decorticate)	3
	Abnormal extension (decerebrate)	2
	No response	1
Total score		15

TABLE 2: Full Outline of UnResponsiveness (FOUR) score.

Eye response	Eyelids open or opened, tracking or blinking to command	4
	Eyelids open but not tracking	3
	Eyelids closed but open to loud voice	2
	Eyelids closed but open to pain	1
	Eyelids remain closed with pain	0
Motor response (upper extremities)	Thumbs up, fist or peace sign	4
	Localizing to pain	3
	Flexion response to pain	2
	Extension response to pain	1
	No response to pain or generalized Myoclonus status	0
Brainstem reflexes	Pupil and corneal reflexes present	4
	One pupil wide and fixed	3
	Pupil or corneal reflex absent	2
	Pupil and corneal reflex absent	1
	Absent pupil, corneal and cough reflexes	0
Respiration pattern	Not intubated, regular breathing pattern	4
	Not intubated, Cheyne–Stokes breathing pattern	3
	Not intubated, irregular breathing	2
	Breathes above ventilatory rate	1
	Breathes at ventilator rate or apnea	0

however, it does not aid in the diagnoses of coma. The GCS grades the severity of coma using eye opening, motor, and verbal responses. It is very easy to use and has good interobserver reliability thus making the admission GCS a good prognostic marker in a number of conditions including traumatic brain injury (TBI), SAH, and bacterial meningitis.

The Full Outline of UnResponsiveness (FOUR) score **(Table 2)**[2] is an alternative scale to assess consciousness and has greater utility than the GCS score for diagnosis of coma, mainly by including a brainstem examination. This score is also useful when the patient is on a ventilator as the score includes respiration as one of the criteria to assess consciousness. The FOUR score basically uses eye response, motor response, brainstem reflexes, and respiration and grades them to give a composite score. FOUR score is however slightly complicated to perform and does not have the long history/track-record that the GCS score has, therefore, making its utility slightly less as compared to the GCS score.

Motor response: The next important step in the neurological examination of a comatose patient is the motor examination. Examination is directed to look for focal deficits and more importantly to look for posturing. Decorticate and decerebrate posturing are important indicators of raised ICP.

Brainstem response: Pupillary examination to assess light reflex is an important step in the neurological examination to assess for herniation syndrome as a consequence of raised ICP.

Coma has many causes; the common etiologies that lead to intensive care unit (ICU) admissions are trauma, cerebrovascular disease, intoxications, infections, and seizures. Increased ICPs are serious complications of these neurological injuries. Successful management of patients with increased ICP mandates that one should recognize elevated ICP and use appropriate monitoring and therapy directed at reducing ICP.

This 74-year-old female presented in the vignette has symptoms of headache and vomiting and has a GCS of E1M1V1. Pupils are asymmetrical and right-sided pupil is dilated. She has a history of hypertension and her presentation of coma is acute in onset. Vital signs demonstrate Cushing's triad. This brief history and examination findings all points to an intracranial catastrophe, raised ICP, and signs of brain tissue displacement and herniation syndrome.

Intracranial pressure: To understand the concept of increased ICP, we need to invoke the Monro–Kellie doctrine, understand the physiology of intracranial compliance, cerebral blood flow (CBF), autoregulations, and cerebral perfusion pressure (CPP).

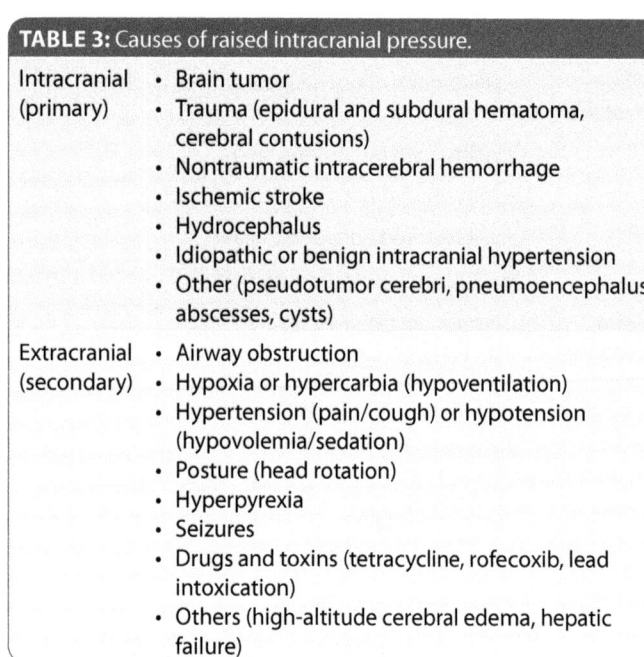

TABLE 3: Causes of raised intracranial pressure.

Intracranial (primary)	• Brain tumor • Trauma (epidural and subdural hematoma, cerebral contusions) • Nontraumatic intracerebral hemorrhage • Ischemic stroke • Hydrocephalus • Idiopathic or benign intracranial hypertension • Other (pseudotumor cerebri, pneumoencephalus, abscesses, cysts)
Extracranial (secondary)	• Airway obstruction • Hypoxia or hypercarbia (hypoventilation) • Hypertension (pain/cough) or hypotension (hypovolemia/sedation) • Posture (head rotation) • Hyperpyrexia • Seizures • Drugs and toxins (tetracycline, rofecoxib, lead intoxication) • Others (high-altitude cerebral edema, hepatic failure)

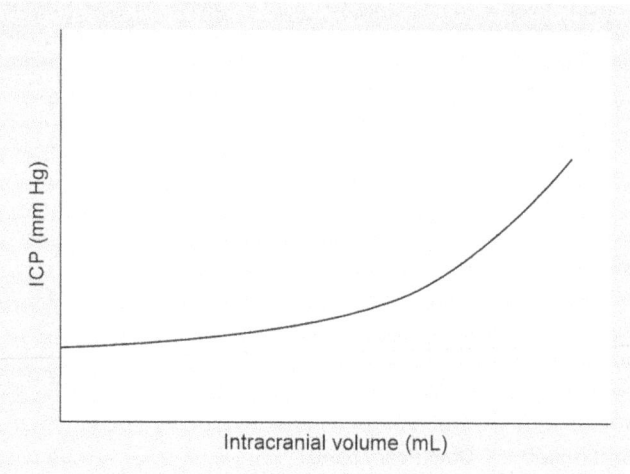

Fig. 1: Langfitt curve—curve with intracranial pressure (ICP) on the Y-axis and intracranial volume on the X-axis. As the volume in the cranium increases, the compartment is compliant and pressure rises slowly, however at a critical juncture, the pressure rises rapidly as volume increases.

The ICP is force per unit area, relative to atmospheric pressure, within the cranial cavity. ICP is generally <15 mm Hg and a pathological rise in pressure/intracranial hypertension is said to be present when the pressures exceed 20 mm Hg. The cranial cavity is occupied by the brain, blood, and cerebrospinal fluid (CSF). Brain is about 88% of the total volume of 1,500 mL, blood is about 7.5%, and CSF is about 4.5% of the total volume. The total of the partial pressures and volumes of these three compartments is the ICP. Thus, when the volume of one compartment increases, the pressure in the cranium increases and to compensate this increase in pressures, the volume of the other compartments decreases to keep ICP constant. This is the Monro-Kellie theory of ICP. Raised ICP can be a result of intracranial and extracranial etiologies. Nontraumatic intracranial causes include intracranial hemorrhages (parenchymal, subarachnoid, and subdural), hydrocephalus, cerebral edema, brain tumor, cerebral venous sinus thrombosis, and infections **(Table 3)**.

Intracranial compliance (Langfitt curve): Intracranial compliance is defined as the change in intracranial volume with increase in ICPs. The reciprocal of this is elastance. If one was to draw a graph with intracranial volume on the X-axis and ICP on the Y-axis as shown in the Langfitt curve **(Fig. 1)**,[3] the graph would demonstrate an initial flat portion, followed by a steep increase in pressure as volume increases in the intracranial cavity. The slope of this curve reflects the compliance of the cranial cavity. Initially as a disease process leads to an increase in the volume of one of the components of the cranium, there is adaptation by the other compartments, which accommodate the volume without an elevation in ICP. Initially this adaptation is mediated by a decrease in the subarachnoid CSF space. As volume in the cranial cavity increases, CSF spaces cannot be displaced any more. Subsequently, the blood vessels act as a point of compliance by eliminating blood out of the cranium, by reducing the venous volume and finally the arterial volume. As the volume reaches a threshold level, the compliance of the system worsens and there is no reserve in the other compartments leading to an abrupt and rapid increase in ICP. Lastly, the brain parenchyma itself will follow the ICP gradient and shift away from the space occupying lesion in the parenchyma. This is called as brain herniation.

Cerebral blood flow: Progressive increase in ICP results in brain cell death due to reduction in CBF or brainstem compression due to herniation syndromes. Determinants of CBF can be derived using the analogy of Ohm's law for electricity. CBF thus depends on the CPP divided by the resistance across the vessels, i.e., cerebral vascular resistance (CVR).

$$CBF = CPP/CVR$$

As CPP is the difference between mean arterial pressure (MAP) and the ICP, the earlier equation can be rewritten as:

$$CBF = (MAP - ICP)/CVR$$

Normal CPP is >60 mm Hg and CBF is >40-50 mL/min per 100 g brain tissue.

Autoregulation: It is the physiologic process by which CBF is maintained constant over a wide range of CPP. The CVR is due to the brain penetrating precapillary cerebral arterioles and its tone is tightly controlled by pressure autoregulation to ensure a constant CBF despite a fluctuating CPP **(Fig. 2)**.

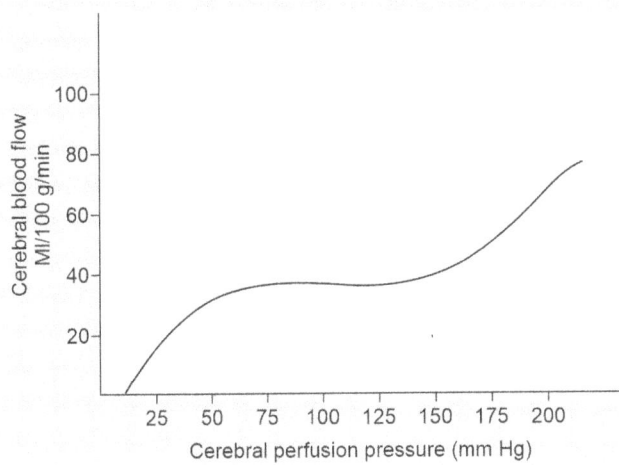

Fig. 2: Autoregulation of cerebral blood flow.

Autoregulation is mediated by chemical mediators between adjacent vascular endothelial cells and neighboring smooth muscles and nerves around the vessels. Autoregulation becomes dysfunctional in certain disease states such as stroke and trauma. In such situations, CBF is entirely dependent on MAP. This is an important concept for understanding cerebral hemodynamics in a patient with raised ICP due to a primary injury.

Another important concept in autoregulation is the change in set-point of autoregulation as seen in patients with chronic hypertension. With chronic hypertension the cerebral vasculature responds by dilatation of the arteries and arterioles. This maintains CPP and prevents the transmission of the elevated BP into the smaller intracranial arteries. This concept is important as acute reductions in BP, even though within normal ranges can produce ischemia in patients with chronic hypertension.

Q2. How do you diagnose raised ICP?

Like systemic hypertension, the diagnosis of raised ICP needs confirmation by direct measurement of pressure. The best method to determine ICP is to place a pressure transmitting or sensing device in the cranial cavity. Indications for ICP monitoring in SAH include a GCS ≤ 8 or neurological worsening, acute hydrocephalus, the development of cerebral edema (either early or delayed), intracranial masses, and the need for perioperative monitoring or CSF drainage. It can provide frequent and accurate estimations of ICP when clinical examination is not sufficient and thus limits the irrational use of therapies aimed at decreasing ICP, which can actually be harmful. ICP monitoring has not been shown to improve outcomes in trauma. In a recent study of patients with TBI, care focused on maintaining ICP < 20 mm Hg was not shown to be superior to care based on imaging and clinical examination.[4] Contraindications of a monitoring device are limited to the risks from the procedural aspect and coagulopathy.

Various techniques available to monitor ICP include:
- *Invasive methods:*
  - Ventriculostomy with external ventricular drainage (EVD) system
  - Subarachnoid bolt
  - Epidural pressure monitor
  - Brain parenchymal strain gauge devices
  - Combination devices.

Ventriculostomy with EVD remains the best technique for ICP monitoring using a fluid-filled manometer or transducer. The biggest advantage of the ventriculostomy is the dual benefit of using the EVD to treat elevated ICP by controlling CSF drainage. Usually the ventricle with less blood is selected to minimize the risk of clogging the device. However, the compartmentalization of ICP must be considered because ICP is often more significant on the side of maximum pathology. However, the device is not easy to insert into the lateral ventricle, especially when the ventricles are not swollen and are compressed. When an EVD is placed before aneurysm occlusion it can protect against sudden rises in ICP if rebleeding occurs. However, careful avoidance of large acute CSF withdrawals before the aneurysm is secured is warranted because this has been associated with a higher incidence of rebleeding.[5-7]

In cases where the ventricles are not accessible then the strain gauge device placed in the brain parenchyma (Codman Microsensor) is the best alternative. The lack of possibility for CSF drainage limits the use of isolated intraparenchymal probes in aneurysmal SAH (aSAH). Because ICP monitoring through an open EVD is unreliable and hence relies on periodic closing,[8] some centers prefer placing both devices routinely, thus allowing continuous CSF drainage and simultaneous monitoring.[9] Moreover, this approach proves helpful when there are technical limitations to intraventricular monitoring, such as a collapsed ventricle around the catheter compromising the accuracy of measurements.[10]

The ICP measurement should not only include values but also the waveform analysis. A normal waveform consists of a percussion wave (P1), tidal wave (P2), and dicrotic waves (P3) **(Fig. 3)**. These waves occur at the same frequency as the heart rate and they correspond to the transmitted arterial BP variations. P2 > P1 indicates poor compliance and tall peaked waves indicate that the compliance curve (*see* **Fig. 1**) is shifting to the right. Abnormal plateau waves lasting from 5 to 20 minutes with pressures as high as 100 mm Hg called as Lundberg A waves are an early sign of worsening ICP.[11]

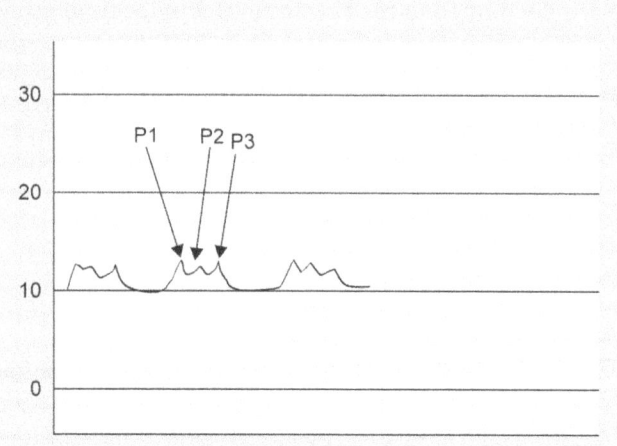

Fig. 3: Normal intracranial pressure (ICP) tracing (10 mm Hg). (P1: percussion wave; P2: tidal wave; P3: dicrotic wave)

- *Noninvasive methods:* When indications are unclear or invasive methods are not available (i.e., low-income countries) or contraindicated (i.e., severe coagulopathy), these methods are used as a "triage" tool to noninvasively discriminate patients who are at risk of developing intracranial hypertension.
  - *Ultrasound evaluation of optic nerve sheath diameter (ONSD):* Because the meninges enclose the optic nerve inside the orbit, and the space between them and the nerve directly connects with the intracranial subarachnoid space, any increase in ICP would transmit along the nerve, thus causing optic nerve sheath dilation. However, probably because of the initial bleeding that stresses the sheath, this technique is not reliable in patients with SAH.
  - *Transcranial Doppler (TCD):* A combination of elevated pulsatility index and low diastolic flow velocity is used to suggest elevated ICP at the bedside. However, its clinical utility is questionable because of its poor precision.

Q3. What are the options for the management of raised ICP?

Intracranial pressure threshold and dose: Stemming from the trauma literature, a "classical" threshold is around an ICP of 20 mm Hg (22 mm Hg as per the Brain Trauma Foundation). Interestingly, the association with poor outcomes occurred at lower ICP values than usually considered.[12-14] Although this might be partially explained by the continuously open EVD resulting in lower ICPs or that ICP elevation is a surrogate marker of underlying mechanisms leading to neurological deterioration, it could also reflect the need to lower our ICP target in SAH further. Of note, Cagnazzo et al.[12] found that ICP significantly influenced the occurrence of delayed cerebral ischemia (DCI)-related cerebral infarction, indicating values of ICP <6.7 mm Hg as protective against cerebral ischemia; they suggested that a lower ICP threshold in patients with SAH might reduce the pressure around capillary vessels, improving nutritive exchanges with brain parenchyma. A recent SAH consensus recommended maintaining a CPP of 70 mm Hg, with the arterial transducer zeroed at the level of the tragus for an accurate estimation.[15]

Rather than referring to just a threshold value, the concept of "dose", reflecting both the intensity and duration of exposure to raised ICP, better quantifies the ICP burden, define the tolerance to intracranial hypertension and more closely correlate with long-term neurological outcomes.

Management of raised ICP in aSAH: Emergency management of raised ICP, like any other medical emergency in the ICU, begins with the management of airway, breathing, and circulation (ABC). In case of raised ICP, ABC management is supplanted with ABCD, wherein decompression of the pressure also takes an important role, to prevent herniation syndromes. Decompression involves keeping head-end of bed (HOB) elevated at 30–45° and using osmotic agents like mannitol at a dose of 1 g/kg of 20% mannitol as intravenous (IV) bolus. The critical care physician should ensure a patent airway, adequate breathing, and an adequate circulation, prior to proceeding to imaging.

Airway management in patients suspected of having an elevated ICP should proceed in an orderly stepwise fashion. Preintubation should include decompression measures as mentioned before, preoxygenation with 100% oxygen to keep saturations [oxygen saturation (SpO_2)] >94%, hyperventilate to PCO_2 of 28–32 mm Hg. Rapid sequence intubation with short-acting agents should be the method of choice for intubating patients with raised ICP. Intubation step includes a fast head down and maintaining MAP >80 mm Hg. Postintubation step should include immediate elevation of HOB immediately to 30–45°, maintaining MAP >80 mm Hg, maintaining SpO_2 >94%, securing the endotracheal tube (ETT) without using circular neckbands and following pupillary responses. Patient should be ventilated with a goal minute ventilation to achieve partial pressure of arterial carbon dioxide ($PaCO_2$) of 35–40 mm Hg and a partial pressure of oxygen (PO_2) >100 mm Hg.

The next step is to obtain an emergent CT of the brain without contrast. An emergent CT scan of the brain aids in identifying the cause of elevated ICP, enabling appropriate further treatment to decrease ICP. In the vignette given, CT brain shows diffuse SAH. This patient should have a stepwise management of raised ICP in the ICU.

Stepwise management of increased ICP: Specific guidelines for treating raised ICP in patients with SAH are missing, and the current recommendations are extrapolated from the TBI population. Although, sufficient research-based literature on individual ICP treatments exists to allow creation of an evidence report,[16] unfortunately, there is insufficient research on the amalgamation of these individual treatments into a management algorithm to allow development of a treatment approach. The Seattle International Severe Traumatic Brain Injury Consensus Conference (SIBICC) guidelines[17] is such an amalgamated tier-driven stepwise approach for treatment of raised ICP, from which suggestions can be extrapolated to ICP treatment in aSAH.

The algorithm consists of four tiers namely tier zero, one, two, and three. Treatments in any given tier are considered equivalent, with selection of one treatment over another based on individual patient characteristics and physician discretion. General clinical management is considered tier zero. Treatment of intracranial hypertension will generally begin at tier one. Movement to higher tiers reflects increasingly aggressive interventions. During any given episode being addressed, multiple items from a single tier can be tried individually or in combination with the goal of a rapid response. The provider should maintain awareness of the duration of any episode and consider moving to more aggressive interventions in a higher tier quickly if the patient is not responding. In some cases, it might be preferable to skip one or more tiers (e.g., choosing to decompress a patient with midline shift due to hemispheric swelling and very high initial ICP).

- *Tier zero:* The goal is to establish a stable, neuroprotective physiologic baseline regardless of eventual ICP readings. Tier-zero sedatives and analgesics target comfort and ventilator tolerance rather than ICP. Temperature management targets avoiding fever (core temperature > 38°C). The minimal CPP threshold is 60 mm hg. Head-end elevated to 30° to facilitate venous return. Transfusion trigger is set at 7 g/dL. Hyponatremia avoided and SpO_2 kept >94%.
- *Tier one:* Tier one represents the first foray into managing intracranial hypertension. Tier-one sedative or analgesic manipulation focuses on lowering ICP, usually with short-acting agents like fentanyl and propofol. CPP target kept between 60 and 70 mm Hg and partial pressure of carbon dioxide (PCO_2) between 35 and 38 mm Hg. PCO_2 is a strong vasomodulator, with a reduction in CO_2 causing vasoconstriction of cerebral arteries, resulting in reduced cerebral blood volume and hence ICP. This vasoconstrictive effect is transient. Therefore, hyperventilation is indicated only as a temporary measure to control ICP and should be terminated once the indication ceases. This strategy needs to be used cautiously in the SAH setting, in which maintaining adequate blood flow in the early stages of the disease is a priority. As subclinical seizure activity can cause intracranial hypertension, electroencephalogram (EEG) monitoring and consideration for 1 week of prophylactic antiepileptic drugs is also suggested in tier one.

Cerebrospinal fluid withdrawal: It is a crucial strategy for controlling ICP and tier-one therapy advocates CSF drainage when EVD in situ. The recommendations are:
- Insert an EVD before securing the aneurysm in patients with a World Federation of Neurological Surgeons score of ≥3 or acute hydrocephalus.
- After EVD placement, set the drainage to high thresholds (>20 mm Hg) or ICP until aneurysm obliteration to prevent aneurysmal transmural pressure reduction and rebleeding.
- After securing the aneurysm, use a continuous EVD drainage approach, leaving the drain open against a gradient of 10–15 mm Hg. Early blood clearance after aSAH has been associated with less DCI. Close the EVD for proper recording of ICP for 10–15 minutes every hour. Monitor the drained volume hourly and aim for a target of around 10 mL/hour. If a parenchymal device is available, record ICP continuously.
- If ICP is not controlled with CSF diversion alone, escalate to ICP management strategies following a stepwise approach. Rule out extracranial confounders, such as fever, high PCO_2 levels, venous drainage disturbances, or low CPP causing vasodilation.

In the vignette presented there is no mention of a hydrocephalus, so there is no role of CSF drainage but ICP monitoring can be considered as GCS is <8, with the goal of maintaining ICP <20 mm Hg and CPP between 60 and 70 mm Hg.

Osmotherapy: It is frequently used in patients with aSAH and the main agents used are mannitol and hypertonic saline (HTS). The supposed mechanism of action is to improve blood rheology and cerebral microvascular flow and create an osmolar gradient across the blood–brain barrier (BBB), favoring cerebral edema reabsorption. Mannitol is an osmotic diuretic, and at doses of 0.25–1 g/kg with a target osmolality of 320 mOsm/L it has been associated with effective ICP reduction. HTS can expand the intravascular volume and increase BP and serum sodium levels. The HTS concentrations reported were between 3 and 23.5%. Equimolar doses decrease ICP similarly. The upper safety limit is often reported as serum sodium level of 155 mEq/L. According to guidelines for treating cerebral edema in SAH, a symptom-based bolus dosing is suggested rather than a sodium-target-based dosing.[18] A recent review[19] on HTS confirmed its efficacy in reducing refractory ICP in patients with SAH, although no recommendation on the dose, volume, and concentration was made. In addition, Bentsen et al.[20] found osmotherapy with HTS to attenuate both static ICP and ICP wave amplitude; of note, they report that in the majority of HTS infusions, the ICP wave amplitude target was not reached even though ICP and CPP targets were, a finding consistent with an unfavorable intracranial compliance state despite normal static values.

- *Tier two:* Administration of neuromuscular blocker and checking for cerebral autoregulation are the two main highlights of tier-two therapy.

  After ensuring adequate analgosedation, a trial of bolus neuromuscular blockage is performed to check for benefits and if found to be efficacious, progression to continuous infusion is made.

  An increasing MAP can lower ICP if autoregulation is intact. When MAP is raised the vasoconstriction attendant to active autoregulation decreases cerebral blood volume and reduce ICP. On the other hand, if autoregulation is disrupted, elevation of MAP may worsen ICP. This can easily be done by a MAP challenge (under stable conditions, initiation or titration of a vasopressor is done to increase the MAP by 10 mm Hg and for 20 minutes; no other active changes in care should be made during the challenge including adjustments in sedation, analgesia, EVD drainage or other physiological parameters). Interaction between MAP, ICP, and CPP are observed at the beginning and end of the test. If the test is positive (autoregulation intact), judgement is required as to whether the benefit of the ICP decrease justifies the risks of raising MAP to the new elevated target, with fluids vasopressors and/or inotropes. If the test is negative (autoregulation disrupted), MAP is adjusted back to baseline and ICP reduction becomes the only mean to optimize CPP.

- *Tier three:* Hypothermia, barbiturate coma, and decompressive craniectomy are the last resorts for raised refractory ICP and are supported at most by anecdotal evidence. In the Intraoperative Hypothermia for Aneurysm Surgery trial, hypothermia during aneurysm surgery, used as a prophylactic neuroprotective strategy, did not improve outcomes.[21] Fever is common and is an independent predictor of poor outcome. Therefore, in the absence of evidence of the beneficial effects of hypothermia, strict normothermia should be targeted.

  Barbiturates prolong sedation, cause metabolic derangement, respiratory and immunological suppression, and associated with cardiovascular adverse events. Hence, their initiation should be based on the response to a test dose and endpoint should be ICP control and not burst suppression in EEG. However, evidence is lacking for routine administration in patients of aSAH with raised refractory ICP.

  Currently, there is insufficient evidence to establish the superiority of decompressive craniectomy over medical management for treating severe raised refractory ICP in patients with SAH. Nevertheless, bilateral decompression remains a viable option as a rescue therapy when maximal medical management has been exhausted. It represents the most promising intervention in situations where clinicians have explored all other available alternatives.

- *Inter-tier recommendations:* Stepping to a higher tier is a potential indicator of increased disease severity. As higher tiers represent interventions with increased associated risks, reassessing the patient's basic intra- and extracranial physiologic status (CPP and ABG values) and reconsidering the surgical status of intracranial mass lesions (e.g., contusions) not previously considered operative, seems reasonable. Repeat clinical examination and assessing need for CT head and/or EEG is also justified. If the patient is at a nonspecialist center at the point of upward tier advancement, consultation and potential need for transfer to a center with increased resources may also be considered. When desired, transfer is best completed before clinical decline precludes it.

Figure 4[22] shows different tier therapies for control of ICP.

Q4. What is the etiology of SAH? What are the clinical manifestations? How do you classify SAH? How do you confirm the diagnosis in patients with SAH?

The SAH results from the sudden rupture of an intracerebral artery into the subarachnoid space. About 85% of the cases are due to rupture of a berry aneurysm; the remaining 15% are nonaneurysmal, perimesencephalic, or pretruncal SAH accounts for 10% of cases. The remaining 5% of all SAH are due to various rare conditions **(Table 4)**.[23]

The clinical findings in patients with SAH range from a classical thunderclap headache ("the worst headache of my life"), vomiting, and change in mental status as presented in the vignette. Headache is sudden in onset and immediately reaches maximal intensity. A warning or sentinel headache that precedes the aSAH-associated presentation occurs in 10–43% of cases. Physicians must maintain a high level of awareness and concern for this diagnosis and pursue

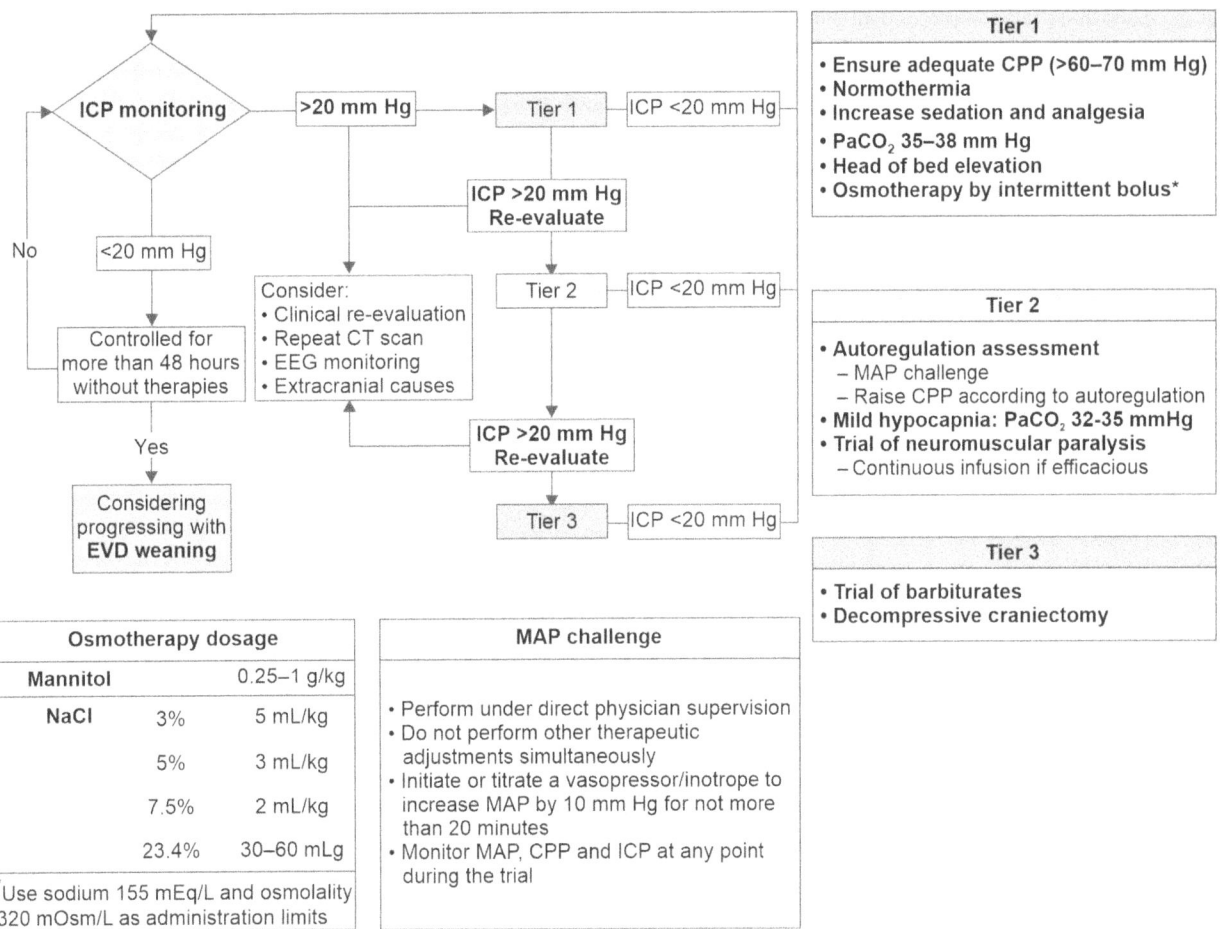

Fig. 4: Strategies for controlling intracranial pressure. (CPP: cerebral perfusion pressure; EEG: electroencephalogram; EVD: external ventricular drainage; ICP: intracranial pressure; MAP: mean arterial pressure; $PaCO_2$: partial pressure of arterial carbon dioxide)

appropriate workup, when necessary, because diagnosis of a sentinel bleed before a catastrophic rupture can be lifesaving. Seizures, focal neurological deficit, and nuchal rigidity are other manifestation of SAH. The severity of SAH is classified based on the clinical presentation and CT findings. It is important to classify the severity of SAH as outcomes correlate well with severity level and the grading also guides the timing of surgery.

The clinical classification by the World Federation of Neurological Surgeons is one of the methods for grading the severity of SAH.[24]

- *Grade 1:* GCS 15, no motor deficit
- *Grade 2:* GCS 14 to 13, no motor deficit
- *Grade 3:* GCS 14 to 13, motor deficit present
- *Grade 4:* GCS 12 to 7, motor deficit may be present or absent
- *Grade 5:* GCS < 6, motor deficit may be present or absent

The other classification for severity of SAH is the Hunt and Hess scale:[25]

- *Grade 1:* Asymptomatic or mild headache
- *Grade 2:* Moderate-to-severe headache, nuchal rigidity with or without motor deficit

TABLE 4: Causes of subarachnoid hemorrhage.

Cerebral aneurysm	• Saccular
	• Mycotic
	• Fusiform
	• Diffuse
	• Globular
Nonaneurysmal	Perimesencephalic
Other	• Trauma
	• Coagulopathy
	• Vasculitis
	• Idiopathic

- *Grade 3:* Confusion, lethargy, or mild focal symptoms
- *Grade 4:* Stupor, hemiparesis, or both
- *Grade 5:* Coma or extensor posturing

The diagnosis of SAH can be obtained with a noncontrast CT scan of the head which is 95% sensitive if performed within the first 24 hours. The Fisher scale[26] categorizes patients according to the CT findings.

- *Grade 1:* No SAH on CT scan
- *Grade 2:* Broad diffusion of subarachnoid blood, no clots, and no layers of blood >1 mm deep

Flowchart 1: Workflow for patients with symptoms concerning for aneurysmal subarachnoid hemorrhage (aSAH).

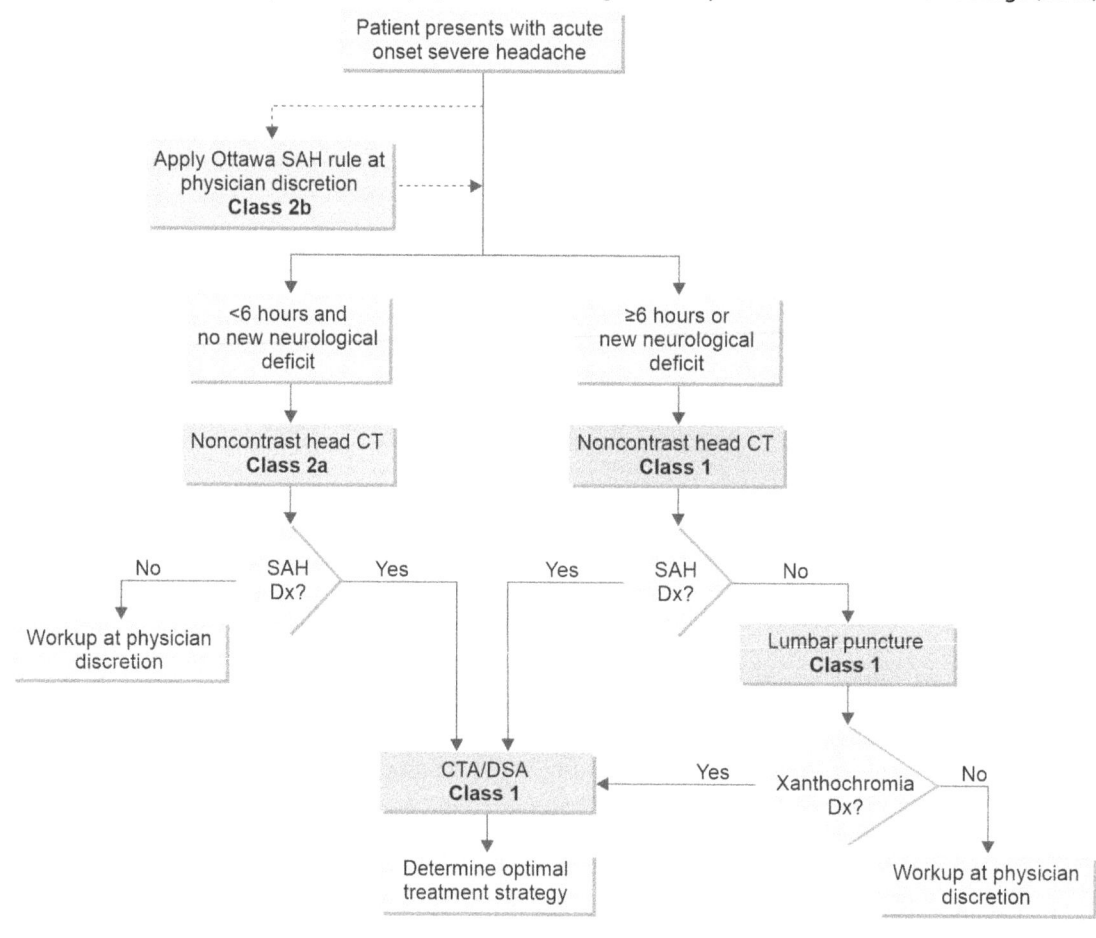

- *Grade 3:* Localized blood clots in the subarachnoid space or layers of blood >1 mm thick
- *Grade 4:* Intraventricular and intracerebral blood present, in the absence of significant subarachnoid blood.

Although noncontrast head CT remains the mainstay of SAH diagnosis, the specific diagnostic workup depends on the time of presentation from symptom onset and the patient's neurological status. **Flowchart 1**[27] outlines a suggested workflow for patients presenting to medical attention with a severe headache or other symptoms concerning for aSAH. Treating physicians will need to exercise judgment on the likelihood that a certain test will alter their clinical management.

The Ottawa SAH rule **(Box 1)**[27] serves as a method to screen out individuals with a low likelihood of aSAH. Application of the rule requires that patients who present with a severe headache and meet any of the criteria outlined in **Box 1** may need to undergo additional testing as directed by the treating physician. The rule is 100% sensitive but the specificity ranges from 7.6 to 15.3% across studies.[27] Use of the Ottawa SAH rule can therefore identify a subset of patients (albeit small) who are unlikely to have aSAH and thereby

BOX 1: Ottawa subarachnoid hemorrhage (SAH) rule.

For alert patients >15 years of age with new severe nontraumatic headache reaching maximum intensity within 1 hour. Patients require additional investigation for SAH if they meet any of the following criteria:
- Age ≥40 years
- Neck pain or stiffness
- Witnessed loss of consciousness
- Onset during exertion
- Thunderclap headache (instantly peaking pain)
- Limited neck flexion on examination

avoid additional imaging and workup that use resources and expose patients to unnecessary risk.

For patients presenting within 6 hours of headache onset and who have no new neurological deficits, the lack of SAH on a noncontrast head CT is likely sufficient to exclude aSAH.

It is important to note that this does not apply to patients with atypical presentations such as primary neck pain, syncope, seizure, or new focal neurological deficit. Therefore, the lack of a classic presentation should still prompt appropriate imaging and workup.

In patients who do not meet criteria for application of the Ottawa SAH rule, additional workup with head CT and, if negative or equivocal, lumbar puncture (LP) for xanthochromia evaluation or CT angiography is necessary. LP is often performed >6-12 hours after symptom onset. No study has evaluated CT angiography versus LP as the next step in the workup. CT angiography does not directly evaluate for SAH, only cerebrovascular pathology, and its sensitivity is ≈97.2%. Not all the centers are equipped with angiography facility and in case of ruptured aneurysms <3 mm its sensitivity decreases to 61%.[27] Given the severe morbidity and potential mortality associated with a missed aSAH diagnosis, these small differences are critical. LP for xanthochromia evaluation should be performed in patients presenting >6 hours from ictus in whom there is a nondiagnostic CT head and a high suspicion for SAH.

On the other hand, CT angiography often becomes the next performed diagnostic test when SAH is diagnosed with noncontrast CT head. It can be performed at the time of the initial CT brain, can detect an aneurysm, especially in certain hemorrhage patterns (diffuse basal cistern and Sylvian fissure SAH vs. small volume focal cortical SAH), and in patients presenting in extremis due to a large intraparenchymal clot that may require urgent surgical evacuation.

Digital subtraction angiography however remains the gold standard for diagnosing aneurysms defining the geometry and choosing optimal treatment modality.

Magnetic resonance imaging (MRI) with fluid-attenuated inversion recovery, proton density, and gradient echo sequences are very sensitive for detecting blood in the subarachnoid spaces but are often not done due to time concerns and dearth of logistic support.

Q5. Discuss the management of subarachnoid hemorrhage.

The patient presented in the vignette has a clinical grade 5 SAH and a Fisher grade 2 based on radiology. Management of SAH should follow a definite chronology with an early phase directed at managing ICP, stabilizing the cardiopulmonary systems as described earlier. The other important consideration in the early phase is preventing early rebleeding. This early phase is followed by a period of vasospasm which aims to prevent DCI and infarction and finally a subacute time period during which various medical and neurological complications of SAH may occur.

Preventing early rebleeding risk: Risk of aneurysm rerupture is about 4-14% in the first 24 hours after SAH. The early phase goal for a patient with SAH is to limit the risk of early rebleeding by (1) BP control, (2) correcting coagulation parameters, and (3) early aneurysm repair.

- *Blood pressure control:* Treatment of hypertension is commonly pursued in practice until the ruptured aneurysm is treated, but the effect of early hypertension control on the risk of rebleeding is not well established.[28-30] Although it is reasonable to treat severe hypertension (>180-200 mm Hg) on presentation, there is insufficient evidence to recommend a particular BP target. Strict avoidance of hypotension (MAP <65 mm Hg) and close neurological monitoring to be ensured while lowering the BP. Beta-adrenergic blockade with labetalol (10-20 mg intravenously every 10-15 minutes as needed) or esmolol (500 mg/kg IV loading dose, then 2.5-200 mg/kg per minute infusion) is the preferred strategy for BP control. Hydralazine (10-20 mg intravenously every 10-15 minutes as needed) is also a good agent for BP control in this situation. When deciding on the target for BP reduction, factors to appraise include BP at presentation, brain swelling, hydrocephalus, and history of hypertension and renal impairment.

- *Correction of coagulation parameters and antifibrinolytic therapy:* It is of paramount importance to correct any coagulation abnormalities, if existing. Though the benefit of emergency reversal of anticoagulation has not been tested in patients with aSAH, yet based on data from other forms of intracranial hemorrhage, the American Heart Association/American Stroke Association (AHA/ASA) strongly recommends immediate anticoagulation reversal according to current published standards for life-threatening bleeding.[27] There is some evidence that aspirin use could be associated with an increased risk of rebleeding and platelet transfusion has got possible harmful effect in patients with spontaneous supratentorial cerebral hemorrhage associated with antiplatelet therapy. Also there is currently very limited evidence on the risks and benefits of platelet transfusion in patients with aSAH, either in general or in patients who require an open surgical intervention. So it might be reasonable to decide on a case-to-case basis before platelet transfusion for reversal of antiplatelet effects.

Administration of antifibrinolytic therapy might reduce the risk of rebleeding, but this effect has not been consistent across trials. Furthermore, it does not improve functional outcomes and there was an increased risk of DCI and venous thromboembolic events (VTEs) in earlier trials. However, the most recent and largest high-quality randomized control trial (RCT) to date evaluating antifibrinolytic therapy in aSAH, the ULTRA (Ultra-Early Tranexamic Acid After Subarachnoid Hemorrhage) trial,[31] concluded that the ultra-early short-term (tranexamic acid was started after a median time of 185 minutes from symptom onset and continued until the aneurysm was secured, up to 24 hours) antifibrinolytic therapy did not show a significant reduction in the rate of rebleeding (10% in tranexamic acid group vs. 14% in control group) and demonstrated no improvement in functional outcomes at 6 months [modified Rankin Scale (mRS) score 0-3 was 60% in tranexamic acid group vs. 64% in control group]. Moreover, the rate of excellent functional outcome (mRS score 0-2) was actually lower in the tranexamic acid arm. This RCT also showed no differences in terms of mortality, cerebral ischemia, and thromboembolic complication rates between patients treated with tranexamic acid or placebo. Consequently, both the Neurocritical Care Society (NCS) and AHA/ASA recommends that antifibrinolytic therapy is not indicated due to lack of benefit. While the NCS strongly advocates against antifibrinolytic therapy in patients with aSAH,[32] AHA/ASA concludes that it is not useful as part of routine management keeping a note that there might still be a possible role of antifibrinolytic therapy in settings where aneurysm obliteration will be delayed beyond 14 hours from symptom onset because of logistic or other medical reasons (median time to aneurysm obliteration was 14 hours from symptom onset in the ULTRA trial).

- *Aneurysm repair:* The best way to prevent rerupture is evaluation by specialists with endovascular and surgical expertise and according to patient and aneurysmal characteristics completely repair the aneurysm, either surgically or by endovascular techniques, as early as possible (preferably within 24 hours of onset). Both techniques have different advantages and disadvantages and choice of treatment depends on different factors such as age, aneurysm geometry and location, severity of SAH and brain injury, and presence of intraparenchymal hemorrhage.

Q6. How will you decide between clipping and coiling of the aneurysm?
Longer life expectancy and better long-term protection from rerupture related to clipping favor consideration of clipping in young patients (<40 years), whereas in older patients (>70 years), there are insufficient data to support a clear benefit of one technique over the other. While primary coiling is preferred for posterior circulation and internal carotid artery aneurysms, clipping is superior in the wide neck aneurysm, and middle cerebral artery (MCA) cohort.

For anterior circulation aneurysm rupture and good grade aSAH (Hunt and Hess/WFNS grade 1-3), the Cochrane review and meta-analysis of four RCTs of clipping versus coiling indicates that primary coiling provides higher odds of functional independence (mRS score 0-2) at 1 year, with an relative risk (RR) 0.77 [95% confidence interval (CI), 0.67-0.87) for death/dependency.[33] However, post hoc analysis of the largest RCT, the International Subarachnoid Aneurysm Trial (ISAT),[34] showed that at 5 years the difference between coiling and clipping was not significant for either death or dependency [RR, 0.88 (95% CI, 0.77-1.02)] or death alone [RR, 0.82 (95% CI, 0.64-1.05)].[35] Long-term data also indicate a small but higher incidence of rebleeding with coiling and a higher incidence of seizures with clipping.[33-37]

All the primary coiling involves balloon-assisted technique. Due to increased thrombogenicity, need for dual antiplatelet therapy and consequent high hemorrhagic complications, stent-assisted coiling should only be used when other treatment options are not feasible. In the acute phase, patients in whom complete obliteration of the aneurysm is not feasible, either technically or due to procedural risks, partial obliteration and retreatment in a delayed fashion seems reasonable.

For older patients (>65 years) and patients with poor grade aSAH (Hunt and Hess/WFNS grade 4-5) may be candidates for aneurysm treatment as long as they do not have irrecoverable and devastating neurological injury. Modifiable medical conditions such as seizures, hydrocephalus, hyponatremia, hypothermia, intraparenchymal bleed, cerebral edema, and raised ICP should be identified and treated first. Treatment to prevent rebleeds needs careful consideration of individual comorbidities and prehemorrhage functional status, and should incorporate shared decision-making and discussion of the likely prognosis with the family or surrogate decision makers. Good outcomes are observed in 39-42%[27] of treated patients as per current literature. In the vignette, the 74-year-old patient has presented with a clinical grade 5 and the aforementioned approach has to be followed.

Q7. Discuss cerebral vasospasm and DCI after subarachnoid hemorrhage.
Historically, arterial narrowing with subsequent downstream low flow and ischemia was considered the sole cause of delayed neurological deterioration in SAH patients with vasospasm. Although the majority of SAH patients develop angiographic vasoconstriction (up to 70%), only around 20-30% develop DCI.[38] DCI occurs mostly between days 4 and 14 after aSAH. Large-vessel narrowing with subsequent low flow might be one of multiple mechanisms of DCI, but the causal framework also includes multiple other independent mechanisms such as early brain injury (EBI), microcirculatory dysfunction with loss of autoregulation, cortical spreading depolarization (CSD), and microthrombosis.[39] Cerebral infarction sometimes develops in the absence of demonstrable vasoconstriction or in a vascular territory unaffected by vasospasm and therapy directed at successful treatment of angiographic

BOX 2: Harmonized definition of delayed cerebral ischemia and cerebral infarction.

Delayed cerebral ischemia
Focal (hemiparesis, aphasia, hemianopia, or neglect) or global (2 points decrease on GCS) neurological impairment lasting for at least 1 hour and/or cerebral infarction, which:
- Is not apparent immediately after aneurysm occlusion
- Is attributable to ischemia
- Is not attributed to other causes (i.e., surgical complication and metabolic derangements) after appropriate clinical, imaging, and laboratory evaluation

Cerebral infarction
Presence of cerebral infarction on CT or MR scan of the brain within 6 weeks after SAH, or on the latest CT or MR scan made before death within 6 weeks, or proven at autopsy; that is:
- Not present on the CT or MR scan between 24 and 48 hours after early aneurysm occlusion
- Not attributable to other causes such as surgical clipping or endovascular treatment
- Not due to a nonischemic lucency related to a ventricular catheter, intraparenchymal hematoma, or brain retraction injury

(CT: computed tomography; GCS: Glasgow Coma Scale; SAH: subarachnoid hemorrhage)

TABLE 5: Grading of vasospasm based on transcranial Doppler.

Degree of vasospasm	Mean flow velocity	Lindegaard ratio
Mild	120–149 cm/s	3–6
Moderate	150–199 cm/s	3–6
Severe	>200 cm/s	>6

vasoconstriction alone does not necessarily lead to a better functional outcome.[3] **Box 2**[40] shows the harmonized definition of DCI and cerebral infarction.

Diagnosis and monitoring of vasospasm and role of TCD: Detection of cerebral vasospasm in aSAH is crucial as this is one of the main determinants of DCI and poor neurological outcome. Diagnosis of DCI is challenging and serial neurological examinations are of limited value in patients with high grade aSAH. CT angiography, CT perfusion imaging, continuous electroencephalography (cEEG), TCD all have been used for diagnosis of vasospasm. CT angiography has a high sensitivity (91%) for central vasospasm but accuracy diminishes in distal territories. CT angiographic vasospasm scores are direct predictors of DCI and poor neurological outcome,[41] and CT perfusion allows early (as early as day 3; vasospasm window) prediction of perfusion abnormalities.[42,43] CT perfusion can therefore aid in the detection of alterations to the microcirculation, in addition to the macroscopic vasospasm that can be detected with CT angiography. CT perfusion has a positive predictive value of 0.67 for DCI. However, there might be logistic issues and lack of expertise for interpretation in real-time. CT angiography is also associated with risks of contrast and radiation exposure. cEEG is not always available and not very useful unless used with quantitative software programs. TCD is a low-cost, noninvasive, and safe bedside neuromonitoring technique that allows repetitive and dynamic assessment of vasospasm after aSAH. Although angiography remains the gold standard, serial TCD examinations [one to two times/day and using quantified acceleration of mean flow velocities (MFVs) as a surrogate of large cerebral vessel narrowing] along with close clinical neuromonitoring can be done to assess vasospasm, to monitor treatment response and to guide additional investigations. In case of clinical suspicion of vasospasm (i.e., neurological deterioration), conventionally an absolute cut off value of MCA MFV >200 cm/s or a rise by 50 cm/s from previous value is used to initiate treatment immediately and perform additional confirmatory imaging like cerebral CT perfusion or angiography. If MFV >120 cm/s but <200 cm/s, MFV in the extracranial internal carotid artery is assessed and the Lindegaard ratio **(Table 5)** (ratio of MCA MFV to extracranial ICA MFV) is calculated to differentiate vasospasm from cerebral hyperemia. Most of the published literature focused on MCA vasospasm and the most recent systematic review and meta-analysis including 17 studies (n = 2,870 patients)[44] shows TCD evidence of vasospasm was found to be highly predictive of DCI. As TCD has a sensitivity of 90% (95% CIs 77–96%), specificity of 71% (95% CI 51–84%), positive predictive value of 57% (95% CI 38–71%), and negative predictive value of 92% (95% CI 83–96%) to diagnose vasospasm of MCA,[44] cerebral CT perfusion or angiography still to be performed in case of clinical suspicion of vasospasm with MFV below <120 cm/s. In another updated meta-analysis of high-quality TCD studies (n = 18),[45] pooled sensitivities for the MCA (66.7%, 55.9–75.9) and the basilar arteries (62.1%, 33.3–84.3) were higher than for the anterior cerebral artery (ACA) (32.7%, 10.9–65.7). The pooled specificities were very similar for these three arteries: MCA 89.5% (80.3–94.7), basilar 84.5% (71.1–92.3), ACA 89.6% (48.2–98.7). The reasons for these wide range of sensitivity may be sonographer-related (wrong vessel, missing peak velocity, and interoperator variability), technology-related (inability to visualize peak velocity, inability to correct for angle of insonation), and/or patient-related (poor temporal bone window, heart rate, and BP). Also retrospective observational studies suggest that the combination of TCD and other neuromonitoring modalities [such as cEEG, CTP, and continuous brain tissue oxygen ($Pbto_2$)][27] may increase the prediction of DCI, this combination may not be possible in majority set ups due to logistic issues. As TCD is performed intermittently (at best one to two times/day) and there is absence of validated MFV cut off values for intracranial vessels other than MCA, it is reasonable to do TCD examinations using MCA MFV values (combining other modalities when possible) for detection of vasospasm and predict DCI.

Prevention and treatment of cerebral vasospasm and DCI
Nimodipine: Delayed cerebral ischemia prevention has been the Holy Grail of SAH research for decades, but few options are available and unfortunately most attempts have yielded disappointing results. Nimodipine, a dihydropyridine calcium channel antagonist, is the only pharmacologic intervention so far associated with better outcome in SAH patients, although it has no impact on large vessel vasospasm. Multiple trials have demonstrated a benefit,[46] with the seminal trial showing an impressive reduction in cerebral infarction, poor neurological outcome, and death with oral nimodipine 60 mg given every 4 hours for 21 days.[47] Other calcium channel blockers and routes for prophylactic use are not recommended presently due to adverse effects.

Enhanced blood clearance: Numerous attempts have been made to accelerate clearance of subarachnoid blood, since it is strongly associated with vasospasm. The only RCT investigating the use of intraoperative administration of recombinant tissue-type plasminogen activator (r-tPA) failed to show any effect on outcome.[48] Lumbar drainage of CSF was also unsuccessful at improving mRS[49] or Glasgow Outcome Scale (GOS)[50] scores at 6 months in two RCTs. Hence, these are not advocated presently.

Avoidance of hypovolemia and hyponatremia: Hyponatremia and hypovolemia is noted frequently after SAH due to either excessive natriuresis and/or inappropriate secretion of antidiuretic hormone (ADH), and have been associated with impending DCI.[51] This has led many experts to recommend continuous monitoring and optimization of adequate circulating blood volume in aSAH. On the other hand, there are consistent signals that liberal fluid administration targeting hypervolemia is associated with a higher risk of pulmonary edema. Early goal-directed treatment using continuous monitoring and optimization of hemodynamic parameters, including cardiac output (CO), preload, and stroke volume variability to guide fluid and hemodynamic management in aSAH during endovascular/surgical therapy and ICU care, can increase the detection and treatment of dehydration/intravascular volume depletion compared with conventional methods and a protocolized isotonic crystalloid fluid therapy targeting euvolemia seems to be a reasonable approach. However, the technique to assess or achieve this goal remains undefined at present and this may not also affect the incidence of vasospasm, DCI, death, or functional outcome.[27]

Hyponatremia, with or without polyuria or natriuresis, is a prominent clinical feature in aSAH but has been inconsistently associated with DCI and poor outcome in cohort studies.[27] Several moderately sized RCTs found fludrocortisone to be effective in reducing the incidence of hyponatremia and natriuresis when started early after aSAH onset and continued for 10-14 days, but fludrocortisone did not consistently reduce DCI or affect outcome.[27]

Induced hypertension and hemodynamic augmentation: Variability in BP is associated with less favorable neurological outcomes in SAH.[52] Clinically, hypotension can precede the development of focal neurological deficits in patients who are neurologically compensated otherwise. The only RCT of induced hypertension in aSAH, HIMALAIA (Hypertension Induction in the Management of Aneurysmal Subarachnoid Hemorrhage with Secondary Ischemia), was discontinued prematurely because of a lack of benefit for cerebral perfusion and poor enrolment, limiting the ability to interpret results. There was no difference in functional outcome, but the study was underpowered.[53] Observational data, including large, multiyear, multicenter retrospective data, indicate an improvement after induced hypertension in ≈80% of symptomatic patients.[53,54] Taken together, these data suggest that induced hypertension and hemodynamic augmentation may be reasonable in patients with DCI but use of these interventions should be judicious and tailored to the patient's individual hemodynamic profile.

The peak risk for DCI and cerebral vasospasm is post-bleed days 6-10 after aSAH and patients treated with prophylactic hemodynamic augmentation had no difference in neurological outcomes but a higher incidence of complications, including congestive cardiac failure, atrial fibrillation, myocardial infarction, and death. So a reactive rather than prophylactic approach to hemodynamic augmentation should be taken to reduce iatrogenic patient harm. Permissive autoregulation seems a reasonable strategy in view of the fact that in patients with aSAH developing DCI, there is a rise in BP values that correlates with developing cerebral vasospasm.

Normal saline as part of protocolized fluid therapy along with noradrenaline remains first-line treatment of choice. Noradrenaline is chosen due to its combination of alpha and beta receptor stimulation, the low frequency of tachycardia, and the reliable hemodynamic response in other scenarios. Depending on patients baseline BP a starting target [either systolic blood pressure (SBP) or MAP; CPP can be targeted where ICP monitoring in place] is usually selected and the target can then be increased every 30 minutes stepwise in a goal-directed fashion and titrated to clinical response. In symptomatic patients with a reliable clinical examination, the goal is resolution of symptoms, whereas, in poor grade aSAH patients, clinicians must rely on available monitoring (TCD and cEEG). Most centers use a maximal target range of around 120 mm Hg for CPP, 140 mm Hg for MAP, and 220 mm Hg for SBP. Complications such as heart failure, arrhythmia, and myocardial demand ischemia should be monitored closely. As far as de-escalation of hypertensive therapy is concerned, the literature is devoid of guidelines. A stable neurological condition for at least 24–48 hours to be obtained and monitoring for recurrence of ischemia to be continued before de-escalating in a stepwise fashion. CO augmentation using a validated monitoring device, such as a transpulmonary thermodilution (PiCCO) or a pulmonary artery catheter, to titrate fluids, pressors, and inotropes[55] and targeting a cardiac index of >4.0 L/min/m^2 can also be done as a second-line hemodynamic intervention once arterial BP has been optimized. The role of milrinone, a selective inhibitor of the phosphodiesterase III isoenzyme, is promising in this regard. It provides more effective inotropy than dobutamine in the setting of neurogenic stunned myocardium, which is associated with beta-receptor desensitization.[56] Available evidence also suggests that the medication is well tolerated as an IV infusion through the period of peak DCI risk and may have a beneficial effect in preventing symptomatic vasospasm or DCI.[57,58]

Hemoglobin optimization: Based on current evidence from randomized clinical trials in the general ICU population a restrictive strategy aiming for a hemoglobin level above 7 g/dL is the favored approach for SAH patients prior to the onset of DCI. It is questionable however, whether this is the appropriate threshold for patients with active and ongoing brain ischemia. Anemia is seen in >50% of SAH patients[59] and is consistently associated with poor outcome.[60] Optimal transfusion strategies and specific hemoglobin thresholds are of clinical relevance because anemia is a potentially modifiable factor influencing secondary brain injury. This makes the use of red blood cell transfusion to optimize cerebral oxygen delivery appealing when facing active brain ischemia refractory to first-line therapies. However, blood transfusions are also associated with medical complications, poor outcome, and even higher mortality in the SAH population.[61] The ongoing RCT aSAH, Red Blood Cell Transfusion and Outcome (SAHaRA Pilot), comparing RBC transfusion triggers from 10 g/dL down to 8 g/dL will hopefully shed light on this debate. In the meantime, a transfusion threshold of 7 g/dL to be followed in SAH patients. However, in cases of DCI unresponsive to first-line therapy, a more aggressive transfusion trigger of 9–10 g/dL can be used as rescue therapy.

Endovascular therapy: When confronted with medically refractory DCI, cases in which significant neurologic deficits exist despite hemodynamic optimization or in the face of complications resulting from heart failure, fluid overload, or myocardial ischemia,[62] endovascular therapy is the next step. It can be subdivided into vasorelaxation/spasmolysis with intra-arterial vasodilators and mechanical stretching and dilatation of vasospastic arteries via percutaneous transluminal coronary angioplasty (PTCA).

Intra-arterial vasodilators allow access to both proximal and distal cerebral vasculature. They have a more diffuse effect, and a better safety profile. A range of agents (papaverine, nicardipine, nimodipine, verapamil, and milrinone), doses, and treatment durations have been evaluated over the years, but no high-quality studies have compared them in a randomized fashion. Disadvantages include recurrent vasospasm due to the short-lasting effect of these agents, increased ICP secondary to vasodilation,[63] and potential hypotension due to systemic effects. Today, the most commonly used agents are intra-arterial nicardipine 10–20 mg or verapamil 20–40 mg, infused over about 1 hour. Doses of up to 720 mg per treatment have been described in refractory severe vasospasm.[64] Vasodilators are most often used with balloon angioplasty for more distal or diffuse vasospasm and intermittent therapy is favored over continuous infusion for both efficacy and complication profiles.

Percutaneous transluminal coronary angioplasty is limited to proximal vessels and has more durable response with occasional cases of recurrence that require repeated procedures. Observational studies suggest that early intervention (<2 hours after neurological decline) results in a better clinical response.[65] The drawback of PTCA is that serious complications can occur in up to 5% of patients, including embolism, thrombosis, dissection, and vessel rupture, although contemporary safety profiles are favorable. Combination therapy with intra-arterial vasodilator infusions allows access to the entire vasculature for diffuse spasm.

When facing evidence of ongoing neurological injury despite the aforementioned measures, the clinician is left with the option of pursuing nonevidence-based therapies. There are anecdotal reports regarding use of intrathecal nicardipine and nitroprusside, use of HTS, use of intra-aortic balloon pump (IABP) counterpulsation, targeted temperature management (TTM) to attain levels between 33 and 36°C, with or without barbiturate coma as rescue therapy in extreme cases of refractory DCI, but these interventions should only be instituted in centers with the appropriate expertise and monitoring, and should be proportionate to the global goals of care.

Role of statins, magnesium, and endothelin antagonists: Routine use of these agents to reduce DCI and improve functional neurological outcome in aSAH patients is not recommended due to lack of benefit and increased risk of adverse events.

Q8. What are the neurological and medical complications of subarachnoid hemorrhage?

Neurological complications typically include seizures and hydrocephalus

Management of seizures: Incidence of aSAH-associated seizures is relatively common and earlier studies reported seizure-like episodes in up to 26% patients with aSAH. However, with improved EEG monitoring capability, more recent studies suggest a lower seizure incidence of 7.8–15.2%.[27] Based on the timing of occurrence, these aSAH associated seizures can be classified as onset (occur at the time of hemorrhage), early (occur during first week), and late (occur either postoperatively or after 1 week) seizures. Despite the absence of randomized data, providing antiseizure medications to patients with aSAH-associated onset seizures for a period of ≤7 days seems reasonable to minimize early complications such as nonconvulsive status epilepticus and rerupture of an unsecured aneurysm and decrease long-term medication side effects. Compared to neurosurgical clipping endovascular coil embolization seems to be associated with a lower incidence of late seizures. In addition to the surgical management of aneurysms, MCA aneurysm location, high clinical/radiological grade (HH grade >3 or Fisher grade III/IV), cortical infarction, or hydrocephalus has been associated with an elevated seizure risk[27] and it may be reasonable to use prophylactic antiseizure medications with cEEG monitoring in these cases or in those with a depressed neurological examination.[27] Nonrandomized data do highlight that although control of identified seizures can be achieved with phenytoin, excess morbidity (poor cognitive function) associated with the use of phenytoin outweighs the benefits of seizure prophylaxis and prompt the use of alternative antiseizure medications.[66] Whether this increased morbidity is related to an effect on DCI through metabolic competition with nimodipine or undiagnosed transaminase elevations is unclear. A single-blinded randomized study of levetiracetam versus phenytoin demonstrated the same outcomes with respect to mortality or seizure control as evaluated by cEEG. Therapy with levetiracetam resulted in a lower incidence of adverse effects as evaluated by the GOS-Extended and Disability Rating Scale.

Early and late seizures are distinct from onset seizures in that they are not the immediate result of the initial hemorrhage and potentially are related to the treatment modality or posthemorrhage infarct. Accordingly, both categories warrant longer term antiseizure medication that should be managed in the postoperative period by a clinician who specializes in seizure management.

Management of hydrocephalus: The risk of acute hydrocephalus after aSAH ranges from 15 to 87% in the acute stage.[67,68] aSAH with associated acute symptomatic hydrocephalus should be managed urgently by CSF diversion (EVD or lumbar drainage) to improve neurological condition (ICP monitoring may be considered in patients with suspected intracranial hypertension even in the absence of hydrocephalus). Adherence to a targeted, bundled EVD management protocol addressing aseptic insertion techniques, need for antibiotic coated catheters, CSF sampling frequency and technique, EVD dressing management, clamping and weaning, nursing education has been identified as a best practice for prevention of ventriculostomy-associated infection and other associated complications However, aSAH associated persistent or chronic shunt-dependent hydrocephalus occurs in 8.9–48% of patients[68] and requires permanent CSF diversion in the form of a ventriculoperitoneal shunt. Significant predictors of shunt dependency include poor admission neurological grade, increased age, acute hydrocephalus, high Fisher grades, presence of intraventricular hemorrhage, rebleeding, ruptured posterior circulation artery aneurysm, anterior communicating artery aneurysm, surgical clipping, endovascular coiling, cerebral vasospasm, meningitis, and a prolonged period of EVD.[67,68] According to a large observational study, clipping and coiling of ruptured and unruptured cerebral aneurysms were associated with similar incidences of ventriculoperitoneal shunt placement for hydrocephalus.[69]

Medical complications are listed in **Table 6**. These include cardiac, pulmonary, infective, and medical complications such as fever, hyperglycemia, hyponatremia, and hypernatremia.

TABLE 6: Medical complications of subarachnoid hemorrhage.

Cardiac complications	• Troponin elevation • Arrhythmias • Left ventricular dysfunction
Pulmonary complications	• Neurogenic pulmonary edema • ARDS
Infective complications	• Fever • Ventilator-associated pneumonia
Endocrine complications	Hyperglycemia
Electrolyte disturbances	• Hyponatremia • Hypernatremia

CONCLUSION

The patient presented in the vignette has coma due to an intracerebral catastrophe. Immediate recognition of increased ICP and ABCD management followed by CT scan are the emergency steps to be followed. A stepwise tier-driven approach to reduce ICP and optimize CPP is the next step. Recognizing SAH, classifying its severity, considering measures to prevent rerupture, and preventing DCI and medical and neurological complications are the mainstay of treatment for this patient. Endovascular treatment results in better functional outcomes as compared to open surgical methods. Open surgical methods are preferred based on certain morphological characteristics and associated hematomas and are preferred in younger patients due to greater durability of the surgical treatment. The patient in the vignette is >65 years of age and has a poor grade aSAH with features of raised ICP. Possibility of good outcome on treatment is ≈40%. Any modifiable medical condition, like raised ICP in the vignette, should be identified and treated first. Thereafter decision regarding coiling or clipping to be taken after careful consideration of her comorbidities and baseline functional status. A shared decision-making approach to be taken after discussion of the likely prognosis with the family members or surrogate decision-maker.

REFERENCES

1. Teasdale G, Jennett B. Assessment of coma and impaired consciousness. A practical scale. Lancet. 1974;2(7872):81-4.
2. Wijdicks EF, Bamlet WR, Maramattom BV, Manno EM, McClelland RL. Validation of a new coma scale: The FOUR score. Ann Neurol. 2005;58(4):585-93.
3. Turner JM. Intracranial pressure. In: Matta BF, Menon DK, Turner JM (Eds). Textbook of Neuroanaesthesia and Critical Care. London: Greenwich Medical Media; 2000. Pp. 53-9.
4. Chesnut RM, Temkin N, Carney N, Dikmen S, Rondina C, Videtta W, et al. A trial of intracranial-pressure monitoring in traumatic brain injury. N Engl J Med. 2012;367(26):2471-81.
5. Hellingman CA, van den Bergh WM, Beijer IS, van Dijk GW, Algra A, van Gijn J, et al. Risk of rebleeding after treatment of acute hydrocephalus in patients with aneurysmal subarachnoid hemorrhage. Stroke. 2007;38:96-9.
6. Heuer GG, Smith MJ, Elliott JP, Winn HR, Leroux PD. Relationship between intracranial pressure and other clinical variables in patients with aneurysmal subarachnoid hemorrhage. J Neurosurg. 2004;101:408-16.
7. McIver JI, Friedman JA, Wijdicks EFM, Piepgras DG, Pichelmann MA, Toussaint LG, et al. Preoperative ventriculostomy and rebleeding after aneurysmal subarachnoid hemorrhage. J Neurosurg. 2002;97:1042-4.
8. Liu X, Grifth M, Jang HJ, Ko N, Pelter MM, Abba J, et al. Intracranial pressure monitoring via external ventricular drain: Are we waiting long enough before recording the real value? J Neurosci Nurs. 2020;52:37-42.
9. Coppadoro A, Citerio G. Subarachnoid hemorrhage: an update for the intensivist. Minerva Anestesiol. 2011;77:74-84.
10. Gigante P, Hwang BY, Appelboom G, Kellner CP, Kellner MA, Connolly ES. External ventricular drainage following aneurysmal subarachnoid haemorrhage. Br J Neurosurg. 2010;24:625-32.
11. Michael DB. Intracranial pressure monitoring. In: Kruse JA, Fink MP, Carlson RW (Eds). Saunders' Manual of Critical Care. The Curtis Center, Independence Square West, Philadelphia: Saunders; 2003.
12. Cagnazzo F, Chalard K, Lefevre P-H, Garnier O, Derraz I, Dargazanli C, et al. Optimal intracranial pressure in patients with aneurysmal subarachnoid hemorrhage treated with coiling and requiring external ventricular drainage. Neurosurg Rev. 2021;44:1191-204.
13. Fugate JE, Rabinstein AA, Wijdicks EFM, Lanzino G. Aggressive CSF diversion reverses delayed cerebral ischemia in aneurysmal subarachnoid hemorrhage: a case report. Neurocrit Care. 2012;17:112-6.
14. Samuelsson C, Hillered L, Enblad P, Ronne-Engström E. Microdialysis patterns in subarachnoid hemorrhage patients with focus on ischemic events and brain interstitial glutamine levels. Acta Neurochir (Wien). 2009;151:437-46.
15. Picetti E, Barbanera A, Bernucci C, Bertuccio A, Bilotta F, Boccardi EP, et al. Early management of patients with aneurysmal subarachnoid hemorrhage in a hospital with neurosurgical/neuroendovascular facilities: a consensus and clinical recommendations of the Italian Society of Anesthesia and Intensive Care (SIAARTI)-Part 1. J Anesth Analg Crit Care. 2022;2:13.
16. Carney N, Totten AM, O'Reilly C, Ullman JS, Hawryluk GW, Bell MJ, et al. Guidelines for the management of severe traumatic brain injury. Neurosurgery. 2017;80:6-15.
17. Hawryluk GWJ, Aguilera S, Buki A, Bulger E, Citerio G, Cooper DJ, et al. A management algorithm for patients with intracranial pressure monitoring: the Seattle International Severe Traumatic Brain Injury Consensus Conference (SIBICC). Intensive Care Med. 2019;45(12):1783-94.
18. Diringer MN, Zazulia AR. Osmotic therapy: fact and fiction. Neurocrit Care. 2004;1:219-33.
19. Pasarikovski CR, Alotaibi NM, Al-Mufti F, Macdonald RL. Hypertonic saline for increased intracranial pressure after aneurysmal subarachnoid hemorrhage: a systematic review. World Neurosurg. 2017;105:1-6.
20. Bentsen G, Stubhaug A, Eide PK. Differential effects of osmotherapy on static and pulsatile intracranial pressure. Crit Care Med. 2008;36:2414-9.
21. Todd MM, Hindman BJ, Clarke WR, Torner JC, Investigators IH for ASTI. Mild intraoperative hypothermia during surgery for intracranial aneurysm. N Engl J Med. 2005;352:135-45.
22. Addis A, Baggiani M, Citerio G. Intracranial Pressure Monitoring and Management in Aneurysmal Subarachnoid Hemorrhage. Neurocrit Care. 2023.
23. Baldiserri MR. Subarachnoid haemorrhage. In: Kruse JA, Fink MP, Carlson RW (Eds). Saunders Manual of Critical Care. Philadelphia: Saunders; 2003.

24. Report of World Federation of Neurological Surgeons Committee on a Universal Subarachnoid Hemorrhage Grading Scale. J Neurosurg. 1988;68(6):985-6.
25. Hunt WE, Hess RM. Surgical risk as related to time of intervention in the repair of intracranial aneurysms. J Neurosurg. 1968;28(1):14-20.
26. Fisher CM, Kistler JP, Davis JM. Relation of cerebral vasospasm to subarachnoid hemorrhage visualized by computerized tomographic scanning. Neurosurgery. 1980;6(1):1-9.
27. Hoh BL, Ko NU, Amin-Hanjani S, Chou SH-Y, Cruz-Flores S, Dangayach NS, et al. 2023 Guideline for the management of patients with aneurysmal subarachnoid hemorrhage: a guideline from the American Heart Association/American Stroke Association. Stroke. 2023;54:e314-70.
28. Wijdicks EF, Vermeulen M, Murray GD, Hijdra A, van Gijn J. The effects of treating hypertension following aneurysmal subarachnoid hemorrhage. Clin Neurol Neurosurg. 1990;92:111-7.
29. Ohkuma H, Tsurutani H, Suzuki S. Incidence and significance of early aneurysmal rebleeding before neurosurgical or neurological management. Stroke. 2001;32:1176-80.
30. Calviere L, Gathier CS, Rafiq M, Koopman I, Rousseau V, Raposo N, A et al. Rebleeding after aneurysmal subarachnoid hemorrhage in two centers using different blood pressure management strategies. Front Neurol. 2022;13:836268.
31. Post R, Germans MR, Tjerkstra MA, Vergouwen MDI, Jellema K, Koot RW, et al. Ultra-early tranexamic acid after subarachnoid haemorrhage (ULTRA): a randomised controlled trial. Lancet. 2021;397(10269):112-8.
32. Treggiari MM, Rabinstein AA, Busl KM, Caylor MM, Citerio G, Deem S, et al. Guidelines for the Neurocritical Care Management of Aneurysmal Subarachnoid Hemorrhage. Neurocrit Care. 2023.
33. Lindgren A, Vergouwen MD, van der Schaaf I, Algra A, Wermer M, Clarke MJ, et al. Endovascular coiling versus neurosurgical clipping for people with aneurysmal subarachnoid haemorrhage. Cochrane Database Syst Rev. 2018;8:CD003085.
34. Molyneux AJ, Kerr RS, Yu LM, Clarke M, Sneade M, Yarnold JA, et al. International subarachnoid aneurysm trial (ISAT) of neurosurgical clipping versus endovascular coiling in 2143 patients with ruptured intracranial aneurysms: a randomised comparison of effects on survival, dependency, seizures, rebleeding, subgroups, and aneurysm occlusion. Lancet. 2005;366(9488):809-17.
35. van Donkelaar CE, Bakker NA, Birks J, Clarke A, Sneade M, Kerr RSC, et al. Impact of treatment delay on outcome in the International Subarachnoid Aneurysm Trial. Stroke. 2020;51:1600-3.
36. Molyneux AJ, Birks J, Clarke A, Sneade M, Kerr RS. The durability of endovascular coiling versus neurosurgical clipping of ruptured cerebral aneurysms: 18 year follow-up of the UK cohort of the International Subarachnoid Aneurysm Trial (ISAT). Lancet. 2015;385:691-7.
37. Molyneux AJ, Kerr RS, Birks J, Ramzi N, Yarnold J, Sneade M, et al. Risk of recurrent subarachnoid haemorrhage, death, or dependence and standardised mortality ratios after clipping or coiling of an intracranial aneurysm in the International Subarachnoid Aneurysm Trial (ISAT): long-term follow-up. Lancet Neurol. 2009;8:427-33.
38. Millikan CH. Cerebral vasospasm and ruptured intracranial aneurysm. Arch Neurol. 1975;32:433-49.
39. Budohoski KP, Guilfoyle M, Helmy A, Huuskonen T, Czosnyka M, Kirollos R, et al. The pathophysiology and treatment of delayed cerebral ischaemia following subarachnoid haemorrhage. J Neurol Neurosurg Psychiatry. 2014;85(12):1343-53.
40. Francoeur CL, Mayer SA. Management of delayed cerebral ischemia after subarachnoid hemorrhage. Crit Care. 2016;20:277.
41. van der Harst JJ, Luijckx GR, Elting JWJ, Lammers T, Bokkers RPH, van den Bergh WM, et al. The predictive value of the CTA Vasospasm Score on delayed cerebral ischaemia and functional outcome after aneurysmal subarachnoid hemorrhage. Eur J Neurol. 2022;29:620-5.
42. Dankbaar JW, Rijsdijk M, van der Schaaf IC, Velthuis BK, Wermer MJ, Rinkel GJ. Relationship between vasospasm, cerebral perfusion, and delayed cerebral ischemia after aneurysmal subarachnoid hemorrhage. Neuroradiology. 2009;51:813-9.
43. Maegawa T, Sasahara A, Ohbuchi H, Chernov M, Kasuya H. Cerebral vasospasm and hypoperfusion after traumatic brain injury: combined CT angiography and CT perfusion imaging study. Surg Neurol Int. 2021;12:361.
44. Kumar G, Shahripour RB, Harrigan MR. Vasospasm on transcranial Doppler is predictive of delayed cerebral ischemia in aneurysmal subarachnoid hemorrhage: a systematic review and meta-analysis. J Neurosurg. 2016;124:1257-64.
45. Mastantuono J-M, Combescure C, Elia N, Tramèr MR, Lysakowski C. Transcranial Doppler in the diagnosis of cerebral vasospasm. Crit Care Med. 2018;46:1665-72.
46. Allen GS, Ahn HS, Preziosi TJ, Battye R, Boone SC, Chou SN, et al. Cerebral arterial spasm—a controlled trial of nimodipine in patients with subarachnoid hemorrhage. N Engl J Med. 1983;308(11):619-24.
47. Pickard JD, Murray GD, Illingworth R, Shaw MDM, Teasdale GM, Foy PM, et al. Effect of oral nimodipine on cerebral infarction and outcome after subarachnoid haemorrhage: British aneurysm nimodipine trial. BMJ. 1989;298:636-42.
48. Amin-Hanjani S, Ogilvy CS, Barker II FG, Dumont AS, Kassell NF, Dempsey RJ, et al. Does intracisternal thrombolysis prevent vasospasm after aneurysmal subarachnoid hemorrhage? A meta-analysis. Neurosurgery. 2004;54(2):326-35.
49. Al-Tamimi YZ, Bhargava D, Feltbower RG, Hall G, Goddard AJ, Quinn AC, et al. Lumbar drainage of cerebrospinal fluid after aneurysmal subarachnoid hemorrhage: a prospective, randomized, controlled trial (LUMAS). Stroke. 2012;43(3):677-82.
50. Park S, Yang N, Seo E. The effectiveness of lumbar cerebrospinal fluid drainage to reduce the cerebral vasospasm after surgical clipping for aneurysmal subarachnoid hemorrhage. J Korean Neurosurg Soc. 2015;57(3):167-73.
51. Hasan D, Wijdicks EF, Vermeulen M. Hyponatremia is associated with cerebral ischemia in patients with aneurysmal subarachnoid hemorrhage. Ann Neurol. 1990;27(1):106-8.

52. Manning L, Hirakawa Y, Arima H, Wang X, Chalmers J, Wang J, et al. Blood pressure variability and outcome after acute intracerebral haemorrhage: a post-hoc analysis of INTERACT2, a randomised controlled trial. Lancet Neurol. 2014;13:364-73.
53. Gathier CS, van den Bergh WM, van der Jagt M, Verweij BH, Dankbaar JW, Muller MC, et al. Induced hypertension for delayed cerebral ischemia after aneurysmal subarachnoid hemorrhage: a randomized clinical trial. Stroke. 2018;49:76-83.
54. Haegens NM, Gathier CS, Horn J, Coert BA, Verbaan D, van den Bergh WM. Induced hypertension in preventing cerebral infarction in delayed cerebral ischemia after subarachnoid hemorrhage. Stroke. 2018;49:2630-6.
55. Taccone FS, Citerio G. Participants in the International Multi-disciplinary Consensus Conference on Multimodality Monitoring. Advanced monitoring of systemic hemodynamics in critically ill patients with acute brain injury. Neurocrit Care. 2014;21(S2):38-63.
56. Naidech A, Du Y, Kreiter KT, Parra A, Fitzsimmons BF, Lavine SD, et al. Dobutamine versus milrinone after subarachnoid hemorrhage. Neurosurgery. 2005;56(1):21-6.
57. Lakhal K, Hivert A, Alexandre PL, Fresco M, Robert-Edan V, Rodie-Talbere PA, et al. Intravenous milrinone for cerebral vasospasm in subarachnoid hemorrhage: the MILRISPASM controlled before-after study. Neurocrit Care. 2021;35:669-79.
58. Bernier TD, Schontz MJ, Izzy S, Chung DY, Nelson SE, Leslie-Mazwi TM, et al. Treatment of subarachnoid hemorrhage-associated delayed cerebral ischemia with milrinone: a review and proposal. J Neurosurg Anesthesiol. 2021;33:195-202.
59. Le Roux PD. Anemia and transfusion after subarachnoid hemorrhage. Neurocrit Care. 2011;15(2):342-53.
60. Naidech AM, Jovanovic B, Wartenberg KE, Parra A, Ostapkovich N, Connolly ES, et al. Higher hemoglobin is associated with improved outcome after subarachnoid hemorrhage. Crit Care Med. 2007;35(10):2383-9.
61. Festic E, Rabinstein AA, Freeman WD, Mauricio EA, Robinson MT, Mandrekar J, et al. Blood transfusion is an important predictor of hospital mortality among patients with aneurysmal subarachnoid hemorrhage. Neurocrit Care. 2013;18(2):209-15.
62. Hollingworth M, Chen PR, Goddard AJP, Coulthard A, Söderman M, Bulsara KR. Results of an international survey on the investigation and endovascular management of cerebral vasospasm and delayed cerebral ischemia. World Neurosurg. 2015;83(6):1120-6.e1.
63. McAuliffe W, Townsend M, Eskridge JM, Newell DW, Grady MS, Winn HR. Intracranial pressure changes induced during papaverine infusion for treatment of vasospasm. J Neurosurg. 1995;83(3):430-4.
64. Albanese E, Russo A, Quiroga M, Willis RN, Mericle RA, Ulm AJ. Ultrahigh-dose intraarterial infusion of verapamil through an indwelling microcatheter for medically refractory severe vasospasm: initial experience. Clinical article. J Neurosurg. 2010;113(4):913-22.
65. Rosenwasser RH, Armonda RA, Thomas JE, Benitez RP, Gannon PM, Harrop J. Therapeutic modalities for the management of cerebral vasospasm: timing of endovascular options. Neurosurgery. 1999;44(5):975-9.
66. Szaflarski JP, Sangha KS, Lindsell CJ, Shutter LA. Prospective, randomized, single-blinded comparative trial of intravenous levetiracetam versus phenytoin for seizure prophylaxis. Neurocrit Care. 2010;12:165-72.
67. Connolly ES, Rabinstein AA, Carhuapoma JR, Derdeyn CP, Dion J, Higashida RT, et al. Guidelines for the management of aneurysmal subarachnoid hemorrhage: a guideline for healthcare professionals from the American Heart Association/American Stroke Association. Stroke. 2012;43:1711-37.
68. Xie Z, Hu X, Zan X, Lin S, Li H, You C. Predictors of shunt-dependent hydrocephalus after aneurysmal subarachnoid hemorrhage? A systematic review and meta-analysis. World Neurosurg. 2017;106:844-860.e6.
69. Hoh BL, Kleinhenz DT, Chi YY, Mocco J, Barker FG. Incidence of ventricular shunt placement for hydrocephalus with clipping versus coiling for ruptured and unruptured cerebral aneurysms in the Nationwide Inpatient Sample database: 2002 to 2007. World Neurosurg. 2011;76:548-54.

CHAPTER 13

Acute Ischemic Stroke

Keyur Shah, Kapil Gangadhar Zirpe, Atul Prabhakar Kulkarni

CASE STUDY

A 65-year-old male, a known hypertensive, also suffering from type 2 diabetes mellitus was brought to the emergency room with complaints of weakness of the right side of the body for 2 hours. He woke up from sleep at 4 AM and was apparently normal. He noticed weakness of the right side of the body and face at 6 AM, which has remained constant. His current medications are tablet (tab) losartan 50 mg BD, tab amlodipine 5 mg with hydrochlorothiazide 12.5 mg OD, tab metformin 500 mg BD, and tab glimepiride 1 mg BD.

On examination, he was drowsy, but obeying commands, and was now complaining of mild-to-moderate headache. His clinical examination revealed mild fever (temperature: 99°F), tachycardia [heart rate (HR) 90 beats/min, regular], hypertension [blood pressure (BP) 190/110 mm Hg], and oxygen saturation (SpO$_2$) 98% while breathing room air. Central nervous system (CNS) examination revealed slurring of speech, right facial palsy, and right dense hemiplegia (power 1/5 in upper limb and 2/5 in lower limb). Pain and touch sensation on the right side of the body were absent. The plantar reflex was upgoing and deep tendon reflexes were mute on the right side. The left side motor and sensory examination was normal.

Later, one of the close relatives gave a history of psychiatric treatment started for known "bipolar disorder." He (relative) showed a strip of lithium carbonate (300 mg), of which he was taking two tablets twice daily.

When asked about any previous investigations, the relative showed a complete blood count (CBC) report from 1 month ago.

Q1. What are the differential diagnoses in this patient?

- *Ischemic stroke:* The presence of focal neurological deficit, upper motor neuron deficit, altered sensorium in the background of old age, diabetes mellitus, and hypertension make an ischemic stroke the most likely diagnosis.
- *Hemorrhagic stroke:* Intracerebral hemorrhage could present with headache, focal neurological deficit, and altered sensorium. Amyloid angiopathy may be a cause of intracerebral hemorrhage in this age group.
- *Brain abscess:* The presence of headache, fever, focal neurological deficit, and altered sensorium may be present in a brain abscess; however, the symptoms would develop gradually over a few days.
- *Hypoglycemia:* Hypoglycemia may present with a focal neurological deficit and is possible in view of history of diabetes, with low serum glucose leading to a decreased level of consciousness.
- *Lithium toxicity:* Lithium toxicity may present with confusion, ataxia, or slurring of speech; however, hemiplegia is rare unless postictal in origin.
- *Hypertensive encephalopathy:* Patients with hypertensive encephalopathy may present with headache, delirium, significant hypertension, cortical blindness, cerebral edema, and seizures.
- *Subarachnoid hemorrhage:* Patients develop sudden severe and usually lateralized headache and meningism in cases of subarachnoid hemorrhage. Lateralizing neurological signs are usually absent at presentation.
- *Neoplasm:* The neurological deficit generally develops over a long period of time. This may be caused occasionally by the raised intracranial pressure (ICP) due to the tumor itself, increasing edema or bleeding in the tumor. This may lead to headaches and sometimes even seizures.
- *Sinus (sagittal) venous thrombosis:* Patients with cortical venous sinus thrombosis usually present with early seizures, headache, and typical risk factors (head or neck trauma, malignancy, diabetes, dehydration, or hypercoagulability).
- *Multiple sclerosis:* These patients present with a subacute onset of symptoms over many days with a waxing and waning course. Rarely they may become suddenly symptomatic and have neurological deficit within a few hours.

- *Postictal paresis/Todd's paralysis:* It is seen after a generalized or focal seizure and usually lasts a few minutes to hours.
- *Migraine:* Patients with a hemiplegic variant of migraine may present with a history of similar events in the past, with preceding aura and headache.
- *Meningitis/vasculitis:* Patients with meningitis usually present with fever, meningism, and altered mental status. Focal neurological deficits are uncommon early in the course but may appear later due to vasculitic infarcts. Typical cerebrospinal fluid (CSF) findings may help in distinguishing these from other causes.
- *Hysteria and other psychiatric illnesses:* Patients with psychiatric causes would have a history of psychiatric illness or similar episodes in the past. They will present without positive cranial nerve findings, or findings nonspecific to a vascular distribution, and will have inconsistent examination. In this patient, objective signs of neurological deficit are present, making this diagnosis less likely.

Q2. Can you distinguish between ischemic and hemorrhagic stroke clinically?

The following features favor a diagnosis of ischemic stroke:
- Absence of onset headache and vomiting
- Rapid onset and offset of symptoms
- Presence of cardiovascular diseases such as chronic hypertension, recent myocardial infarction, atrial fibrillation (AF), valvular heart disease, and peripheral vascular disease
- Clinical findings such as murmurs, carotid bruits, and AF.

The following features favor a diagnosis of hemorrhagic stroke:
- Presence of onset headache and vomiting, especially associated with subarachnoid hemorrhage
- Absence of neurological deficit at onset
- Altered mental status and seizures are more common in hemorrhagic stroke
- Progression of neurological deficit over few hours and absence of early improvement
- Severe uncontrolled hypertension and cocaine use.

Q3. Describe in brief the Cincinnati Prehospital Stroke Scale.

The Cincinnati Prehospital Stroke Scale is a clinical tool used to identify potential stroke patients in the prehospital setting. It has been derived from the National Institutes of Health Stroke Scale (NIHSS) for use in the prehospital setting. It has also been used to predict severe stroke and large vessel occlusion.

Criteria: Assign one point for each of the three criteria:
1. *Facial droop:* Patient shows teeth or smiles
   a. *Abnormal:* If one side moves less or does not move at all
   b. *Normal:* Bilateral symmetrical facial movements
2. *Arm drift:* Patient holds arms straight out in front, with palms facing up, with eyes closed for 10 seconds
   a. *Abnormal:* If one arm is unable to be raised or drifts from the starting position.
   b. *Normal:* Both arms move equally
3. *Dysarthria:* When the patient is asked to repeat a sentence like "you can't teach an old dog new tricks," he will have either slurred speech or use inapt words or may not respond at all verbally. When the person is normal, he will use correct words without slurring.

A score of 1 predicts stroke with a probability of 75%, whereas a score of 3 predicts stroke with a probability of >85%.[1,2]

Q4. Describe the NIHSS in brief.

The NIHSS can be used in the initial assessment as a clinical tool to quantify the severity of a stroke. It is used to evaluate and document neurological status in stroke patients. It has been validated for predicting lesion size and measuring stroke severity. The NIHSS has been shown to be a predictor of both short-term and long-term outcomes of stroke patients. It also helps in choosing the appropriate treatment modality.[3]

The NIHSS has 11 different components that evaluate specific abilities of the brain (**Table 1**). Each component has a maximum score of 4 and a minimum score of 0, 0 being normal functioning and 4 being completely impaired. The total score is calculated by adding the number for each element of the scale. The higher the score, the more impaired is the stroke patient. 42 is the highest score possible (**Table 2**).

The NIHSS also has a few limitations; it may be difficult to implement in patients with prior neurologic deficits, endotracheal intubation, or language barrier.

Q5. What is the role of imaging in the initial management of a stroke patient?

For confirmation of diagnosis of stroke, imaging is important along with history and clinical examination. Neuroimaging in the form of computed tomography (CT)/diffusion-weighted (DW) magnetic resonance imaging (MRI) is urgently required. The first step is the performance of a noncontrast enhanced CT scan. Door-to-CT imaging time should be ≤25 minutes.

Nonenhanced computed tomography (NECT) brain

Nonenhanced computed tomography definitively excludes parenchymal hemorrhage, can be used to assess other

TABLE 1: The National Institutes of Health Stroke Scale (NIHSS).		
Component of NIHSS		Score range
Level of consciousness	Responsiveness	0–3
	Questions	0–2
	Commands	0–2
Horizontal eye movement		0–2
Visual field test		0–3
Facial palsy		0–3
Motor arm	Left	0–4
	Right	0–4
Motor leg	Left	0–4
	Right	0–4
Limb ataxia		0–2
Sensory		0–2
Language		0–3
Speech		0–2
Extinction, inattention		0–2
Total score		0–42

TABLE 2: Interpretation of the National Institutes of Health Stroke Scale (NIHSS) score.	
Severity of stroke	NIHSS score
No stroke	0
Minor stroke	1–4
Moderate stroke	5–15
Moderate-to-severe stroke	16–20
Severe stroke	21–42

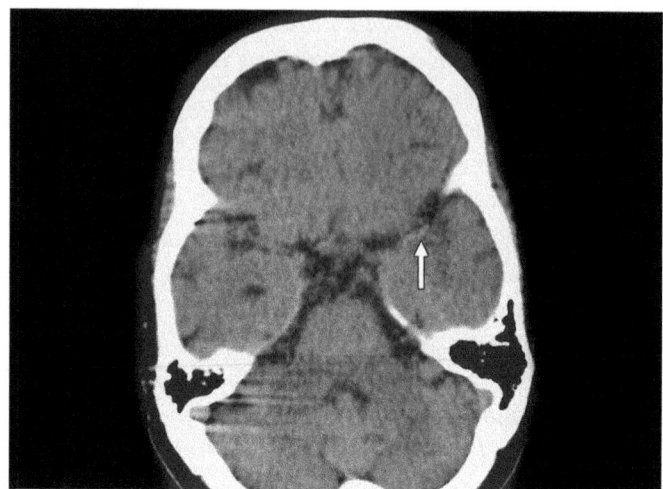

Fig. 1: Case of carcinoma of breast on neoadjuvant chemotherapy (NACT). Acute onset of right hemiplegia, plain computed tomography (CT) brain reveals middle cerebral artery (MCA) sign. Arrow suggests hyperdense MCA sign.

exclusion criteria for intravenous (IV) recombinant tissue plasminogen activator (rtPA) like extensive area of hypoattenuation, and may demonstrate subtle visible parenchymal damage within 3 hours. NECT is correctly able to identify most causes of intracranial bleeding and can help to diagnose other causes of neurological symptoms such as brain tumors.[4-10]

Nonenhanced computed tomography will be unable to pick up acute infarcts and small posterior fossa lesions. It is also not useful when the patient has small cortical or subcortical infarctions.[11] NECT is the most common modality used in acute ischemic stroke imaging due to easy availability, faster scan time, and easy interpretation.

With the widespread use of thrombolytic therapy in ischemic stroke, there is growing interest in using NECT to identify subtle, early signs of ischemic brain injury (loss of gray-white differentiation) or arterial occlusion (hyperdense vessel sign) that might affect decisions about treatment.[12-16] Loss of gray-white differentiation can be seen as a loss of difference among the basal ganglia nuclei (lenticular obscuration) or as a merging of the densities of the cortex and white matter below in the insula (known as insular ribbon sign) and over the convexities (cortical ribbon sign). The swelling of the gyri that produce sulcal effacement also suggests the presence of cerebral ischemia. The faster these signs appear, the higher the degree of ischemia. The ability of observers to pick up the signs early on NECT is quite variable and low and occurs in ≤67% of imaging performed within 3 hours. The size of the infarct, the severity of ischemia, and the time between symptom onset and imaging affect the detection.[17,18]

A large-vessel occlusion may be seen on the CT as increased density within the occluded artery, for example, the hyperdense middle cerebral artery (MCA) sign **(Fig. 1)**.

Occlusion of a large vessel causes severe stroke, and it independently predicts a poor neurological outcome.[19-21] It is a stronger predictor of "neurological deterioration" **(Figs. 2 and 3)** [91% positive predictive value (PPV)] than early CT evidence of >50% MCA involvement (75% PPV).[21,22] The hyperdense MCA sign is seen only in about 30-50% of patients in whom thrombosis is proven by angiography; thus, it is diagnostic of the presence of thrombus when seen.[22,23]

The hyperdense MCA "dot" sign **(Fig. 4)** seen on CT denotes a thrombus in a branch of the MCA, suggesting a volume of thrombus in the MCA. This is a better target for treatment with IV rtPA.[24] Probably because of the smaller burden of thrombus, the patients with MCA dot sign alone had better outcomes than those who had a hyperdense MCA sign.[24] Both the hyperdense MCA sign and the hyperdense basilar artery sign have similar clinical significance.[25,26] The risk of hemorrhagic transformation of an infarct after administration of fibrinolytic drugs is higher and correlates

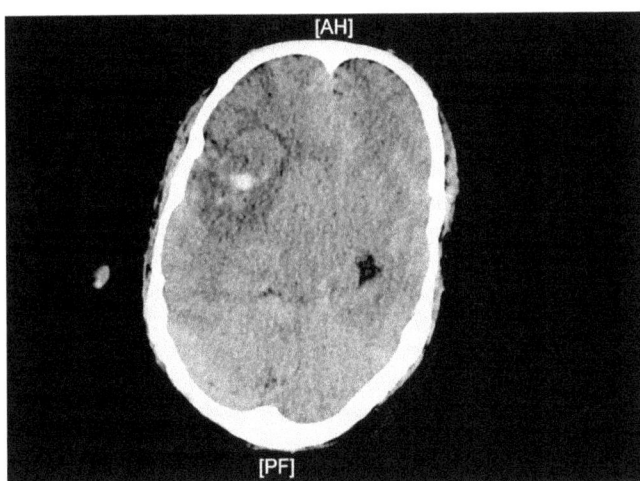

Fig. 2: Right middle cerebral artery territory infarct with hemorrhagic transformation. (AH: anterior hemosphere, PF: posterior fossa)

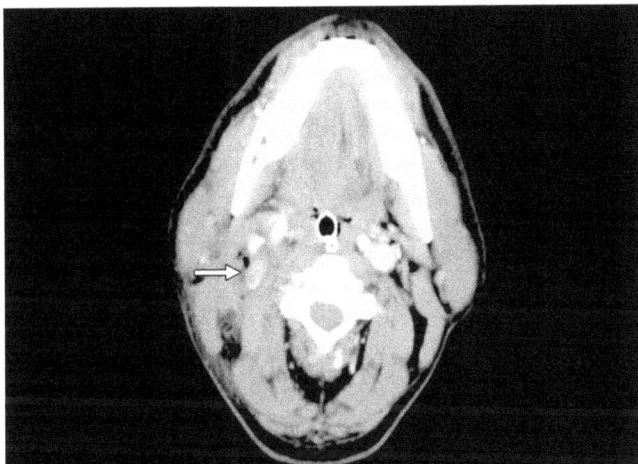

Fig. 3: Computed tomography (CT) angiography with thrombus in the right internal carotid artery (arrow).

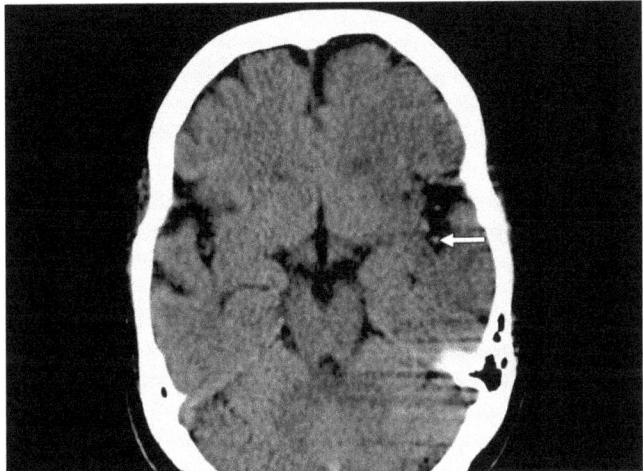

Fig. 4: Case of carcinoma of breast on neoadjuvant chemotherapy (NACT). Acute onset of hemiplegia, plain computed tomography (CT) brain reveals middle cerebral artery (MCA) sign/Sylvian fissure sign (arrow).

well with the findings of NECT depicting the extent of ischemia and infarction. A pooled data analysis of two trials of IV rtPA given in <3 hours of symptom onset showed that if there was a presence of early hypodensity on NECT or a presence of mass effect, the risk of subsequent symptomatic hemorrhage was eight times higher.[27]

Another analysis showed that the presence of subtle early infarct signs involving >30% of the MCA was not associated with an increased risk of adverse outcomes and the administration of IV rtPA still benefited these patients.[10]

Further, a European trial demonstrated that fibrinolytic therapy within 6 hours benefited those with lower involvement of MCA (less than a third) as compared to those with areas of higher involvement, who also had an increased risk of intracranial bleed.[6,28] This led to the exclusion of patients with involvement of more than one-third of the territory of the MCA in the pivotal trial, which later confirmed the benefit of IV fibrinolytic therapy in the 3–4.5-hour window and also the trials of intra-arterial fibrinolysis up to 6 hours.[29-31]

Alberta Stroke Program Early CT Score (ASPECTS):
The ASPECTS is a 10-point CT scan score, used in patients with MCA stroke. A segmental assessment of the MCA area is made and 1 point is deducted from the initial score of 10 for every region involved:

1. Caudate
2. Putamen
3. Internal capsule
4. Insular cortex
5. *M1:* "Anterior MCA cortex" corresponding to frontal operculum
6. *M2:* "MCA cortex lateral to insular ribbon" corresponding to anterior temporal lobe
7. *M3:* "Posterior MCA cortex" corresponding to posterior temporal lobe
8. *M4:* "Anterior MCA territory immediately superior to M1"
9. *M5:* "Lateral MCA territory immediately superior to M2"
10. *M6:* "Posterior MCA territory immediately superior to M3".

A variant of the ASPECTS scoring system has been described for use in the posterior circulation stroke and referred to as pc-ASPECTS.[32]

As is the case for the anterior circulation, the pc-ASPECTS is a 10-point scale, where points are lost for each region affected. Unlike ASPECTS, the pons and the midbrain are worth 2 points each (regardless of whether or not the changes are bilateral; any involvement of the pons, e.g., deducts 2 points).

The points as per the area affected are as follows:
- Thalamus (1 point)
- Occipital lobes (1 point each)
- Midbrain (2 points)

- Pons (2 points)
- Cerebellar hemispheres (1 point each)

An ASPECTS score ≤7 predicts a worse functional outcome at 3 months as well as symptomatic hemorrhage. According to the study performed by Aviv et al., patients with ASPECTS score <8 treated with thrombolysis did not have a good clinical outcome.[33]

Computed tomography perfusion imaging is a CT-based modality, which utilizes quantitative analysis of kinetics of a bolus of CT contrast passing through the brain to obtain a perfusion map of the brain and predict whether tissue will die or survive.

Magnetic resonance imaging

Magnetic resonance imaging techniques can help define subgroups of stroke patients who may benefit from thrombolysis or mechanical thromboaspiration. MRI with gradient echo (GRE) sequences is equivalent to CT to detect acute intracerebral bleeds. MRI protocols combining T1 and T2 imaging with diffusion-weighted imaging (DWI), perfusion-weighted imaging (PWI), and GRE can reliably diagnose both intracerebral bleeds and acute ischemic stroke without causing treatment delays.[34] DWI is currently the most sensitive (88-100%) and specific (95-100%) imaging technique for diagnosis of an acute ischemic infarct very early, i.e., within minutes of symptom onset.[35-44] It allows identification of the lesion size, site, and age. DWI can detect relatively small cortical lesions and small deep or subcortical lesions, including those in the brainstem or cerebellum, areas often poorly or not visualized with standard MRI sequences and NECT scan techniques.[45-48] DWI can identify subclinical satellite ischemic lesions that provide information on stroke mechanism.[36,39,42,49-60]

Diffusion-weighted imaging in combination with apparent diffusion coefficient (ADC) can differentiate between vasogenic and cytotoxic edema. In acute ischemic stroke, cytotoxic edema is seen as hyperintense on DWI and as hypointense on ADC, whereas vasogenic edema appears hyperintense in both DWI and ADC imaging.

Diffusion-weighted imaging denotes the presence of ischemic injury, whereas PWI measures perfusion of brain tissue with contrast agent and hence measures ischemia itself. The diffusion–perfusion mismatch may help identify the ischemic penumbra, which may represent areas at risk of infarction or possibility of salvage by reperfusion techniques. Diffusion–perfusion mismatch correlates well with the initial NIHSS score and may predict early neurologic deterioration.[61,62]

Q6. Compare the utility of CT versus MRI in acute stroke.

Advantages of MRI:
- DWI is highly sensitive and specific in diagnosing acute ischemic stroke.
- It has the ability to distinguish acute, small cortical, small deep, and posterior fossa infarcts.
- It has the ability to distinguish acute from chronic ischemia.
- It can identify subclinical satellite ischemic lesions that provide information on stroke mechanism.
- It avoids exposure to ionizing radiation.
- It has greater spatial resolution.
- The GRE is as good as CT to detect intraparenchymal bleed.

Limitations of MRI (in the acute setting):
- Cost
- Relatively limited availability of the test
- Relatively long duration of the test
- Increased vulnerability to motion artifact
- Patient contraindications such as claustrophobia, cardiac pacemakers, patient confusion, or metal implants.

Advantages of the CT scan over MRI:
- Detection of bleeding
- Less time consuming
- Cost
- Widespread availability
- Less artifacts.

Q7. Which other investigations are required during the initial assessment of a suspected stroke patient?
- Blood glucose
- SpO_2
- Serum electrolytes/renal function tests*
- CBC, including platelet count*
- Markers of cardiac ischemia*
- Prothrombin time (PT)/international normalized ratio (INR)*
- Activated partial thromboplastin time (aPTT)*
- Electrocardiography (ECG)*
- CT angiography/MR angiography/digital subtraction angiography
- Carotid Doppler
- Two-dimensional (2D) echocardiography

In selected patients:
- Thrombin time (TT) and/or ecarin clotting time (ECT) if it is suspected the patient is taking direct thrombin inhibitors or direct factor Xa inhibitors.

---

*Although it is desirable to know the results of these tests before giving IV rtPA, fibrinolytic therapy should not be delayed while awaiting the results unless (1) there is clinical suspicion of a bleeding abnormality or thrombocytopenia, (2) the patient has received heparin or warfarin, or (3) the patient has received other anticoagulants (direct thrombin inhibitors or direct factor Xa inhibitors).

- Hepatic function tests
- Toxicology screen
- Blood alcohol level
- Pregnancy test
- Arterial blood gas tests (if hypoxia is suspected)
- Chest radiography (if lung disease is suspected)
- Lumbar puncture (if subarachnoid hemorrhage is suspected and CT scan is negative for blood)
- Electroencephalogram (if seizures are suspected).

Q8. Describe in brief various clinical features to identify the mechanism of stroke.

The mechanism of stroke can often be determined by typical findings on history taking and clinical examination. The typical clinical features of various mechanisms of stroke are as follows:

Microangiopathic or lacunar stroke

The onset and clinical course of lacunar infarcts differ from those infarcts coming from elsewhere.

- Presence of transient ischemic attacks (TIAs) (15–20%) shortly (several days) before the infarction. TIAs occur in clusters and are more stereotypical as compared to large-vessel TIAs.
- Occur insidiously, gradually, and have a stammering course.
- The lesions are small but may be symptomatic if they involve regions full of high-density axons having multiple extensions, such as the cerebral peduncles and the brainstem.
- The presentation may vary: Pure motor stroke, pure sensory stroke, sensory–motor stroke, ataxic hemiparesis, and dysarthria-clumsy-hand syndrome.

Systemic embolism

- Presence of preexisting organic cardiovascular disease such as mechanical valve or cardiac valve dysfunction, AF, left atrial and/or ventricular thrombus, dilated cardiomyopathy, recent myocardial infarction (<4 weeks), left ventricular aneurysm, sick sinus syndrome, infective myocarditis, or atrial myxoma.
- Sudden in onset, with maximal severity at onset
- They usually occur in awakened state and during activity. A presentation on awakening is not common.
- Recurrent TIAs can be seen involved in various anatomical areas.

Large artery thrombosis

This may occur by one of the three mechanisms:
1. Poststenotic perfusion deficit in a major vessel
2. Sudden occlusion by atherothrombosis
3. Arterioarterial embolism. The clinical picture may be similar to that in systemic embolism.

At the same time, there will be history suggestive of the following:
- Typical atherogenic risk factors such as hypertension, diabetes mellitus, obesity, smoking, male sex
- Frequent TIAs, e.g., amaurosis fugax [internal carotid artery (ICA) stenosis], in the same arterial territory
- Onset often during sleep or atherothrombotic stroke during activity, a gradual progression or stepwise course over minutes to hours is characteristic (attributable to gradual accumulation of thrombus or to lowering of BP, e.g., following antihypertensive therapy).

Dissection of cervical arteries

The (typically younger) patient's history may reveal risk factors such as:
- Recent trauma
- Previous infection
- Signs of connective tissue abnormalities (hyperextensible joints, Marfan syndrome, known as mitral valve prolapse)

The characteristic clinical presentation is a focal neurological syndrome in combination with a unilateral headache or neck pain, pulsatile tinnitus, and an ipsilateral Horner syndrome in the case of ICA dissection.

Q9. What is the typical clinical presentation seen in case of various arterial territories?

The typical clinical features of involvement of various arterial territories are as follows:

- *ICA:*
  - Hemiplegia (face = arm = leg)
  - Hemisensory loss (face = arm = leg)
  - Hemianopia
- *Infarcts of the MCA territory:*
  - Contralateral motor and/or sensory deficit of face and arm more than leg
  - Higher cerebral dysfunction (aphasia, apraxia)
  - Conjugated ipsilateral eye deviation in large infarcts
  - Homonymous visual field defects, alone or in combination with above
- *Infarcts of the anterior cerebral artery territory:*
  - Contralateral hemiparesis with emphasis on the lower limb
- *Infarcts of the posterior cerebral arterial territory:*
  - Hemianopia
- *Infarcts of the vertebrobasilar arterial territory:*
  - Altered consciousness
  - Ipsilateral cranial nerve palsy with contralateral motor and/or sensory deficit
  - Disorder of conjugate eye movement (vertical = midbrain, horizontal = pons)
  - Bilateral motor and/or sensory deficit

- Dysarthrophonia, dysphagia
- Cerebellar dysfunction without ipsilateral long-tract deficit
- *Lacunar infarcts:*
  - Hemiplegia (face = arm = leg)
  - Hemisensory loss (face = arm = leg).

Q10. Describe in brief the initial prehospital and emergency room management of a patient with acute ischemic stroke.

The goals of the initial management of a stroke patient include:
- Ensuring physical stability including airway, breathing, and circulation
- Preventing further neurological injury
- Determining the optimal modality for reperfusion if indicated.

Assessment and stabilization of vital signs is an integral part of the initial management of all critically ill patients including those with stroke. Patients with altered sensorium and bulbar dysfunction, who might be unable to protect the airway, may require endotracheal intubation to protect them against aspiration. Patients with hypoxemia should receive oxygen supplementation to maintain acceptable oxygenation. Patients who are not hypoxemic should not receive oxygen supplementation. Patients with aspiration and hypoxemia may require mechanical ventilation. Patients with altered sensorium and hypoventilation may need mechanical ventilation to prevent hypercapnia, which may cause cerebral vasodilation and worsen raised ICP.

Hypotension should be immediately treated with fluids and vasopressors as it may worsen ischemic injury. Hypertension should not be treated unless BP is >185/110 mm Hg and thrombolysis is planned. A brief neurological assessment with Glasgow Coma Scale (GCS) and NIHSS score should be performed. Measures for control of raised ICP should be initiated in patients with signs of raised ICP. Seizures if present should be promptly controlled. There is no benefit of prophylactic antiepileptic drugs. Euthermia and glycemia should be maintained to prevent further neurological injury.[63]

Neuroimaging and other investigations should be performed, and an appropriate modality for reperfusion if indicated should be chosen.

Q11. What are the common indications for admission to intensive care unit (ICU) in a patient with acute ischemic stroke?

A stroke patient may require ICU for various physiological alterations as described below:
- Altered sensorium, brainstem dysfunction requiring airway protection
- Respiratory dysfunction to aspiration
- Severe bradyarrhythmias or tachyarrhythmias
- Severe hypotension or hypertension
- Patients with signs of raised ICP or seizures
- Stroke patients with high-risk lesions
  - Basilar occlusion/brainstem infarction
  - Large hemispheric infarction, especially in younger patients
  - Large territorial cerebellar infarction prone to swelling
- Patients treated by thrombolytics who need monitoring if no bed is available in the stroke unit.

Q12. Give an overview of IV thrombolysis for reperfusion in an ischemic stroke.

The important factors that determine the outcome after reperfusion therapy are appropriate patient selection and early treatment. The short-term goal of reperfusion is to restore blood flow to the ischemic areas of the brain, which can be salvaged, whereas limiting disability and mortality in the long term.

Alteplase (rtPA) is the mainstay of a thrombolytic agent approved for thrombolysis in acute ischemic stroke. It is indicated in patients with suspected diagnosis of acute ischemic stroke, with a persistent measurable neurological deficit and with treatment commencing within 4.5 hours of symptom onset after ruling out contraindications to IV thrombolysis. It is administered in a dose of 0.9 mg/kg of actual body weight with a maximum dose of 90 mg. 10% of the dose is given as a slow IV bolus followed by infusion of the remaining drug over 1 hour.[63]

Tenecteplase is a type of rtPA (modified version of alteplase); these modifications make it longer acting and more fibrin specific compared to alteplase. Meta-analysis of randomized controlled trials (RCTs) has shown it to be equivalent to alteplase.[64]

Tenecteplase is administered as a single bolus at 0.25 mg/kg (maximum 25 mg); this easier dosing can translate into faster door-to-needle time when compared with alteplase.

EXTEND-IA TNK trial suggested higher reperfusion rates and a better functional outcome with tenecteplase [0.25 mg/kg (maximum 25 mg)] than with alteplase before mechanical recanalization with large-vessel occlusion,[65] while the NOR-TEST study showed no advantage for tenecteplase (0.4 mg/kg) compared to the standard alteplase with regard to the modified Rankin scale (mRS) after 3 months when used in patients with minor strokes (median NIHSS score was 4).[66] NOR-TEST 2, Part A, which included patients with moderate-to-severe ischemic stroke (the median NIHSS was 11) within 4.5 hours of onset, randomly assigned patients to tenecteplase 0.4 mg/kg or alteplase 0.9 mg/kg, suggested worse favorable functional outcomes at 3 months in addition to a higher rate of intracranial hemorrhage (ICH) and mortality.[67]

As per American Heart Association (AHA)/American Stroke Association (ASA) guidelines, tenecteplase should be used as an alternative to alteplase (but only as a bridging thrombolysis before mechanical recanalization in case of large-vessel occlusion).[68]

Hemorrhage (intracranial and/or extracranial) is the main complication of thrombolytics, used for ischemic stroke. Symptomatic hemorrhagic complication is 6–7%.[27] Angioedema is another dreaded complication with IV thrombolytic agents.

Enumerate the contraindication to thrombolysis.[63]
- Time of onset from 0 to 4.5 hours in patients presenting with mild non disabling stroke (NIHSS score 0–5).
- CT suggestive of acute ICH
- CT showing extensive areas of hypoattenuation
- Ischemic stroke within 3 months
- Severe head trauma within 3 months
- Intracranial or intraspinal surgery within 3 months
- History of ICH
- Clinical features consistent with subarachnoid hemorrhage
- Presence of a structural gastrointestinal (GI) malignancy or GI bleed within 21 days
- Patients with coagulopathy defined as platelets <100,000/mm^3, INR >1.7, aPTT >40 seconds, or PT >15 seconds
- Patients who have received therapeutic low-molecular-weight heparin (LMWH) within 24 hours
- Current use of direct thrombin inhibitors or direct factor Xa inhibitors or glycoprotein (Gp) IIb/IIIa inhibitors
- Clinical features consistent of infective endocarditis
- Aortic arch dissection
- Intra-axial intracranial neoplasm.

Q13. Describe the role of antiplatelet agents in the management of acute ischemic stroke.

All patients with ischemic stroke should receive aspirin within 24–48 hours of onset. Aspirin administration may be delayed by 24 hours in patients receiving IV thrombolysis. Administration of Gp IIb/IIIa inhibitor abciximab in acute ischemic stroke is potentially harmful and may increase the risk of ICH.[63] The Clopidogrel in High-Risk Patients with Acute Nondisabling Cerebrovascular Events (CHANCE) trial showed that short-term dual antiplatelet therapy with clopidogrel and aspirin for 21 days reduced early secondary stroke without causing an increase in major bleeding. However, a recent trial, the Platelet-Oriented Inhibition in New TIA and Minor Ischemic Stroke (POINT) trial showed that dual antiplatelet therapy although decreased major ischemic events but nearly doubled the chance of major bleeding at 90 days. It is recommended that in patients presenting with minor noncardioembolic ischemic stroke (NIHSS score ≤3) who did not receive IV alteplase, treatment with dual antiplatelet therapy (aspirin and clopidogrel) started within 24 hours after symptom onset and continued for 21 days is effective in reducing recurrent ischemic stroke for a period of up to 90 days from symptom onset.[68] However, the role of dual antiplatelet therapy in acute ischemic stroke is controversial at present and should be definitely avoided in patients at increased risk of bleeding.[69,70]

Q14. What is the role of a combination anticoagulant with antiplatelet therapy in the management of acute ischemic stroke?

A meta-analysis, restricted to patients with an acute cardioembolic stroke, showed that anticoagulants given within 48 hours of clinical onset were associated with a nonsignificant reduction in recurrence of ischemic stroke but with no substantial reduction in death or disability. The recent ELAN trial that randomized patients (>2,000 patients) with AF and acute ischemic stroke in early direct oral anticoagulant (DOAC) therapy (<48 hours of minor/moderate stroke and 6–7 days after major stroke) and late DOAC therapy (3–4 days of minor stroke, 6–7 days of moderate stroke, and 12–14 days of major stroke) suggested a nonsignificant trend of benefit toward early DOAC therapy, which was not associated with an increased rate of symptomatic ICH.[71]

Despite the lack of evidence, some experts recommend full-dose heparin in selected patients, such as those with cardiac sources of embolism and high risk of re-embolism, e.g., AF particularly if too early in the acute illness to start warfarin, arterial (carotid/vertebral) dissection, sinus vein thrombosis, fresh thrombus in carotid artery/heart, or high-grade arterial stenosis prior to surgery.

Today, there are few indications for heparin treatment in stroke care; contraindications include large infarcts (e.g., >50% of MCA territory), uncontrollable arterial hypertension, and advanced microvascular changes in the brain as in amyloid angiopathy.

Q15. What is the target BP in this patient? How will you control BP?

Potential approaches to arterial hypertension in acute ischemic stroke patients who are candidates for acute reperfusion therapy include the following:

Patient otherwise eligible for acute reperfusion therapy except that BP is >185/110 mm Hg:
- Labetalol 10–20 mg IV over 1–2 minutes; or
- Nicardipine 5 mg/h IV, titrate up by 2.5 mg/h every 5–15 minutes, maximum 15 mg/h; or

- Clevidipine 1–2 mg/h IV, titrate by doubling the dose every 2–5 minutes until desired BP reached; maximum 21 mg/h; or
- Other agents (hydralazine, enalaprilat, etc.) may be considered when appropriate.

If BP is not maintained at or below 185/110 mm Hg, do not administer rtPA.

Monitor BP every 15 minutes for 2 hours from the start of rtPA therapy, then every 30 minutes for 6 hours, and then every hour for 16 hours and maintain at or below 185/110 mm Hg.

If systolic BP is higher than 180–230 mm Hg or diastolic BP >105–120 mm Hg.

Labetalol 10 mg IV followed by continuous IV infusion 2–8 mg/min; or nicardipine 5 mg/h IV, titrate up to desired effect by 2.5 mg/h every 5–15 minutes, maximum 15 mg/h. If BP is not controlled or diastolic BP is higher than 140 mm Hg, consider IV sodium nitroprusside.[63]

Q16. What are the indications for thrombolysis after 3 hours of acute ischemic stroke?

The European Cooperative Acute Stroke Study-3 (ECASS-3) trial in 2008 demonstrated that IV thrombolysis up to 4.5 hours is beneficial. It has to be understood that an extended time window must not lead to delayed therapy. Thrombolysis is more effective the earlier it is applied.[30] It cannot be performed after 3 hours if any one of the following criteria is present (these are the exclusion criteria for ECASS-3):

- Age >80 years
- History of prior stroke and diabetes
- NIHSS >25
- Any active anticoagulation (even with INR 1.7)
- CT showing multilobar infarction (hypodensity higher than one-third cerebral hemisphere).

Q17. What are the indications for thrombolysis of patients after 4.5 hours of onset of stroke?

Analysis of trials of IV thrombolysis indicates that there is a decrease in benefit from IV thrombolysis when used after 4.5 hours of onset. Certain patients have good collateral circulation; this makes reversibility extend beyond the known limit possible.

Now imaging tools are able to identify patients with unknown time of onset of stroke or patients who wake up with neurodeficit.

In the WAKE-UP trial, patients with an undetermined onset of stroke but >4.5 hours underwent MRI brain. The patient who had diffusion–fluid-attenuated inversion recovery (FLAIR) mismatch (diffusion abnormality was present without a corresponding hyperintensity on FLAIR imaging, which suggests that the true time of onset of stroke is within 3 hours) were randomized to standard-dose IV tPA or placebo. Result suggested an 11.5% greater favorable outcome in the tPA group.[72]

The EXTEND trial randomized patients to IV tPA or placebo if they were 4.5–9 hours since last seen well and if there was a mismatch between the ratio of perfusion abnormality and core infarct volume of at least 1.2 using CT or MR perfusion using RAPID automated software. The tPA group had more patients who had a favorable outcome at 90 days.[73]

Based on these trials, it is suggested to administer IV alteplase in patients with acute ischemic stroke who awake with stroke symptoms or have unclear time of onset >4.5 hours from last known well or at baseline state and who have a DW-MRI lesion smaller than one-third of the MCA territory and no visible signal change on FLAIR.[68]

Q18. Describe in brief the utility of mechanical thrombectomy in acute ischemic stroke.

Mechanical thrombectomy is a reperfusion modality used in patients with acute ischemic stroke due to large artery occlusion in the anterior circulation. It has been proven to be beneficial if used within 24 hours of symptom onset with or without using alteplase in the 4.5-hour window. Mechanical thrombectomy if indicated should be initiated as early as possible without waiting for response to IV rtPA.

Prerequisites for mechanical thrombectomy include:
- Neuroimaging evidence of small infarct core and exclusion of hemorrhage
- Angiographical evidence of proximal large arterial anterior circulation stroke
- Patient has persistent disabling neurodeficit
- Expertise and facilities for mechanical thrombectomy with second-generation stent retrievers are available
- No significant prestroke disability (mRS ≤ 1)
- Femoral puncture can be achieved within 24 hours from the last known neurologic baseline.

Mechanical thrombectomy <6 hours from onset

It can be done if there is angiographic evidence of occlusion of distal ICA, M1, M2 segments of MCA, or A1, A2 segments of the anterior cerebral artery. A Randomized Trial of Intra-arterial Treatment for Acute Ischemic Stroke (MR CLEAN) trial, the Stent-Retriever Thrombectomy after Intravenous t-PA vs. t-PA Alone in Stroke (SWIFT PRIME) trial, the Thrombectomy within 8 Hours after Symptom Onset in Ischemic Stroke (REVASCAT) trial, the Endovascular Therapy for Ischemic Stroke with Perfusion-Imaging Selection (EXTEND IA) trial, and the Randomized Assessment of Rapid Endovascular Treatment of Ischemic Stroke (ESCAPE) trial are the major trials showing improved outcomes with early mechanical thrombectomy in patients with acute ischemic stroke.[74-78]

Mechanical thrombectomy from 6 to 24 hours of symptom onset

It can be done in cases of failed or contraindicated thrombolysis, intracranial occlusion of ICA or M1 segment of MCA, and a clinical–radiological mismatch. The thrombectomy 6-24 hours after stroke with a mismatch between deficit and infarct (DAWN) trial and the thrombectomy for stroke at 6-16 hours with selection by perfusion imaging (DEFUSE 3) trial have shown benefit of late mechanical thrombectomy in patients with acute ischemic stroke.[79,80]

These benefits in outcome have been seen with second-generation stent retriever devices only.

Q19. What are the mechanical interventions feasible for clot extraction/dissolution?

First-generation devices:
- Mechanical Embolus Removal in Cerebral Ischemia (MERCI) retriever
- Penumbra System®

Second-generation devices:
- Solitaire stent retriever system
- Stryker neurovascular Trevo stent retriever

The patient developed generalized tonic–clonic seizures and on examination was found to have a drop in GCS to 10/15 (E2M5V3) and unequal pupils sluggishly reacting to light.

Q20. What are the possible causes for this deterioration? How will you manage it?

The possible clinical condition leading to a fall in GCS could be the consequence of one of the following:
- Progression of ischemic infarct with midline shift causing a drop in GCS
- Recurrent ischemic stroke
- Hemorrhagic transformation of ischemic infarct or intraparenchymal bleed
- Developing edema around previous infarct causing mass effect
- Postictal state, subclinical seizure activity
- Metabolic causes (hyponatremia, hypernatremia, hypercalcemia, hypoglycemia, hyperglycemia, sepsis, uremia, hyperammonemia)
- Drug overdose, sedative use.

Management:
Given the complexity of severe stroke and potential complications, a multidisciplinary care team composed of neurologists, neurointensivists, and neurosurgeons, as well as dedicated stroke nursing, are required to optimally manage these complex patients.

- As features are suggestive of possible raised ICP, initiate measures to control raised ICP including head-end elevation, sedation, analgesia, and osmotherapy and start ICP monitoring and CSF drainage. Intubation and mechanical ventilation and maintain normocapnia.
- Antiepileptics should be initiated to treat seizures and prevent further neurological damage.
- Continue with general neuroprotective measures (head-end elevation 30–45°, euvolemia, euglycemia, euthermia, treat hypoxemia if present, maintain cerebral perfusion pressure)
- Neuroimaging of brain to look for progression of infarct, recurrence of infarct, edema, and mass effect or hemorrhagic transformation
- If worsening despite medical measures to control ICP, neurosurgical intervention such as decompressive craniectomy might be needed.

Q21. When should you offer decompressive craniectomy to the patient and what is its rationale?

- Decompressive craniectomy is a controversial therapy for malignant MCA stroke.
- Malignant MCA stroke is indicated by:
  - MCA territory stroke of higher than 50% on CT
  - Perfusion deficit of >66% on CT
  - Infarct volume higher than 82 mL within 6 hours of onset (on MRI)
  - Infarct volume >145 mL within 14 hours of onset (on MRI)

Rationale:
- Malignant MCA infarction is a devastating event with substantial morbidity and mortality, due to:
  - Involvement of a large amount of brain tissue, resulting in cerebral edema and increased ICP
  - Risk of hemorrhagic transformation
  - Midline shift resulting in compression of medial cerebral structures
  - Potential for transtentorial herniation, with compression of the posterior cerebral artery
  - Poor perfusion of the contralateral cerebral hemisphere due to increased ICP.

Decompressive craniectomy may have the following effects, which could lead to improved morbidity and mortality:
- Can decrease ICP by increasing cranial compliance
- Prevent transtentorial herniation
- Improve perfusion in the penumbra of the stroke

Advantages:
- Face validity based on theoretical rationale
- Decreased mortality in age below 60 years within 48 hours of onset of malignant MCA stroke

- Well tolerated even after thrombolysis (though apparently antiplatelet drugs tend to increase the risk of bleeding)
- Craniectomy and evacuation of clot may be required for hemorrhagic transformation anyway.

Disadvantages:
- Highly invasive procedure
- Resource intensive (monetary cost, neurosurgeons, operating room, ICU care)
- Craniectomy has to be large enough to extend past the margins of the infarct.
- Evidence base is limited by small trials and potential for systematic bias (e.g., due to lack of allocation concealment).
- It should only be considered if age is below 60 years and <48 hours since stroke onset.

Though DESTINY trial (2007), DECIMAL trial (2007), and HAMLET trial (2009) showed favorable results with decompressive craniectomy in terms of mortality, the neurological outcomes were not good, a finding which was later confirmed by the DESTINY II trial.[81-85]

Therefore, decompressive craniectomy can be considered in patients below 60 years of age within 48 hours of stroke onset, although outcomes are still likely to be poor. It should not be performed in malignant MCA stroke patients aged >60 years as survivors would have increased disability.

Two days later, a repeat CT showed a bleed into the infarcted area with the surrounding edema and midline shift. The daughter of the patient questions the cause of deterioration after initial improvement and blames that the thrombolytic agent injection led to his clinical deterioration. Her father's condition has deteriorated; GCS has dropped to 10/15.

Q22. What are the complications associated with thrombolytic therapy and how will you manage post-thrombolysis ICH and how will you counsel the daughter?
- Introduce yourself to ask her which language she is comfortable in speaking.
- As a treating physician of the patient, try to understand the situation and emotions of patients' relatives and respect their concerns.
- Avoid leading questions; ask relatives of the patient whether they understood the explanation given and give them the opportunity to ask further questions if they wish.
- Arrange a multidisciplinary meeting of the family with the specialists involved in the treatment of the patient.
- Inform the relatives that "deterioration following initial improvement after ischemic stroke is well known, occurring in around 13% of patients due to reocclusion, hemorrhage, or edema."[86] It can also occur as one of the complications related to thrombolysis, which has been mentioned to them and other family members during informed consent.
- *Complications of thrombolytic therapy:* Thrombolytic therapy has been associated with the following complications:
  - Intracerebral hemorrhage = asymptomatic or symptomatic
  - Systemic bleeding
  - Angioedema
  - Post-thrombolysis reperfusion injury.

The most feared complication of thrombolytic therapy in stroke is symptomatic intracerebral hemorrhage.

Post-thrombolysis intracerebral hemorrhage[68]
It has been seen with the incidence ranging from 2 to 7% with the greatest risk seen in patients with most severe strokes after the use of IV thrombolytics.

Usually, asymptomatic intracerebral hemorrhage is seen within 36 hours of the use of IV thrombolytics with around half occurring within 10 hours; any hemorrhage occurring after 36 hours of thrombolytics is unlikely to be caused by the use of IV thrombolytics.

Symptomatic intracerebral hemorrhage is classified based on two main factors:
1. *Radiographic appearance of hemorrhage:* This has been graded as:
   a. HI1 = Petechial hemorrhage along infarct tissue margin
   b. HI2 = Confluent petechial hemorrhage within the infarcted tissue
   c. PH1 = Parenchymal hematoma involving <30% of infarct tissue with slight mass effect
   d. PH2 = Parenchymal hematoma involving >30% of infarct tissue with significant mass effect
2. Presence of associated neurological deterioration

Definition of symptomatic intracerebral hemorrhage:
- NINDS trial definition = Any hemorrhagic transformation temporally associated with neurological worsening
  - This is an overly inclusive definition as it may include patients with small petechial hemorrhage with subtle neurological deterioration, which may not have significant long-term impact on a patient's functional outcomes.
- ECASS-2, ECASS-3, and SITS-MOST trial definition = Intracerebral hemorrhage with significant neurological worsening (defined by drop in NIHSS score ≥4).

Risk factors for the development of symptomatic ICH:
- Older age
- Greater stroke severity
- Higher baseline glucose

- Hypertension
- Congestive heart failure
- Renal impairment
- Diabetes mellitus
- Ischemic heart disease
- AF
- Baseline antiplatelet use
- Cerebral microbleeds
- Visible acute infarction on neuroimaging
- Leukoaraiosis.

Risk scores and scoring systems for prediction of risk of ICH in patients treated with IV thrombolytics:
- HAT score
- DRAGON score
- SEDAN score
- SPAN-100 index
- SITS SICH score
- Stroke-thrombolytic predictive instrument.

Management of symptomatic ICH after IV thrombolytics:
- If the patient develops neurological worsening after initiation of IV thrombolytics, consider possibility of ICH.
- Immediately stop thrombolytic drug infusion.
- Get urgent noncontrast computed tomography (NCCT) brain/MRI.
- Draw and send blood samples for CBC, coagulation profile, fibrinogen, and cross-matching.
- If symptomatic hemorrhage is confirmed on imaging:
  - Give 10 units of cryoprecipitate over 10–30 minutes or more to achieve S. fibrinogen level of 150–200 mg/dL.
  - Consider tranexamic acid 10–15 mg/kg IV over 10–15 minutes/aminocaproic acid 5 g IV over 1 hour followed by 1 g/h infusion for 8 hours till bleeding is controlled.
  - Patient prior on warfarin therapy = Consider prothrombin complex concentrate (PCC)/fresh frozen plasma (FFP) with vitamin K
  - Patient receiving unfractionated heparin (UFH) = Administer 1 mg of protamine for each 100 U of UFH
  - Patient with platelet count < 100,000/μL = Transfuse —six to eight units of platelets
- Obtain neurosurgery and hematology consultation.

REFERENCES

1. Kothari R, Hall K, Brott T, Broderick J. Early stroke recognition: developing an out-of-hospital NIH Stroke Scale. Acad Emerg Med. 1997;4:986-90.
2. Sinz E, Navarro K, Soderberg ES. Advanced Cardiovascular Life Support. Provider Manual. Dallas, TX: American Heart Association; 2011.
3. Adams HP, Davis PH, Leira EC, Chang KC, Bendixen BH, Clarke WR, et al. Baseline NIH Stroke Scale score strongly predicts outcome after stroke: a report of the Trial of Org 10172 in Acute Stroke Treatment (TOAST). Neurology. 1999;53:126-31.
4. von Kummer R, Bourquain H, Bastianello S, Bozzao L, Manelfe C, Meier D, et al. Early prediction of irreversible brain damage after ischemic stroke at CT. Radiology. 2001;219:95-100.
5. The European Stroke Organisation (ESO) Executive Committee, ESO Writing Committee. Guidelines for management of ischaemic stroke and transient ischaemic attack 2008. Cerebrovasc Dis. 2008;25:457-507.
6. Larrue V, von Kummer R, del Zoppo G, Bluhmki E. Hemorrhagic transformation in acute ischemic stroke. Potential contributing factors in the European Cooperative Acute Stroke Study. Stroke. 1997;28:957-60.
7. Wahlgren N, Ahmed N, Eriksson N, Aichner F, Bluhmki E, Dávalos A, et al. Multivariable analysis of outcome predictors and adjustment of main outcome results to baseline data profile in randomized controlled trials: Safe Implementation of Thrombolysis in Stroke-Monitoring STudy (SITS-MOST). Stroke. 2008;39:3316-22.
8. Demchuk AM, Hill MD, Barber PA, Silver B, Patel SC, Levine SR, et al. Importance of early ischemic computed tomography changes using ASPECTS in NINDS rtPA Stroke Study. Stroke. 2005;36:2110-5.
9. Dzialowski I, Hill MD, Coutts SB, Demchuk AM, Kent DM, Wunderlich O, et al. Extent of early ischemic changes on computed tomography (CT) before thrombolysis: prognostic value of the Alberta Stroke Program Early CT Score in ECASS II. Stroke. 2006;37:973-8.
10. Patel SC, Levine SR, Tilley BC, Grotta JC, Lu M, Frankel M, et al. Lack of clinical significance of early ischemic changes on computed tomography in acute stroke. JAMA. 2001;286:2830-8.
11. Kidwell CS, Alger JR, Di Salle F, Starkman S, Villablanca P, Bentson J, et al. Diffusion MRI in patients with transient ischemic attacks. Stroke. 1999;30:1174-80.
12. Noguchi K, Ogawa T, Inugami A, Toyoshima H, Sugawara S, Hatazawa J, et al. Acute subarachnoid hemorrhage: MR imaging with fluid-attenuated inversion recovery pulse sequences. Radiology. 1995;196:773-7.
13. Sames TA, Storrow AB, Finkelstein JA, Magoon MR. Sensitivity of new-generation computed tomography in subarachnoid hemorrhage. Acad Emerg Med. 1996;3:16-20.
14. Tomura N, Uemura K, Inugami A, Fujita H, Higano S, Shishido F. Early CT finding in cerebral infarction: obscuration of the lentiform nucleus. Radiology. 1988;168:463-7.
15. Truwit CL, Barkovich AJ, Gean-Marton A, Hibri N, Norman D. Loss of the insular ribbon: another early CT sign of acute middle cerebral artery infarction. Radiology. 1990;176:801-6.
16. von Kummer R, Meyding-Lamadé U, Forsting M, Rosin L, Rieke K, Hacke W, et al. Sensitivity and prognostic value of early CT in occlusion of the middle cerebral artery trunk. AJNR Am J Neuroradiol. 1994;15:9-15.
17. Barber PA, Demchuk AM, Zhang J, Buchan AM. Validity and reliability of a quantitative computed tomography score in predicting outcome of hyperacute stroke before thrombolytic therapy. ASPECTS Study Group. Alberta Stroke Programme Early CT Score. Lancet. 2000;355:1670-4.

18. Demchuk AM, Coutts SB. Alberta Stroke Program Early CT Score in acute stroke triage. Neuroimaging Clin N Am. 2005;15:409-19.
19. Moulin T, Cattin F, Crépin-Leblond T, Tatu L, Chavot D, Piotin M, et al. Early CT signs in acute middle cerebral artery infarction: predictive value for subsequent infarct locations and outcome. Neurology. 1996;47:366-75.
20. Manno EM, Nichols DA, Fulgham JR, Wijdicks EF. Computed tomographic determinants of neurologic deterioration in patients with large middle cerebral artery infarctions. Mayo Clin Proc. 2003;78:156-60.
21. Smith WS, Tsao JW, Billings ME, Johnston SC, Hemphill 3rd JC, Bonovich DC, et al. Prognostic significance of angiographically confirmed large vessel intracranial occlusion in patients presenting with acute brain ischemia. Neurocrit Care. 2006;4:14-7.
22. Tomsick T, Brott T, Barsan W, Broderick J, Haley EC, Spilker J, et al. Prognostic value of the hyperdense middle cerebral artery sign and stroke scale score before ultraearly thrombolytic therapy. AJNR Am J Neuroradiol. 1996;17:79-85.
23. Flacke S, Urbach H, Keller E, Träber F, Hartmann A, Textor J, et al. Middle cerebral artery (MCA) susceptibility sign at susceptibility-based perfusion MR imaging: clinical importance and comparison with hyperdense MCA sign at CT. Radiology. 2000;215:476-82.
24. Barber PA, Demchuk AM, Hudon ME, Pexman JH, Hill MD, Buchan AM. Hyperdense sylvian fissure MCA "dot" sign: a CT marker of acute ischemia. Stroke. 2001;32:84-8.
25. Arnold M, Nedeltchev K, Schroth G, Baumgartner RW, Remonda L, Loher TJ, et al. Clinical and radiological predictors of recanalisation and outcome of 40 patients with acute basilar artery occlusion treated with intra-arterial thrombolysis. J Neurol Neurosurg Psychiatr. 2004;75:857-62.
26. Goldmakher GV, Camargo EC, Furie KL, Singhal AB, Roccatagliata L, Halpern EF, et al. Hyperdense basilar artery sign on unenhanced CT predicts thrombus and outcome in acute posterior circulation stroke. Stroke. 2009;40:134-9.
27. The National Institute of Neurological Disorders and Stroke rt-PA Stroke Study Group. Tissue plasminogen activator for acute ischemic stroke. N Engl J Med. 1995;333:1581-7.
28. Hacke W, Kaste M, Fieschi C, Toni D, Lesaffre E, von Kummer R, et al. Intravenous thrombolysis with recombinant tissue plasminogen activator for acute hemispheric stroke. The European Cooperative Acute Stroke Study (ECASS). JAMA. 1995;274:1017-25.
29. Furlan A, Higashida R, Wechsler L, Gent M, Rowley H, Kase C, et al. Intra-arterial prourokinase for acute ischemic stroke. The PROACT II study: a randomized controlled trial. Prolyse in Acute Cerebral Thromboembolism. JAMA. 1999;282:2003-11.
30. Hacke W, Kaste M, Bluhmki E, Brozman M, Dávalos A, Guidetti D, et al. Thrombolysis with alteplase 3 to 4.5 hours after acute ischemic stroke. N Engl J Med. 2008;359:1317-29.
31. Ogawa A, Mori E, Minematsu K, Taki W, Takahashi A, Nemoto S, et al. Randomized trial of intraarterial infusion of urokinase within 6 hours of middle cerebral artery stroke: the Middle Cerebral Artery Embolism Local Fibrinolytic Intervention Trial (MELT) Japan. Stroke. 2007;38:2633-9.
32. Puetz V, Sylaja PN, Coutts SB, Hill MD, Dzialowski I, Mueller P, et al. Extent of hypoattenuation on CT angiography source images predicts functional outcome in patients with basilar artery occlusion. Stroke. 2008;39:2485-90.
33. Aviv RI, Mandelcorn J, Chakraborty S, Gladstone D, Malham S, Tomlinson G, et al. Alberta Stroke Program Early CT Scoring of CT perfusion in early stroke visualization and assessment. AJNR Am J Neuroradiol. 2007;28:1975-80.
34. Kang DW, Chalela JA, Dunn W, Warach S, NIH-Suburban Stroke Center Investigators. MRI screening before standard tissue plasminogen activator therapy is feasible and safe. Stroke. 2005;36:1939-43.
35. Barber PA, Darby DG, Desmond PM, Gerraty RP, Yang Q, Li T, et al. Identification of major ischemic change. Diffusion-weighted imaging versus computed tomography. Stroke. 1999;30:2059-65.
36. Fiebach JB, Schellinger PD, Jansen O, Meyer M, Wilde P, Bender J, et al. CT and diffusion-weighted MR imaging in randomized order: diffusion-weighted imaging results in higher accuracy and lower interrater variability in the diagnosis of hyperacute ischemic stroke. Stroke. 2002;33:2206-10.
37. González RG, Schaefer PW, Buonanno FS, Schwamm LH, Budzik RF, Rordorf G, et al. Diffusion-weighted MR imaging: diagnostic accuracy in patients imaged within 6 hours of stroke symptom onset. Radiology. 1999;210:155-62.
38. Ay H, Buonanno FS, Rordorf G, Schaefer PW, Schwamm LH, Wu O, et al. Normal diffusion-weighted MRI during stroke-like deficits. Neurology. 1999;52:1784-92.
39. Barber PA, Darby DG, Desmond PM, Yang Q, Gerraty RP, Jolley D, et al. Prediction of stroke outcome with echoplanar perfusion- and diffusion-weighted MRI. Neurology. 1998;51:418-26.
40. Lee LJ, Kidwell CS, Alger J, Starkman S, Saver JL. Impact on stroke subtype diagnosis of early diffusion-weighted magnetic resonance imaging and magnetic resonance angiography. Stroke. 2000;31:1081-9.
41. Lövblad KO, Laubach HJ, Baird AE, Curtin F, Schlaug G, Edelman RR, et al. Clinical experience with diffusion-weighted MR in patients with acute stroke. AJNR Am J Neuroradiol. 1998;19:1061-6.
42. Lutsep HL, Albers GW, DeCrespigny A, Kamat GN, Marks MP, Moseley ME. Clinical utility of diffusion-weighted magnetic resonance imaging in the assessment of ischemic stroke. Ann Neurol. 1997;41:574-80.
43. van Everdingen KJ, van der Grond J, Kappelle LJ, Ramos LM, Mali WP. Diffusion-weighted magnetic resonance imaging in acute stroke. Stroke. 1998;29:1783-90.
44. Warach S, Chien D, Li W, Ronthal M, Edelman RR. Fast magnetic resonance diffusion-weighted imaging of acute human stroke. Neurology. 1992;42:1717-23.
45. Albers GW, Lansberg MG, Norbash AM, Tong DC, O'Brien MW, Woolfenden AR, et al. Yield of diffusion-weighted MRI for detection of potentially relevant findings in stroke patients. Neurology. 2000;54:1562-7.
46. Bryan RN, Levy LM, Whitlow WD, Killian JM, Preziosi TJ, Rosario JA. Diagnosis of acute cerebral infarction: comparison of CT and MR imaging. AJNR Am J Neuroradiol. 1991;12:611-20.

47. Perkins CJ, Kahya E, Roque CT, Roche PE, Newman GC. Fluid-attenuated inversion recovery and diffusion- and perfusion-weighted MRI abnormalities in 117 consecutive patients with stroke symptoms. Stroke. 2001;32:2774-81.
48. Wiener JI, King Jr JT, Moore JR, Lewin JS. The value of diffusion-weighted imaging for prediction of lasting deficit in acute stroke: an analysis of 134 patients with acute neurologic deficits. Neuroradiology. 2001;43:435-41.
49. Arauz A, Murillo L, Cantú C, Barinagarrementeria F, Higuera J. Prospective study of single and multiple lacunar infarcts using magnetic resonance imaging: risk factors, recurrence, and outcome in 175 consecutive cases. Stroke. 2003;34:2453-8.
50. Ay H, Oliveira-Filho J, Buonanno FS, Ezzeddine M, Schaefer PW, Rordorf G, et al. Diffusion-weighted imaging identifies a subset of lacunar infarction associated with embolic source. Stroke. 1999;30:2644-50.
51. Baird AE, Lövblad KO, Schlaug G, Edelman RR, Warach S. Multiple acute stroke syndrome: marker of embolic disease? Neurology. 2000;54:674-8.
52. Caso V, Budak K, Georgiadis D, Schuknecht B, Baumgartner RW. Clinical significance of detection of multiple acute brain infarcts on diffusion weighted magnetic resonance imaging. J Neurol Neurosurg Psychiatr. 2005;76:514-8.
53. Etgen T, Gräfin von Einsiedel H, Röttinger M, Winbeck K, Conrad B, Sander D. Detection of acute brainstem infarction by using DWI/MRI. Eur Neurol. 2004;52:145-50.
54. Gerraty RP, Parsons MW, Barber PA, Darby DG, Desmond PM, Tress BM, et al. Examining the lacunar hypothesis with diffusion and perfusion magnetic resonance imaging. Stroke. 2002;33:2019-24.
55. Keir SL, Wardlaw JM, Bastin ME, Dennis MS. In which patients is diffusion-weighted magnetic resonance imaging most useful in routine stroke care? J Neuroimaging. 2004;14:118-22.
56. Mullins ME, Schaefer PW, Sorensen AG, Halpern EF, Ay H, He J, et al. CT and conventional and diffusion-weighted MR imaging in acute stroke: study in 691 patients at presentation to the emergency department. Radiology. 2002;224:353-60.
57. Seifert T, Enzinger C, Storch MK, Pichler G, Niederkorn K, Fazekas F. Acute small subcortical infarctions on diffusion weighted MRI: clinical presentation and aetiology. J Neurol Neurosurg Psychiatr. 2005;76:1520-4.
58. Takahashi K, Kobayashi S, Matui R, Yamaguchi S, Yamashita K. The differences of clinical parameters between small multiple ischemic lesions and single lesion detected by diffusion-weighted MRI. Acta Neurol Scand. 2002;106:24-9.
59. Wessels T, Röttger C, Jauss M, Kaps M, Traupe H, Stolz E. Identification of embolic stroke patterns by diffusion-weighted MRI in clinically defined lacunar stroke syndromes. Stroke. 2005;36:757-61.
60. Wityk RJ, Goldsborough MA, Hillis A, Beauchamp N, Barker PB, Borowicz Jr LM, et al. Diffusion- and perfusion-weighted brain magnetic resonance imaging in patients with neurologic complications after cardiac surgery. Arch Neurol. 2001;58:571-6.
61. Beaulieu C, De Crespigny A, Tong DC, Moseley ME, Albers GW, Marks MP. Longitudinal magnetic resonance imaging study of perfusion and diffusion in stroke: evolution of lesion volume and correlation with clinical outcome. Ann Neurol. 1999;46:568-78.
62. Lövblad KO. Diffusion-weighted MRI: back to the future. Stroke. 2002;33:2204-5.
63. Powers WJ, Rabinstein AA, Ackerson T, Adeoye OM, Bambakidis NC, Becker K, et al. 2018 guidelines for the early management of patients with acute ischemic stroke: a guideline for healthcare professionals from the American Heart Association/American Stroke Association. Stroke. 2018;49:e46-99.
64. Thelengana A, Radhakrishnan DM, Prasad M, Kumar A, Prasad K. Tenecteplase versus alteplase in acute ischemic stroke: systematic review and meta-analysis. Acta Neurol Belg. 2018;119:359-67.
65. Campbell BC, Mitchell PJ, Churilov L, Yassi N, Kleinig TJ, Dowling RJ, et al. Tenecteplase versus alteplase before thrombectomy for ischemic stroke. N Engl J Med. 2018;378:1573-82.
66. Logallo N, Novotny V, Assmus J, Kvistad CE, Alteheld L, Rønning OM, et al. Tenecteplase versus alteplase for management of acute ischaemic stroke (NOR-TEST): a phase 3, randomised, open-label, blinded endpoint trial. Lancet Neurol. 2017;16(10):781-8.
67. Kvistad CE, Næss H, Helleberg BH, Idicula T, Hagberg G, Nordby LM, et al. Tenecteplase versus alteplase for the management of acute ischaemic stroke in Norway (NOR-TEST 2, part A): a phase 3, randomised, open-label, blinded endpoint, non-inferiority trial. Lancet Neurol. 2022;21(6):511-9.
68. Warner JJ, Harrington RA, Sacco RL, Elkind MSV. Guidelines for the early management of patients with acute ischemic stroke: 2019 update to the 2018 guidelines for the early management of acute ischemic stroke. Stroke. 2019;50(12):3331-2.
69. Wang Y, Wang Y, Zhao X, Liu L, Wang D, Wang C, et al. Clopidogrel with aspirin in acute minor stroke or transient ischemic attack. N Engl J Med. 2013;369:11-9.
70. Johnston SC, Easton JD, Farrant M, Barsan W, Conwit RA, Elm JJ, et al. Clopidogrel and aspirin in acute ischemic stroke and high-risk TIA. N Engl J Med. 2018;379:215-25.
71. Fischer U, Koga M, Strbian D, Branca M, Abend S, Trelle S, et al. Early versus later anticoagulation for stroke with atrial fibrillation. N Engl J Med. 2023;388(26):2411-21.
72. Thomalla G, Simonsen CZ, Boutitie F, Andersen G, Berthezene Y, Cheng B, et al. MRI-guided thrombolysis for stroke with unknown time of onset. N Engl J Med. 2018;379(7):611-22.
73. Ma H, Campbell BCV, Parsons MW, Churilov L, Levi CR, Hsu C, et al. Thrombolysis guided by perfusion imaging up to 9 hours after onset of stroke [published correction appears in N Engl J Med. 2021;384(13):1278]. N Engl J Med. 2019;380(19):1795-1803.
74. Berkhemer OA, Fransen PS, Beumer D, Van Den Berg LA, Lingsma HF, Yoo AJ, et al. A randomized trial of intraarterial treatment for acute ischemic stroke. N Engl J Med. 2015;372:11-20.
75. Saver JL, Goyal M, Bonafe A, Diener HC, Levy EI, Pereira VM, et al. Stent-retriever thrombectomy after intravenous t-PA vs. t-PA alone in stroke. N Engl J Med. 2015;372:2285-95.

76. Jovin TG, Chamorro A, Cobo E, de Miquel MA, Molina CA, Rovira A, et al. Thrombectomy within 8 hours after symptom onset in ischemic stroke. N Engl J Med. 2015;372:2296-306.
77. Campbell BC, Mitchell PJ, Kleinig TJ, Dewey HM, Churilov L, Yassi N, et al. Endovascular therapy for ischemic stroke with perfusion-imaging selection. N Engl J Med. 2015;372:1009-18.
78. Goyal M, Demchuk AM, Menon BK, Eesa M, Rempel JL, Thornton J, et al. Randomized assessment of rapid endovascular treatment of ischemic stroke. N Engl J Med. 2015;372:1019-30.
79. Nogueira RG, Jadhav AP, Haussen DC, Bonafe A, Budzik RF, Bhuva P, et al. Thrombectomy 6 to 24 hours after stroke with a mismatch between deficit and infarct. N Engl J Med. 2018;378:11-21.
80. Albers GW, Marks MP, Kemp S, Christensen S, Tsai JP, Ortega-Gutierrez S, et al. Thrombectomy for stroke at 6 to 16 hours with selection by perfusion imaging. N Engl J Med. 2018;378(8):708-18.
81. Jüttler E, Schwab S, Schmiedek P, Unterberg A, Hennerici M, Woitzik J, et al. Decompressive surgery for the treatment of malignant infarction of the middle cerebral artery (DESTINY): a randomized, controlled trial. Stroke. 2007;38:2518-25.
82. Vahedi K, Vicaut E, Mateo J, Kurtz A, Orabi M, Guichard JP, et al. Sequential-design, multicenter, randomized, controlled trial of early decompressive craniectomy in malignant middle cerebral artery infarction (DECIMAL Trial). Stroke. 2007;38:2506-17.
83. Hofmeijer J, Kappelle LJ, Algra A, Amelink GJ, van Gijn J, van der Worp HB. Surgical decompression for space-occupying cerebral infarction (the Hemicraniectomy After Middle Cerebral Artery infarction with Life-threatening Edema Trial [HAMLET]): a multicentre, open, randomised trial. Lancet Neurol. 2009;8:326-33.
84. Vahedi K, Hofmeijer J, Juettler E, Vicaut E, George B, Algra A, et al. Early decompressive surgery in malignant infarction of the middle cerebral artery: a pooled analysis of three randomised controlled trials. Lancet Neurol. 2007;6:215-22.
85. Jüttler E, Bösel J, Amiri H, Schiller P, Limprecht R, Hacke W, et al. DESTINY II: DEcompressive Surgery for the Treatment of malignant INfarction of the middle cerebral arterY II. Int J Stroke. 2011;6:79-86.
86. Grotta JC, Welch KM, Fagan SC, Lu M, Frankel MR, Brott T, et al. Clinical deterioration following improvement in the NINDS rt-PA Stroke Trial. Stroke. 2001;32(3):661-8.

CHAPTER 14

Spontaneous Intracerebral Hemorrhage

Keyur Shah, Atul Prabhakar Kulkarni

CASE STUDY

*A 56-year-old man with history of hypertension and ischemic heart disease presented to emergency room (ER) with complaint of sudden-onset nausea, vomiting, and weakness involving right side of face and right arm and leg. The patient is currently on aspirin 75 mg and atorvastatin 40 mg and amlodipine 10 mg and telmisartan 40 mg for abovementioned medical conditions. On presentation to hospital, time of onset of symptoms was established as 60 minutes before arrival. Quick Cincinnati Prehospital Stroke Scale assessment shows right side of weakness involving face, arm, and leg and Glasgow Coma Scale (GCS) of 12. Vitals signs were as follow: heart rate (HR)—78 beats/min, blood pressure (BP)—210/110 mm Hg, respiratory rate of 24/min, and fingerstick blood glucose was 164 mg/dL. Under stroke protocol, he underwent initial noncontrast computed tomography (NCCT) brain which showed left basal ganglia hemorrhage (**Fig. 1**).*

Q1. What are the risk factors for development of ICH?

Intracerebral hemorrhage (ICH) accounts for approximately 10% of all strokes with mortality ranging from 35 to 45% in 30 days. Hypertension is the most common risk factor for ICH, by causing vasculopathy known as lipohyalinosis.[1] Most commonly affected area by hypertensive ICH is *putamen* (basal ganglia) followed by *thalamus*.

Other risk factors for ICH:[2]

- Advanced age
- African–American race/Japanese ethnicity
- Drug abuse like cocaine and methamphetamine
- Arteriovenous malformations (typically in young ICH)
- Anticoagulation (vitamin K antagonists, novel oral anticoagulants)
- Altered coagulation profile (liver/renal disease, thrombocytopenia)
- Thrombolysis
- Tumor bleeding
- Hemorrhagic infarcts (seen frequently in cerebral venous sinus thrombosis)
- Excessive alcohol abuse
- Vasculitis.

Q2. What is the Cincinnati Stroke Scale?

The most commonly used scales for prehospital stroke assessment by the first responders are "The Cincinnati Prehospital Stroke Scale" (CPSS) and the FAST (Facial drooping, Arm weakness, Speech difficulties, and Time) algorithm or the "Face, Arm, Speech Test", both of which give points for physical findings to diagnose stroke, while "The Los Angeles Prehospital Stroke Screen (LAPSS)" is used to diagnose causes of altered mentation.

The CPSS uses three variables (and gives a score ranging from 0 to 3), i.e., facial droop, dysarthria (slurred speech), and arm drift (weakness of the upper extremity) to confirm stroke probability. A score >2 predicts need for thrombolysis in ischemic stroke.

The FAST algorithm, which was mainly for use by laypersons, advocated by the American Stroke Association (ASA), is not very accurate since one study found it to be positive in patients with stroke mimics.

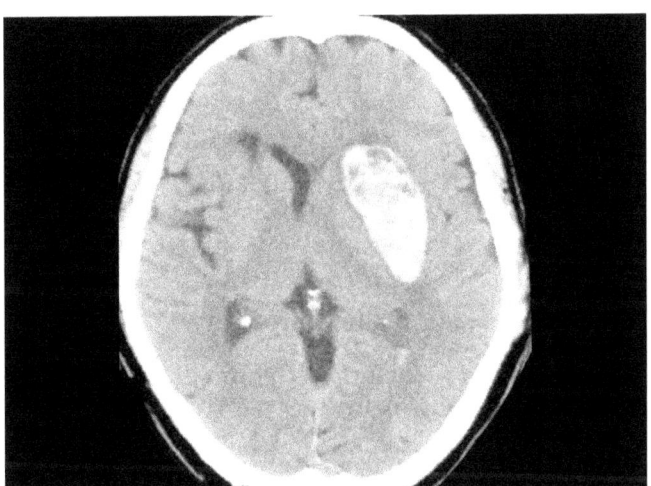

Fig. 1: Left basal ganglia hemorrhage.

The LAPSS uses the following screening criteria to assess stroke probability:
- Age ≥45 years
- Patient ambulatory at baseline
- No prior history of seizures
- Blood glucose levels 60 and 400 mg%
- New-onset neurologic symptoms in last 24 hours
- Looking for obvious asymmetry of the face (droop on either side), grip (weak grip), or arm strength (drifting or dropping down).

If any of these tests are positive or the function cannot be ascertained, it is taken as positive.

Q3. What are the most common small vessel diseases causing ICH?

These so called primary and spontaneous ICH are not truly primary but represent the consequences of underling conditions. Two most common vascular pathologies leading to majority of ICH are arteriosclerosis (lipohyalinosis) and cerebral amyloid angiopathy (CAA).

Arteriosclerosis is detected as concentric hyalinized vascular wall thickening which mainly affects penetrating arterioles of basal ganglia, thalamus, deep cerebellar nuclei, and brainstem.[1] Lipohyalinosis is strongly associated with hypertension and also associated with diabetes, with advanced age.

In CAA, there is deposition of beta-amyloid protein in arterioles and capillaries of cerebral cortex and cerebellar hemispheres (lobar territories).[3] Primary risk factors of CAA are age and apolipoprotein E2 and E4 alleles. CAA is characterized by small and often asymptomatic cerebral microbleeds in T2-weighted magnetic resonance imaging (MRI), multiple strictly lobar ICHs, and cortical superficial siderosis.

Q4. How can we establish the diagnosis of ICH?

Clinical features such as rapid-onset neurological dysfunction and signs and symptoms of raised intracranial pressure (ICP) like headache, vomiting, and altered sensorium suggest the diagnosis of ICH, but this can also occur in ischemic stroke. Clinical features of ICH are as per area involved by hemorrhage; these make diagnosis of ICH solely based on history and clinical examination untrustworthy.

Noncontrast computed tomography brain (being the gold standard) can help achieve at rapid diagnosis of ICH with hematoma volume (as per ABC/2 method[4]), surrounding edema, intraventricular extension. Hyperacute blood on CT brain will appear as hyperdense except in rare case of some anemia where it appears isodense.

Conditions can mimic ICH on NCCT brain as blood and calcium both appear white on CT scan. The following may be mistaken for hemorrhage:

- Basal calcification (Fahr's disease, hyperparathyroidism)
- Calcified choroid plexus
- Calcified tumors (e.g., oligodendrocytoma).

Neuroimaging in ICH[5,6]
- CT brain and MRI brain (echo planar gradient echo or susceptibility weighted sequences) are equally effective for diagnosing or ruling out acute ICH. MRI is slightly more sensitive than CT for detecting small intraventricular hemorrhage (IVH) and more accurate for detecting chronic ICH.[7]
- Serial CT brain after initial scan is useful to evaluate for development of hematoma expansion (HE), hydrocephalus, or perihematomal edema, particularly in patients whose neurological status deteriorates and in those with impaired level of consciousness in whom examination is limited.[8]
- HE usually occurs within 24 hours and it is extremely rare after 24 hours of development of ICH. HE is associated with poor outcome and mortality. Follow-up CT scan done at 6 hours and 24 hours of onset are usually adequate to exclude HE and document final ICH volume. CT scan signs suggestive of HE are hypodensities, fluid level, swirl, black hole, blend, island, or satellite signs in NCCT,[9] while spot sign in CT angiography (CTA).[10]
- In patients with (1) lobar spontaneous ICH and age <70 years, (2) deep/posterior fossa ICH and age <45 years, or (3) deep/posterior fossa and age 45–70 years without history of hypertension → acute CTA plus consideration of venography is recommended to exclude macrovascular causes or cerebral venous thrombosis → if CTA ± venography and MRI/MRA (magnetic resonance angiography) are negative then catheter intra-arterial digital subtraction angiography (DSA) is reasonable to exclude a macrovascular cause.[11,12]
- In patients with spontaneous ICH with a negative CTA/venography → MRI and MRA to establish a nonmacrovascular cause of ICH (such as CAA, deep perforating vasculopathy, cavernous malformation, or malignancy) → if CTA or MRA suggestive of a macrovascular cause, catheter intra-arterial DSA should be performed as soon as possible to confirm and manage underlying intracranial vascular malformations.[12]

Q5. Describe in brief the initial steps to manage this patient.

If a patient is deteriorating rapidly, optimization of his airway, breathing, and circulation should be done and a battery of investigations including hematological, biochemical, electrocardiogram (ECG), coagulation profile, and chest radiograph[13] need to be performed.

Optimization of airway, breathing, and circulation
Patient with depressed level of consciousness and GCS of <8 or a patient with brainstem stroke who is at risk of aspiration, endotracheal intubation to protect airway should be performed using rapid sequence intubation. During intubation, short-acting agents such as intravenous (IV) fentanyl (2-3 µg/kg) or IV lidocaine (1-1.5 mg/kg) can be given to block the increase in ICP from tracheal stimulation due to laryngoscopy and intubation.

Acute BP control
Patients with acute spontaneous ICH usually present with hypertension, which if uncontrolled can lead to HE and so it should be carefully managed to ensure continuous smooth and sustained control of BP, avoiding peaks, and large variability in systolic blood pressure (SBP).[14] Several studies have shown that high variation in SBP during acute phase of ICH is associated with worse outcome and so sustained control of BP is recommended.

In patients with *mild to moderately severe ICH (GCS score ≥5, excluding massive ICH) who present with SBP between 150 and 220 mm Hg*, acute lowering of BP to target 140 mm Hg (range of 130-150 mm Hg) improves functional outcome. This acute lowering of BP should be initiated within 2 hours of ICH onset and target BP should be achieved within 1 hour to reduce risk of HE and to improve functional outcomes.[15]

In patients who present with *large ICH (>30 mL) requiring ICP monitoring or severe IVH requiring external ventricular drainage (EVD)*, early intensive BP lowering (EIBPL) is not associated with improved outcome, so such patients should be managed with individualized approach to maintain cerebral perfusion pressure (CPP) of 60 to ≥70 mm Hg.[16]

These recommendations are based on data from the two largest trials [INTERACT2 (Intensive Blood Pressure Reduction in Acute Cerebral Hemorrhage Trial 2)[17] and ATACH-2 (Antihypertensive Treatment of Acute Cerebral Hemorrhage 2)][16] for EIBPL after ICH.

Intravenous calcium channel blockers (e.g., nicardipine) and β-blockers (i.e., labetalol) are the drugs of choice for early BP reduction, given their short half-life and ease of titration. Nitrates should be avoided given their potential for cerebral vasodilation and elevated ICP. Thiazides have potential to cause hyponatremia and worsen cerebral edema. Oral antihypertensive agents should be started as soon as possible.

Q6. How to prevent further neurological deterioration in patient with ICH?

Admission to ICU or similar settings is beneficial in first 24 hours during which time the risk of neurological deterioration is highest. Use of invasive arterial BP and central venous pressure invasive modalities should be individualized on case-to-case basis.

ICP monitoring
Use of ICP monitoring is not well defined but when used in patients with moderate-to-severe ICH/IVH with reduced levels of consciousness (those with GCS scores of 9-12) or patients with GCS score ≤8, it reduces mortality and improves outcomes.[18] In patients with spontaneous ICH/IVH with hydrocephalus, EVD placement is a lifesaving procedure that can help reduce ICP rapidly.[19] Guidelines suggest maintenance of an *ICP <22 mm Hg and a CPP of 50-70 mm Hg*, depending on capacity for cerebral autoregulation.[5]

Osmotherapy
Prophylactic use of osmotherapy is not recommended.[19] Comparison of hypertonic saline with mannitol in equiosmolar dose for osmotherapy, hypertonic saline is more effective as per 2011 meta-analysis of RCTs over wide range of neuropathologies.[20]

Hyperosmolar therapy is usually administered in bolus doses in 4-6 hours intervals.[5]

Simultaneously, other basic treatment measures to reduce ICP should be continued such as neutral-midline neck position, bed-head elevation to 30°, mild sedation, and avoidance of hypotonic fluids for maintenance. For treatment of transiently raised ICP—osmotherapy can be combined with transient hyperventilation.

Antiseizure treatment
In patients with ICH, antiseizure treatment should only be administered if there is clinically evident seizure or impaired consciousness with electrographically confirmed seizure (nonconvulsive status epilepticus).[21] Patients with impaired or fluctuating consciousness, with primary diagnosis of ICH, warrant use of continuous electroencephalogram (EEG) monitoring for 24 hours.[22]

There is no role of prophylactic antiseizure treatment in patients with ICH as per current guidelines.[23]

Routine care in patients with ICH:
- *Temperature management:* Fever in patients with ICH is associated with worse prognosis, and treating fever improves functional outcomes.[24] Therapeutic hypothermia, though physiologically sounds reasonable since it is likely to reduce perihematomal edema, has not been demonstrated to be clinically beneficial.[25]
- *Glucose management:* Admission hyperglycemia is a potent predictor of 30 days mortality in both diabetic and not diabetic patients with ICH. Episodes of hypoglycemia are also associated with increased mortality and worse neurological outcomes. It is recommended to treat hypoglycemia (40-60 mg/dL) and keep the sugar levels between 180 and 200 mg/dL to improve functional outcomes.[5,26]

- *Thromboprophylaxis:* In nonambulatory patients with ICH, it is recommended to use intermittent pneumatic compression devices (IPCDs) on the day of diagnosis, while graduated compression stockings are not useful for venous thromboembolism (VTE) prophylaxis.[27,28] There is insufficient evidence to use low-molecular-weight heparin (LMWH)/unfractionated heparin (UFH) prophylaxis in first 48 hours after ICH onset due to complication of HE. It is reasonable to use low-dose UFH/LMWH prophylaxis after 48 hours of ICH onset after documentation of hematoma stabilization on repeat scan.[29]
- *Nutrition:* As for all critically ill neurological patients, enteral feeding should be started early (<48 hours) to avoid protein catabolism and malnutrition.
- *Stress ulcer prophylaxis:* Patients with acute ICH are at increased risk of aspiration pneumonia, hospital-acquired pneumonia, *Clostridium difficile* infection and so use of routine stress ulcer prophylaxis is not suggested. It should be used in high-risk patients who are on mechanical ventilation or with history of recent gastrointestinal (GI) bleed.

Case continued: The patient was on aspirin.

Q7. What is the role of platelet transfusion in this patient? If the patient is on anticoagulation, how should it be reversed?

Prophylactic platelet transfusion should only be used in case where emergency neurosurgery is required, as it has been associated with reduced postoperative rate and volume of hemorrhage.[30] One unit of single donor platelets (SDP) can be given before surgery.

The PATCH trial has shown increased odds of death or dependence at 3 months in patients who received prophylactic platelet transfusion who were receiving antiplatelet therapy before development of ICH, so prophylactic transfusion of platelet should be avoided.[31] Effect of ticagrelor is not reversed by platelet transfusion.[32] Role of desmopressin in antiplatelet-related hemorrhage is uncertain, while role of recombinant factor VIIa in spontaneous ICH is also unclear.[33,34]

Tranexamic acid: The TICH-2 (Tranexamic Acid for Hyperacute Primary Intracerebral Haemorrhage) trial suggested that administration of tranexamic acid led to modest reduction in HE and early death (within 7 days), but no significant effect on functional status at 90 days.[35]

Anticoagulation-related hemorrhage
Patients who develop ICH on anticoagulation therapy are at higher risk of HE, rapid neurological deterioration, and poorer outcomes. Immediate discontinuation and *emergency reversal of anticoagulation* is required for management of these patients.[36]

Flowchart 1 shows the approach to guide management of such patients as per 2022 American Heart Association (AHA)/ASA guidelines for management of ICH.[5]

Q8. What is the role of surgical therapy in a patient with ICH?

The role of surgery in a patient with acute ICH differs with the site of bleed.

Cerebrospinal fluid (CSF) drainage for obstructive hydrocephalus

Obstructive hydrocephalus can occur with ICH occurring in:
- Thalamic ICH with third ventricular compression
- Cerebellar hemorrhage with fourth ventricular compression
- ICH with intraventricular extension.

Ventricular drainage with EVD is recommended to reduce ICP in patients with spontaneous ICH with hydrocephalus and decreased level of consciousness.[5]

Craniotomy for posterior fossa hemorrhage
Spontaneous cerebellar hemorrhage is frequently associated with hydrocephalus, brainstem compression, and herniation in the confined space of the posterior fossa and so despite lack of randomized evidence, hematoma evacuation is recommended.

Patients with cerebellar ICH who are deteriorating neurologically, have brainstem compression and/or hydrocephalus from ventricular obstruction, or have cerebellar ICH volume ≥15 mL should undergo *urgent surgical hematoma evacuation* with or without EVD as recommended compared with conservative management to reduce mortality.[37]

Surgical management in supratentorial hemorrhage
Surgical hematoma evacuation for supratentorial ICH is controversial as potential benefits of hematoma evacuation may be offset by surgical morbidity.

For patients with supratentorial ICH of >20- to 30-mL volume with GCS scores in the moderate range (5–12),
- Minimally invasive hematoma evacuation with endoscopic or stereotactic aspiration with or without thrombolytic use can be useful to reduce mortality, however current data suggests that the functional outcomes are not improved.[38]
- Optimal time to surgical treatment with minimally invasive surgery (MIS) is controversial, observational data suggest that early MIS (<12 or 24 hours) may reduce secondary brain injury and improve outcomes with no effect on bleeding risk.[5]

Flowchart 1: Approach for management of patient with anticoagulation-related intracerebral hemorrhage (ICH) (2022 American Stroke Association (ASA)/American Heart Association (AHA) guidelines for management of patients with spontaneous ICH).[5]

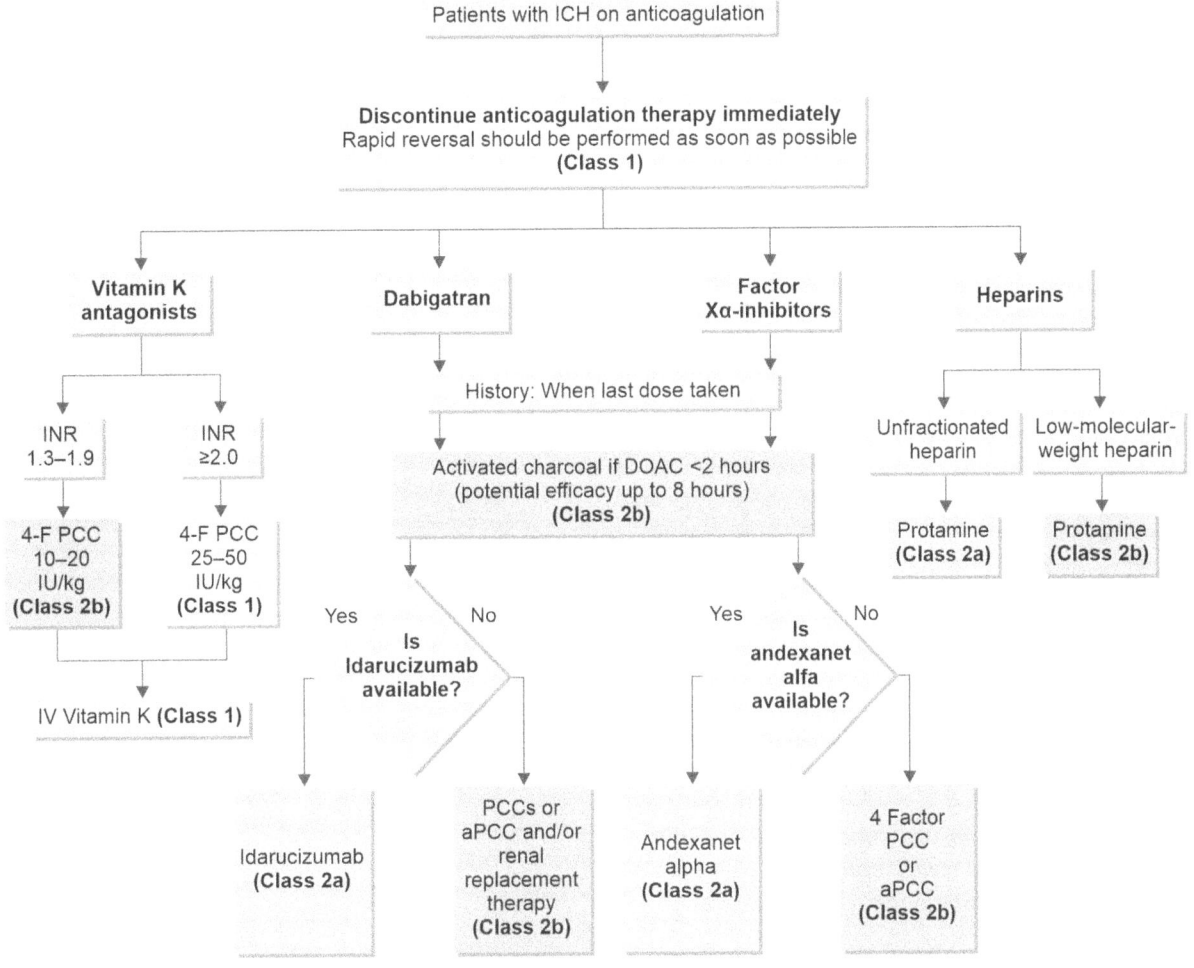

(aPCC: activated prothrombin complex concentrate; DOAC: direct oral anticoagulant; INR: international normalized ratio; IV: intravenous; PCCs: prothrombin complex concentrates)

Minimally Invasive Surgery with Thrombolysis in Intracerebral hemorrhage Evacuation (MISTIE) phase 3 trial enrolled patients with supratentorial ICH and randomized them to stereotaxic placement of a catheter in the hematoma and instillation of tissue plasminogen activator (tPA) for up to 72 hours or medical management.[39] Results suggested lower mortality in surgical group.

The STICH 1 (Surgical Trial in Intracerebral Haemorrhage 1) trial showed increasing likelihood of achieving a good outcome among patients assigned to early surgery (median time to surgery 30 hours after hemorrhage onset) who had craniotomy as opposed to alternate techniques, and in those with hematoma located 1 cm or less from the cortical surface.[40]

The STICH 2 trial enrolled conscious patients with superficial lobar ICH of 10-100 mL and no IVH within 48 hours, and showed trend toward better survival in surgical group.[41]

Patients with supratentorial ICH who are in a coma have large hematomas with significant midline shift or have elevated ICP refractory to medical management; decompressive craniectomy with or without hematoma evacuation may be considered to reduce mortality, however its impact on improving functional outcome is uncertain.[5]

Surgical management of IVH
Approximately 30-50% patients with ICH have intraventricular extension of hemorrhage, which is associated with worse prognosis as it predisposes to development of hydrocephalus and blood breakdown products that promote inflammatory meningitis.

External ventricular drainage (EVD) insertion can be used to treat raised ICP as well as to drain blood products which will improve survival. The addition of thrombolytic irrigation with alteplase or urokinase hastens intraventricular clot removal and results in further mortality reduction.[5]

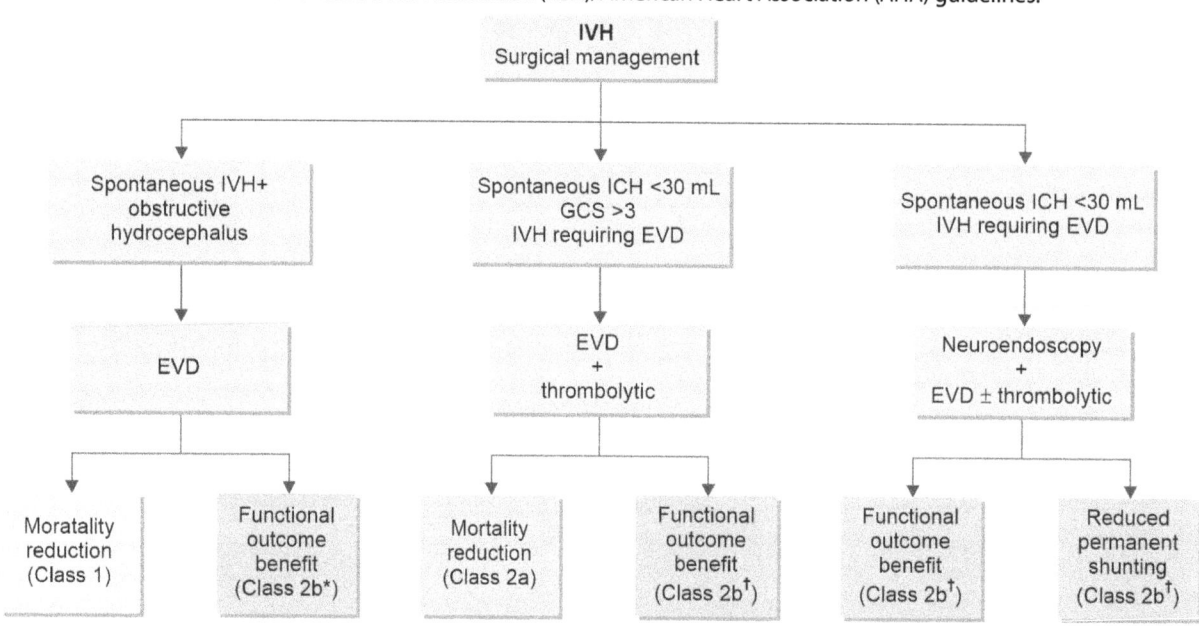

Flowchart 2: Management of intraventricular hemorrhage (IVH) based on recommendations from 2022 American Stroke Association (ASA)/American Heart Association (AHA) guidelines.[5]

*Not well established. †Uncertain.
(EVD: external ventricular drainage; GCS: Glasgow Coma Scale; ICH: intracerebral hemorrhage)

The CLEAR III trial[42] (Clot Lysis: Evaluating Accelerated Resolution of Intraventricular Hemorrhage), which randomized patients with IVH and compared treatment with 1 mg alteplase (tPA) or placebo injected through an EVD every 8 hours, showed lower mortality in patients who received intraventricular thrombolysis **(Flowchart 2)**.

Q9. How do you prognosticate the outcomes of patients with ICH?

Multiple clinical scores have been developed to know risk of 30-day mortality or likelihood of good functional recovery.

Intracerebral hemorrhage (ICH) score **(Table 1)**:[41]
- Six-point clinical and radiographic grading scale
- Predicts 30-day mortality after ICH

30-day mortality rates linearly with increased with ICH score:
- ICH score 1 = 13% mortality
- ICH score 2 = 26% mortality
- ICH score 3 = 72% mortality
- ICH score 4 = 97% mortality
- ICH score 5 = 100% mortality

FUNC (Functional Outcome in Patients with Primary Intracerebral Hemorrhage) score

It is a functional outcome risk stratification scale, which rates prognosis for good functional outcome at 90 days. It has 11 components which consist of age, ICH volume and location, GCS score, history of prior cognitive impairment.

TABLE 1: Intracerebral hemorrhage (ICH) score.

Component	ICH score points
Glasgow Coma Scale (GCS) at presentation	
3–4	2
5–12	1
13–15	0
ICH volume on initial imaging	
>30 cm³	1
<30 cm³	0
Intraventricular extension of ICH	
Present	1
Absent	0
Infratentorial origin of ICH	
Yes	1
No	0
Age	
>80 years	1
<80 years	0
Total	0–6

Q10. How will you prevent recurrent ICH or how do you reduce the risk if recurrent ICH?

Patients with ICH are at increased risk of recurrent hemorrhage, with risk ranging from 1.2 to 3% per year, with the highest event rate in the first year after the first hemorrhage.[43]

Risk factors for recurrent ICH are as follows:
- Lobar location of the initial ICH
- Older age
- Presence, number, and lobar location of microbleeds on MRI
- Presence of disseminated cortical superficial siderosis on MRI
- Poorly controlled hypertension
- Asian or Black race
- Presence of apolipoprotein E ε2 or ε4 alleles
- Control of hypertension is recommended for prevention of recurrent of spontaneous ICH. It is preferred to maintain SBP <130 mm Hg and diastolic blood pressure (DBP) <80 mm Hg in these patients.[5,44]

REFERENCES

1. Garcia JH, Ho KL. Pathology of hypertensive arteriopathy. Neurosurg Clin N Am. 1992;3(3):497-507.
2. Meretoja A, Strbian D, Putaala J, Curtze S, Haapaniemi E, Mustanoja S, et al. SMASH-U: a proposal for etiologic classification of intracerebral hemorrhage. Stroke. 2012;43(10):2592-7.
3. Weber SA, Patel RK, Lutsep HL. Cerebral amyloid angiopathy: diagnosis and potential therapies. Expert Rev Neurother. 2018;18(6):503-13.
4. Kothari RU, Brott T, Broderick JP, Barsan WG, Sauerbeck LR, Zuccarello M, et al. The ABCs of measuring intracerebral hemorrhage volumes. Stroke. 1996;27:1304-5.
5. Greenberg SM, Ziai WC, Cordonnier C, Dowlatshahi D, Francis B, Goldstein JN, et al; American Heart Association/American Stroke Association. 2022 Guideline for the Management of Patients With Spontaneous Intracerebral Hemorrhage: A Guideline From the American Heart Association/American Stroke Association. Stroke. 2022;53(7):e282-e361.
6. Romanova AL, Nemeth AJ, Berman MD, Guth JC, Liotta EM, Naidech AM, et al. Magnetic resonance imaging versus computed tomography for identification and quantification of intraventricular hemorrhage. J Stroke Cerebrovasc Dis. 2014;23:2036-40.
7. Linfante I, Llinas RH, Caplan LR, Warach S. MRI features of intracerebral hemorrhage within 2 hours from symptom onset. Stroke. 1999;30:2263-7.
8. Kazui S, Naritomi H, Yamamoto H, Sawada T, Yamaguchi T. Enlargement of spontaneous intracerebral hemorrhage: incidence and time course. Stroke. 1996;27:1783-7.
9. Morotti A, Boulouis G, Dowlatshahi D, Li Q, Barras CD, Delcourt C, et al; International NCCT ICH Study Group. Standards for detecting, interpreting, and reporting noncontrast computed tomography markers of intracerebral hemorrhage expansion. Ann Neurol. 2019;86:480-92.
10. Dowlatshahi D, Brouwers HB, Demchuk AM, Hill MD, Aviv RI, Ufholz LA, et al. Predicting intracerebral hemorrhage growth with the spot sign: the effect of onset-to-scan time. Stroke. 2016;47:695-700.
11. Hilkens NA, van Asch CJJ, Werring DJ, Wilson D, Rinkel GJE, Algra A, et al; DIAGRAM Study Group. Predicting the presence of macrovascular causes in non-traumatic intracerebral haemorrhage: the DIAGRAM prediction score. J Neurol Neurosurg Psychiatry. 2018;89:674-9.
12. van Asch CJ, Velthuis BK, Rinkel GJ, Algra A, de Kort GA, Witkamp TD, et al; DIAGRAM Investigators. Diagnostic yield and accuracy of CT angiography, MR angiography, and digital subtraction angiography for detection of macrovascular causes of intracerebral haemorrhage: prospective, multicentre cohort study. BMJ. 2015;351:h5762.
13. Al-Shahi Salman R, Labovitz DL, Stapf C. Spontaneous intracerebral haemorrhage. BMJ. 2009;339:b2586.
14. Moullaali TJ, Wang X, Martin RH, Shipes VB, Robinson TG, Chalmers J, et al. Blood pressure control and clinical outcomes in acute intracerebral haemorrhage: a preplanned pooled analysis of individual participant data. Lancet Neurol. 2019;18:857-64.
15. Li Q, Warren AD, Qureshi AI, Morotti A, Falcone GJ, Sheth KN, et al. Ultra-early blood pressure reduction attenuates hematoma growth and improves outcome in intracerebral hemorrhage. Ann Neurol. 2020;88:388-95.
16. Qureshi AI, Foster LD, Lobanova I, Huang W, Suarez JI. Intensive blood pressure lowering in patients with moderate to severe grade acute cerebral hemorrhage: post hoc analysis of Antihypertensive Treatment of Acute Cerebral Hemorrhage (ATACH)-2 Trial. Cerebrovasc Dis. 2020;49(3):244-52.
17. Arima H, Heeley E, Delcourt C, Hirakawa Y, Wang X, Woodward M, et al; INTERACT2 Investigators. Optimal achieved blood pressure in acute intracerebral hemorrhage: INTERACT2. Neurology. 2015;84:464-71.
18. Chen CJ, Ding D, Ironside N, Buell TJ, Southerland AM, Testai FD, et al; ERICH Investigators. Intracranial pressure monitoring in patients with spontaneous intracerebral hemorrhage. J Neurosurg. 2019;132:1854-64.
19. Sun S, Li Y, Zhang H, Wang X, She L, Yan Z, et al. The effect of mannitol in the early stage of supratentorial hypertensive intracerebral hemorrhage: a systematic review and meta-analysis. World Neurosurg. 2019;124:386-96.
20. Kamel H, Navi BB, Nakagawa K, Hemphill JC 3rd, Ko NU. Hypertonic saline versus mannitol for the treatment of elevated intracranial pressure: a meta-analysis of randomized clinical trials. Crit Care Med. 2011;39:554-9.
21. Mehta A, Zusman BE, Shutter LA, Choxi R, Yassin A, Antony A, et al. The prevalence and impact of status epilepticus secondary to intracerebral hemorrhage: results from the US Nationwide Inpatient Sample. Neurocrit Care. 2018;28:353-61.
22. Claassen J, Jetté N, Chum F, Green R, Schmidt M, Choi H, et al. Electrographic seizures and periodic discharges after intracerebral hemorrhage. Neurology. 2007;69:1356-65.
23. Angriman F, Tirupakuzhi Vijayaraghavan BK, Dragoi L, Lopez Soto C, Chapman M, Scales DC. Antiepileptic drugs to prevent seizures after spontaneous intracerebral hemorrhage. Stroke. 2019;50:1095-9.
24. Hervella P, Rodríguez-Yáñez M, Pumar JM, Ávila-Gómez P, da Silva-Candal A, López-Loureiro I, et al. Antihyperthermic

treatment decreases perihematomal hypodensity. Neurology. 2020;94:e1738-48.
25. Kollmar R, Staykov D, Dörfler A, Schellinger PD, Schwab S, Bardutzky J. Hypothermia reduces perihemorrhagic edema after intracerebral hemorrhage. Stroke. 2010;41:1684-9.
26. NICE-SUGAR Study Investigators; Finfer S, Chittock DR, Su SY, Blair D, Foster D, Dhingra V, et al. Intensive versus conventional glucose control in critically ill patients. N Engl J Med. 2009;360:1283-97.
27. CLOTS (Clots in Legs Or sTockings after Stroke) Trials Collaboration; Dennis M, Sandercock P, Reid J, Graham C, Forbes J, Murray G. Effectiveness of intermittent pneumatic compression in reduction of risk of deep vein thrombosis in patients who have had a stroke (CLOTS 3): a multicentre randomised controlled trial. Lancet. 2013;382:516-24.
28. Yogendrakumar V, Lun R, Khan F, Salottolo K, Lacut K, Graham C, et al. Venous thromboembolism prevention in intracerebral hemorrhage: a systematic review and network meta-analysis. PLoS One. 2020;15:e0234957.
29. Pan X, Li J, Xu L, Deng S, Wang Z. Safety of prophylactic heparin in the prevention of venous thromboembolism after spontaneous intracerebral hemorrhage: a meta-analysis. J Neurol Surg A Cent Eur Neurosurg. 2020;81:253-60.
30. Li X, Sun Z, Zhao W, Zhang J, Chen J, Li Y, et al. Effect of acetylsalicylic acid usage and platelet transfusion on postoperative hemorrhage and activities of daily living in patients with acute intracerebral hemorrhage. J Neurosurg. 2013;118:94-103.
31. Baharoglu MI, Cordonnier C, Al-Shahi Salman R, de Gans K, Koopman MM, Brand A, et al; PATCH Investigators. Platelet transfusion versus standard care after acute stroke due to spontaneous cerebral haemorrhage associated with antiplatelet therapy (PATCH): a randomised, open-label, phase 3 trial. Lancet. 2016;387:2605-13.
32. Kaufman RM, Djulbegovic B, Gernsheimer T, Kleinman S, Tinmouth AT, Capocelli KE, et al; AABB. Platelet transfusion: a clinical practice guideline from the AABB. Ann Intern Med. 2015;162:205-13.
33. Mengel A, Stefanou MI, Hadaschik KA, Wolf M, Stadler V, Poli K, et al. Early administration of desmopressin and platelet transfusion for reducing hematoma expansion in patients with acute antiplatelet therapy associated intracerebral hemorrhage. Crit Care Med. 2020;48:1009-17.
34. Mayer SA, Brun NC, Begtrup K, Broderick J, Davis S, Diringer MN, et al; FAST Trial Investigators. Efficacy and safety of recombinant activated factor VII for acute intracerebral hemorrhage. N Engl J Med. 2008;358:2127-37.
35. Sprigg N, Flaherty K, Appleton JP, Al-Shahi Salman R, Bereczki D, Beridze M, et al; TICH-2 Investigators. Tranexamic acid for hyperacute primary IntraCerebral Haemorrhage (TICH-2): an international randomised, placebo-controlled, phase 3 superiority trial. Lancet. 2018;391:2107-15.
36. Hanger HC, Geddes JA, Wilkinson TJ, Lee M, Baker AE. Warfarin-related intracerebral haemorrhage: better outcomes when reversal includes prothrombin complex concentrates. Intern Med J. 2013;43:308-16.
37. Singh SD, Brouwers HB, Senff JR, Pasi M, Goldstein J, Viswanathan A, et al. Haematoma evacuation in cerebellar intracerebral haemorrhage: systematic review. J Neurol Neurosurg Psychiatry. 2020;91:82-7.
38. Akhigbe T, Okafor U, Sattar T, Rawluk D, Fahey T. Stereotactic-guided evacuation of spontaneous supratentorial intracerebral hemorrhage: systematic review and meta-analysis. World Neurosurg. 2015;84:451-60.
39. Hanley DF, Thompson RE, Rosenblum M, Yenokyan G, Lane K, McBee N, et al; MISTIE III Investigators. Efficacy and safety of minimally invasive surgery with thrombolysis in intracerebral haemorrhage evacuation (MISTIE III): a randomised, controlled, open-label, blinded endpoint phase 3 trial. Lancet. 2019;393:1021-32.
40. Mendelow AD, Gregson BA, Fernandes HM, Murray GD, Teasdale GM, Hope DT, et al; STICH Investigators. Early surgery versus initial conservative treatment in patients with spontaneous supratentorial intracerebral haematomas in the international Surgical Trial in Intracerebral Haemorrhage (STICH): a randomised trial. Lancet. 2005;365:387-97.
41. Gregório T, Pipa S, Cavaleiro P, Atanásio G, Albuquerque I, Castro Chaves P, et al. Original intracerebral hemorrhage score for the prediction of short-term mortality in cerebral hemorrhage: systematic review and meta-analysis. Crit Care Med. 2019;47:857-64.
42. Hanley DF, Lane K, McBee N, Ziai W, Tuhrim S, Lees KR, et al; CLEAR III Investigators. Thrombolytic removal of intraventricular haemorrhage in treatment of severe stroke: results of the randomised, multicentre, multiregion, placebo-controlled CLEAR III trial. Lancet. 2017;389:603-11.
43. Azarpazhooh MR, Nicol MB, Donnan GA, Dewey HM, Sturm JW, Macdonell RA, et al. Patterns of stroke recurrence according to subtype of first stroke event: the North East Melbourne Stroke Incidence Study (NEMESIS). Int J Stroke. 2008;3:158-64.
44. Hilkens NA, Greving JP, Algra A, Klijn CJ. Blood pressure levels and the risk of intracerebral hemorrhage after ischemic stroke. Neurology. 2017;88:177-81.

CHAPTER 15

Meningoencephalitis and Status Epilepticus

Kushal Rajeev Kalvit, Atul Prabhakar Kulkarni

CASE STUDY

A 36-year-old male is brought to the casualty with complaints of fever and altered sensorium of 2 days' duration. In the casualty, he is disoriented and restless. He is febrile (101°C), tachycardic [heart rate (HR)—120 beats/min, regular], tachypneic [respiratory rate (RR)—26 beats/min], and normotensive [blood pressure (BP)—130/86 mm Hg], and his Glasgow Coma Scale (GCS) is 11 (E3M5V3). His systemic examination is unremarkable except for nuchal rigidity.

Q1. What are the main principles of management in a patient presenting with fever and altered sensorium?

Assessment of airway, breathing, and circulation (ABC) is the first priority in any patient who presents with altered sensorium. Endotracheal intubation is warranted for airway protection in case the patient has lower cranial nerve palsy, recurrent seizures, vomiting, or if GCS is <8 or is higher but rapidly falling. If the patient has signs of raised intracranial pressure (ICP), measures to lower ICP should be instituted immediately. This patient has a GCS of 11 and is breathing at 26 breaths/min and he will probably not need intubation immediately. He has tachycardia but his BP is 130/86 mm Hg. His hemodynamics are not a cause of concern for now. He also does not have any signs to suggest critically elevated ICP or impending brain herniation. The patient will need to undergo investigations to determine the cause of his fever and altered sensorium. The patient is suffering from a potentially life-threatening condition; therefore, immediate empiric treatment must begin even before a definite diagnosis is made.

Q2. What are the differential diagnoses?

In this young patient, with a relatively short history of fever, altered sensorium, and neck stiffness, bacterial meningitis is the most likely cause. The differential diagnoses are as follows:[1]

- Bacterial meningitis (pneumococcal, meningococcal, *Listeria*, *Legionella*, *Mycoplasma*, Lyme disease)
- Rickettsial meningitis
- Tuberculous (TB) meningitis
- Fungal (cryptococcal) meningitis
- Parasitic meningitis (malaria, toxoplasmosis, schistosomiasis)
- Other causes of meningitis—carcinomatous meningitis, lymphomatous meningitis, vasculitis
- Acute viral encephalitis (neck stiffness usually absent)—herpes simplex virus type 1 (HSV1), herpes simplex virus type 2 (HSV2), varicella-zoster virus (VZV), cytomegalovirus (CMV), Epstein–Barr virus (EBV), adenovirus, measles, mumps, rubella, arboviruses, enterovirus, rabies, human immunodeficiency virus (HIV)
- Autoimmune encephalitis, paraneoplastic encephalitis
- Acute disseminated encephalomyelitis (ADEM)
- Brain abscess, subdural/epidural empyema
- Sepsis-associated encephalopathy (SAE)
- Drug toxicity (cocaine, amphetamine, ecstasy, salicylate, thyroxine, anticholinergics, serotonin syndrome)
- Noninfectious hyperthermic syndromes (neuroleptic malignant syndrome, malignant hyperthermia, heat stroke).

Q3. Discuss the epidemiology of meningoencephalitis.

A recent systemic review and meta-analysis revealed that the incidence of bacterial meningitis varies widely depending on the country. The mortality ranges from 17 to 40% and depends on the causative organism and country income status. Overall, global meningitis-related mortality has reduced by 21% in the last 25 years. Meningococcus is no longer the most common causative bacteria for meningitis mortality owing to the increased vaccination against meningococcus (A, C, W135, and Y). *Streptococcus pneumoniae*, meningococcus serogroup B, and *Haemophilus influenzae* type b are the most common organisms implicated in bacterial meningitis currently. The recent multinational EURECA study evaluated 589 patients admitted to the intensive care unit (ICU) with a clinical diagnosis of meningoencephalitis. They found that 42% had bacterial meningitis, 23% had infective meningoencephalitis of viral/fungal/parasitic etiology, 6% had autoimmune encephalitis, 2% had neoplastic/toxic encephalitis, and 26% had encephalitis of unknown origin.[2,3]

Q4. How will you investigate this case?
Although specific tests would be required to pinpoint the diagnosis from the extensive list of differentials, any patient with febrile encephalopathy will need the following basic set of investigations:
- Complete blood count (CBC) and differential blood count with peripheral blood smear examination
- Biochemical tests—glucose, blood urea nitrogen (BUN), creatinine, liver function test (LFT), electrolyte panel, arterial blood gas (ABG)
- Blood culture
- Lumbar puncture (LP) for cerebrospinal fluid (CSF) analysis
- Neuroimaging [computed tomography (CT) or magnetic resonance imaging (MRI) brain] to demonstrate meningeal enhancement
- Chest X-ray.

Q5. Is it mandatory to obtain a CT scan of the head prior to LP?
In patients with a raised ICP or space-occupying lesions, a lumbar tap with CSF sampling (which causes a craniocaudal pressure gradient) can cause brain herniation. It is, therefore, important to identify patients who are at risk of this complication prior to performing an LP.

A CT scan of the head prior to lumbar tap is necessary in patients with:
- New-onset seizures
- Immunocompromised condition
- Focal neurologic deficits (excluding cranial nerve palsies)
- Moderate-to-severe impairment of consciousness (GCS < 10)

If none of these factors is present, a CT scan before LP is not needed.

Q6. What empiric treatment would you give to this patient?
In patients with suspected bacterial meningitis, antibiotics need to be administered as soon as possible (preferably within 1 hour), after collection of blood culture; however, antibiotic administration should not be delayed for performing LP. This, of course, may lead to negative CSF cultures if antibiotics are administered before LP, but outcomes are clearly better if antibiotics are given quickly. The empiric antibiotic of choice in this patient would be ceftriaxone and vancomycin. If viral encephalitis is suspected, intravenous (IV) acyclovir must also be administered empirically.

Q7. Why have these antibiotics been chosen?
The most common organisms causing community-acquired bacterial meningitis are pneumococcus, meningococcus, and *H. influenzae*. Ceftriaxone has good CSF penetration and is effective against these organisms. Until recently, penicillin-resistant pneumococcal infections were almost unknown in India. There have, however, been recent reports of increasing resistance in pneumococci. Third-generation cephalosporins (ceftriaxone or cefotaxime), therefore, need to be added to cover penicillin-resistant pneumococci and meningococci till sensitivity reports become available. Vancomycin is used to cover cephalosporin-resistant pneumococci.

Q8. How are antibiotics tailored as per the organism and susceptibility testing?

• Penicillin-sensitive pneumococcus • Penicillin-sensitive meningococcus • Beta-lactamase *H. influenzae* • *Listeria monocytogenes*	Ampicillin/amoxicillin
• Penicillin-resistant pneumococcus • Penicillin-resistant meningococcus • Beta-lactamase positive *H. influenzae*	Ceftriaxone/cefotaxime
Cephalosporin-resistant pneumococcus	Vancomycin + ceftriaxone OR vancomycin + rifampicin OR rifampicin + ceftriaxone
Beta-lactamase negative ampicillin-resistant *H. influenzae*	Ceftriaxone/cefotaxime + meropenem
• Methicillin-sensitive *Staphylococcus aureus* (MSSA) • Methicillin-resistant *S. aureus* (MRSA) • Vancomycin-resistant *S. aureus* (VRSA)	• Flucloxacillin/nafcillin/oxacillin • Vancomycin • Linezolid

Q9. What are the special considerations in empirical antibiotic therapy?

Allergy to penicillin/ampicillin/amoxicillin	Administer chloramphenicol (except for *Listeria*)
Allergy to cephalosporins	Administer fluoroquinolones (moxifloxacin/ciprofloxacin)
Allergy to penicillin/ampicillin/amoxicillin for *Listeria* infection	Trimethoprim-sulfamethoxazole OR meropenem
Indications for empirical *Listeria* coverage	Age >50 years OR Age <50 years with cancer/immunosuppression/diabetes
Empirical meropenem therapy	Covers penicillin-resistant pneumococcus, penicillin-resistant meningococcus, penicillin-resistant *H. influenzae*, and *Listeria*

Q10. What is the minimum duration of antibiotic therapy?

Meningococcus	7 days
H. influenzae	7–10 days
Pneumococcus	7–14 days
S. aureus	At least 14 days
Culture-negative	At least 14 days
Listeria	At least 21 days

Q11. What is the role of steroids in patients with suspected meningitis?

In a Cochrane meta-analysis, steroids have been shown to decrease the incidence of overall hearing loss and neurologic sequelae. However, mortality reduction was observed only in a subgroup of patients with pneumococcal meningitis. Steroids should ideally be administered just before or along with the first dose of antibiotics and should be continued for 4 days. In case the antibiotic has been already administered, steroids can be given up to 4 hours after the initiation of antibiotic therapy (based on expert consensus). The recommended dose in children is 0.15 mg/kg of dexamethasone 6 hourly and in adults, it is 10 mg 6 hourly. Steroid therapy should be stopped if the etiological agent is other than pneumococcus or *H. influenzae*.

Q12. What is the role of therapeutic hypothermia and seizure prophylaxis in meningitis?

Therapeutic hypothermia for neuroprotection in bacterial meningitis is contraindicated as a French multicenter randomized controlled trial (RCT) demonstrated excess mortality due to the same. Similarly, there is no role of prophylactic antiepileptics in meningoencephalitis.

Q13. How will you carry out the CSF analysis for acute bacterial meningitis?

Lumbar puncture should ideally be done before the administration of antibiotics. However, this is not feasible in many instances. CSF sterilization even for sensitive organisms takes at least 4–6 hours. Hence, LP should be performed even if antibiotics have been administered in the preceding few hours. At least 5–6 mL of CSF needs to be collected for analysis, of which 1 mL is sent for biochemical tests and 4–5 mL is sent for bacteriological/virological tests. Simultaneous blood glucose is to be done at the bedside to correlate it with the CSF glucose. The CSF opening pressure should be recorded at the time of LP, whenever possible. The following tests need to be sent:[4]

- CSF total cell count, differential count, glucose, protein
- CSF Gram staining, acid-fast bacteria (AFB) staining, culture.

In case of immunocompromised patients, the etiological agents are diverse and need more extensive evaluation in addition to the basic tests.

- CSF multiplex polymerase chain reaction (PCR) [detects bacteria causing community-acquired meningitis, *Cryptococcus*, viruses such as HSV-1, HSV-2, CMV, VZV, human herpesvirus 6 (HHV-6), and enterovirus]
- CSF adenosine deaminase (ADA) and GeneXpert for TB—a negative CSF PCR is not reliable to rule out tubercular meningitis.
- CSF culture for mycobacteria and fungi
- India ink staining and cryptococcal antigen testing.

Q14. How can CSF analysis differentiate between the etiology of meningitis?

	Normal	Bacterial	Viral	TB	Fungal
Opening pressure	6–20 cmH$_2$O	20–50 cmH$_2$O	6–30 cmH$_2$O	20–40 cmH$_2$O	20–100 cmH$_2$O
Color	Clear	Cloudy	Clear	Cloudy/yellow	Clear/cloudy
Cells	<5/mm^3	High (>1,000/mm^3)	10–1,000/mm^3	10–1,000/mm^3	10–1,000/mm^3
Differential	Lymphocytes	Neutrophils	Lymphocytes	Lymphocytes	Lymphocytes
CSF/blood glucose	50–66%	<40%	Normal	<30–40%	Normal-low
Protein	<0.45 g/L	>1 g/L	0.5–1 g/L	1–5 g/L	0.5–5 g/L

Q15. When should we suspect meningitis/ventriculitis in the presence of CSF shunts/drains or recent neurosurgery?

Organisms causing shunt/drain infections typically present with a milder and protracted course of symptoms as compared to acute bacterial community-acquired meningitis. Meningitis/ventriculitis should be suspected in the presence of the following:

- New-onset fever, headache, lethargy, or worsening of mental status
- Abdominal tenderness in the presence of ventriculoperitoneal (VP) shunt (in the absence of a clear etiology)
- Signs of pleuritis in the presence of ventriculopleural shunt (in the absence of a clear etiology)
- Bacteremia and/or glomerulonephritis in the presence of ventriculoatrial shunt (in the absence of a clear etiology)

- Erythema and/or tenderness over subcutaneous shunt tubing.

Q16. What is the role of CSF analysis in suspected healthcare-associated ventriculitis or meningitis?

Cerebrospinal fluid sampling in a patient after neurosurgery or in the presence of devices such as CSF shunts or external ventricular drain (EVD) should be done after consultation with the neurosurgeon. Abnormalities in the routine parameters such as CSF cell count, cell type, glucose, and protein are unreliable indicators of infection in this setting. Spillage of blood into CSF, handling of the meninges, and ventricular cavities may lead to CSF pleocytosis and an increased protein content, but it does not always indicate an infection. A positive CSF culture is the only definitive test to diagnose meningitis/ventriculitis in the presence of devices or after neurosurgery. However, there are a few caveats that need to be kept in mind while interpreting the CSF cultures:

- A positive CSF culture may indicate only colonization or contamination. Hence, it should be treated as an infection only in the presence of clinical symptoms/signs.
- A negative CSF culture does not exclude infection and should be repeated if the clinical suspicion persists.
- A CSF culture may be reported as negative if the infection is due to indolent organisms such as coagulase-negative *Staphylococcus* or *Propionibacterium* acnes. It is recommended to monitor for growth for at least 10 days before reporting as negative.
- If the CSF shunts/drains are removed because of suspected infection, it is recommended to send the device components for culture.
- If the CSF drains/shunts are removed for reasons other than suspected infection, routine culture of device components is not recommended.[5]

Q17. What is the role of biomarkers in the diagnosis of healthcare-associated meningitis/ventriculitis?

Cerebrospinal fluid lactate and CSF procalcitonin are being evaluated for diagnosis of bacterial meningitis in patients after neurosurgery, head trauma, and device-related meningitis. Meta-analyses have shown that a CSF lactate >3.5–4.2 mmol/L is helpful in differentiating bacterial meningitis from aseptic meningitis with sensitivity >90% and specificity >95%. Among the postneurosurgery patients, a cut-off of 4 mmol/L can reliably identify bacterial infections with a sensitivity of 88% and a specificity of 98%. However, one must be aware that the production of CSF lactate is affected by many confounders. Subarachnoid hemorrhage, traumatic brain injury, and seizures themselves may elevate CSF lactate, while benzodiazepines and opiates may reduce CSF lactate production. CSF procalcitonin has been shown to identify postneurosurgical bacterial meningitis using a cut-off of 0.075 ng/mL. However, these studies need further validation with larger sample sizes.[6,7]

Q18. Which are the organisms implicated in healthcare-associated meningitis/ventriculitis?

Coagulase-negative staphylococci (*Staphylococcus epidermidis*), *Propionibacterium acnes*, *S. aureus*, and gram-negative bacilli (*Escherichia coli, Pseudomonas, Acinetobacter, Enterobacter, Citrobacter*).

Q19. What is the empirical antibiotic of choice and duration of therapy in healthcare-associated meningitis/ventriculitis?

Vancomycin in combination with antipseudomonal beta-lactam (cefepime, ceftazidime, or meropenem) is recommended as an empirical therapy till culture results are available. The antibiotics then may be tailored based on the culture report. The antibiotics are continued for 10–14 days for most organisms, except in infections with gram-negative bacilli, where at least 21 days of therapy is recommended. Daily CSF cultures or analysis is not recommended; however, CSF culture at the end of antimicrobial therapy should be done. In patients with repeatedly positive CSF cultures, antimicrobial therapy is to be continued for 14 days after the last positive culture.

Q20. What is the role of intraventricular antibiotics in healthcare-associated meningitis/ventriculitis?

Antibiotics that can be administered via the intraventricular/intrathecal route are vancomycin, aminoglycosides, colistin, polymyxin B, and tigecycline. A recent systematic review has shown that administration of intraventricular antibiotics in postneurosurgical meningitis leads to significantly reduced mortality in addition to IV antibiotics. Intraventricular antibiotics are recommended only when IV antibiotic therapy fails to demonstrate improvement in the patient's clinical status and/or culture results. A combination of IV and intraventricular antibiotic is specifically recommended for healthcare-associated meningitis/ventriculitis caused by carbapenem-resistant *Acinetobacter* spp. After administration of an antibiotic via EVD, the drain should be clamped for 15–60 minutes. If the patient has a VP shunt, it is advised to administer intraventricular antibiotic through a separately implanted shunt reservoir. The dose of intraventricular antibiotic has to be further adjusted based on the ventricle size, output from the EVD, and the minimum inhibitory concentration (MIC) for the organism.[8,9]

Q21. What are the diagnostic criteria for viral encephalitis?

Major criteria:

Altered mental status lasting >24 hours without an alternative cause.

Minor criteria:
- Fever >100.4°F within 72 hours before or after presentation
- Seizures (partial or generalized)
- New-onset focal neurologic deficit
- CSF white blood cell (WBC) count >5/mm^3
- Neuroimaging suggestive of encephalitis (MRI is the modality of choice)
- Electroencephalography (EEG) suggestive of encephalitis
  - Possible encephalitis—one major + two minor required
  - Probable encephalitis—one major + three minor required.[10]

Q22. Which viral etiological agents are of particular concern for encephalitis in India?

The most common etiological agent with high endemicity is mosquito-borne Japanese encephalitis caused by a flavivirus. The incidence is decreasing due to vaccination campaigns; it is still reported mainly from West Bengal, Bihar, and eastern districts of Uttar Pradesh (UP). The case fatality rate is 25–30%, while 50% of affected patients have neurological sequelae. Detection of immunoglobulin M (IgM) antibodies in CSF or serum is required for the diagnosis, while MRI brain may show thalamic hyperintensities.

Dengue virus may cause encephalitis, although it has been traditionally considered a non-neurotropic virus. The dengue ribonucleic acid (RNA) or antibodies in CSF may not always be present making the diagnosis more difficult. Hence, dengue encephalitis should be kept as a differential in any patient presenting with clinical features of encephalopathy and documented dengue (based on serum IgM). MRI features (thalamic or brainstem hyperintensities) are nondiagnostic and are similar to those caused by many other organisms.

Similarly, chikungunya encephalitis, Nipah virus encephalitis, Zika virus encephalitis, and Chandipura encephalitis are the ones that have been seen in India in association with outbreaks in some states. None of these have any targeted treatment available, and the long-term morbidity remains high. Intensive monitoring and organ-supportive therapy is the only treatment.[11]

Q23. Which are the viral encephalitides for which specific therapy targeting the causative organisms is available?

Herpes simplex virus encephalitis: IV acyclovir 10 mg/kg 8 hourly given as slow infusion and hydration with dose modification for renal failure. The duration of therapy is 14 days for immunocompetent patients and 21 days for immunocompromised patients. If the initial CSF is negative but the suspicion of HSV encephalitis remains high (temporal lobe involvement on imaging), a repeat LP within 3–7 days is warranted with the continuation of empirical acyclovir. A repeat CSF PCR at the end of therapy is advised with continuation of acyclovir for another week if it is persistently positive.[12]

Varicella-zoster virus encephalitis: IV acyclovir 10 mg/kg for 7–14 days. Testing for both viral deoxyribonucleic acid (DNA) by PCR and antibodies to VZV in CSF is recommended as the antibodies seem to have greater sensitivity. Corticosteroids are to be reserved only for cases with significant cerebral edema and/or mass effect.

Cytomegalovirus encephalitis: Reduction of immunosuppression with IV ganciclovir.

Enterovirus: No specific therapy is available but intravenous immunoglobulin (IVIG) is widely used in cases of encephalitis due to enterovirus 71, especially if the patient is hypogammaglobulinemic. Diagnosis of enterovirus encephalitis has a better yield if both CSF and non-CSF (throat and stool) samples are tested by PCR.

Human immunodeficiency virus: Highly active antiretroviral therapy

Rabies encephalitis: Consider Milwaukee protocol in consultation with an infectious disease specialist.

West Nile encephalitis: IVIG, interferon alpha, and/or ribavirin may be tried.[13]

Back to the patient: The patient remained in the ICU for further management. He later developed generalized tonic-clonic seizures and IV midazolam was given. However, after 15 minutes, another episode of seizures occurred. The patient did not regain consciousness in between seizures.

Q24. Is this status epilepticus (SE)? How do you define SE?

The patient did not recover consciousness between the two seizures; this would, therefore, qualify as SE. SE is defined as 5 minutes or more of:
- Continuous clinical and/or electrographic seizure activity
- Recurrent seizure activity without recovery (returning to baseline) between seizures.

Q25. What are the causes of SE?

In this patient, bacterial meningitis is the cause of SE. The other causes of SE are as follows:
- Other CNS infections (encephalitis, brain abscess, cerebral malaria)
- CNS tumors
- Stroke (ischemia, hemorrhage, SAH, cortical venous thrombosis)

- Metabolic abnormalities (hypoglycemia, hyponatremia, hypocalcemia, hypomagnesemia, uremic, hypoxic)
- Systemic infections
- Traumatic brain injury
- Drug overdose or withdrawal
- Autoimmune encephalitis.

Q26. What are refractory status epilepticus (RSE) and superrefractory status epilepticus (SRSE)?

Refractory status epilepticus is defined in two ways:[14-16]

1. A seizure lasting for >60 minutes either continuously or intermittently without returning to baseline mental status
2. A seizure that fails to respond to at least ≥2 antiseizure medications (ASMs) including at least one nonbenzodiazepine ASM (preferred definition).

Super-refractory status epilepticus is defined as seizure activity that persists beyond 24 hours, despite treatment with an anesthetizing dose of ASM OR seizure that recurs on attempted weaning of an anesthetic regimen.

Q27. How would you manage a case of SE?

The mainstay of therapy is the stabilization of ABC, administration of anticonvulsant medications, EEG monitoring in case of RSE, investigating the cause for seizures, and cause-specific therapy.

Phase	Duration	Intervention
Stabilization	0–5 minutes	Stabilize ABC. Time the seizure from its onset and monitor vitals. Perform fingerstick blood glucose. Secure IV access and collect blood for CBC, electrolytes, toxicology screen, and anticonvulsant drug levels (if applicable)
Initial therapy	5–20 minutes	Administer benzodiazepine if the seizure continues beyond 5 minutes. Any ONE of the following three can be given: Intramuscular (IM) midazolam 10 mg single dose OR IV lorazepam 0.1 mg/kg/dose up to max 4 mg/dose (may repeat once) OR IV diazepam 0.15 mg/kg/dose up to max 10 mg/dose (may be repeated once)
Second therapy	20–40 minutes	Administer ONE of the following as a SINGLE dose if the seizures continue beyond 20 minutes despite two doses of lorazepam/diazepam or one full dose of IM midazolam.

Contd...

Contd...

Phase	Duration	Intervention
		There is no evidence to prefer one over the other. IV levetiracetam 60 mg/kg up to max 4,500 mg/dose OR IV fosphenytoin 20 mg PE/kg up to max 1,500 mg PE/dose OR IV valproic acid 40 mg/kg up to max 3,000 mg/dose If none of the above are available, IV phenobarbital 15 mg/kg max dose may be given once
Third therapy	40–60 minutes	• No clear evidence to guide further therapy. Options include: • Repeat second-line therapy and/or anesthetic infusions of either thiopental, midazolam, pentobarbital, or propofol or a combination of these drugs (all with continuous EEG monitoring) • Consider immunotherapy (steroids, IVIG, plasmapheresis) if seizures due to autoimmune encephalitis or ADEM • Ketogenic diet/pyridoxine/epilepsy surgery

Q28. What is the target of the therapy for RSE and SRSE?

The target of the therapy for RSE is complete suppression of seizure activity (clinical and electroencephalographic) along with the achievement of around 70% burst suppression pattern (BSP) in EEG (never <50%). This BSP is to be maintained for at least 24–48 hours before attempting weaning of anesthetic drugs. If the infusions were ongoing for <48 hours, they need to be weaned over 6–12 hours. If they were ongoing for >48 hours, they need even slower weaning with dose reductions every 6–12 hours. Scheduled benzodiazepines and maintenance ASMs are needed for infusions that lasted for >5 days.

Q29. What is burst suppression?

The electroencephalographic BSP consists of high-amplitude bursts interrupted by low-amplitude suppressions. Head trauma, stroke, coma, anoxia, and hypothermia can present with BSP. The BSP represents an interaction between neuronal dynamics and brain metabolism. Each series of successive bursts can be viewed as an attempted recovery of basal cortical dynamics. So, the BSP can be seen as a defined "reference point" during the administration of anesthetic or sedative agents and is considered a reliable indicator of adequate cerebral protection during the management of RSE.

Q30. What is new-onset refractory status epilepticus (NORSE) and febrile infection-related epilepsy syndrome (FIRES)?

New-onset refractory status epilepticus is the de novo onset of RSE without any active/acute structural, toxic, or metabolic cause.

Febrile infection-related epilepsy syndrome is a subset of NORSE that requires the presence of a febrile illness 2 weeks and 24 hours before the onset of RSE with or without fever at the time of SE.

Both NORSE and FIRES can occur in any age group and require extensive evaluation to find the etiology. The initial treatment principles remain the same as for any other SE case. However, immunotherapy has a major role in treatment as it is recommended to start pulse dose methylprednisolone and/or IVIG within the first 72 hours. A ketogenic diet needs to be started within the first week. In case of autoimmune encephalitis not responding to immunotherapy, rituximab may be administered.[17]

Q31. Is there any role for chemoprophylaxis for the contacts of patients with meningitis?

Prophylaxis is suggested for contacts of persons with meningococcal meningitis (e.g., household contacts, close medical personnel) and has to be started within 24 hours of identification. Rifampicin (600 mg PO every 12 hourly for 2 days) is the usual recommended agent. It should be used with caution in India due to the high prevalence of *Mycobacterium tuberculosis*. Ceftriaxone 250 mg IM in a single dose or oral ciprofloxacin (500 mg in a single dose) is equally effective.

Q32. Is there any role of vaccination for survivors of bacterial meningitis?

Vaccination with pneumococcal vaccine is recommended for all patients after an episode of pneumococcal meningitis and also in patients with CSF leakage after dura repair. Vaccination with *H. influenzae* type b and meningococcal vaccine (either serogroup C, serogroup B, or quadrivalent A/C/Y/W135) can be considered in patients with meningitis associated with CSF leakage.

REFERENCES

1. van de Beek D, Cabellos C, Dzupova O, Esposito S, Klein M, Kloek AT, et al. ESCMID guideline: diagnosis and treatment of acute bacterial meningitis. Clin Microbiol Infect. 2016;22 Suppl. 3:S37-62.
2. GBD 2016 Meningitis Collaborators. Global, regional, and national burden of meningitis, 1990-2016: a systematic analysis for the Global Burden of Disease Study 2016. Lancet Neurol. 2018;17(12):1061-82.
3. Sonneville R, de Montmollin E, Contou D, Ferrer R, Gurjar M, Klouche K, et al. Clinical features, etiologies, and outcomes in adult patients with meningoencephalitis requiring intensive care (EURECA): an international prospective multicenter cohort study. Intensive Care Med. 2023;49(5):517-29.
4. Meyfroidt G, Kurtz P, Sonneville R. Critical care management of infectious meningitis and encephalitis. Intensive Care Med. 2020;46(2):192-201.
5. Tunkel AR, Hasbun R, Bhimraj A, Byers K, Kaplan SL, Scheld WM, et al. 2017 Infectious Diseases Society of America's clinical practice guidelines for healthcare-associated ventriculitis and meningitis. Clin Infect Dis. 2017;64(6):e34-65.
6. Xiao X, Zhang Y, Zhang L, Kang P, Ji N. The diagnostic value of cerebrospinal fluid lactate for post-neurosurgical bacterial meningitis: a meta-analysis. BMC Infect Dis. 2016;16(1):483.
7. Li Y, Zhang G, Ma R, Du Y, Zhang L, Li F, et al. The diagnostic value of cerebrospinal fluids procalcitonin and lactate for the differential diagnosis of post-neurosurgical bacterial meningitis and aseptic meningitis. Clin Biochem. 2015;48(1-2):50-4.
8. Florez-Perdomo WA, Escobar-Cardona D, Janjua T, Agrawal A, Vasquez H, Lozada-Martinez ID, et al. Antibiotic therapy by intrathecal or intraventricular approach for postsurgical meningitis or ventriculitis: a systematic review and meta-analysis. Egypt J Neurosurg. 2023;38:20.
9. Nau R, Blei C, Eiffert H. Intrathecal antibacterial and antifungal therapies. Clin Microbiol Rev. 2020;33(3):e00190-19.
10. Britton PN, Eastwood K, Paterson B, Durrheim DN, Dale RC, Cheng AC, et al. Consensus guidelines for the investigation and management of encephalitis in adults and children in Australia and New Zealand. Intern Med J. 2015;45(5):563-76.
11. Sapra H, Singhal V. Managing meningoencephalitis in Indian ICU. Indian J Crit Care Med. 2019;23(Suppl. 2):S124-8.
12. Bradshaw MJ, Venkatesan A. Herpes simplex virus-1 encephalitis in adults: pathophysiology, diagnosis, and management. Neurotherapeutics. 2016;13(3):493-508.
13. Venkatesan A, Tunkel AR, Bloch KC, Lauring AS, Sejvar J, Bitnun A, et al. Case definitions, diagnostic algorithms, and priorities in encephalitis: consensus statement of the international encephalitis consortium. Clin Infect Dis. 2013;57(8):1114-28.
14. Glauser T, Shinnar S, Gloss D, Alldredge B, Arya R, Bainbridge J, et al. Evidence-based guideline: treatment of convulsive status epilepticus in children and adults: report of the Guideline Committee of the American Epilepsy Society. Epilepsy Curr. 2016;16(1):48-61.
15. Ochoa JG, Dougherty M, Papanastassiou A, Gidal B, Mohamed I, Vossler DG. Treatment of super-refractory status epilepticus: a review. Epilepsy Curr. 2021;21(6):1535759721999670.
16. Trinka E, Leitinger M. Management of status epilepticus, refractory status epilepticus, and super-refractory status epilepticus. Continuum (Minneap Minn). 2022;28(2):559-602.
17. Wickstrom R, Taraschenko O, Dilena R, Payne ET, Specchio N, Nabbout R, et al. International NORSE Consensus Group. International consensus recommendations for management of New Onset Refractory Status Epilepticus (NORSE) including Febrile Infection-Related Epilepsy Syndrome (FIRES): summary and clinical tools. Epilepsia. 2022;63(11):2827-39.

CHAPTER 16

Traumatic Brain Injury

Rakesh Mohanty, Amit Madhukar Narkhede, Kapil Sharad Borawake, Kapil Gangadhar Zirpe

CASE STUDY

A 40-year-old gentleman was found unconscious after a possible hit and run road traffic accident. He was brought to the emergency department and examination revealed a Glasgow Coma Scale (GCS) of 6 (E2M2V2). His pupils were 4 mm in size, bilaterally equal, and fixed. He had cerebral spinal fluid otorrhea on the left side.

A computed tomography (CT) scan of the head showed subarachnoid hemorrhage with left temporal subdural hemorrhage, a left temporal and parietal hematoma with mass effect causing an 8-mm shift of midline. On examination, his heart rate was 42 beats/min, regular, and blood pressure was 168/108 mm Hg. Primary survey also revealed fracture of right 3rd to 9th ribs with no evidence of hemothorax, pneumothorax, or hemoperitoneum.

Q1. Describe the emergency department management of a patient with traumatic brain injury (TBI).

The management of a patient with TBI should always begin with assessment of the airway. The decision to intubate should be based on the following factors:
- GCS <9
- Peripheral capillary oxygen saturation (SpO$_2$) <92% despite oxygen supplementation
- Signs of cerebral herniation
- Signs of aspiration
- Compromised airway

Traumatic brain injury is commonly associated with cervical spine injury and cervical spine stability should be maintained throughout with manual inline stabilization or cervical collar. Rapid sequence intubation with manual in-line stabilization is the recommended technique for securing the airway as it reduces sympathetic response, agitation, and transient increases in intracranial pressure (ICP) and cervical spine injury. Mechanical ventilation should be initiated to attain normocapnia [partial pressure of carbon dioxide (pCO$_2$) between 35 and 40 mm Hg].

Hypoventilation leading to hypercapnia will cause an increase in ICP and hyperventilation leading to hypocapnia would cause decreased cerebral perfusion through cerebral vasoconstriction. Maintain adequate oxygenation with an oxygen saturation (SpO$_2$) >90% or PaO$_2$ >60 mm Hg to achieve adequate oxygenation of cerebral tissues. Therapeutic hyperventilation (pCO$_2$ around 30 mm Hg) should be only reserved for short periods with acute neurological deterioration due to cerebral herniation or rise in ICP refractory to medical management.

Sustained hypoxia (PaO$_2$ <60 mm Hg) and hypotension [systolic blood pressure (SBP) <90 mm Hg] should be promptly treated as both are known to be strongly associated with worse outcomes in patients with traumatic brain injury. Hypotension (SBP <100 mm Hg) should be promptly corrected with isotonic fluids and blood products as required. Vasopressors may be used if hypotension is not responding to fluids and blood products. Maintaining SBP at >100 mm Hg for patients between 50 and 69 years of age or at >110 mm Hg for patients between 15 and 49 or >70 years old may be considered to decrease mortality and improve outcomes.[1] Any systemic injuries (hemothorax, hemoperitoneum, cardiac tamponade, and tension pneumothorax) should be promptly managed to improve circulation. There is no role of permissive hypotension or hypotensive resuscitation in patients with TBI as trials of permissive hypotension/hypotensive resuscitation and restricted/controlled resuscitation (Dutton in 2002 and Morrison in 2011) have excluded TBI patients as permissive hypotension will cause or exacerbate secondary brain injury.[2,3]

A brief neurologic examination should be performed including GCS, pupillary signs, and symmetry of limb movements. Any signs of increased ICP and impending herniation like significant papillary asymmetry, fixed and dilated pupils, decorticate or decerebrate posturing and the "Cushing triad" of irregular respiration, bradycardia, and hypertension should prompt immediate institution of measures to control ICP. Emergency neurosurgical intervention may be required in such situations. Neurological assessments should be repeated regularly.

Complete blood count, blood glucose, serum electrolytes, coagulation profile, blood alcohol level, and urine toxin screen should be done in patients with TBI. The patient should be transferred to a center with neurosurgical facilities soon after stabilization.

Q2. What are the indications for CT brain in TBI?
- All patients with moderate and severe head injury
- Patients with suspected mild head injury (i.e., witnessed loss of consciousness, definite amnesia, or witnessed disorientation in a patient with a GCS score of 13-15) *and* any one of the following factors:
  - *High risk for neurosurgical intervention:*
    - GCS score <15 at 2 hours after injury
    - Suspected open or depressed skull fracture
    - Any sign of basilar skull fracture (e.g., hemotympanum, raccoon eyes, CSF otorrhea or rhinorrhea, Battle's sign)
    - Vomiting (more than two episodes)
    - Age >65 years
    - Anticoagulant use
  - *Moderate risk for brain injury on CT:*
    - Loss of consciousness (>5 minutes)
    - Amnesia before impact (>30 minutes)
    - Dangerous mechanism (e.g., pedestrian struck by motor vehicle, occupant ejected from motor vehicle, fall from height >3 feet or five stairs)

The CT scan findings along with GCS and other neurological signs may prompt a neurosurgical intervention. CT scan may also be useful for detecting secondary brain injuries such as cerebral edema, infarcts, and herniation. Follow-up CT scan may be required in case of neurological deterioration.

Q3. What is the pathophysiology of traumatic brain injury?
The pathophysiology of TBI is discussed under the two distinct but interrelated categories: (1) primary brain injury and (2) secondary brain injury **(Flowchart 1)**.

Primary brain injury: It is the injury that occurs at the time of trauma, resulting from various external mechanical forces transferred to intracranial structures leading to bone fractures, contusions, hematomas, and axonal injury. The mechanisms commonly implicated in primary brain injury include direct impact, rapid deceleration–acceleration, penetrating injuries, shearing forces, and blast waves. The primary brain injury leads to disruption of blood–brain barrier and loss of cerebral autoregulation, causing

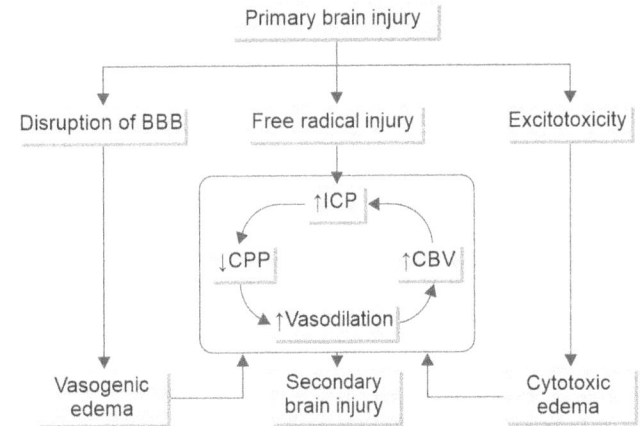

Flowchart 1: Mechanism of primary and traumatic brain injury.

(BBB: blood–brain barrier; CBV: cerebral blood volume; CPP: cerebral perfusion pressure; ICP: intracranial pressure)

worsening of cerebral edema, increase in ICP, and decrease in cerebral perfusion pressure (CPP).

Morphologically, it may be divided into cranial and intracranial injuries. Cranial injuries include various skull fractures due to direct contact force applied to the skull. Skull fractures by themselves are inconsequential; however, damage to underlying neurovascular structures leads to various consequences such as epidural hematoma, cerebrospinal fluid (CSF) rhinorrhea or otorrhea, contusions, facial, and auditory nerve injuries. Intracranial injuries include intra-axial injuries such as cerebral contusions, diffuse axonal injury, and intracerebral hemorrhage; extra-axial injuries such as epidural, subdural, and subarachnoid hemorrhage; and intraventricular hemorrhage (IVH).

Secondary brain injury: The primary trauma triggers a cascade of molecular mechanisms within hours to days causing further neuronal damage called secondary brain injury. The various mechanisms leading to secondary brain injury include:
- *Excitotoxicity:* It is a series of events occurring secondary to activation of neurotransmitters leading to excessive stimulation of neuronal cells and increasing neuronal damage. Glutamate is the major excitatory neurotransmitter which acts through N-methyl-D-aspartate (NMDA) and α-amino-3-hydroxy-5-methyl-4-isoxazolepropionic acid (AMPA) receptors. Cellular membrane disruption due to initial injury leads to increased flux of sodium causing excitatory neurotransmitter release. Excessive calcium affects cellular functions leading to neuronal injury and death.
- *Free oxygen radical injury:* Activation of mitochondrial enzymes leads to development of free radicals such as superoxide ion and nitric oxide. Lipid peroxidation also contributes to free radicals-induced neuronal damage.

- Activation of proteases leads to disruption of neuronal cytoskeleton and axonal damage. Calpains are a family of protease enzymes, the activation of which is implicated in neuronal injury.
- Dysregulation of cell cycle and apoptotic pathways mediated through caspase enzymes also plays important role in neuronal damage after traumatic brain injury.
- Disruption of blood-brain barrier may lead to inflammatory response and vasogenic edema leading to neuronal damage.
- Loss of cellular autoregulation may lead to increase in ICP and decrease in CPP.
- Stress response to TBI may lead to catecholamine surge and organ dysfunction as also lead to hyperglycemia and worsen neurological outcomes.[4]

Q4. Describe the pathoanatomic classification of primary traumatic brain injury.[5]

As described above, the primary TBI results from direct impact of mechanical forces on cranial and intracranial structures, leading to various morphological types of TBI **(Table 1)**.

Skull fractures result from considerable contact force applied directly to the cranium. They may be open or closed, depressed or nondepressed, and stellate or linear. Skull fractures by themselves are inconsequential; however, damage to underlying structures can cause life-threatening injuries. Temporal bone fractures may be associated with middle meningeal artery injury causing epidural hematomas. Basilar fractures may be associated with damage to olfactory, facial, or auditory nerves. They may also be associated with CSF rhinorrhea or otorrhea which may act as a portal of infection leading to bacterial meningitis. Open fractures due to breach of scalp barrier are associated with increased risk of infection.

Cerebral contusions are heterogeneous lesions consisting of areas of hemorrhage, edema, and necrosis. They are commonly found in TBI and could be the only lesions in cases of mild TBI. They commonly result from acceleration-deceleration mechanism of TBI. Based on the mechanism of injury, contusions could be subdivided as coup or contrecoup lesions. As described by Omaya and colleagues in 1971, coup lesions are cerebral contusions that occur directly below the site of an impact to the head whereas contrecoup lesions are contusions located on the side of the brain opposite to the point of impact.[6]

Diffuse axonal injury (DAI) consists of diffuse punctate lesions at the gray mater-white mater interface due to axonal damage resulting from shearing forces caused by rotational or translational forces. Initially, DAI was considered to be purely a primary brain injury, but DAI may also result from biochemical and histological changes, which evolve over a period and be related to secondary brain injury.

Epidural/extradural hematoma (EDH) is an intracranial hematoma located between the inner table of skull bone and the dura mater. It is lenticular in shape and does not cross suture lines as the dura mater is tightly attached to the skull bones. It commonly results from rupture of the middle meningeal artery or its branches associated with squamous temporal bone fractures.

Subdural hematomas (SDHs) are hematomas which develop between the inner surface of dura mater and arachnoid mater and are crescentic in shape. It results from rupture of bridging veins of the cerebral surface or the dural venous sinuses.

Subarachnoid hemorrhage (SAH) occurs due to bleeding into subarachnoid space which lies between the arachnoid and pia mater. It does not cause mass effect but leads to significant mortality and morbidity due to increased risk of cerebral vasospasm. Trauma is a common cause of SAH and is usually associated with other lesions such as cerebral contusion or skull fractures.

Intracerebral hemorrhage (ICH) results from hemorrhage into the substance of the brain and is associated with mass effect and surrounding edema.

Intraventricular hemorrhage results from rupture of subependymal vessels or extension from ICH. Acute hydrocephalus is a common complication.

Q5. What is cerebral perfusion pressure (CPP)? What are factors affecting CPP? Describe in brief Monro-Kellie doctrine.

The CPP is defined as the difference between the mean arterial pressure (MAP) and the ICP and is a clinically measurable determinant of adequacy of the cerebral perfusion.

$$CPP = MAP - ICP$$

Cerebral blood flow (CBF) is regulated by cerebrovascular autoregulation of cerebrovascular resistance and is maintained in a normal range over a wide range of

TABLE 1: Incidence and mortality of lesions associated with traumatic brain injury (n = 13962).[7]

Lesion	Incidence	Mortality
EDH	22.5%	27.7%
SDH	30.1%	32.8%
ICH	21.8%	31.8%
SAH	21.7%	40.4%
No bleed	53.8%	14.6%

(EDH: epidural/extradural hematoma; ICH: intracerebral hemorrhage; SAH: subarachnoid hemorrhage; SDH: subdural hemorrhage)

CPP (50-100 mm Hg). TBI adversely affects cerebral autoregulation and hence CBF is maintained over a narrow range of CPP. Increase in CPP leads to increased ICP due to increased CBF and decreased CPP leads to decreased CBF and ischemic injury to the brain.

Cerebral perfusion pressure is affected by the factors affecting MAP and ICP:
- Mass effect due to intracranial hemorrhage
- *Edema:* Cytotoxic and vasogenic
- Increased resistance to cerebral venous outflow
- Acute hydrocephalus
- Increased central venous pressure (CVP)
- Polytrauma with hemorrhagic shock
- Systemic inflammatory response
- *Factors affecting cerebral vascular tone:* Partial pressure of carbon dioxide, partial pressure of oxygen, and alkalosis. The Brain Trauma Foundation Guidelines for traumatic brain injury recommend to maintain CPP between 60 and 70 mm Hg.[1]

The Monro-Kellie doctrine: The cranium is a rigid structure, with a fixed volume. The intracranial contents include—(1) brain parenchyma (80% by volume), (2) cerebrospinal fluid (CSF) (10% by volume), and (3) blood (10% by volume). The compliance relationship between the intracranial contents is nonlinear, and compliance worsens as volume of intracranial contents increases. Initially, ICP is maintained by the displacement of CSF to thecal sac and decrease in cerebral venous blood volume by venoconstriction and drainage. But as these compensatory mechanisms get exhausted, even minor increases in intracranial contents lead to significant increase in ICP **(Fig. 1)**.

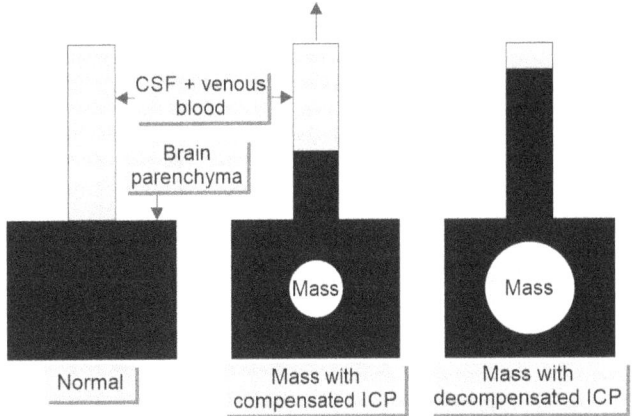

Fig. 1: The Monro-Kellie doctrine. (CSF: cerebrospinal fluid; ICP: intracranial pressure)

TABLE 2: Glasgow Coma Scale.[8]

Best motor response (M)	Verbal response (V)	Eye opening (E)	Score
Obeys commands	–	–	6
Localizing	Oriented	–	5
Normal flexion	Confused	Spontaneous	4
Abnormal flexion	Words	To sound	3
Extension	Sounds	To pressure	2
None	None	None	1

Traumatic brain injury (TBI): *mild:* <8, *moderate:* 9–12, *severe:* 13–15

Q6. Describe the various severity scoring systems used in patients with TBI.

The various severity scoring systems used in TBI include:
- Glasgow Coma Scale
- The FOUR (Full Outline of UnResponsiveness) score
- The Marshall CT classification
- The Rotterdam CT score

1. *Glasgow Coma Scale* **(Table 2)**:[8] Traditionally, the assessment of severity of TBI has been based upon the GCS. It has three components: (1) best motor response (scored from 1 to 6), (2) eye opening (scored from 1 to 4), and (3) verbal response (scored from 1 to 5). The maximum score is 15 and minimum score is 3. It classifies TBI as mild: GCS 13–15, moderate: GCS 9–12, and severe: GCS < 8. It is a universally accepted, simple, practical, easy to use and reproducible clinical tool to assess severity of TBI with a good prognostic value. However, certain factors such as intoxication, sedation, paralysis, and endotracheal intubation may limit its accuracy and practical application. It does not test brainstem reflexes.[8]

2. *The FOUR score* **(Table 3)**:[9] The FOUR score has four components: (1) eye responses, (2) motor response, (3) brainstem reflexes, and (4) respiration. Each component is scored from 0 to 4. It has a minimum score of 0 to a maximum score of 16 (total 17 points). It is a new and more comprehensive tool for assessing the level of consciousness in patients with traumatic brain injury. It is not affected by endotracheal intubation unlike the GCS.[9]

3. *The Marshall computed tomography classification* **(Table 4)**:[10] The Marshall computed tomography (CT) classification was first described in 1991 by Marshall et al. and is the most commonly used CT classification system. It classifies TBI into six categories based on three variables—(1) presence of mass lesion, (2) appearance of perimesencephalic cisterns, and (3) the extent of midline shift on CT scans.[10] It is used as a descriptive as well as a prognostic tool.

TABLE 3: The FOUR score.

Score	Eye response	Motor response (upper extremity)	Brainstem reflexes	Respiration
4	Eyelids open or opened, tracking, or blinking to command	Thumbs-up, fist, or peace sign	Pupil and corneal reflexes present	Not intubated, regular breathing pattern
3	Eyelids open but not tracking	Localizing to pain	One pupil wide and fixed	Not intubated, Cheyne–Stokes breathing pattern
2	Eyelids closed but open to loud voice	Flexion response to pain	Pupil or corneal reflexes absent	Not intubated, irregular breathing
1	Eyelids closed but open to pain	Extension response to pain	Pupil and corneal reflexes absent	Breathes above ventilator rate
0	Eyelids remain closed with pain	No response to pain or generalized myoclonus status	Absent pupil, corneal, and cough reflex	Breathes at ventilator rate or apnea

TABLE 4: The Marshall computed tomography (CT) classification.

Marshall CT class	CT findings
Diffuse injury I	No visible intracranial pathology seen on CT scan
Diffuse injury II	Cisterns are present with midline shift 0–5 mm and/or lesion densities present; No high or mixed density lesion >25 cm^3 may include bone fragments and foreign bodies
Diffuse injury III	Cisterns compressed or absent with midline shift of 0–5 mm No high or mixed density lesions >25 cm^3
Diffuse injury IV	Midline shift >5 mm No high or mixed density lesions >25 cm^3
Evacuated mass lesion	Any surgically evacuated lesion
Nonevacuated mass lesion	High or mixed density lesion >25 cm^3; not surgically evacuated

TABLE 5: The Rotterdam computed tomography score.

Score	CT characteristic			
	Basal cisterns	Midline shift	Epidural mass lesion	IVH or tSAH
0	Normal	None or ≤5 mm	Present	Absent
1	Compressed	>5 mm	Absent	Present
2	Absent	–	–	–

TABLE 6: The Rotterdam score and outcome at 6 months.[11]

Rotterdam score	1	2	3	4	5	6
Predicted 6-month mortality (%)	0	6.8	16	26	53	61

4. *The Rotterdam computed tomography score* **(Table 5)**:[11] It was developed in 2005 using data from 2,269 TBI patients from Europe and North America by Maas et al. It utilizes various CT characteristics such as status of basal cisterns, midline shift, traumatic subarachnoid hemorrhage (tSAH) and/or IVH, and presence/absence of epidural mass lesions to classify TBI and is a prognostication tool. It can reliably predict 6-month mortality outcome in TBI patients.[11]

Add plus 1 to the above score to get the Rotterdam CT score which is used to predict 6-month mortality as stated below **(Table 6)**. The score range of 1–6 also makes it consistent with Marshall CT classification and motor component of GCS.

Q7. What are the indications for monitoring ICP? Describe various modalities for ICP monitoring.

As per the Brain Trauma Foundation guidelines for management of severe TBI,[1] indications for monitoring ICP include:

- All salvageable patients with a severe TBI (GCS <8) and an abnormal CT scan. An abnormal CT scan of the head is defined as having hematomas, contusions, swelling, herniation, or compressed basal cisterns.
- Patients with severe TBI with a normal CT scan if two or more of the following are present at admission:
  • Age over 40 years
  • Unilateral or bilateral motor posturing
  • Systolic blood pressure <90 mm Hg

Intracranial pressure is normally <15 mm Hg in adults and intracranial hypertension is defined as persistent elevation in ICP >20 mm Hg. An ICP target of <22 mm Hg is recommended by guidelines in TBI.[1] The CPP cannot be reliably measured without measuring the ICP. Monitoring ICP continuously enables clinicians to estimate the CPP and hence optimize cerebral blood flow and oxygenation. This helps to reduce the secondary brain injury. ICP can be monitored using various invasive and noninvasive techniques.

Invasive techniques include:

- *Intraventricular catheter with external drainage:* It is the gold standard for ICP monitoring. It consists of a catheter placed in one of the lateral ventricles via a surgical approach. The catheter is transduced and continuous ICP monitoring initiated. Its advantages include simplicity, accuracy, and ability to drain CSF in order to lower ICP. Disadvantages include:
  - *Risk of infection:* The risk increases as the duration of catheter placement increases; routine catheter changes are not protective against infection.
  - Bleeding during insertion.
  - Difficulty or failure of insertion in ventricular compression due to hemorrhage or edema.
- *Epidural monitor:* It consists of a fiberoptic transducer which passes through the skull bone and rests against the dura mater. Advantage is lesser risk of bleeding and simplicity of insertion. Disadvantage is inaccuracy as the dura mater damps the pressure changes in the parenchyma.
- *Subarachnoid bolt:* It consists of a hollow screw placed through the skull into the subarachnoid space through the dura mater. The CSF transmits pressure changes to the fluid-filled column in the screw and transducer. Advantages include low risk of hemorrhage and infection. Disadvantages include inaccuracy, likelihood of blockage by debris.
- *Intraparenchymal monitor:* It consists of a fiberoptic transducer placed through the skull into brain parenchyma. Advantages include lower risk of hemorrhage, infection, and ease of placement. Disadvantages include less accuracy, loss of accuracy over time, and inability to drain CSF.

Various noninvasive techniques of ICP monitoring include:

- *Transcranial Doppler (TCD):* It measures blood flow velocities in proximal cerebral circulation. It estimates raised ICP by assessing changes in blood flow velocities in response to in vascular resistance. Advantage is due to its noninvasive nature. Disadvantage is inaccuracy.
- *Optic nerve sheath diameter:* Ultrasonographic measurement of optic nerve sheath diameter is a noninvasive method of diagnosing raised ICP. An optic nerve sheath diameter of >5-6 mm correlates with raised ICP in TBI.

Other techniques such as optic tonometry, tissue resonance analysis, and tympanic membrane displacement lack accuracy and reproducibility and are not used in clinical practice.

Q8. Describe in brief the various ICP waveforms.[12]

Intracranial pressure waveforms are dynamic and show cyclic variation with arterial pulsations, respiratory variation, and intracranial compliance. The C waves are the smallest in amplitude and are related to the variations in ICP associated with the arterial waveform/cardiac cycle. The C waves are smaller in amplitude 1-4 mm Hg and a higher frequency (as per the heart rate). The ICP pulse waveform can be further divided into three waves: P1, P2, and P3. P1 wave or percussion wave represents the arterial pulse transmitted through the choroid plexus. P2 wave or tidal wave represents a reflection of the arterial pulse from cerebral tissues. P3 waves or dicrotic waves represent the dicrotic notch of the arterial pulse and are related to the closure of the aortic valve. With therapeutic measures to decrease ICP, the P1 amplitude remains the same, while P2 and P3 decrease in amplitude. The B waves are related to the respiratory variation in ICP waveform. They have larger amplitude (2-10 mm Hg) and lesser frequency (as per respiratory rate). A-waves are pathological and they are seen when there is profound and sustained elevation in ICP. The A waves indicate loss of autoregulatory and compensatory mechanisms warranting urgent intervention to reduce ICP **(Table 7; Figs. 2 and 3)**.

Q9. Describe advanced techniques of neuromonitoring in TBI.

Brain tissue oxygen tension, jugular venous oximetry, and cerebral microdialysis are the commonly studied advanced neuromonitoring techniques.

TABLE 7: Interpretation of intracranial pressure (ICP) waveform.[12]

ICP waveform changes	Conditions
Increase mean ICP and ICP waveform amplitude	Acutely presenting mass lesion, increase in CSF volume, severe arterial hypertension, hypercapnia, hypoxemia, and decreased venous return
Decrease mean ICP, and ICP waveform amplitude	Arterial hypotension (especially P1), decreased CSF volume, hyperventilation
Prominent P2	Cerebral edema (ICP), cerebral vasospasm (decreased P1 amplitude)
Blunting of respiratory variation	Increased ICP

(CSF: cerebrospinal fluid)

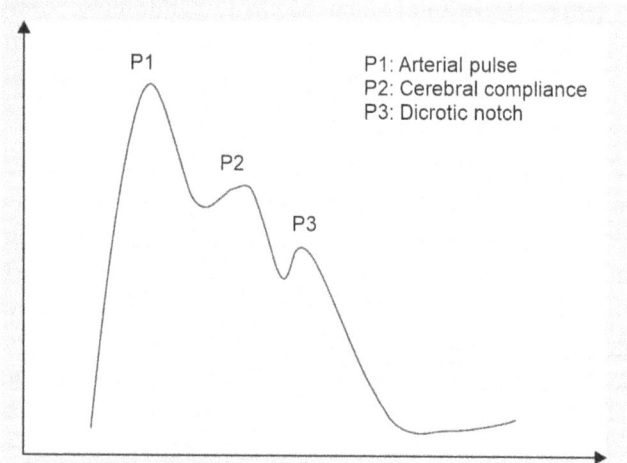

Fig. 2: Intracranial pressure (ICP) waveforms related to arterial pulse.

P1: Arterial pulse
P2: Cerebral compliance
P3: Dicrotic notch

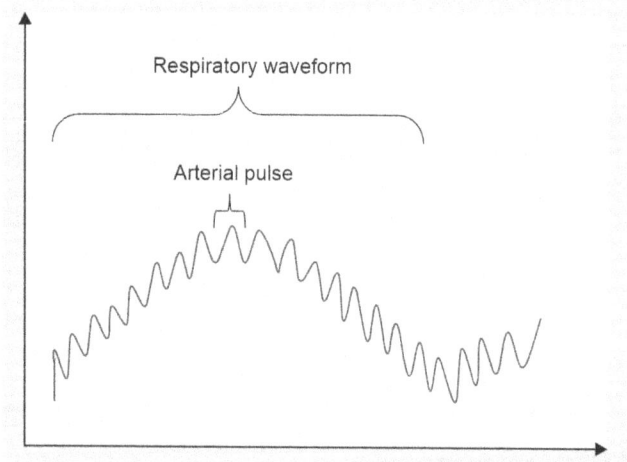

Fig. 3: Respiratory variation in intracranial pressure (ICP) waveform.

- *Brain tissue oxygen monitoring:* It involves placement of a polarographic microelectrode in the brain parenchyma through a fixed cranial bolt which measures brain tissue oxygen tension (PbO_2).

  Generally, a continuous brain tissue oxygen ($PbtO_2$) level <15 mm Hg is associated with >50% mortality. Drawbacks associated with $PbtO_2$ monitoring include the fact that $PbtO_2$ is a focal measure, influenced by probe location, and invasive and may be affected by arterial partial pressure of oxygen.

- *Jugular venous oximetry:* Measurement of the oxygen saturation of the jugular venous blood ($SjvO_2$) provides a measure of global cerebral oxygen delivery of the sampling side. It also provides a way of estimating the relation between global oxygen flow and metabolism thereby detecting cerebral hypoperfusion and helps in preventing secondary brain injury. It is measured by placing a catheter in a retrograde manner via the internal jugular vein at the jugular venous bulb to measure oxygen saturation. It also helps to calculate the arteriovenous oxygen difference [(a-v)DO_2]. [(a-v) DO_2] and $SjvO_2$ are inversely related. Normal $SjvO_2$ is 60 mm Hg. A $SjvO_2$ of <50 indicates breach of cerebral ischemic threshold and needs urgent intervention. Causes of low $SjvO_2$ include low CBF, low CPP, fever, and seizures. Limitations include: it is invasive, it may be influenced by hemoglobin levels, it is a global indicator, and regional ischemic changes may be missed.

- *Cerebral microdialysis:* It utilizes a capillary to sample metabolites from brain parenchyma with a goal of detecting neurochemical changes indicative or predictive of brain injury. The commonly measured metabolites include glucose, lactate, pyruvate, glutamate, and glycerol. A decrease in glucose level, increase in lactate:pyruvate ratio(>30), and increase in glutamate may indicate ischemia. Increased glycerol may be a sign of cell membrane breakdown. The catheter is placed at the penumbra and not in the injured brain parenchyma. It is an intermittent technique, has a lag period of approximately 20 minutes, and has variable results based on location of catheter.

Q10. How will you manage raised ICP in this patient?
Intracranial hypertension is defined as ICP >20 mm Hg. Maintaining an ICP <22 mm Hg or CPP of 60–70 mm Hg has been recommended by the Brain Trauma Foundation guidelines.[1] Maintaining higher CPP may not be beneficial and may increase risk of hypoxemic respiratory failure[13] **(Flowchart 2).**

Measures at reducing ICP should begin with elevation of head of bed by 30–45° to allow adequate venous drainage as well maintain cerebral perfusion. Neck should be maintained in neutral position, endotracheal/tracheostomy tube ties, and cervical braces be loosened if too tight to facilitate venous drainage.

Provision of adequate analgesia and sedation helps to ameliorate sympathetic response, decrease cerebral metabolic rate, and improve endotracheal tube tolerance and patient–ventilator dyssynchrony. Short-acting agents such as propofol, dexmedetomidine, and fentanyl are commonly used and allow frequent neurological assessment. Neuromuscular blocking agents are generally discouraged but may be used in selected patients to avoid patient–ventilator dyssynchrony.

Both hypercapnia and hypocapnia can be deleterious. Ventilation should be managed to maintain normocapnia with pCO_2 targeted within a range of 35–40 mm Hg. Hyperventilation may be used as a temporary measure to treat intracranial hypertension. It is desirable to monitor

Flowchart 2: The management of severe traumatic brain injury guided by intracranial pressure measurements.

Tier 1

- Maintain CPP 60–70 mm Hg
- Increase analgesia to lower ICP
- Increase sedation to lower ICP
- Maintain P_aCO_2 at low end of normal (35–38 mm Hg/4.7–5.1 kPa)
- Mannitol by intermittent bolus (0.25–1.0 g/kg)
- Hypertonic saline by intermittent bolus*
- CSF drainage if EVD in situ
- Consider placement of EVD to drain CSF if parenchymal probe used initially
- Consider anti-seizure prophylaxis for 1 week only (unless indication to continue)
- Consider EEG monitoring

Principles for Using Tiers:
- When possible, use lowest tier treatment
- There is no rank order within a tier
- It is not necessary to use all modalities in a lower tier before moving to the next tier
- If considered advantageous, tier can be skipped when advancing treatment

Tier 2

- Mild hypocapnia range 32–35 mm Hg/4.3–4.6 kPa)
- Neuromuscular paralysis in adequately sedated patients if efficacious**
- **Perform MAP Challenge to assess cerebral autoregulation and guide MAP and CPP goals in individual patients**†
  - Should be performed under direct supervision of a physician who can assess response and ensure safety
  - No other therapeutic adjustments (i.e., sedation) should be performed during the MAP challenge
  - Initiate or titrate a vasopressor or inotrope to increase MAP by 10 mm Hg for not more than 20 minutes
  - Monitor and record key parameters (MAP, CPP, ICP and $P_{bt}O_2$) before during and after the challenge
  - Adjust vasopressor/inotrope dose based on study findings
- Raise CPP with fluid boluses, vasopressors and/or inotropes to lower ICP when autoregulation is intact

- Re-examine the patient and consider repeat CT to re-evaluate intracranial pathology
- Reconsider surgical options for potentially surgical lesions
- Consider extracranial causes of ICP elevation
- Review that basic physiologic parameters are in desired range (e.g., CPP, blood gas values)
- Consider consultation with higher level of care if applicable for your health care system

Tier 3

- Pentobarbital or thiopentone coma titrated to ICP control if efficacious‡
- Secondary decompressive craniectomy
- Mild hypothermia (35–36°C) using active cooling measures

*We recommend using sodium and osmolality limits of 155 mEq/L and of 320 mEq/L respectively as administration limits for both mannitol and hypertonic saline.
**We recommend a trial dose of neuromuscular paralysis and only proceeding to a continuous infusion when efficacy is demonstrated.
†Rosenthal G, et al. 2011
‡Barbiturate administration should only be continued when a beneficial effect on ICP is demonstrated. Titrate barbiturate to achieve ICP control but do not exceed the dose which achieves burst suppression. Hypotension must be avoided when barbiturates are administered.
(CPP: cerebral perfusion pressure; ICP: intracranial pressure; MAP: mean arterial pressure)

jugular venous saturation during hyperventilation to monitor oxygen delivery to brain.[1]

Cerebrospinal fluid drainage using an external ventricular drainage (EVD) is an easy way to reduce ICP in patients with EVD and ICP monitoring. An EVD system zeroed at the level of the midbrain/external auditory meatus with continuous drainage more effectively normalizes ICP than intermittent drainage.[1]

Osmotic therapy with agents such as mannitol and hypertonic saline removes water from the brain parenchyma by creating an osmotic gradient across the blood–brain barrier, leading to a decrease in ICP. Mannitol should be used in a dose of 0.25–1 g/kg to control raised ICP. While doing so, arterial hypotension (SBP < 90 mm Hg) should be avoided. Prior to ICP monitoring, mannitol should be restricted to patients with signs of transtentorial herniation or progressive neurological deterioration not attributable to extracranial causes. Hypertonic saline has been used in various concentrations from 3 to 23.5%. 3% saline is commonly used as an infusion to target serum sodium levels of 145-155 mEq/L, whereas 23.4% saline is used as intermittent boluses. It has a theoretical advantage over mannitol in patients with hypovolemia, ongoing bleeding with less likelihood of leakage into brain tissue, and renal failure. However, there is no convincing clinical evidence of superiority of hypertonic saline over mannitol in severe TBI.[14] Effect of treatment diminishes over time; hence, prolonged use is not recommended. Also, osmotic agents should not be abruptly stopped due to the risk of rebound cerebral edema.

Therapeutic hypothermia has been proposed to manage raised ICP after severe TBI on account of its potential to reduce ICP, cerebral metabolic rate, and secondary brain injury. A recently conducted large randomized control trial (RCT)—the Eurotherm3235 Trial (2015), however, failed to show any benefit in improving outcomes.[15] The Prophylactic Hypothermia Trial to Lessen Traumatic Brain Injury-Randomized Clinical Trial (POLAR-RCT, 2018) by Cooper and colleagues was a recently conducted large RCT which evaluated therapeutic hypothermia in patients with TBI and failed to show any benefit.[16] The trial also demonstrated possible harm of prophylactic hypothermia due to likelihood of increased incidence of pneumonia, bradycardia, noradrenaline, and trend toward increased ventilation days. Hyperthermia is harmful and should be avoided and promptly treated.

Induced barbiturate coma has been used in severe TBI to reduce ICP and cerebral metabolic rate to reduce secondary brain injury and it is expected to improve outcomes. Barbiturate coma is achieved with pentobarbital infusion with a target to achieve burst suppression on electroencephalography. Although barbiturate coma reduces ICP, it also causes hypotension and has not shown to improve outcomes.[17] Prophylactic use of barbiturates is discouraged; however, they may be used in patients with refractory intracranial hypertension with stable hemodynamics.[1]

Decompressive craniectomy, in refractory intracranial hypertension following TBI, has been proposed and commonly practiced. Although propofol is recommended for the control of ICP, it is not recommended for improvement in mortality or 6-month outcomes. Caution is required as high-dose propofol can produce significant morbidity.[18,19] However, two large RCTs—the DECRA trial (2011) and the RESCUEicp trial (2016)—had conflicting findings. The DECRA trial showed that early bi-fronto-temporo-parietal decompressive craniectomy reduces ICP in patients with severe TBI without mass lesions but worsens 6-month functional outcome and overall unfavorable outcome (death, vegetative state, and severe disability).

The RESCUEicp trial, on the other hand, found that use of decompressive craniectomy in patients with sustained elevation in ICP despite conventional medical therapy reduced mortality but increased the risk of long-term severe disability.

The difference in finding can be explained by the design of the trial. In DECRA trial, craniectomy was used much earlier (as soon as 15 minutes of elevated ICP) while in RESCUEicp, craniectomy was used later (more of a last line modality).

Based on findings of these trials, the 2020 updates of BTF on decompressive craniectomy has made the following recommendations:
- Secondary DC performed for *late* refractory ICP elevation is recommended to improve mortality and favorable outcomes.
- Secondary DC performed for *early* refractory ICP elevation is not recommended to improve mortality and favorable outcomes.
- Secondary DC, performed as a treatment for either early or late refractory ICP elevation, is suggested to reduce ICP and duration of intensive care.
- A large fronto-temporo-parietal DC (not less than 12 × 15 cm or 15 cm in diameter) is recommended over a small fronto-temporo-parietal DC for reduced mortality and improved neurological outcomes in patients with severe TBI.

Hemodynamic management involves maintaining CPP 60–70 mm Hg. It can be achieved using fluids and vasopressors as indicated. Normal saline is the preferred fluid as balanced salt solutions may be relatively hypotonic. Colloids including albumin should be avoided.[20] Hypertension should be treated only if it appears to be causing raised ICP with a high CPP.

Q11. What are the risk factors for post-traumatic seizures and how will you prevent it?

The post-traumatic seizures (PTS) could be early-occurring within 7 days or late-occurring after 7 days. The incidence of clinical PTS may be as high as 12% while that of subclinical PTS may be as high as 20–25%. The risk factors for early PTS include:
- GCS of less than or equal to 10
- Immediate seizures
- Post-traumatic amnesia for >30 minutes
- Linear or depressed skull fracture
- Penetrating head injury
- Subdural, epidural, or intracerebral hematoma
- Cortical contusion
- Age ≤65 years
- Chronic alcoholism

Routine seizure prophylaxis for post-traumatic seizures is commonly utilized. Seizure prophylaxis has been shown to reduce early PTS whereas not affecting late PTS. Thus, guidelines recommend use of phenytoin for seizure prophylaxis for early PTS and not for late PTS. There has been increasing use of levetiracetam for the above indication; however, there is no strong evidence to support its use over phenytoin.[1]

Q12. Describe in brief the role of steroids in traumatic brain injury (TBI).

Earlier, steroids were postulated to restore increased vascular permeability, decrease CSF production, decrease free radical-induced injury, and thereby possibly improve outcomes in TBI. However, there was no strong data to support this practice. In the year 2004, the MRC-CRASH trial was published which studied the effect of methylprednisolone on 14-day mortality in patients with TBI. The study showed increased 14-day mortality in the study group as compared to placebo.[21] A 6-month follow-up study also showed increased mortality in patients who received methylprednisolone.[22] Guidelines strongly recommend against the use of steroids in patients with TBI.[1]

Q13. Describe in brief the neurosurgical management of traumatic brain injury (TBI).

Epidural hematoma: An EDH >30 cm³ should be surgically evacuated regardless of the GCS score. An EDH <30 cm³ *and* with <15-mm thickness *and* with <5-mm midline shift in patients with a GCS score >8 *without* focal deficit can be managed nonoperatively with serial CT scanning and close neurological observation in a neurosurgical center. Patients with an acute EDH in coma (GCS score < 9) with anisocoria should undergo surgical evacuation as soon as possible.[23]

Subdural hematoma: An acute SDH with a thickness >10 mm *or* a midline shift of >5 mm on CT scan should be surgically evacuated, regardless of the patient's GCS score. All patients with acute SDH in coma (GCS < 9) should undergo ICP monitoring. A comatose patient with an SDH <10-mm thick and a midline shift <5 mm should undergo surgical evacuation of the lesion if the GCS score decreased between the time of injury and hospital admission by two or more points on the GCS and/or the patient presents with asymmetric or fixed and dilated pupils and/or the ICP exceeds 20 mm Hg. Surgical evacuation should be performed using a craniotomy with or without bone flap removal and duraplasty.[24]

The following patients with parenchymal hematomas should undergo neurosurgical intervention:

- Patients with mass lesions with progressive neurological deterioration, refractory intracranial hypertension, or mass effect on CT scan
- Patients with GCS 6–8 with frontal or temporal contusions >20 cm³ with midline shift ≥5 mm and/or cisternal compression on CT scan
- Patients with any lesion of >50 cm³ in volume. Patients with parenchymal mass lesions, who do not show evidence for neurological compromise, have controlled ICP, and no significant signs of mass effect on CT scan may be managed nonoperatively with intensive monitoring and serial imaging.

Craniotomy with evacuation of focal mass lesion, bifrontal decompressive craniectomy for refractory intracranial hypertension, and decompressive procedures (subtemporal decompression, temporal lobectomy, and hemispheric decompressive craniectomy) for refractory intracranial hypertension with impending transtentorial herniation are various neurosurgical interventions recommended in parenchymal hematomas.[25].

Q14. What steps should be taken for infection control in traumatic brain injury (TBI)?

1. Early tracheostomy is recommended to reduce mechanical ventilation days when the overall benefit is thought to outweigh the complications associated with such a procedure.
2. Antimicrobial-impregnated catheters may be considered to prevent catheter-related infections during external ventricular drainage.
3. The use of povidone iodine oral care is not recommended to reduce ventilator-associated pneumonia and may cause an increased risk of acute respiratory distress syndrome.
4. Transgastric jejunal feeding is recommended to reduce the incidence of ventilator-associated pneumonia.

Q15. Describe in brief prognostic prediction models employed in traumatic brain injury (TBI) prognostication.

There are two main prognostic prediction models utilized in the management of TBI patients: (1) the IMPACT prognostic model and (2) the CRASH prognostic model.

1. *The IMPACT prognostic model:* The International Mission for Prognosis and Analysis of Clinical Trials (IMPACT) study database has pooled data of 9,205 TBI patients from eight RCTs and three observational studies. The IMPACT prognostic model uses patient admission characteristics to predict 6-month outcomes as assessed by the GOS, which is an ordered outcome measure with five categories: (1) dead, (2) vegetative state, (3) severe disability, (4) moderate disability, and (5) good recovery. The IMPACT prognostic model has three models depending on the number and complexity of variables. The core model has three variables and consists of age, motor score, and pupillary reaction to light. The extended model has six variables including hypoxia, hypotension, and CT characteristics in addition to the core model. The laboratory model has eight variables with hemoglobin and blood glucose levels in addition to the extended model. The performance of the model improves with increasing numbers of variables.[26]

2. *The CRASH prognostic model:* The Medical Research Council–Corticosteroid Randomization After Significant Head Injury (MRC–CRASH) trial investigated the role of corticosteroids in 10,008 patients with TBI enrolled from 1994 to 2004. The CRASH prognostic model is based on data obtained from the MRC–CRASH trial. The CRASH prognostic model predicts 14-day mortality and 6-month neurological outcome on the GOS based on certain admission characteristics. It also has two models. The basic model has four variables incorporating age, GCS, pupillary reaction to light, and presence of major extracranial injury. The extended model has five variables including CT scan characteristics in addition to the basic model. It has separate models for low-income and high-income countries.[27]

REFERENCES

1. Carney N, Totten AM, O'reilly C, Ullman JS, Hawryluk GW, Bell MJ, et al. Guidelines for the management of severe traumatic brain injury. Neurosurgery. 2017;80:6-15.
2. Dutton RP, Mackenzie CF, Scalea TM. Hypotensive resuscitation during active hemorrhage: impact on in-hospital mortality. J Trauma. 2002;52:1141-6.
3. Morrison CA, Carrick MM, Norman MA, Scott BG, Welsh FJ, Tsai P, et al. Hypotensive resuscitation strategy reduces transfusion requirements and severe postoperative coagulopathy in trauma patients with hemorrhagic shock: preliminary results of a randomized controlled trial. J Trauma. 2011;70:652-63.
4. Greve MW, Zink BJ. Pathophysiology of traumatic brain injury. Mt Sinai J Med. 2009;76:97-104.
5. Saatman KE, Duhaime AC, Bullock R, Maas AI, Valadka A, Manley GT. Classification of traumatic brain injury for targeted therapies. J Neurotrauma. 2008;25:719-38.
6. Ommaya AK, Grubb RLJr, Naumann RA. Coup and contre-coup injury: observations on the mechanics of visible brain injuries in the rhesus monkey. J Neurosurg. 1971;35:503-16.
7. Perel P, Roberts I, Bouamra O, Woodford M, Mooney J, Lecky F. Intracranial bleeding in patients with traumatic brain injury: a prognostic study. BMC Emerg Med. 2009;9:15.
8. Teasdale G, Jennett B. Assessment of coma and impaired consciousness: a practical scale. Lancet. 1974;304:81-4.
9. Wijdicks EF, Bamlet WR, Maramattom BV, Manno EM, McClelland RL. Validation of a new coma scale: the FOUR score. Ann Neurol. 2005;58:585-93.
10. Marshall LF, Marshall SB, Klauber MR, Clark MV, Eisenberg HM, Jane JA, et al. A new classification of head injury based on computerized tomography. J Neurosurg. 1991;75:S14-20.
11. Maas AI, Hukkelhoven CW, Marshall LF, Steyerberg EW. Prediction of outcome in traumatic brain injury with computed tomographic characteristics: a comparison between the computed tomographic classification and combinations of computed tomographic predictors. Neurosurgery. 2005;57:1173-82.
12. Kirkness CJ, Mitchell PH, Burr RL, March KS, Newell DW. Intracranial pressure waveform analysis: clinical and research implications. J Neurosci Nurs. 2000;32:271-7.
13. Contant CF, Valadka AB, Gopinath SP, Hannay HJ, Robertson CS. Adult respiratory distress syndrome: a complication of induced hypertension after severe head injury. J Neurosurg. 2001;95:560-8.
14. Berger-Pelleiter E, Émond M, Lauzier F, Shields JF, Turgeon AF. Hypertonic saline in severe traumatic brain injury: a systematic review and meta-analysis of randomized controlled trials. CJE Med. 2016;18:112-20.
15. Andrews PJ, Sinclair HL, Rodriguez A, Harris BA, Battison CG, Rhodes JK, et al. Hypothermia for intracranial hypertension after traumatic brain injury. N Engl J Med. 2015;373:2403-12.
16. Cooper DJ, Nichol AD, Bailey M, Bernard S, Cameron PA, Pili-Floury S, et al. Effect of early sustained prophylactic hypothermia on neurologic outcomes among patients with severe traumatic brain injury: the POLAR randomized clinical trial. JAMA. 2018;320:2211-20.
17. Roberts I, Sydenham E. Barbiturates for acute traumatic brain injury. Cochrane Database Syst Rev. 2012;(12):CD000033.
18. Cooper DJ, Rosenfeld JV, Murray L, Arabi YM, Davies AR, D'urso P, et al. Decompressive craniectomy in diffuse traumatic brain injury. N Engl J Med. 2011;364:1493-502.
19. Hutchinson PJ, Kolias AG, Timofeev IS, Corteen EA, Czosnyka M, Timothy J, et al. Trial of decompressive craniectomy for traumatic intracranial hypertension. N Engl J Med. 2016;375:1119-30.
20. Myburgh J, Cooper DJ, Finfer S, Bellomo R, Norton R, Bishop N, et al. Saline or albumin for fluid resuscitation in patients with traumatic brain injury. N Engl J Med. 2007;357:874-84.
21. Roberts I, Yates D, Sandercock P, Farrell B, Wasserberg J, Lomas G, et al. Effect of intravenous corticosteroids on death within 14 days in 10008 adults with clinically significant head injury (MRC CRASH trial): randomised placebo-controlled trial. Lancet. 2004;364:1321-8.
22. Edwards P, Arango M, Balica L, Cottingham R, El-Sayed H, Farrell B, et al. Final results of MRC CRASH, a randomised placebo-controlled trial of intravenous corticosteroid in adults with head injury—outcomes at 6 months. Lancet. 2005;365:1957-9.
23. Chesnut R, Ghajar J, Gordon D. Surgical management of acute epidural hematomas. Neurosurgery. 2006;583:S2-7.
24. Bullock MR, Chesnut R, Ghajar J, Gordon D, Hartl R, Newell DW, et al. Surgical management of acute subdural hematomas. Neurosurgery. 2006;58:S2-16.
25. Bullock MR, Chesnut R, Ghajar J, Gordon D, Hartl R, Newell DW, et al. Surgical management of traumatic parenchymal lesions. Neurosurgery. 2006;58:S2-25.
26. Marmarou A, Lu J, Butcher I, McHugh GS, Mushkudiani NA, Murray GD, et al. IMPACT database of traumatic brain injury: design and description. J Neurotrauma. 2007;24:239-50.
27. Collaborators MRC CRASH Trial, Perel P, Arango M, Clayton T, Edwards P, Komolafe E, et al. Predicting outcome after traumatic brain injury: practical prognostic models based on large cohort of international patients. BMJ. 2008;336:425-9.

CHAPTER 17: Polytrauma

*Jacob George Pulinilkunnathil, Balkrishna D Nimavat, Pradnya Atul Kulkarni,
Atul Prabhakar Kulkarni, Kapil Gangadhar Zirpe*

CASE STUDY

A 33-year-old gentleman is being shifted to the intensive care unit (ICU) from the casualty with a history of car crashing into a tree in the early morning. The casualty admission notes 2 hours before show a heart rate (HR) of 140 beats/min, regular with feeble volume, and blood pressure (BP) of 80/60 mm Hg. He was tachypneic with a respiratory rate of 40 breaths/min. His temperature was 36°C, Glasgow Coma Scale (GCS) 8 (E2M3V3). The e-FAST (extended focused abdominal sonography for trauma) done in the casualty showed free fluid in the abdomen with doubtful perisplenic and perihepatic collection or bleed and a collection in the left pleural space. He had a fracture of shaft of right femur also. He was given 3 L normal saline in casualty and the arterial blood gas (ABG) at hospital admission showed pH—7.10, partial pressure of carbon dioxide (PCO_2)—46 mm Hg, partial pressure of oxygen (PO_2)—80 mm Hg, bicarbonate (HCO_3)—14 mEq/L, base excess (BE)—10, sodium (Na)—138 mEq/L, and chloride—111 mEq/L. His complete blood count (CBC) and coagulation profile revealed hemoglobin (Hb)—4.2 g/dL, platelet count—80,000 cm^3, international normalized ratio (INR)—1.76, prothrombin time (PT)—28 seconds, activated partial thromboplastin time (aPTT)—50 seconds, and fibrinogen—70 mg/dL. On arrival to the ICU, he was still disoriented, drowsy, and tachycardic (HR—156 beats/min) with peripheral oxygen saturation (SpO_2) of 89% with 6 L oxygen by a simple face mask. His BP was 78/50 mm Hg.

Q1. How to define polytrauma? Is my patient having polytrauma injuries?

Definition of polytrauma

Definition of polytrauma evolves over time.

According to Berlin definition of polytrauma (2014), polytrauma is defined as "a significant injury of three or more points in two or more body regions with one or more variables from five physiological parameters, namely:

1. Unconsciousness (GCS score ≤8)
2. Acidosis (BE ≤–6.0)
3. Coagulopathy (partial thromboplastin time ≥40 seconds or INR ≥1.4)
4. Age (≥70 years)
5. Hypotension [systolic blood pressure (SBP) ≤90 mm Hg]

Q2. How will you assess and resuscitate a polytrauma patient?

This is a case of polytrauma and has presented in hemorrhagic shock (**Table 1**). Shock is defined as a state

TABLE 1: Classification of hemorrhagic shock.

Physiologic parameters	Class 1	Class 2	Class 3	Class 4
Heart rate	Mild tachycardia	Tachycardia	Tachycardia	Tachycardia
Pulse pressure	Normal	Decreased	Decreased	Decreased
Hypotension	Absent	Absent	Present	Present
Tachypnea	Absent	Absent	Present	Present
Glasgow Coma Scale (GCS)	Normal	Normal	Decreased	Decreased
Oliguria	Absent	Absent	Present	Present
Base excess (base deficit)	0 to –2 mEq/L	–2 to –6 mEq/L	–6 to 10 mEq/L	–10 mEq/L or less
Estimated blood loss	<15% of blood volume	15–30% of blood volume	30–40% of blood volume	>40% of blood volume
Need for blood	Unlikely	Likely, coalesce with surgeon	Call for matched blood products	Activate massive transfusion protocol

where the cardiac output is inadequate to meet the body's demands, which results in inadequate organ perfusion and tissue oxygenation. Management of this patient requires a team approach that is rapid, focused, and structured with the aim of simultaneous resuscitation and treatment. A multidisciplinary trauma team with a team leader should be formed and each member should be assigned a specific role. The trauma team will then undertake the primary survey, secondary survey, and tertiary survey as per Advanced Trauma Life Support (ATLS) protocols.[1]

Usually, the resuscitation for stable medical patients follows the sequence of a good history-taking, detailed and meticulous head-to-toe physical examination after which a differential diagnosis is derived, which is further validated by investigations to arrive at the final diagnosis. However, in trauma, this approach is abandoned, and the primary aim is to prevent death from whatever cause. The ATLS has been recently modified and updated. **Box 1** summarizes the changes that have been suggested in the 10th edition of Advanced Trauma Life Support (ATLS).

Out of the multiple issues that the patient might have, the one that is of the greatest threat to life is addressed first and treatment is not withheld because the diagnosis is uncertain. An in-depth history is not essential and along with primary survey, resuscitation should take place simultaneously. Two large-bore cannulas should be used to secure the intravenous (IV) access. Blood samples should be collected for CBC, blood grouping and cross-matching, renal and liver function tests, ABG, and electrolytes.

The primary survey is designed to assess and treat any life-threatening injuries in a prioritized sequence. In practice, these steps are frequently accomplished simultaneously **(Table 2)**. Continuous electrocardiography (ECG) and saturation measurement by pulse oximetry, and extended focused abdominal sonography for trauma (e-FAST) are also used as adjuncts to primary survey.

Once the patient is stabilized, a detailed head-to-toe examination is carried out along with appropriate radiographic studies. This is followed by tertiary assessment for any injuries missed during primary and secondary survey. The patient should be evaluated for possible complications of polytrauma according to the mechanism of injury. For example, a patient presenting with a history of fall from height is usually associated with axial spine injury, calcaneal injury/bilateral lower limb injury, and pelvic injury. Head-on collisions in motor vehicle accidents are associated with steering injury/dashboard injury (flail chest, traumatic aortic injury, pneumothorax, and myocardial contusion) and windscreen injury (facial injury and head injury). Side injury in motor vehicle accidents is associated with diaphragmatic

BOX 1: Changes in the revised edition of Advanced Trauma Life Support (ATLS).

- Emphasis on team management of trauma
- Limits the volume of initial resuscitation to 1 L of crystalloids
- Early recognition of shock and emphasis on early initiation of massive transfusion protocols, if needed
- New emphasis of the concept of base excess (base deficit) in hemorrhagic shock classification
- Tranexamic acid 1 g to be bolused at site and followed up with 1 g over 10 minutes after 8 hours
- Use of tourniquet to control bleeding
- Increased importance on the concept of damage control surgery
- Drug-assisted intubation suggested instead of rapid sequence intubation
- Use of ultrasound to rule out pneumothorax
- Shift of the preferred position for needle thoracostomy to fifth intercostal space slightly anterior to midaxillary line (except in pediatrics)
- Preference of smaller chest tube sizes for drainage of pneumothorax or hemopneumothorax
- Addition of a new algorithm for traumatic cardiac arrest
- Early management for aortic injury, with addition of beta blocker, if permissible
- Affirmation that prostate examination not sensitive to diagnose urethral injury
- To consider preperitoneal packing
- Use of exclusion rules for imaging of cervical spine (NEXUS criteria and Canadian C-Spine rule)
- Clarification of terms in Glasgow Coma Scale
- Specific targets for resuscitation of traumatic brain injury (blood pressure, temperature, hemoglobin, INR, platelets, serum sodium, glucose, PaO_2, $PaCO_2$, pH, cerebral perfusion pressure, intracranial pressure, pulse oximetry, $PbtO_2$)
- Use of PECARN rule in pediatric head trauma
- Spinal immobilization changed to spinal motion restriction
- Time on spinal boards to be reconsidered during resuscitation to prevent pressure ulcers
- Lower threshold to image elderly victims
- In case of referral to another hospital is required—to avoid unnecessary investigation, and unnecessary procedures
- Use of ABC–SBAR for communication

(ABC–SBAR: airway, breathing, circulation followed by situation, background, assessment, and recommendation; INR: international normalized ratio; NEXUS: National Emergency X-Radiography Utilization Study; PaO_2: partial pressure of arterial oxygen; $PaCO_2$: partial pressure of arterial carbon dioxide; $PbtO_2$: brain tissue oxygenation; PECARN: Pediatric Emergency Care Applied Research Network; pH: potential of hydrogen)

injury, abdominal visceral injury, and pelvic and lower limb fractures. Injury with impact from behind leads to head injury and cervical spine (C-spine) injury. Penetrating injury/gunshot injury depends on area involved and the underlying structures, i.e., thoracic area (hemothorax and pneumothorax) and abdomen (solid organ injury such as

TABLE 2: Primary survey: the Airway, Breathing, Circulation, Disability and Exposure (ABCDE) approach.

Steps	Significance	In our patient	Comment
Airway with cervical spine clearance	• The airway is assessed for patency, with precaution for cervical spine immobilization • Apply chin lift or jaw thrust maneuver, if airway is obstructed • Search for foreign bodies, secretions, and remove them, if present (and burns in case of thermal injuries) • Look for facial fractures or airway lacerations • Apply a cervical spine collar that is to be opened only when airway management is necessary • Provide manual in-line stabilization of the spine, if intubation is required	• Start oxygen and prepare for a difficult airway—anatomically and physiologically. Two operators, with the senior most person to intubate • Start vasopressors, if needed • Drug-assisted intubation—etomidate, fentanyl and rocuronium or succinylcholine	• Our patient does not seem to be a fluid responder as there is no improvement in hemodynamics after 3 L of crystalloids. Call for blood • Ketamine may not increase the intracranial pressure (ICP) as considered previously. Rather, it might reduce the ICP and improve cerebral perfusion pressure and systemic blood pressure.[2] As the patient is already hypotensive, propofol or benzodiazepines is not preferred. Selection of drugs depends upon availability and experience of the operator with the aim of avoiding further hypotension during intubation
Breathing and ventilation	• Assess for adequate ventilation. Expose the neck and chest of the patient. Assess for jugular venous distention, tracheal shift, and chest wall movements. Perform percussion and auscultation • Rule out a tension pneumothorax, massive hemothorax, open pneumothorax, and airway injuries	• e-FAST scan in our patient has revealed left-sided pleural effusion—most probably hemothorax. Prepare for ICD insertion urgently • Liaise with cardiothoracic surgeon for indications of emergent thoracotomy	Indication for urgent thoracotomy after ICD insertion includes an intercostal drain output of approximately 1,500 mL blood on insertion, or a drain output of >250 mL of blood drainage/hour for 3 consecutive hours
Circulation	Assess for adequacy of circulation—assess for any blood loss and adequacy of cardiac output	Common causes of hypotension in trauma include bleeding, cardiac tamponade, and tension pneumothorax	• Once obstructive shock and neurogenic shock are ruled out, the common areas of internal hemorrhage such as the thorax, abdomen retroperitoneum, pelvis, and long bones should be rechecked for blood collection. Physical examination and imaging [e.g., chest X-ray, pelvic X-ray, extended focused abdominal sonography for trauma (e-FAST), and diagnostic peritoneal lavage (DPL)] might be used as adjuncts to diagnose occult bleeding • IV crystalloids should be administered either prewarmed to 37°C or through fluid warming devices. After administration of a bolus of 1 L of an isotonic solution, the response must be assessed, and if the patient is unresponsive to initial crystalloid therapy, he or she should receive a blood transfusion
Disability	Assess the patient for level of consciousness, pupillary size and reaction, presence of lateralizing signs, and spinal cord injury level, if any	Primary injury to the brain and other causes such as hypoxia, hypotension, and drugs such as narcotics need to be ruled out, if the GCS is low	Recheck the blood glucose level, consider dextrose, naloxone, oxygen, and thiamine as per the situation, especially if the patient is drowsy. If traumatic brain injury is suspected, inform a neurosurgeon immediately and care should be taken to prevent secondary brain injury from hypoxia, hypotension, and hypo- or hyperglycemia

Contd...

Contd...

Steps	Significance	In our patient	Comment
Exposure and environment control	Measure the patients' body temperature and try to maintain normothermia	Exposure to cold environment, hypovolemic shock, and resuscitation with cold fluids and blood products all can result in hypothermia	Measures need to be taken to prevent unnecessary exposure to hypothermic environment. After proper examination, ensure that the patient is covered adequately so that he is kept warm. Resuscitation fluids should be prewarmed before administering to the patient

(GCS: Glasgow Coma Scale; IV: intravenous)

splenic, liver, or hollow viscera injury). Lower limb fractures lead to complications, such as crush injury, compartment syndrome, rhabdomyolysis, fat embolism syndrome (FES), thromboembolic events, and vascular injury.

Q3. What are the scoring systems commonly used in trauma?

Scoring systems in the early clinical setting of trauma aid as a guide to clinical management and prognostication and inpatient triage. Some scoring systems also predict the estimated hospital length of stay and patient morbidity. Though not specific to trauma, the GCS is commonly used and it aids in decision-making like the need for airway control. The commonly described specific injury scoring systems are the Injury Severity Score (ISS), Trauma score, Revised Trauma score, APACHE (Acute Physiology and Chronic Health Evaluation) score, Acute Trauma Index, Abbreviated Injury Scale, Modified Injury Severity Score, Trauma and Injury Severity Score, A Severity Characteristic of Trauma (ASCOT), etc.[3]

Q4. What are the indications of cervical protection with cervical collar? Does the abovementioned patient require cervical collar or evaluation of spine?

The evidence for cervical cord protection for preventing C-spine injury is vague. Of all patients admitted with brain injury, about 5% will have an added spinal cord injury and about 2.5% will have a cervical cord injury.[4] In these patients, spinal cord movements can worsen the neurological damage, apart from the ongoing damage from ischemia or edema progression. However, if the cervical collar is not fixed properly, it can still permit spinal cord injury to happen while the treating personnel might be under a false impression of security. Cervical collars are not without complications and cause severe discomfort for the patients. They can impair the attempts to secure the airway and delay intubations. The cervical collar can also cause pressure ulcers, hamper proper examination of the patient, compress the neck veins reducing venous return, and significantly increase the intracranial pressure (ICP). Hence, cervical collar should be retained only in patients in whom a cervical cord injury cannot be ruled out even after adequate clinicoradiological examination.

In conscious patients, without any other distracting injuries, the absence of any neurological deficit, pain or tenderness along the spine, and during a full range of voluntary movements rule out spinal cord injury. However, in patients who are unconscious, or those who have neurological deficits, ruling out a cervical cord injury is more difficult. A comprehensive radiological imaging, interpreted by an expert, is required and the cervical collar is retained until a comprehensive clinical evaluation of the C-spine including a complete neurological assessment, palpation, and voluntary movement in all planes have been checked and found to be normal.

Radiographic evaluation of the C-spine is done with either a multidetector computed tomography (MDCT) from the occiput to T1 or by ordering for lateral, anteroposterior (AP), and open-mouth odontoid X-rays. These radiological evaluations should be done only by a person qualified for the same. To identify the patents in whom C-spine imaging can be safely avoided, the National Emergency X-radiography Utilization Study (NEXUS) Low-risk Criteria, or Canadian C-Spine Rule (CCR) have been put forward **(Table 3)**.[5]

In view of persistent shock, hypoxia, and tachypnea, it was decided to intubate the patient with drug-assisted intubation (DAI), resuscitate the patient with blood and blood products, and insert a left-sided intercostal drain.

Q5. How do you classify fluid responders in trauma and why?

Control of external bleeding and resuscitation should occur simultaneously. Resuscitation of trauma victim starts with the administration of 1 L of warmed crystalloid after which the response to fluids is assessed. Accordingly, they are classified as fluid responders, transient responders, and nonresponders[1] **(Table 4)**. In the case of a lack of adequate response to fluid, large-volume fluid resuscitation is not recommended, and these patients may require early administration of blood and blood products or surgical or

TABLE 3: Exclusion rules for cervical spine (C-spine) imaging.

The National Emergency X-radiography Utilization Study (NEXUS) Criteria	The Canadian C-Spine Rule
[N—neurodeficit, E—EtOH intoxication, X—extremity injury, U—unable to provide history (altered level of consciousness), S—spinal tenderness (midline)] Radiologic imaging is not required, if there is: • No cervical spine tenderness • Patient is fully conscious with no signs of intoxication (no smell of alcohol) • Fully alert (Glasgow Coma Scale score >14, oriented to person, place, time, or events, intact recent memory, prompt and appropriate response to external stimuli) • No neurological deficits and no injuries which might distract the patient during clinical examination Another mnemonic—NSAID: • Neurodeficit • Spinal tenderness (in C-spine) • Alertness • Intoxication • Distracting injury	Radiologic imaging is not required in a cooperative patient, if: • Absence of high-risk factors such as age <65 years, absent paresthesia or neurological defects, absent dangerous mechanism of injury • Presence of any low-risk factors such as low-risk collision, ambulatory patient who can sit with no immediate neck pain or spinal tenderness • The patient can rotate their head without significant pain to 45°

radiologic procedures to control the bleeding. Large-volume infusion of >1.5 L of crystalloid fluid has been associated with increased mortality in trauma victims—while up to 1 liter of crystalloid is probably safe.[6] Hence, the current ATLS recommends considering early blood and blood products, if 1 L of crystalloid fails to attain adequate hemodynamic response.

The patient had a coagulation profile showing an INR—1.76, PT—28 seconds, aPTT—50 seconds, and fibrinogen—70 mg/dL.

Q6. How will you manage/approach this patient? Briefly describe trauma-induced coagulopathy (TIC) and massive transfusion.

During trauma, the internal milieu of inflammation, anticoagulation, and cellular dysfunction gives rise to TIC. TIC occurs due to tissue hypoperfusion from blood loss and severe anatomical tissue injury and is classically described in three phases by Cap and Hunt.[7] Initially as tissue injury and/or tissue hypoperfusion occurs, there is activation of hemostatic pathways and increased fibrinolysis. This phase is called the phase of acute traumatic coagulopathy. This is followed by the second phase where iatrogenic factors during resuscitation can worsen coagulopathy (dilutional coagulopathy), and the third phase ensues—which is a prothrombotic state predisposing to venous thromboembolism.[8] The first phase of TIC is acute traumatic coagulopathy, which is independent of iatrogenic factors. It in early, within minutes after the injury and is seen even at admission to emergency room in up to 25–35% of trauma patients.[9] The key processes of TIC development include dysfunction of natural anticoagulant mechanisms, platelet dysfunction, fibrinogen consumption, and

TABLE 4: Types of responders to fluids.

Types of responders	Vital signs	Estimated blood loss	Need for blood	Other interventions required
Rapid responders	Return to normal	<15%	Urgent need for blood is unlikely	Discuss with the surgeon in case an operative intervention is required
Transient responders	Return to normal and then fall back to the previous or worse values	15–40%, ongoing bleed is a possibility	Might need blood transfusion—arrange preferably group-specific blood	Urgent discussion with interventional radiologist and surgeon regarding further investigation and management of a possible ongoing bleed
Nonresponders or minimal responders	Remains abnormal always	>40%, unless other etiologies of shock are present Rule out obstructive shock and neurogenic shock	Call for urgent blood—if cross-matched blood is unavailable, type O packed red blood cells (pRBCs) and AB plasma are given. Rh-negative pRBCs are preferred for young females	Urgent surgical intervention; use further monitoring such as echo and ultrasound to differentiate the type of shock

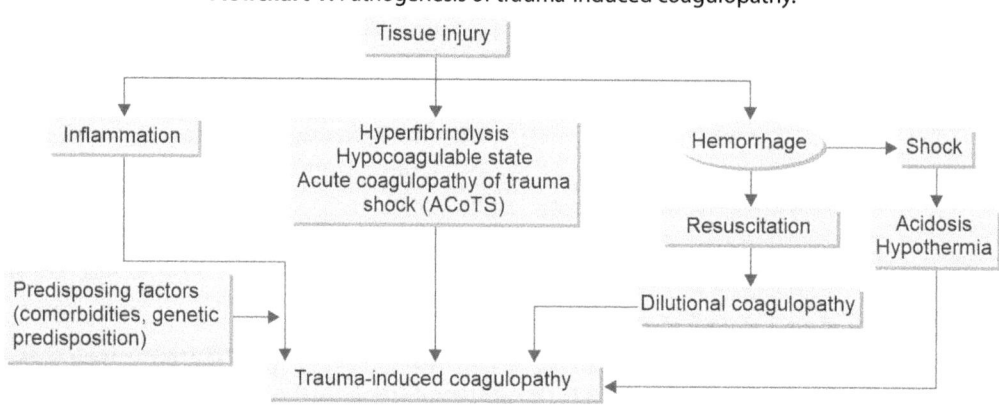

Flowchart 1: Pathogenesis of trauma-induced coagulopathy.

hyperfibrinolysis, which are further worsened by dilution of blood from resuscitation fluids. Environmental hypothermia and acidosis can modulate clot formation, adding more layers of complexity to TIC. When present, TIC is strongly associated with a four- to fivefold increased risk of mortality **(Flowchart 1)**.[8,10]

Q7. What can be done to prevent TIC?

In patients who do not require massive transfusion, transfusion may be guided by coagulation studies, along with fibrinogen and platelet levels. In cases where there is a doubt or strong history of using a newer anticoagulant agent or antiplatelet agents, coagulation should be monitored with bedside measures like thromboelastography (TEG) or rotational thromboelastometry (ROTEM) (if available) apart from the normal coagulation tests. Early administration of packed red blood cells (pRBCs), plasma, and platelets in a balanced ratio helps to minimize excessive crystalloid administration and may improve patient survival.[11] This approach has been termed as "balanced", "hemostatic" resuscitation. Efforts should be made to rapidly control the bleeding and reduce the detrimental effects of coagulopathy, hypothermia, and acidosis.

The European guideline on management of major bleeding and coagulopathy put forward the following recommendations for managing patients presenting with TIC. On admission, do a rapid initial assessment and assess the extent of traumatic hemorrhage. Patients presenting with shock should be identified early and urgent attempts to identify the source of bleeding should be made. For all patients, the coagulation profile, hematocrit, serum lactate, and base deficit should be assessed, and any significant history of anticoagulant therapy should be elicited. Patients should be resuscitated while preventing hypothermia, until bleeding has stopped and the Hb level of 7–9 g/dL is attained. Tranexamic acid (TXA)—1 g should be initiated and, if bolused on site, a second bolus may be added in 8 hours.

In the absence of traumatic brain injury, a target SBP of 80–90 mm Hg should be achieved. If a surgical intervention is required to control the bleed or to attend any life-threatening emergencies, then preferably only a damage control surgery should be performed. For massive bleeding, the massive transfusion protocol (MTP) should be activated, and target fibrinogen level and platelet level should be maintained.[12]

Q8. What is massive transfusion (in trauma)?

A subset of patients with shock will require massive transfusion, defined as "requirement of >10 units of pRBCs within the first 24 hours of admission" or "requirement of more than four packed cells in an hour with anticipation of ongoing need" or "the requirement to replace >50% of the estimated blood volume with blood and blood products within 3 hours of admission".[13,14] Massive transfusion aims not only at replacement of the depleted intravascular volume, but also to prevent further blood loss by achieving homeostasis early and preventing or treating TIC. Early identification of patients requiring massive transfusion is important as they may rapidly progress to coagulopathy. Implementation of MTP guidelines decreases both the mortality and the overall amount of blood requirement due to better resuscitation. Significant difference in mortality was demonstrated by improving the compliance with timely activation and type of the product given.[15] Cotton et al. found that both the short-term and long-term survivals are increased when MTP is initiated early in the course—in the emergency room rather than in the operating room.[16] Massive transfusion though lifesaving is also associated with severe complications **(Box 2)**.[17] Initiation of MTP requires precision—either using scoring systems or by the clinical gestalt. Pommerening et al. showed that the clinical gestalt has a sensitivity and specificity of roughly 66% and a positive predictive value (PPV) of 35% and a negative predictive value (NPV) of 86%.[18,19] Clinical gestalt, therefore, should be considered as a poor screening test for massive transfusion that may result in overtransfusion but is a fair predictor of predicting patients who might not require one. Several scoring systems have been proposed to predict the need for massive transfusion, but each has its own limitations. The assessment of blood consumption (ABC) score was developed by Cotton et al. as a simple bedside tool, which gives one point for each of the following: mechanism of trauma—penetrating or not, SBP <90 mm Hg or not, presence of tachycardia >120 beats/min, and a positive scan on e-FAST examination.[20] An ABC score of ≥2 points had a sensitivity of 75–90%, and specificity of 67–86% to predict the need of massive transfusion within 24 hours. The advantage of ABC score over other scores is that it requires no laboratory data, can be determined within minutes of patient arrival, and can be easily recalculated over time. Various other scoring systems **(Table 5)** have been proposed but none of them have shown good reliability in

BOX 2: Complications of massive transfusion.

- Transfusion-associated acute lung injury (TRALI)
- Acute respiratory distress syndrome (ARDS)
- Transfusion-associated cardiac overload (TACO)
- Transfusion-associated immunomodulation (TRIM)
- Transmission of infections
- Electrolyte abnormalities—hypokalemia, hyperkalemia, hypocalcemia
- Citrate toxicity
- Hypothermia
- Compartment syndrome
- Dilutional coagulopathy
- Hemolytic transfusion reactions
- Post-transfusion graft-versus-host disease

TABLE 5: Scores used to predict need for massive transfusion (MT).

Score	Parameters assessed
Trauma-Associated Severe Hemorrhage (TASH) score	Fractures of the extremity or pelvis, heart rate, systolic blood pressure, gender, hemoglobin, base excess (BE), a positive e-FAST examination; a TASH score ≥16 points indicates the probability of requiring MT is >50%
Assessment of Blood Consumption (ABC)	• Mechanism of injury—penetrating injury or not tachycardia with a heart rate of 120 beats/min or greater • Hypotension with systolic blood pressure of 90 mm Hg or less; a positive result on e-FAST scan
Emergency Transfusion Score (ETS)	Age 20–60 or >60 years, admission from scene, mechanism of injury (road traffic accident or fall from a height of >3 meters), systolic blood pressure greater or <90 mm Hg, e-FAST positive, unstable pelvic ring fracture on clinical examination
Prince of Wales Hospital score (Rainer score)	• Tachycardia >120 beats/min, hypotension with systolic blood pressure ≤90 mm Hg, a low Glasgow Coma Scale (GCS) <8; presence of a displaced pelvic fracture, a positive radiologic imaging (CT scan or ultrasound) positive for fluid, base deficit >5 mmol/L and anemia with hemoglobin (Hb) ≤7 g/dL (10 points) • A score >6 indicates the possibility for MT
Trauma-Induced Coagulopathy Clinical Score (TICCS)	TICCS is based on the severity of injury with points assigned for severity of injury, blood pressure, and extent of body injury
Traumatic Bleeding Severity Score (TBSS)	Ranges from 0 to 57, with points assigned for age, gender, systolic blood pressure, positive e-FAST scan, presence of a pelvic fracture and serum lactate
Shock Index	Ratio of heart rate to systolic blood pressure
Leemann et al.	Based on coagulation parameters such as ROTEM, based on the values obtained—such as A5, A10, maximum clot firmness, etc.
Massive Transfusion score	Derived from the PROMMTT data, with points scored for each of the seven variables such as tachycardia >120 beats/min, an INR >1.5, systolic blood pressure <90 mm Hg, a Hb level <11 g/dL, a base deficit of >6, a positive e-FAST report, and mechanism of trauma (penetrating trauma); score ranges from 0 to 7 and a value <2 is unlikely to require a blood transfusion
The Vandromme score	Clinical parameters on admission including a blood lactate of >5 mmol/L, baseline tachycardia >105 beats/min, an elevated INR >1.5, Hb <11 g/dL, and hypotension with systolic blood pressure <110 mm Hg
Code red	Simple bedside tool consisting of three variables—suspicion or evidence of active hemorrhage, hypotension with systolic blood pressure <90 mm Hg, and failure of hypotension to respond to fluids
Larson score	Consists of four variables—admission systolic blood pressure, heart rate, Hb, and base deficit
McLaughlin score	Uses a complex mathematical equation using the variables such as tachycardia >105 beats/min, hypotension with systolic blood pressure <110 mm Hg, ABG showing a pH <7.2 and hematocrit <32.0%
The coagulopathy of severe trauma (COAST) score	Points are given for entrapment of body, hypothermia, hypotension, injury to abdominal or pelvic content, and chest decompression

(ABG: arterial blood gas; e-FAST: extended focused abdominal sonography for trauma; INR: international normalized ratio; PROMMTT: Prospective, Observational, Multicenter, Major Trauma Transfusion; ROTEM: rotational thromboelastometry)

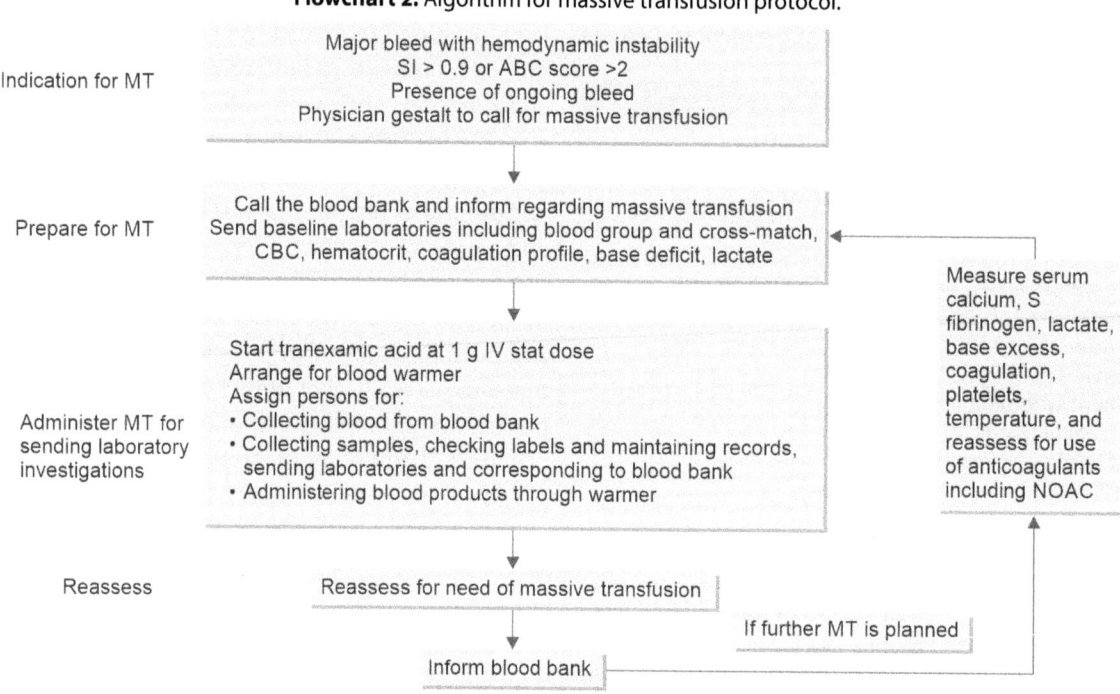

Flowchart 2: Algorithm for massive transfusion protocol.

(CBC: complete blood count; IV: intravenous; MT: massive transfusion; NOAC: newer oral anticoagulant; SI: Shock Index; S fibrinogen: serum fibrinogen)

predicting the need of massive transfusion in day-to-day practice. In research settings, complex scoring systems might show an increased efficacy; however, they lack utility in a busy trauma care system.[19,21,22] Once MTP is initiated, a team work is initiated with every team member having assigned roles **(Flowchart 2)**.

This definition of massive transfusion is currently being replaced by other terminologies, such as resuscitation intensity, the critical administration threshold (CAT), and substantial bleeding. This is because massive transfusion does not consider the critically ill patient having a higher mortality, requiring fluid resuscitation, transfusions of other blood products, or transfusion of pRBCs, but not meeting the definition of massive transfusion. The CAT is defined as the requirement of at least three units of pRBC in *any* 1 hour time period during the initial 24 hours of trauma. CAT is a more sensitive predictor of mortality than the older MTP definition, can be obtained prospectively, can be used as a marker of mortality, and can suggest the need for abbreviated instead of definitive laparotomy.[23]

Substantial bleeding is defined as the need of one red blood cell (RBC) unit within 2 hours and five RBC units or death from hemorrhage within 4 hours of admission.[22] This implies the severity of blood loss rather than a preset transfusion volume. The advantage of this definition is that it includes patients requiring large-volume transfusion early in their resuscitation and also those who do not meet the conventional transfusion definitions. However, this term also does not consider transfusion of colloids, crystalloids, or other blood products, such as fresh frozen plasma or platelets and transfusion amounts.

Resuscitation intensity is defined as the number of all resuscitative units infused within half an hour of patient arrival.[24] As per this criteria, 1 L of crystalloid, half liter of colloid, one unit of packed cells, one unit of plasma, and every unit of apheresis platelets are all considered as resuscitation fluid. Patients requiring more than four units of resuscitation fluid within 30 minutes of arrival had a twofold increase in mortality that remained elevated even after 24 hours.[24]

Fixed ratio transfusion: The evidence for a 1:1 transfusion ratio stems from a landmark study 2007 by Borgman et al. In this retrospective chart review at a military hospital, they found that those patients who received transfusions with a high plasma to RBC ratio had higher survival rates compared with those who received transfusions with a low plasma to RBC ratio.[25] However, this study was criticized for high risk of bias and noncomparable baseline variables. Similar data from civilian trauma also endorsed a high plasma to pRBCs transfusion ratio although the flaws of this trial remain the same.[26] The Pragmatic Randomized Optimal Platelet and Plasma Ratios (PROPPR) trial in 2015 that randomized patients to 1:1:1 or 1:2:1 transfusion protocol showed similar 30-day mortality although there was more exsanguination deaths in the low-ratio group.[27] The treatment group did not report an increase in transfusion-related complications also suggesting the safety of high fixed transfusion ratios.

TABLE 6: Comparison of PROMMTT (Prospective, Observational, Multicenter, Major Trauma Transfusion) and PROPPR (Pragmatic Randomized Optimal Platelet and Plasma Ratios) trials.

	PROMMTT, 2013	PROPPR, 2015
Study design	Prospective observational study	Randomized control study
Plasma:RBC	1:1 versus 1:2	1:1:1 versus 1:2:1
Number of patients	905	680
Results	The ratio of plasma to red blood cells (RBCs) and platelet to RBCs ratios were not constant in the initial 24 hours. An increased plasma to RBCs and platelet to RBCs ratios were associated with reduced 6-hour mortality, after 24 hours, these ratios were not associated with mortality.	No significant differences in mortality at 24 hours or at 30 days; exsanguination was significantly decreased in the 1:1:1 group; no differences in complications across both groups
Conclusion	Higher ratio of plasma to RBC reduces 6-hour mortality although there was no difference in 24-hour mortality in patients who required more than three blood products.	• No difference in 24-hour or 30-day mortality; no increased complications due to transfusion • Patients who received blood products in the ratio 1:1:1 had early hemostasis and less death from exsanguination in 24 hours.

A comparison of PROPRR and Prospective, Observational, Multicenter, Major Trauma Transfusion (PROMMTT) 2013 is given in **Table 6**.

In our patient, who is a nonresponder and has coagulopathy, it was decided to call for blood and activate the MTP. Fixed ratio blood products were called for and a simultaneous call to the surgeons was made for damage control surgery.

Q9. As resuscitation is ongoing, what adjunct treatment may be tried in addition to massive transfusion?

Adjuncts to massive transfusion: In addition to a balanced hemostatic resuscitation, other pharmacologic adjuncts such as TXA, supplemental fibrinogen, recombinant factor VII (rFVIIa), and prothrombin complex concentrate (PCC, also known as factor IX complex, containing clotting factors II, IX, and X) have been suggested to reduce bleeding and transfusion-related complications.

Tranexamic acid is a lysine analog that reversibly binds to the lysine receptor sites on plasminogen causing a competitive inhibition of plasminogen, resulting in inhibition of fibrinolysis and stabilization of the clot. CRASH-2 (Clinical Randomization of Antifibrinolytics in Significant Hemorrhage 2) trial demonstrated an improvement in all-cause mortality and mortality attributed to hemorrhage when TXA was used in adult patients with traumatic hemorrhage within 3 hours from time of injury.[28] Similar reports have also been reported from the MATTERs (Military Application of Tranexamic Acid in Trauma Emergency Resuscitation) and PED-TRAX (Pediatric Trauma and Tranexamic Acid) trials.[29,30] TXA should be administered early, within 3 hours and preferably in the subset of patients who present with the lethal triad of acidosis, hypothermia, coagulopathy, with an absolute or relative thrombocytopenia or those with a lysis at 30 minutes (LY30) >3% in TEG, and those with a severe hemorrhagic shock with SBP <75 mm Hg.[31] As the hemostatic abnormalities change from the hyperfibrinolysis in the early phase to fibrinolytic shutdown in the late stages, administration of TXA after the initial 3 hours of trauma may be counterproductive.[32] Rapid administration of TXA might result in hypotension and should be avoided as it might further accentuate hypotension.[33]

Apart from TXA, the use of fibrinogen, rFVIIa, and PCC has also been studied in massive transfusion. Factor VIIa may be administered on a case-by-case basis when the hemorrhage continues even after hemostasis has been achieved by surgical and/or radiological means and the other hematologic parameters such as hematocrit, platelets, coagulation studies, calcium levels, and pH are normalized. Overall, treatment with rFVIIa is associated with a reduced requirement for blood and blood products and reduced incidence of multiorgan failure. Similarly, PCC may be considered in case of patients who are on novel anticoagulants, or those who are exsanguinating in spite of best medical measures, although the routine use cannot be recommended.

Q10. Does the age of transfused RBC make a difference in outcome of critically ill patients or patients with trauma? What are storage lesions?

Storage of RBC results in significant structural and biochemical changes collectively called as storage lesion. With storage, the 2,3-diphosphoglycerate (2,3-DPG) in RBC is progressively depleted, and this results in an increased affinity of Hb for oxygen, which shifts the oxygen Hb curve to the left. This hampers the release of oxygen to the tissues till the 2,3-DPG stores are replenished. During storage, RBC also undergoes membrane changes that make it more prone for sequestration and hemolysis, as it flows across

TABLE 7: Biochemical abnormalities on storage of packed red blood cells (RBCs).

Variables		Duration of blood storage		
Biochemical abnormalities on storage	Immediate	Within a week	Within 2 weeks	By 6 weeks
Potassium (mmol/L)	3.9 ± 0.6	13.6 ± 1.7	24.5 ± 2.1	46.6 ± 4.1
Lactate (mmol/L)	3.6 ± 0.4	7.8 ± 0.7	17.2 ± 2.5	34.5 ± 4.4
pH	6.8 ± 0.03	6.74 ± 0.03	6.64 ± 0.02	6.37 ± 0.04
Iron (µmol/L)	3.8 ± 0.9	6.8 ± 2.9	7.6 ± 1.6	14.2 ± 2.9
% of irreversible deformed RBC	—	8.4 ± 1.6	14.7 ± 2.6	29.9 ± 4.0

Source: Adapted and modified from Aubron et al.[34]

TABLE 8: Trials comparing transfusion of old versus fresh blood.

Author, trial, year	Number of subjects	% of patients with trauma	Comparison	Result
Steiner et al., RECESS trial, 2015[38]	1,098 patients of postoperative CTVS patients CTVS including CPB	Nil	<10 days versus >21 days	No difference in MODS
Lacroix et al., ABLE trial, 2015[39]	2,430	15% patients with trauma	Fresh blood of <8 days compared with older blood	No mortality benefit
Heddle et al., INFORM trial, 2016[40]	20,858	13% patients with trauma	Freshest available blood versus the oldest available	No mortality benefit
Cooper et al., TRANSFUSE, 2017[41]	4,919	10% patients with trauma	Freshest available RBC versus standard issue	No difference in 90-day mortality

(ABLE: Age of Blood Evaluation; CPB: cardiopulmonary bypass; CTVS: cardiothoracic valvular surgery; INFORM: Informing Fresh versus Old Red Cell Management; MODS: multiple organ dysfunction syndrome; RECESS: Red-Cell Storage Duration Study; RBC: red blood cell; TRANSFUSE: Transfusion versus Fresher Red-Cell Use in Intensive Care)

microcapillaries. Adenosine triphosphate (ATP) depletion, lipid peroxidation, lactic acidosis, and hyperkalemia are other significant changes that occur with storage.[34] The biochemical changes that occur in pRBCs during storage are shown in **Table 7**.[34]

A retrospective study done in postoperative cardiac surgery patients, suggested significantly increased postoperative complications, and an increased short-term and long-term mortality in patients who received blood stored for >2 weeks. However, this finding could not be replicated in prospective trials in various patient populations.[35]

In premature infants, the ARIPI (Age of Red Blood Cells in Premature Infants) trial concluded that RBCs stored for 7 days or less, as compared with the standard of care, had no difference with respect to major nosocomial infection or organ dysfunction among premature infants with birth weights <1,250 g.[36] The data regarding age of pRBCs transfused in patients with trauma remain sparse and the evidence so far does not support fresh blood over old blood.[37]

A summary of the similar trials in critical care patients that compared fresh versus old blood has been summarized in **Table 8**.

Q11. What is lethal triad in trauma patient?
As early as in 1982, it was proposed that hypothermia, acidosis, and coagulopathy might be a triad of complicating factors in patients with traumatic injuries that resulted in poor patient outcome; warranting the same attention as for management of injuries and shock.[42] This observation was later confirmed by numerous researchers naming it as the lethal triad of death. A description of the lethal triad of death is given in the **Table 9**.

As described, it is important to control hypothermia, acidosis, and the coagulopathy along with other surgical or medical interventions. Care should be taken to use warm blood and blood products as well as warm crystalloids for resuscitation. Avoid unnecessarily prolonged exposure to the environment and cover all patients once the primary survey is over. Lactic acidosis is prevented and treated by adequate,

TABLE 9: The lethal triad.		
Pathology	**Cause**	**Effect**
Hypothermia	• Hypovolemic (hemorrhagic) shock, loss of ability to regulate the core temperature, e.g., traumatic brain injuries, alcohol intoxication, extremes of age, etc. • Prolonged exposure to cold environment; loss of protective skin—burns • Resuscitation with fluids that are hypothermic to the patient core temperature	• It affects the temperature-dependent enzymatic reactions of the coagulation system—predisposing to coagulopathy and hemorrhage • It reduces the myocardial performance and cardiac output. It reduces the response to catecholamines • It increases the vulnerability to arrhythmias such as atrial fibrillation and atrial flutter • It reduces the phagocytic efficacy of the neutrophils predisposing to infections and sepsis
Acidosis	• Increased lactate from tissue hypoperfusion due to anemia (hemorrhage), vasoconstriction (hypothermia-induced), and impaired cardiac output • Hyperchloremic metabolic acidosis due to large-volume resuscitation with normal saline (pH 5.5); type 4 respiratory failure (hypoperfusion of respiratory muscles in patients in shock)	• Severe acidosis decreases the cardiac output and blunts the heart response to catecholamines, and predisposes to the development of malignant arrhythmias including ventricular fibrillation • The acidosis increases the respiratory load as the body tries to compensate via respiratory alkalosis and eventually type 4 respiratory failure ensues • Acidosis inhibits the pH-dependent enzymatic reactions of the coagulation system—predisposing to coagulopathy and hemorrhage
Coagulopathy	Medicines that the patient might be taking can have anticoagulant effect, loss of clotting factors via hemorrhage, consumptive coagulopathy, and dilutional coagulopathy	Ongoing bleeding with worsening of dilutional and consumptive coagulopathy results in a vicious circle

appropriate resuscitation and damage control resuscitation (DCR) (see question 19), and avoiding overzealous fluid resuscitation. Coagulopathy needs to be corrected by early administration of TXA along with fixed ratio blood and blood products. Practical targets for resuscitation include a core temperature >35°C, INR <1.5, fibrinogen >1.5–2 g/L, platelets >50,000/mm^3, and pH 7.35–7.45. The serum calcium level needs to be monitored and hypocalcemia should be avoided.

Q12. In view of deteriorating hemodynamic status, the decision to simultaneously intubate the patient is taken. How will you manage airway and breathing? What is DAI?

Drug-assisted intubation is the new term that is currently being used for all intubations that are being facilitated with the use of sedatives and/or paralytic agents. It is a broad term that also includes rapid sequence intubation (intubation aided by neuromuscular blockade) and sedation-facilitated intubation (intubation aided by sedatives or hypnotics). DAI is indicated in all patients with intact gag reflex but needing intubation for either airway control or oxygenation. Common indications for securing the airway include:

- Inability to maintain airway patency either due to drugs or local injuries
- Persistent hypoxia even after oxygen supplementation or the presence of apnea
- Low GCS due to cerebral trauma or cerebral hypoperfusion or status epilepticus or in anticipation to protect the airway from vomitus or blood.

Once the decision to secure the airway is taken, necessary precautions should be arranged for. Ambu mask, oropharyngeal or nasopharyngeal airway, laryngoscopes with different sizes of blades, stylets, and Eschmann tracheal tube introducer (gum elastic bougie—GEB) should be kept ready along with endotracheal tubes of various sizes. Facility of airway suctioning should be available, and oxygen reserve for ventilation before and during intubation attempts should be ensured. A backup plan—including the possibility of performing a surgical airway—should be considered in the event of facing difficulty to oxygenate or ventilate the patient due to any reason. After appropriate preparation, start preoxygenation of the patient with 100% oxygen while maintaining cricoid pressure. The induction agent (etomidate, ketamine, fentanyl, and propofol) may be used as per the local protocols and patient indication. Muscle relaxation, if needed, is achieved with IV succinylcholine. After adequate relaxation, the patient is intubated via the oral route under vision/with aid of GEB and the tube placement is confirmed by end-tidal carbon dioxide monitor and auscultation. The cricoid pressure is then released, and the patient is ventilated. Any complication that arises during the procedure (including hypotension) is then managed.

Q13. Which drugs would you prefer for intubation in this case and why?

With the introduction of hypnotic agents such as propofol, alfentanil, and remifentanil that have rapid onset of action, the role for additional paralytic agents during intubation has undergone re-evaluation. Neuromuscular blockade improves the quality of intubating conditions, reduces the requirement of additional sedatives, thereby facilitating tracheal intubation and avoiding hypotension. Neuromuscular blockade reduces the time of success at tracheal intubation, reduces the incidence of laryngeal trauma, with reduced possibility of aspiration, and improves the success rates of intubation. Hence, it would be judicious to attempt intubation with moderate sedation and neuromuscular paralysis. Succinylcholine is used in most of the cases except for conditions such as hyperkalemia, burns, oliguric renal failure, etc., where rocuronium may be used. Neuromuscular paralysis after sedation reduces the chance of rise in ICP associated with patient fighting or coughing during intubation. The major concern with neuromuscular blockade is an apneic situation that can arise in case we cannot ventilate the patient. With the shorter duration of action, succinylcholine has the theoretical advantage over rocuronium. However, a retrospective study of intubation in patients with traumatic brain injury seemed to suggest an association between the use of succinylcholine and increased mortality as compared to rocuronium.[43]

The choice of hypnotic would depend on the personal choice of the rescuer. Care should be taken to reduce the incidence of hypotension by starting fluids and vasopressors high, using drugs that cause minimal myocardial depression. Care should also be taken to avoid drugs that might increase ICP in case a traumatic brain injury is suspected. Hence in this patient, after coloading him with fluids, etomidate, fentanyl, or low dose of propofol in combination with neuromuscular blockade may be attempted. If using etomidate, adrenal suppression needs to be watched out for. See **Table 10** for the commonly used drugs for rapid sequence intubation and their dosages.

Q14. What is the concept of using hypertonic saline (HTS) as resuscitation fluid in trauma patient? What is the evidence supporting this concept?

Hypertonic saline has been an attractive option in managing patients with hemorrhagic shock as it is stable at warm temperature, small-volume boluses result in blood volume expansion, and it may help to lower the ICP in patients with traumatic brain injury.[44] HTS is also proposed to have beneficial effects on neutrophil migration and permeability of the blood–brain barrier. The administration of HTS + dextran combination early in hemorrhagic shock of trauma

TABLE 10: Drug dosages for commonly used drugs for rapid sequence intubation.

Drugs	Dose
Ketamine	1.5–2 mg/kg ideal body weight
Etomidate	0.3–0.4 mg/kg total body weight
Fentanyl	2–10 µg/kg total body weight
Midazolam	0.1–0.3 mg/kg total body weight
Propofol	1.5 mg/kg × total body weight
Thiopentone	3–5 mg/kg total body weight
Succinylcholine (suxamethonium)	1–2 mg/kg total body weight
Rocuronium	0.6–1.2 mg/kg total body weight

may improve the biomarkers of brain injury. However, at this point of time, the evidence base for HTS/HTS + dextran combination for managing hemorrhagic shock in trauma is scarce.[45] HTS + dextran administered during out-of-hospital resuscitation of patients with blunt trauma and a prehospital SBP ≤90 mm Hg had no impact on the survival without acute respiratory distress syndrome at 28 days. Similarly, a small study (n = 34) on prehospital resuscitation of traumatic hemorrhagic shock with hypertonic solutions (HTS and HTS + dextran) showed worsening of coagulation parameters as compared to 0.9% saline. Meta-analysis of the trials that have investigated hyperosmolar therapies including HTS also found no added advantage in the setting of hemorrhagic shock and trauma.[46-48]

Q15. After intubation, the patient's BP dropped requiring increase in the dose of vasopressor agents. What are the causes of hypotension in this patient? What will be your blood pressure target for resuscitation in this patient? What is the principle of permissive hypotension?

Hypotension in trauma can be multifactorial and it needs to be addressed immediately. The most common causes of hypotension in trauma patients are mentioned in **Table 11**. In cases of penetrating trauma, if the tissues are well perfused then aggressive resuscitative efforts targeting a specific BP target may not be required. This requires a closely monitored balanced approach with frequent re-evaluation. This is commonly referred to permissive hypotension and should be considered as a bridge to definitive hemostasis.

Permissive hypotension is also known as hypotensive resuscitation and low-volume resuscitation, and is part of DCR. It aims to achieve hemostasis rather than attaining a fixed target of BP. The tissues continue to be perfused but with the lowest BP required to maintain tissue perfusion. This approach limits the chance of dilutional coagulopathy and favors clot formation and stabilization internally.

TABLE 11: Causes of hypotension in trauma.		
Type of shock	Etiology	Diagnosis and management
Hypovolemic shock	• Ongoing bleeding • Inadequate resuscitation • Fluid sequestration in abdomen	Look for ongoing external or internal bleeding. Sites for occult bleeding include thorax, abdomen, retroperitoneum, pelvis, and long bones, which need to be actively searched by clinical examination and imaging. Over-resuscitation of these patients can lead to third spacing due to underlying inflammation resulting in intra-abdominal hypertension and abdominal compartment syndrome
Cardiogenic shock	• Myocardial depression • Myocardial contusion • Arrhythmias	Cardiogenic shock can be due to direct myocardial contusion, myocardial depression due to drugs used for sedation or arrhythmias. Arrhythmias need to be managed as per ACLS protocols, while the rest can be observed by vasopressors and inotropes
Distributive shock	• Neurogenic shock • Anaphylaxis	• Injury to the cervical or upper thoracic spinal cord (T6 and above) causes impairment of the descending sympathetic pathways resulting in vasodilation of visceral and peripheral blood vessels, venous pooling of blood, and hypotension. A compensatory tachycardia might not manifest due to denervation of sympathetic nervous system and the patient may even develop bradycardia • This should not be confused with spinal shock, which is the flaccid areflexia that occurs due to spinal cord injury. While neurogenic shock is due to the loss of vasomotor tone and sympathetic innervation to the heart • In case where anaphylaxis is suspected, adrenalin should be administered, and patient should be managed accordingly
Obstructive shock	Tension pneumothorax, cardiac tamponade, etc.	Tension pneumothorax and cardiac tamponade are common causes of hypotension during trauma that can lead to obstructive shock. This is a medical emergency and requires urgent evacuation with either needle aspiration or pigtail insertion.

(ACLS: advanced cardiac life support)

However, it must be remembered that hypotension is not the end target but a compromise till hemostasis is achieved. Once hemostasis is achieved normal targets of hemodynamics should be followed. The data supporting permissive hypotension is of low quality and this should not be accepted as a compromise in case of obstructive shock. This may also not be acceptable in cases where traumatic brain injury might be present or in patents with underlying hypertension in which the target BP may vary as per case.

The patient is currently stabilized with noradrenaline 0.2 µg/kg/min, maintaining an HR of 140 beta/min and mean arterial pressure (MAP) of 60 mm Hg. The peripheries remain cold and urine output is 0.3 mL/kg/h for the past 6 hours. The abdominal girth has increased by 2 cm although the hematocrit and ABG show no worsening. During discussion, the surgical team suggests whole body imaging followed by surgical exploration and definitive surgery. The surgical team feels a whole-body computed tomography (WBCT) will help them to proceed with definitive surgery.

Q16. What is the role of WBCT over selected computed tomography (SCT) in trauma?

The SCT approach relies upon correlation of the history, initial physical examination findings, and findings on conventional imaging [X-ray and ultrasonography (USG)] to decide upon the need for CT. This approach depends heavily on the clinical gestalt of the physician and significant injuries may be missed (incidence of injuries missed due to SCT varies from study to study with literature reporting ranges of 1.3–39% out of which 15–22.3% being significant). However, these studies were conducted at various time periods and were not standardized, limiting its applicability to the current scenario of improved diagnostics and awareness.[49] As SCT is usually ordered after patient evaluation and at times on re-evaluation, it might result in significant delay in the diagnosis. These disadvantages of SCT can be minimized with WBCT. But there are no current protocols or clear-cut decision criteria for WBCT so far. By limiting the number of CT scans, SCT avoids the risk of transporting a hemodynamically unstable patient to a far-off CT room, and reduces the risk of radiation exposure to patient without increasing the mortality.

On the other hand, the WBCT approach includes plain CT scans of the head and cervical region and contrast-enhanced images for chest, abdomen, and pelvis for all patients coming with trauma, especially severe trauma. The pickup rate of incidental findings is higher with WBCT although their clinical significance is not clear. Data from retrospective trials and meta-analysis seem to suggest a mortality benefit with WBCT, however, the REACT-2 trial did not show any mortality benefit of WBCT.[50] REACT-2 trial was criticized for its nonblinded nature and increased exclusions postrandomization that might have biased the result. The sample size for REACT-2 was calculated to detect a mortality benefit of 5% when the existing data suggested a mortality benefit of 3%.[51] Although the REACT-2 trial showed no difference as per the sample size calculation, possibility of a type 2 error still exists. Few WBCT studies including unstable multitrauma patients have reported a lower mortality rate with WBCT, but the data is not robust. Although the risk of radiation exposure is significantly higher in WBCT group, incorporation of adaptive dose-reduction algorithms can reduce the radiation exposure. As of the current prevailing evidence, WBCT cannot be recommended as the standard of care for all victims of trauma.[52]

Q17. In view of the positive e-FAST, should a diagnostic peritoneal lavage (DPL) be attempted in this patient? Mention the indications and contraindications of DPL.

Diagnostic peritoneal lavage is a cheap minimally invasive bedside procedure that is easy to perform and provides rapid results in patients with suspected abdominal injury. DPL, however, is nontherapeutic, does not identify the source of injury, and has significant false-positive or false-negative results. Although safe, it can still cause damage to underlying organs and can be technically difficult in obese patients, pregnant patients, or those with prior abdominal surgery. Hence, once considered as the gold standard for the evaluation of abdominal trauma, DPL has currently fallen out of favor and has given way to imaging technologies, such as e-FAST and CT scan.

Currently DPL is indicated in:
- The evaluation of the hemodynamically unstable trauma patient to detect or rule out intra-abdominal hemorrhage in case there are limitations for e-FAST examination or abdominal CT
- The detection of hollow viscus injury and mesenteric injury
- The detection of abdominal hemorrhage in patients with blunt abdominal injury with CT suggestive of free abdominal fluid with no obvious source of hemorrhage
- The detection of diaphragmatic injury, if the lavage fluid is seen exiting from a chest tube.

A clear indication for immediate laparotomy is a contraindication for DPL. Apart from that, relative contraindications for DPL include prior abdominal surgeries, presence of coagulopathy, known case of advanced cirrhosis, and morbid obesity. Pregnancy and suspected pelvic trauma are not contraindications for DPL although the technique of DPL must be modified.

The DPL is done under local anesthesia after complete evacuation of the stomach and bladder by insertion of nasogastric tube and Foley's catheter. DPL kits or a rigid peritoneal dialysis catheter may be used to gain access into the peritoneal cavity. The incision is made 2 cm below the umbilicus except in the case of a pregnant trauma patient or in case of a pelvic fracture where supraumbilical insertion is preferred. After insertion, direct fluid aspiration is performed gently. Presence of >10 mL of blood or enteric contents is considered positive and further instillation of fluid for lavage is not necessary. If <10 mL fluid is aspirated then lavage is done by instilling 1 L of warm saline into the abdomen, and immediately allowing it to drain out passively. The returned fluid is then analyzed for RBCs, white blood cells (WBCs), amylase, bacteria, and enteric contents. RBC count of >100,000/mm^3, WBC count >500/mm^3, an elevated amylase level, or the presence of enteric contents or bacteria is considered as a positive DPL. False-positive results can occur, if the catheter is directly placed into a pelvic hematoma or if a pelvic hematoma has ruptured into the peritoneal cavity. False-negative DPL is usually due to technical errors with the catheter being placed into an extraperitoneal location or if the injury is retroperitoneal. Most complications of DPL are due to the catheter placement. Bowel, vascular bladder, and stomach (if not decompressed prior to the procedure) injuries can occur as a part of DPL.

Here, the patient is still hypotensive, persistently tachypneic, and tachycardic. e-FAST has already showed features of hemoperitoneum and splenic injury. An increase in abdominal girth by 2 cm is also ominous, although it can be a warning sign for bowel edema and intra-abdominal hypertension. DPL is not necessary with this information and it might be risky in view of coagulopathy. This patient needs to be taken up urgently for a damage control surgery.

Q18. What are the advantages and disadvantages of CT in abdominal trauma patient?

A multidetector helical CT can give information regarding intra-abdominal injury rapidly with very high sensitivity and specificity. The advantages of CT scan include its noninvasive nature, better identification of organ injury, the potential for conservative management of injuries, and detection of the source of hemoperitoneum and its quantification. It can also be clubbed with screening of other body parts that may also provide significant information. CT scans have a high NPV, so that negative imaging virtually rules out a clinically significant injury. Hence, in hemodynamically stable patients with suspicion of abdominal injury, a helical MDCT can provide valuable information rapidly with minimal added risks. However, as MDCT is associated with significant radiation exposure and expense, the patients should be selected carefully. The disadvantages of CT scan include its high cost, the associated radiation, and contrast exposure, need to shift from ICU to CT console, and its poor sensitivity for mesenteric, bowel, and pancreatic duct injuries.

In view of the hemodynamically unstable state and risk of coagulopathy, it was decided to take up the patient for a damage control surgery.

Q19. What do you mean by DCR?
Damage control resuscitation is a systematic approach of resuscitation for a patient with exsanguinating trauma. It consists of balanced hemostatic resuscitation, avoiding hypothermia and acidosis, and at the same time maintaining an effective circulation till the patient is fit enough for a definitive intervention. DCR is initiated in the emergency room and later continued in the ICU and operating theater as damage control surgery.

Damage control surgery is a series of minimal surgeries or surgical interventions aiming to control the bleeding and minimize the contamination temporarily, till the patient recovers sufficiently to tolerate the physiological consequences of definitive interventions. This approach stresses on maintaining physiological homeostasis and hemostasis before any definitive procedure is undertaken. After a bare minimum surgical intervention to control the bleeding and minimize the contamination, attempts are made to rewarm body cavities and the patient is transferred back to the ICU for ongoing balanced hemostatic resuscitation. The definitive surgery is planned after the initial stabilization, usually within 24–36 hours. This approach has shown better benefits in view of better temperature control and control of coagulopathy with lesser blood and blood products.

As the patient is about to be shifted to the operating room, the nurse informs you that the urine output has dropped significantly, and the calf has become swollen up and tense. A crush injury with compartment syndrome is suspected and the workup for the same is sent.

Q20. How do you diagnose crush injury and compartment syndrome? What are the possible complications? How will you manage the patient?
Crush injury develops in individuals who have sustained a compression to the muscle, usually at the thigh or calf. There is a direct muscle injury, muscle ischemia, and cell death resulting in release of large quantities of myoglobin. The urine turns amber-colored and the serum creatine kinase levels rise—usually >10,000 U/L. Rhabdomyolysis can lead to systemic effects, such as metabolic acidosis, hyperkalemia, hypocalcemia, disseminated intravascular coagulation, acute renal failure, and shock.

Q21. When to administer antibiotic and which antibiotic to prefer in traumatic open/contaminated wound?
According to ATLS guideline: If wound is <1 cm plus minimal soft tissue damage/contamination: First generation of cephalosporin will suffice (if penicillin allergy selects clindamycin). If wound is >1 cm (and <10 cm) with moderate soft tissue damage/contamination/communication of fracture add clindamycin. If any vascular injury with soft tissue damage add aminoglycoside. Farmyard, soil, or water contamination of wound irrespective of size or severity receives Piperacillin + Tazobactam (Pip + Taz) as broad-spectrum antibiotic.

Q22. Is any role of steroid or TXA in traumatic brain injury patient?
The CRASH study, which investigated the use of corticosteroids after severe traumatic brain injury in >10,000 patients, found an increased mortality rate in the corticosteroids group and no difference in the incidence of pneumonia.

CRASH-3 results show that TXA is safe in patients with traumatic brain injury and that treatment within 3 hours of injury reduces head injury-related death. Patients should be treated as soon as possible after injury.

Q23. What are the options for endovascular trauma and bleeding management (EVTM)? Nonoperative options for abdominal blunt trauma/What are the options for severe pelvic injuries?
According to World Journal of Emergency Surgery I–III (WSES I–III) for splenic and liver injury patients (those who are hemodynamically stable, fluid responder) and where imaging shows positive blush, endovascular intervention is very helpful. WSES IV grade injuries/hemodynamically unstable patient or transient responder should be approached by laparotomy.

Resuscitative thoracotomy with aortic cross-clamping represents an acute measure of temporary bleeding control for unresponsive patients "in extremis" with exsanguinating pelvic traumatic hemorrhage (Grade 1A)

Resuscitative Endovascular Balloon Occlusion of the Aorta (REBOA) technique may provide a valid innovative alternative to aortic cross-clamping (Grade 2B) in hemodynamic unstable patients with suspected pelvic bleeding

Q24. What is the role of viscoelastic hemostatic assays (VHAs) compared to conventional coagulation tests (CCTs) in trauma patients?
Conventional plasma-based coagulation tests, such as PT, aPTT, INR, fibrinogen, and platelet number, only reflect the initiation of the hemostatic process; the tests cannot be used to evaluate the amplification of propagation or increased fibrinolysis. Whole blood assays, such as TEG or ROTEM, provide rapid evaluation of clot formation, strength, and lysis, which reflect the entire hemostatic process.

According to ITACTIC trial published in 2021, there was no difference in overall outcomes between VHA- and CCT-augmented major hemorrhage protocols. To summarize, viscoelastic assay seems quite promising on physiological basis, but evidences are still not so strong in major trauma patients.

Q25. How do you diagnose limb (myofascial) compartment syndrome? How is it managed? What are its complications?

During trauma, the pressure in a myofascial compartment increases either due to swelling of the injured muscles or hematoma formation due to a closed fracture inside a closed compartment. As the intracompartmental pressure goes above 20 mm Hg, the capillary flow ceases and at pressures of 30–40 mm Hg muscle and nerve ischemia occur. If the intracompartmental pressure is measured then an absolute difference between diastolic BP and intracompartmental pressure <30 mm Hg is suggestive of compartment syndrome. Compartment syndrome is a medical emergency, as it results in ischemia and loss of the limb, if not treated quickly. It is commonly associated with trauma and fractures although it can also be seen with crush injury, prolonged immobilization, snake bite, burns, etc. Clinically, the limb becomes swollen, tense, and tender on palpation. On passive movements, the pain is exacerbated and is considered as the most sensitive sign. The presence of distal pulses, a normal capillary refill or a pulse oximetry trace are insensitive indicators of loss of capillary perfusion and not recommended in the detection of compartment syndrome. Imaging has no role in the diagnosis of compartment syndrome and management includes removing all constrictive dressings, limb elevation, optimization of traction in case of fractures, and emergency fasciotomy may be needed, if the limb is not improving. These patients should be monitored for rhabdomyolysis, acute kidney injury, and hyperkalemia.

After the damage control surgery and fasciotomy, it was decided to manage the fractures with an open reduction after 2 days. He was shifted to the ICU for further observation. His hemodynamics were stabilizing, urine output had increased, and the acidosis was improving gradually. However, after 12 hours, the patient became disoriented and the HR increased up to 150 beats/min and respiratory rate increased up to 40 breaths/min. He remained hemodynamically stable with a BP of 130/76 mm Hg. His saturation now dropped to 84% and with 6 L oxygen given via face mask, it improved to 96%.

Q26. What are the differential diagnoses of acute desaturation in this patient?

The differentials of acute desaturation in these patients are given in **Box 3**. Given the clinical scenario, a thorough

BOX 3: Differential diagnoses of desaturation in trauma patients.
- Pulmonary contusion
- Pulmonary edema—cardiogenic
- Massive pleural effusion
- Pneumothorax/tension pneumothorax
- Pneumonia/sepsis
- Massive pleural effusion/hemothorax
- Thromboembolism—venous or fat embolism
- Acute respiratory distress syndrome
- Transfusion-associated lung injury (TRALI)

clinical examination investigation including measurement of temperature, BP, pulse volume and pulse pressure, chest X-ray, ECG, ABG analysis, screening bedside echocardiography with BLUE (bedside lung ultrasound in emergency) protocol, N-terminal pro-brain natriuretic peptide (NT-ProBNP), cardiac enzymes, and a CT scan of the brain and CT pulmonary angiogram might have to be done.

The sensorium dropped further with a GCS of E2M3V2. Even with 10-liter oxygen via a nonrebreathing mask, the saturation was not maintained. The bedside screening ultrasound and X-ray chest ruled out effusion or pneumothorax and ABG showed type 1 respiratory failure with a widened alveolar to arterial (A-a) gap and respiratory alkalosis. Cardiac enzymes and 2D echocardiography are normal [no right atrial (RA) or right ventricular (RV) dilatation, no regional wall motion abnormalities (RWMA)]. ECG showed sinus tachycardia. There were no signs of any wound infection. CT brain was reported as normal, with no evidence of intraparenchymal bleed. A diagnosis of fat embolism was made, and the patient was intubated for type 1 respiratory failure.

Q27. Discuss briefly about the etiopathogenesis of FES.

Fat embolism syndrome is a clinical syndrome characterized by a constellation of pulmonary and neurological symptoms along with other system involvement, such as thrombocytopenia and fever. Fat embolism is usually associated with trauma of the long bones. It has also been reported after surgeries involving intramedullary reaming, during arthroplasty, after administration of fluid intraosseously with the use of lipid-soluble radiocontrast, during liposuction, and during bone marrow harvesting and transplant. Noniatrogenic causes of fat embolism reported in literature include sickle cell crisis, pancreatitis, fat necrosis of omentum, hepatic steatosis, osteomyelitis, and bone tumor lysis. The exact pathophysiology is unclear and can neither be fully explained by the physical properties of the circulating fat globules nor the biochemical changes accompanying it. Clinical features include disorientation, delirium, agitation or coma having an onset within 24–72 hours following injury. Pulmonary involvement is characterized by poor

TABLE 12: Pathogenesis of fat embolism syndrome (FES).	
Theory	**Pathogenesis**
Mechanical theory (Gauss et al.)[54]	This suggests that the physical properties of the dissolved fat droplets blocked in the pulmonary circulation are responsible for the symptoms of FES. The workload of the right heart increases and, at times, acute cor pulmonale may ensue. However, this theory can neither explain the changes in the neurological system nor the time lag of occurrence of fat embolism to fat embolism syndrome
Biochemical theory (Lehman et al.)[55]	It suggests that the circulating free fatty acids and glycerol (formed as a result of hydrolysis of fatty acids by lipase secreted from the lung) cause an increase in the permeability of the capillary bed of lungs, a destruction of the alveolar architecture, and damage to lung surfactant to cause pulmonary symptoms
Combination	As both theories cannot explain the entire spectrum of manifestations, a combined theory of both mechanical and biochemical causation for FES has been proposed. The initial symptoms are attributed to the physical properties of the fat globules followed by activation of the biochemical cascade, which is responsible for the rest of the symptoms
Coagulation theory[56]	It proposes tissue thromboplastin released with marrow elements to activate the complement system and extrinsic coagulation cascade via direct activation of factor VII, which in turn leads to production of intravascular coagulation by fibrin and fibrin degradation products.

TABLE 13: Diagnostic criteria for fat embolism syndrome (FES).	
Criteria	**Description**
Gurd's criteria (one major + four minor criteria)[57]	• *Major criteria:* Presence of any respiratory symptoms, neurological symptoms or petechial rash • *Minor criteria:* Fever, tachycardia, anemia or thrombocytopenia, raised ESR, and detection of fat globules in urine or retina
Lindeque's criteria: In patients with history of trauma, presence of any one of the following suggests FES[58]	Dyspnea, tachycardia, anxiety, sustained hypoxia <60 mm Hg, or a pH <7.3 and a sustained respiratory rate >35 breaths/min despite sedation
Schonfeld criteria (a score of 5 or more)[59]	One point each for confusion, pyrexia, tachycardia (>120 beats/min), tachypnea (>30 breaths/min) and confusion, three points for hypoxia with PaO_2 <70 mm Hg, four points for diffuse alveolar infiltrates on chest radiography, and five points for petechiae

(ESR: erythrocyte sedimentation rate; PaO_2: partial pressure of arterial oxygen)

partial pressure of arterial oxygen (PaO_2)/fraction of inspired oxygen (FiO_2) ratio with a widened A-a gradient that may progress to acute respiratory distress syndrome.[53]

It is not clear and why only some people with fat embolism go on to develop FES, and various theories on the etiopathogenesis of fat embolism have been proposed, which are summarized in the **Table 12**. The diagnosis is mainly clinical, although circulating fat globules detected in the urine, retina, or bronchoalveolar lavage fluid may help.

Q28. What are the clinical features and investigation results in a patient with FES?

Fat embolism syndrome is mainly a clinical diagnosis and no diagnostic investigation is sufficiently sensitive or specific to diagnose or exclude FES. The classic triad of clinical features including the respiratory manifestations, neurological symptoms, and petechiae in the appropriate setting can be used to diagnose FES. The common laboratory abnormalities include unexplained anemia, thrombocytopenia, elevated erythrocyte sedimentation rate (ESR) deranged PT, hypofibrinogenemia, hypocalcemia, and an elevated serum lipase. ABGs will show type 1 respiratory failure with a low PO_2 and PCO_2 resulting in respiratory alkalosis and widened A-a oxygen gradient. The chest radiology appearance is called the snow storm appearance, which is rare and not pathognomonic. Echocardiography might show features of right heart strain and RV dysfunction. CT brain is nonspecific while brain MRI shows spotty areas of high intensity on T2-weighted images. The different criteria used for diagnosis of fat embolism are summarized in **Table 13**.

Q29. How will you manage a case of FES?

The management of FES is nonspecific and is directed toward general ICU care. Treatment includes maintenance of adequate oxygenation and ventilation, stabilizing the hemodynamics and management of RV failure, transfusion of blood products as indicated, prophylaxis of deep venous thrombosis and stress-related gastrointestinal bleeding and adequate nutrition. Initial stages of acute type 1 respiratory failure might require intubation and lung-protective ventilation. Various therapies have been tried to treat FES but without success. These include corticosteroids, aspirin, heparin and N-acetylcysteine, and IV ethanol. Surgical management includes early fixation of fractures and some surgical steps whose description is beyond the scope of this chapter. The role of albumin seems promising due to its ability to bind with fatty acids and may decrease the extent of FES. The role of corticosteroids for prophylaxis of FES and hyperbaric oxygen remains to be proven.[53]

This patient was managed with lung protective ventilation sedation and analgesia. His oxygenation and sensorium showed signs of improvement and he was extubated to high flow nasal oxygen in 2 days. Oxygen also was later weaned and stopped and the patient was discharged to home.

REFERENCES

1. American College of Surgeons. ATLS-Advanced Trauma Life Support: Student Course Manual, 10th edition. [online] Available from https://cirugia.facmed.unam.mx/wp-content/uploads/2018/07/Advanced-Trauma-Life-Support.pdf [Last accessed August, 2023].
2. Zeiler FA, Teitelbaum J, West M, Gillman LM. The ketamine effect on ICP in traumatic brain injury. Neurocrit Care. 2014;21(1):163-73.
3. Senkowski CK, McKenney MG. Trauma scoring systems: a review. J Am Coll Surg. 1999;189(5):491-503.
4. Sundstrøm T, Asbjørnsen H, Habiba S, Sunde GA, Wester K. Prehospital use of cervical collars in trauma patients: a critical review. J Neurotrauma. 2014;31(6):531-40.
5. Andrew E. Overview and Comparison of NEXUS and Canadian C-Spine Rule. Am J Clin Med. 2006;3:12-5.
6. Ley EJ, Clond MA, Srour MK, Barnajian M, Mirocha J, Margulies DR, et al. Emergency department crystalloid resuscitation of 1.5 L or more is associated with increased mortality in elderly and nonelderly trauma patients. J Trauma. 2011;70(2):398-400.
7. Cap A, Hunt B. Acute traumatic coagulopathy. Curr Opin Crit Care. 2014;20(6):638-45.
8. Kushimoto S, Kudo D, Kawazoe Y. Acute traumatic coagulopathy and trauma-induced coagulopathy: an overview. J Intensive Care. 2017;5:6.
9. Giordano S, Spiezia L, Campello E, Simioni P. The current understanding of trauma-induced coagulopathy (TIC): a focused review on pathophysiology. Intern Emerg Med. 2017;12(7):981-91.
10. Pidcoke HF, Aden JK, Mora AG, Borgman MA, Spinella PC, Dubick MA, et al. Ten-year analysis of transfusion in Operation Iraqi Freedom and Operation Enduring Freedom. J Trauma Acute Care Surg. 2012;73(6 Suppl 5):S445-52.
11. Zink KA, Sambasivan CN, Holcomb JB, Chisholm G, Schreiber MA. A high ratio of plasma and platelets to packed red blood cells in the first 6 hours of massive transfusion improves outcomes in a large multicenter study. Am J Surg. 2009;197(5):565-70.
12. Rossaint R, Bouillon B, Cerny V, Coats TJ, Duranteau J, Fernández-Mondéjar E, et al. The European guideline on management of major bleeding and coagulopathy following trauma: fourth edition. Crit Care. 2016;20:100.
13. Patil V, Shetmahajan M. Massive transfusion and massive transfusion protocol. Indian J Anaesth. 2014;58:590-5.
14. Pham HP, Shaz BH. Update on massive transfusion. Br J Anaesth. 2013;111:i71-82.
15. Bawazeer M, Ahmed N, Izadi H, McFarlan A, Nathens A, Pavenski K. Compliance with a massive transfusion protocol (MTP) impacts patient outcome. Injury. 2015;46(1):21-8.
16. Cotton BA, Dossett LA, Au BK, Nunez TC, Robertson AM, Young PP. Room for (performance) improvement: provider-related factors associated with poor outcomes in massive transfusion. J Trauma. 2009;67(5):1004-12.
17. Sihler KC, Napolitano LM. Complications of massive transfusion. Chest. 2010;137(1):209-20.
18. Pommerening MJ, Goodman MD, Holcomb JB, Wade CE, Fox EE, Del Junco DJ, et al; MPH on behalf of the PROMMTT Study Group. Clinical gestalt and the prediction of massive transfusion after trauma. Injury. 2015;46(5):807-13.
19. Tonglet ML. Early prediction of ongoing hemorrhage in severe trauma: presentation of the existing scoring systems. Arch Trauma Res. 2016;5:e33377.
20. Nunez TC, Voskresensky IV, Dossett LA, Shinall R, Dutton WD, Cotton BA. Early prediction of massive transfusion in trauma: simple as ABC (assessment of blood consumption)? J Trauma. 2009;66:346-52.
21. Fredericks C, Kubasiak JC, Mentzer CJ, Yon JR. Massive transfusion: an update for the anesthesiologist. World J Anesthesiol. 2017;6:14-21.
22. Cantle PM, Cotton BA. Prediction of massive transfusion in trauma. Crit Care Clin. 2017;33(1):71-84.
23. Savage SA, Zarzaur BL, Croce MA, Fabian TC. Redefining massive transfusion when every second counts. J Trauma Acute Care Surg. 2013;74:396-400; discussion 400-2.
24. Rahbar E, Fox EE, del Junco DJ, Harvin JA, Holcomb JB, Wade CE, et al; PROMMTT Study Group. Early resuscitation intensity as a surrogate for bleeding severity and early mortality in the PROMMTT study. J Trauma Acute Care Surg. 2013;75(1 Suppl1):S16-23.
25. Borgman MA, Spinella PC, Perkins JG, Grathwohl KW, Repine T, Beekley AC, et al. The ratio of blood products transfused affects mortality in patients receiving massive transfusions at a Combat Support Hospital. J Trauma. 2007;63:805-13.
26. Holcomb JB, del Junco DJ, Fox EE, Wade CE, Cohen MJ, Schreiber MA, et al; PROMMTT Study Group. The prospective, observational, multicenter, major trauma transfusion (PROMMTT) study: comparative effectiveness of a time-varying treatment with competing risks. JAMA Surg. 2013;148:127-36.
27. Holcomb JB, Tilley BC, Baraniuk S, Fox EE, Wade CE, Podbielski JM, et al; PROPPR Study Group. Transfusion of plasma, platelets, and red blood cells in a 1:1:1 vs a 1:1:2 ratio and mortality in patients with severe trauma. JAMA. 2015;313:471-82.
28. Roberts I, Shakur H, Coats T, Hunt B, Balogun E, Barnetson L, et al. The CRASH-2 trial: a randomised controlled trial and economic evaluation of the effects of tranexamic acid on death, vascular occlusive events and transfusion requirement in bleeding trauma patients. Health Technol Assess. 2013;17:1-79.
29. Morrison JJ, Dubose JJ, Rasmussen TE, Midwinter MJ. Military application of tranexamic acid in trauma emergency resuscitation (MATTERs) study. Arch Surg. 2012;147:113-9.
30. Eckert MJ, Wertin TM, Tyner SD, Nelson DW, Izenberg S, Martin MJ. Tranexamic acid administration to pediatric trauma patients in a combat setting. J Trauma Acute Care Surg. 2014;77:852-8.

31. Napolitano LM, Cohen MJ, Cotton BA, Schreiber MA, Moore EE, Arbor A. Tranexamic acid in trauma: How should we use it? J Trauma Acute Care Surg. 2013;74:1575-86.
32. Nishida T, Kinoshita T, Yamakawa K. Tranexamic acid and trauma-induced coagulopathy. J Intensive Care. 2017;5:5.
33. Pabinger I, Fries D, Schöchl H, Streif W, Toller W. Tranexamic acid for treatment and prophylaxis of bleeding and hyperfibrinolysis. Wien Klin Wochenschr. 2017;129:303-16.
34. Aubron C, Nichol A, Cooper DJ, Bellomo R. Age of red blood cells and transfusion in critically ill patients. Ann Intensive Care. 2013;3:2.
35. Koch CG, Li L, Sessler DI, Figueroa P, Hoeltge GA, Mihaljevic T, et al. Duration of red-cell storage and complications after cardiac surgery. N Engl J Med. 2008;358:1229-39.
36. Fergusson DA, Hébert P, Hogan DL, LeBel L, Rouvinez-Bouali N, Smyth JA, et al. Effect of fresh red blood cell transfusions on clinical outcomes in premature, very low-birth-weight infants: the ARIPI randomized trial. JAMA. 2012;308:1443-51.
37. George JP, Myatra SN. Blood transfusion in the critically ill patient. Bangladesh Crit Care J. 2018;6:40-6.
38. Steiner ME, Ness PM, Assmann SF, Triulzi DJ, Sloan SR, Delaney M, et al. Effects of red-cell storage duration on patients undergoing cardiac surgery. N Engl J Med. 2015;372:1419-29.
39. Lacroix J, Hébert PC, Fergusson DA, Tinmouth A, Cook DJ, Marshall JC, et al; ABLE Investigators; Canadian Critical Care Trials Group. Age of transfused blood in critically Ill adults. N Engl J Med. 2015;372:1410-8.
40. Heddle NM, Cook RJ, Arnold DM, Liu Y, Barty R, Crowther MA, et al. Effect of short-term vs. long-term blood storage on mortality after transfusion. N Engl J Med. 2016;375:1937-45.
41. Cooper DJ, McQuilten ZK, Nichol A, Ady B, Aubron C, Bailey M, et al; TRANSFUSE Investigators and the Australian and New Zealand Intensive Care Society Clinical Trials Group. Age of red cells for transfusion and outcomes in critically ill adults. N Engl J Med. 2017;377:1858-67.
42. Kashuk JL, Moore EE, Millikan JS, Moore JB. Major abdominal vascular trauma—a unified approach. J Trauma. 1982;22:672-9.
43. Patanwala AE, Erstad BL, Roe DJ, Sakles JC. Succinylcholine is associated with increased mortality when used for rapid sequence intubation of severely brain injured patients in the emergency department. Pharmacotherapy. 2016;36:57-63.
44. Angle N, Cabello-Passini R, Hoyt DB, Loomis WH, Shreve A, Namiki S, et al. Hypertonic saline infusion: can it regulate human neutrophil function? Shock. 2000;14(5):503-8.
45. MacDonald RD. Articles that may change your practice: hypertonic fluid resuscitation in trauma. Air Med J. 2018;37(1):18-9.
46. Delano MJ, Rizoli SB, Rhind SG, Cuschieri J, Junger W, Baker AJ, et al. Prehospital resuscitation of traumatic hemorrhagic shock with hypertonic solutions worsens hypocoagulation and hyperfibrinolysis. Shock. 2015;44:25-31.
47. de Crescenzo C, Gorouhi F, Salcedo ES, Galante JM. Prehospital hypertonic fluid resuscitation for trauma patients. J Trauma Acute Care Surg. 2017;82:956-62.
48. Wu MC, Liao TY, Lee EM, Chen YS, Hsu WT, Lee MG, et al. Administration of hypertonic solutions for hemorrhagic shock. Anesth Analg. 2017;125:1549-57.
49. Pfeifer R, Pape HC. Missed injuries in trauma patients: a literature review. Patient Saf Surg. 2008;2(1):20.
50. Sierink JC, Treskes K, Edwards MJR, Beuker BJA, den Hartog D, Hohmann J, et al; REACT-2 study group. Immediate total-body CT scanning versus conventional imaging and selective CT scanning in patients with severe trauma (REACT-2): a randomised controlled trial. Lancet. 2016;388:673-83.
51. Huber-Wagner S, Lefering R, Qvick LM, Körner M, Kay MV, Pfeifer KJ, et al; Working Group on Polytrauma of the German Trauma Society. Effect of whole-body CT during trauma resuscitation on survival: a retrospective, multicentre study. Lancet. 2009;373:1455-61.
52. Çorbacıoğlu ŞK, Aksel G. Whole body computed tomography in multi trauma patients: review of the current literature. Turkish J Emerg Med. 2018;18:142-7.
53. George J, George R, Dixit R, Gupta RC, Gupta N. Fat embolism syndrome. Lung India. 2013;30:47-53.
54. Gauss H. The pathology of fat embolism. Arch Surg. 1924;9:593-605.
55. Lehman EP, Moore RM. Fat embolism including experimental production without trauma. Arch Surg. 1927;14:621-62.
56. Soloway HB, Robinson EF. The coagulation mechanism in experimental pulmonary fat embolism. J Trauma. 1972;12:630-1.
57. Gurd AR, Wilson RI. The fat embolism syndrome. J Bone Joint Surg Br. 1974;56B:408-16.
58. Lindeque BG, Schoeman HS, Dommisse GF, Boeyens MC, Vlok AL. Fat embolism and the fat embolism syndrome. J Bone Joint Surg. 1987;69B:128-31.
59. Schonfeld SA, Ploysongsang Y, DiLisio R, Crissman JD, Miller E, Hammerschmidt DE, et al. Fat embolism prophylaxis with corticosteroids. A prospective study in high-risk patients. Ann Intern Med. 1983;99:438-43.

CHAPTER 18: Snake and Scorpion Bites

Niteen D Karnik, Priyanshu D Shah

CASE STUDIES

Case 1

A 55-year-old male residing in a village area presented to the emergency room around 1 PM with history of snake bite to the left leg around 9 AM while he was working in his farm. The snake was apparently half-a-feet long and brownish in color as per the patient and escaped after the bite. The patient went to a nearby peripheral health center, where he was administered tetanus toxoid injection, his wound was bandaged and referred to a tertiary care hospital. During the journey to the hospital, he developed pain at the bite site. He presented to our emergency 3 hours later with intense pain, swelling, and oozing of blood from the site of the bite. Patient even had difficulty in walking due to the pain. There was no history of convulsions, drooping of eyelid, or limb weakness. Also, there was no history of bleeding from any other site or hematuria. There was no family history of any blood disorders. Patient was a known case of hypertension since the last 5 years and was on tablet Telmisartan 40 mg once a day. There was no other significant past or personal history.

On presentation in emergency, patient was conscious and oriented with a pulse rate of 100 beats/min, blood pressure of 120/72 mm Hg, and respiratory rate of 18 breaths/min. Body temperature was 37.2°C. On local examination of the left leg, there were two fang marks along with tenderness, redness, and swelling just above the lateral malleolus with persistent oozing of blood from bite site. Systemic examination was normal. His investigations are given in **Table 1**.

Over the next 48 hours, the patient developed decreased urine output (oliguria) with rise in serum creatinine levels to 4.5 mg% and whole blood clotting time (WBCT) remained >20 minutes, but oozing from the bite site had stopped. Early blackish discoloration was noticed in the left leg second and third toes.

Q 1. What is your diagnosis?
It is a case of vasculotoxic snake bite with disseminated intravascular coagulation (DIC).

TABLE 1: Investigations chart.

Hemoglobin	12.1 g%	Total protein	6.8 g%
Leukocyte count	9,500/mm³	Serum albumin	4.1 g%
Platelet count	85,000/mm³	Serum Na⁺/K⁺	141/4.2 mEq/L
Prothrombin time	48 (control 11.5 seconds)	Serum Calcium	9.2 mg%
INR	4.5	Serum Magnesium	2.4 mg%
aPTT	98 seconds	Total bilirubin	0.6 mg%
WBCT	>20 minutes	SGOT/SGPT	21/26 U/L
		BUN/Creatinine	16/0.7 mg%
Chest X-ray	Normal	ECG	Normal

(aPTT: activated partial thromboplastin time; BUN: blood urea nitrogen; ECG: electrocardiogram; INR: international normalized ratio; SGPT: serum glutamic pyruvic transaminase; SGOT: serum glutamic oxaloacetic transaminase; WBCT: whole blood clotting time)

Q2. If the snake is identified, how do you differentiate a poisonous snake from a non-poisonous snake (Table 2)?

TABLE 2: Differences between poisonous and non-poisonous snake.

Trait	Poisonous snake	Non-poisonous snake
General	Stout, dull colored, abruptly tapering tail	Slender, bright colored, gradually tapering tail
Head	Usually triangular in shape	Usually rounded or oval
Head scales	Usually small, but some have large scales	Usually large
Fangs	Long and canalized like hypodermic needle	Short and solid
Belly scales	Broad or large and extend across entire width of the belly	Small and do not extend across the entire width
Tail	Compressed, rounded, or flattened	Not markedly compressed, always rounded
Fang marks	Two fang marks with or without small marks of other teeth	Number of small teeth marks in a row
Habits	Usually nocturnal	No specific habits

Q3. How would you manage this case?
- Reassure the patient, give tetanus toxoid injection to prevent tetanus.
- Next step is to administer anti-snake venom (ASV) preferably after a test dose (since ASV is prepared in equine serum, medicolegally it is always safe to give a test dose).

There are two regimens of ASV therapy which can be used for vasculotoxic snake bite:
1. *Low-dose infusion therapy:* 10 vials for Russell's viper or six vials for saw-scaled viper envenomations as stat dose given as an intravenous (IV) infusion over 30 minutes followed by two vials every 6 hours as infusion in 100 mL of normal saline till clotting time normalizes or for 3 days, whichever is earlier.
2. *High-dose intermittent bolus therapy:* 10 vials of polyvalent ASV as stat dose over 30 minutes given as an IV infusion followed by six vials every 6 hours as bolus therapy till clotting time normalizes and/or local swelling subsides.

The dose of venom injected per bite varies from 5 mg to 147 mg. So, the total dose required ranges from 10 to 30 vials as each vial neutralizes 6 mg of Russell's viper venom. A lack of adequate response may warrant additional vials.

Q4. How do you monitor and titrate the ASV dose?
Monitoring and titration of ASV dose are shown in **Flowchart 1**.

Q5. Why do you think the patient is in DIC?
Points in favor of DIC:
- Oozing of blood from bite site with presence of two fang marks (confirms bite by a poisonous snake)
- Deranged WBCT, aPTT, INR and low platelet counts

Q6. How do you manage DIC in this case?
Management of DIC: Fresh frozen plasma (FFP) and platelets are used respectively in cases with deranged INR or aPTT

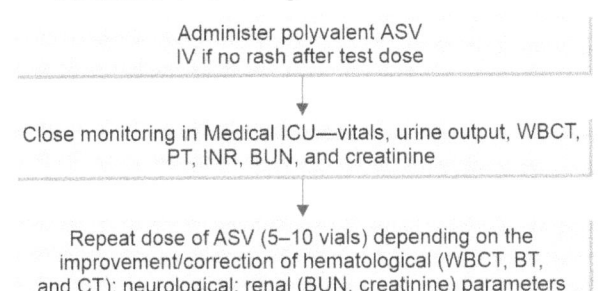

Flowchart 1: Monitoring and titration of ASV dose.

(ASV: antisnake venom; BT: bleeding time; BUN: blood urea nitrogen; CT: clotting time; ICU: intensive care unit; INR: international normalized ratio; PT: prothrombin time; WBCT: Whole blood clotting time)

and thrombocytopenia (platelet counts <10,000/mm^3 or >10,000/mm^3 with evidence of bleeding). Cryoprecipitate is indicated for low fibrinogen levels in cases of intractable bleeding.

Q7. What complication has occurred in this case?
The complication which has occurred in this case is acute renal failure (ARF).

Q8. What other complications do you expect in this case?
Other complications which can occur in this case include intractable bleeding due to DIC presenting as hematuria, hemoptysis, epistaxis, hematemesis or hematochezia. The most dreaded complication would be retinal hemorrhage or intracranial (IC) bleed. Rarely, the thrombotic DIC complication may present with stroke or pulmonary embolism, altered sensorium or cutaneous and peripheral gangrene.

Q9. What are the causes of ARF in patients with snake bite?
ARF also known as acute kidney injury (AKI) can occur in patients with vasculotoxic snake bites, particularly those caused by certain venomous snakes. The venom of these snakes contains various toxins that can directly or indirectly affect the kidneys, leading to kidney injury. Here are some of the main causes of ARF in patients with vasculotoxic snake bites:
- *Direct nephrotoxicity:* Some snake venoms contain toxins that can damage the renal tubules and impair the kidney's ability to filter and excrete waste products, resulting in acute tubular necrosis (ATN), i.e., injury or destruction of renal tubular cells.
- *Hemolysis:* Certain venomous snake bites can lead to intravascular hemolysis, causing the breakdown of red blood cells. The released hemoglobin can overwhelm the kidneys' ability to filter and process it, leading to acute tubular injury and ARF.
- *Hypotension:* Some snake venoms can cause systemic effects, including hypotension which leads to diminished blood flow to the kidneys, compromising renal function, and causing ischemic injury.
- *Coagulation abnormalities:* Venomous snake bites can result in coagulation abnormalities such as DIC which can lead to microvascular thrombosis, causing inadequate blood flow to the kidneys and contributing to ARF.
- *Rhabdomyolysis:* In some cases, snake venom can cause rhabdomyolysis where damaged muscle cells release their contents, including myoglobin, into the bloodstream. Myoglobin can be toxic to the kidneys, leading to acute tubular injury and renal dysfunction.
  - *Immune complex deposition:* The venom of some snakes can trigger an immune response, leading to the formation of immune complexes. These immune

complexes can deposit in the kidneys, causing inflammation and renal injury.
- *Pre-existing conditions*: Patients with pre-existing kidney disease or other co-morbidities may be at higher risk for ARF following a vasculotoxic snake bite due to decreased kidney reserve and compromised renal function.

Q10. How do you manage renal failure with DIC in vasculotoxic snake bites?

Management and outcome of ARF with DIC in vasculotoxic snake bite cases: It is essential to recognize and manage ARF promptly in patients with vasculotoxic snake bites, as it can lead to serious complications and even be life-threatening. Treatment may involve supportive measures, such as hydration, use of diuretics, correction of coagulation abnormalities—DIC corrected with FFP or platelet transfusion, low fibrinogen levels are treated with cryoprecipitate and management of hypertension or hypotension. In severe cases, renal replacement therapy—hemodialysis (usually heparin free) may be required to support renal function until recovery occurs. Renal cortical necrosis comes with a guarded prognosis. Majority of such patients need alternate day hemodialysis for up to 3-4 weeks. Recovery is heralded by rise in urine output followed by falling trends in serum creatinine levels. Rarely, the patient may require lifelong dialysis or renal transplantation.

Early administration of ASV when available and indicated may also help mitigate the kidney injury caused by snake venom. Timely and appropriate medical intervention can significantly improve the patient's prognosis and reduce the risk of long-term renal damage.

Case 2

A 50-year-old male came to our casualty around 11 AM with history of snake bite on his right hand under influence of alcohol while trying to scare it away at a public park. The snake was killed by his friends and brought to the casualty as well. His friends also tied a piece of cloth just above the bite site on his right hand. Patient has a history of ischemic heart disease for 5 years. Patient also underwent PTCA 4 years ago.

Patient was immediately taken by his friends to a peripheral hospital initially where the patient was anxious with a pulse rate of 88 beats/min and blood pressure of 124/76 mm Hg. On local examination of the bite, they had mentioned that there was a puncture wound with 2 fang marks on the first web space between the thumb and index finger on the dorsal aspect of right hand along with redness and swelling. Systemic examination was normal. Patient was administered tetanus toxoid injection along with 4 vials of ASV and was referred to a tertiary care hospital for further management. On reaching our emergency room 1 hour later, patient had developed drooping of eyelids and neck flexor weakness. He also complained of weakness of the limbs. The piece of cloth tied above the bite site was removed.

*Investigations are summarized in **Table 3**.*

Q1. What is your clinical impression and which snake envenomations can cause the above clinical features?

It is a case of neurotoxic snake bite. Cobra, krait, and sea snake bite patients commonly present with neurological manifestations.

Q2. What are the features of neurotoxic snake bite?

Neurotoxic snake bite features include ptosis, double vision, paralysis of external ocular muscles, bulbar palsy, weakness of muscles of the neck with neck lag, or respiratory muscles weakness due to neuromuscular junction involvement needing invasive mechanical ventilation. Other manifestations include convulsions, altered sensorium, or unconsciousness.

TABLE 3: Investigations chart.

Hemoglobin	14.2 g%	Total protein	6.2 g%
Leukocyte count	7,650 /mm^3	Serum albumin	3.9 g%
Platelet count	264,000/mm^3	Serum Na$^+$/K$^+$	137/3.9 mEq/L
Prothrombin time	12.5 (control 11.5 seconds)	Serum Calcium	9.0 mg%
INR	1.09	Serum Magnesium	2.2 mg%
aPTT	27 seconds	Total bilirubin	0.4 mg%
WBCT	<20 minutes	SGOT/SGPT	11/14 U/L
		BUN/Creatinine	14.6/0.9 mg%
Chest X-ray	Normal	ECG	Normal

(aPTT: activated partial thromboplastin time; BUN: blood urea nitrogen; ECG: electrocardiogram; INR: international normalized ratio; SGPT: serum glutamic pyruvic transaminase; SGOT: serum glutamic oxaloacetic transaminase; WBCT: whole blood clotting time)

Q3. Is it possible to get both paralytic and bleeding manifestations in a snake bite victim?

Yes. Russell's viper bite victims can present with hematological, renal, and neurological clinical features.

Q4. What things should have been avoided in this patient prior to getting the patient to the hospital?

Things which should not be done or to be avoided in a snake bite case are as follows:

- Application of tight tourniquets proximal to bite site, incision around bite site, oral suctioning, application of ice packs and chemicals or herbal remedies can worsen the localized tissue damage and even lead to infection and gangrene.
- Also, there is no need to kill or handle the snake and bring it to the emergency department. Only mobile phone camera pictures of the same are sufficient for identification and planning further management.

Q5. What are the complications of neurotoxic snake bite?

Neurotoxic snake bites can be life-threatening and lead to various complications due to the venom's effects on the nervous system as it interferes with nerve cell function and transmission, leading to paralysis and other neurological manifestations. The severity of the complications depends on factors such as the type of snake, the amount of venom injected and the time elapsed before receiving appropriate medical treatment. Here are some of the main complications that can occur in neurotoxic snake bites:

- *Respiratory paralysis:* It is one of the most critical complications of neurotoxic snake bites. The venom can affect the nerves that control respiration, leading to weakness or paralysis of the respiratory muscles. This can result in tachypnea, dyspnea, or respiratory distress, and, if not promptly managed, even lead to respiratory failure.
- *Bulbar paralysis:* Some neurotoxic venoms can cause paralysis of the muscles involved in swallowing and speaking, leading to dysphagia and speech difficulties.
- *Cranial nerve dysfunction:* Neurotoxic venom can affect various cranial nerves, leading to a range of neurological deficits resulting in visual disturbances, diplopia, ptosis, and other cranial nerve-related symptoms.
- *Generalized muscle weakness:* Neurotoxic envenomations can cause generalized muscle weakness, which can progress to paralysis if not treated promptly.
- *Autonomic nervous system dysfunction:* Few neurotoxic venoms can interfere with the autonomic nervous system, leading to fluctuations in heart rate or arrhythmias, fluctuation in blood pressure (hypotension or hypertension) and sudden onset profuse sweating.
- *Neurological impairments*: In severe cases, neurotoxic snake bites can lead to neurological impairments, including altered mentation, confusion and loss of consciousness.
- *Organ failure*: In extremely severe cases, the paralysis and systemic effects of neurotoxic venom can lead to multiorgan failure, including respiratory failure, cardiovascular collapse, and renal failure.
- *Long-term disability*: Delayed or inadequate treatment of neurotoxic snake bites can lead to long-term neurological deficits and disabilities.

It is important to seek immediate medical attention in the event of a suspected or confirmed neurotoxic snake bite. Early administration of specific ASV and supportive care is essential to prevent or minimize complications and improve the chances of a favorable outcome. Rapid transport to a medical facility equipped to manage snake bites is crucial, especially in regions where venomous snakes are prevalent. In some cases, mechanical ventilation or other supportive measures may be required to manage respiratory distress and other complications associated with neurotoxic snake bites.

Q6. What are the differential diagnoses of neurotoxic snake bite cases?

Occasionally, patients are brought with an alleged history of "unknown" bite, especially during sleep, followed by varying degree of neurological symptoms. Some of these have been referred to as "neuroparalytic syndrome" in "jhuggi dwellers".[1] Some of the differential diagnoses to consider apart from neurotoxic snake envenomation include:

- Stings by poisonous wasps and bees
- Tick paralysis
- Myasthenic crisis especially on background of a febrile illness
- Bite may be a "red herring" and the patient may have:
  - Hypokalemic periodic paralysis
  - Fulminant Guillain–Barré syndrome (GBS)
  - Organophosphate poisoning—predominantly nicotinic features

Q7. How do you manage neuroparalytic snake bite?

- Reassure the patient, give tetanus toxoid injection to prevent tetanus.
- Next step is to administer ASV preferably after a test dose (since ASV is prepared in equine serum, medicolegally it is always safe to give a test dose).
  - *Dose of ASV for neuroparalytic snake bite*—10 vials stat dose as IV infusion over 30 minutes followed by second dose of 10 vials after 1 hour if there is no improvement in symptoms.

- Also, IV neostigmine is administered after preloading with IV atropine (0.6 mg) to prevent the cholinergic side effects of neostigmine on the heart.

Q8. What is the prognosis of this patient with neurotoxic snake bite?

Prognosis of a patient with a neurotoxic snake bite can vary widely based on several factors, including the type of snake, the amount of venom injected, the time elapsed before receiving medical treatment, the patient's age and overall health, and the availability and effectiveness of ASV therapy. Generally, early recognition and prompt medical intervention are crucial in improving the prognosis of neurotoxic snake bites.

Favorable prognostic factors:
- *Timely medical treatment*: Seeking medical attention promptly after a neurotoxic snake bite is essential. Early administration of ASV can significantly improve the patient's chances of recovery.
- *Adequate antivenom therapy*: If the ASV if available and is administered in sufficient quantities, it can effectively neutralize the venom's neurotoxic effects and lead to a positive outcome.
- *Good respiratory muscle function*: If the respiratory muscles are not severely affected, the risk of respiratory failure can be minimized.
- *Absence of severe systemic effects*: If the venom's systemic effects, such as cardiovascular collapse or multiorgan failure, can be managed effectively, the prognosis improves.
- *Supportive care*: Adequate supportive care, including maintaining airway and breathing, managing blood pressure and hydration, and treating any complications, is vital in improving the prognosis.

Unfavorable prognostic factors:
- *Delayed medical treatment*: Delay in seeking medical attention can lead to a worsened prognosis, especially if the patient experiences significant paralysis or respiratory distress before receiving ASV therapy.
- *Severe respiratory paralysis*: If the respiratory muscles are severely affected it can to respiratory failure and the prognosis may be guarded.
- *Inadequate or unavailable ASV*: The lack of access to ASV or its insufficient availability can hinder successful management and worsen the prognosis.
- *Advanced age and co-morbidities*: Older age and pre-existing medical conditions can complicate the clinical course and reduce the patient's ability to tolerate the venom's effects.
- *Delayed recovery*: Prolonged paralysis or neurological deficits may indicate more severe envenomation and could result in a more prolonged recovery period.

It is important to note that the prognosis of neurotoxic snake bites can vary significantly depending on the geographic region and the particular species of venomous snakes involved. Some snakes may have highly potent neurotoxic venoms, which can be lethal even in small quantities. Intensive medical management in specialized medical facilities can significantly improve the chances of survival and recovery in patients with neurotoxic snake bites.

Q9. What progress has been made in ASV production?

The initial ASV consisted of the serum itself which was derived from equine blood; source being hyperimmunized by sublethal doses of snake venom. Advances in production technology allowed immunoglobulins or their fragments (Fab) to be marketed instead of serum ASV.[2]

These immunoglobulins are obtained by plasmapheresis of equine/ovine blood, allowing the red blood cells to be re-injected into the donor animals, thereby, preventing anemia in them. Thus, the ideal term should be "ASV immunoglobulin".

At present, polyvalent-refined immunoglobulin (equine) prepared from the serum of hyperimmunized horses is available in India. "CroFab" is another polyvalent ASV obtained from sheep which is used for the treatment of "crotalid" group of snake bites. This group includes snakes from the "pit viper" family found in the North American subcontinent which are rattlesnakes, pit vipers, and copperheads' species.

Special situations

Management of snake bite in pregnancy— Snake bites during pregnancy can be a serious medical emergency, especially if the snake is venomous and has vasculotoxic effects. The snake venom can also be fatal to the fetus. It can lead to abruptio placenta due to DIC. The venom can provoke uterine contractions leading to premature delivery and fetal loss. Both the snake venom as well as the ASV have the potential to cause anaphylaxis, leading to maternal shock.

The ability of the ASV to cross the placenta varies as per its type and molecular weight. Fab ASV with a molecular weight of approximately 50,000 daltons may not be able to cross the placenta.[3] In such a setting, hemorrhages could occur in the fetus even in the absence of maternal DIC with fetal wastage.

Snake envenomations in pregnancy are associated with a maternal mortality rate of 10% and a fetal mortality rate of 10% as well. Management of vasculotoxic snake bites in pregnancy is a complex medical decision that requires a multidisciplinary approach involving physician, obstetricians, general surgeon, toxicologists, and neonatologist.

Reported maternal complications in vasculotoxic snake bite cases in pregnancy are ante-partum hemorrhage, placental abruption, preterm labor, post-partum hemorrhage, DIC, hypotension, hypovolemic shock, anemia AKI and posterior reversible encephalopathy syndrome.

Fetal complications reported include miscarriage, fetal distress, intrauterine death, prematurity, hydrocephalus and polydactyly.

Therefore, prompt and appropriate medical attention is crucial to ensure the best possible outcome for both the mother and the baby.

- *First aid and immobilization*: If possible, immediately seek help and avoid unnecessary movement to prevent the venom from spreading quickly. Keep the affected limb immobilized and at or below the level of the heart to slow down the venom's spread.
- *Immediate medical care*: Seek emergency medical care at a hospital or healthcare facility with expertise in managing snake bites and high-risk pregnancies. Time is critical in managing the complications of vasculotoxic snake bites.
- *Monitoring*: Frequent monitoring of the mother and the fetus is essential to detect any adverse reactions or changes in the condition preferably in the intensive care unit (ICU). This may include monitoring vital signs, fetal heart rate, and coagulation parameters such as prothrombin time (PT), activated partial thromboplastin time (aPTT), and platelet count, is necessary to assess the extent of coagulopathy and plan appropriate treatment.
- *ASV administration*: It is crucial to identify the snake responsible for the bite, as different snake venoms can have varying effects on the coagulation system and may require ASV administration. ASV is the most effective treatment for venomous snake bites and generally considered safe in pregnancy. Potential risks and benefits must be carefully weighed by the medical team based on the severity of envenomation.
- *Supportive care*: Pregnant women with vasculotoxic snake bites may require additional supportive care, such as pain management, fluid resuscitation, transfusion of blood and blood products, correction of coagulopathy with the help of FFP and cryoprecipitate, platelet transfusions and management of any complications that may arise. In patients nearing term for delivery, in the setting of a coagulopathy following snake envenomation, empirical administration of uterine relaxants such as isoxsuprine or nifedipine is warranted till the coagulopathy is corrected.
- *Delivery*: In cases with DIC or impending bleeding risks where the mother's life is at risk or when the pregnancy is near term, delivery of the baby may be considered to improve the mother's condition and facilitate further treatment.
- *Potential risks*: The potential risks of vasculotoxic snake bites in pregnancy include preterm labor, fetal distress, and maternal complications related to venom effects. These risks may vary depending on the specific venom of the snake and the severity of envenomation.
- *Prevention*: Whenever it is possible, try to avoid areas where snakes are prevalent. Wear protective clothing and footwear in snake-prone regions. Be cautious when walking or sitting outdoors, especially in tall grass or near water bodies.

Gupta A et al.[4] reported a successful outcome of managing a female with coagulopathy following a snake bite during the third trimester of pregnancy, the patient was treated with IV fluids, blood products and anticoagulants along with steroids for fetal maturity followed by timely labor induction. They transfused fresh whole blood and FFP along with packed red blood cells for a successful outcome without consumption coagulopathy. They also highlighted the point that in peripheral institutes where there is a scarcity of blood products, fresh whole blood could be used as an alternative to clotting factors, particularly when there is presence of or an impending risk of anemia. They also demonstrated the importance of early intervention, symptomatic management and intensive monitoring in managing snake bite in pregnancy. Bolliger et al.[5] also reviewed and revealed that prevention of consumption coagulopathy is possible by transfusion of packed RBCs along with FFP, cryoprecipitate, fibrinogen concentrate and factor XIII concentrate.

Similarly, two case reports of vasculotoxic snake bite in pregnancy with successful outcomes were reported by Singh S et al.[6] First case was a pregnant female bitten by a vasculotoxic snake in her first trimester (8 weeks) who presented with WBCT >20 minutes. She was treated with just ASV and antibiotics and her coagulation parameters normalized. She was followed-up on OPD basis for the rest of her pregnancy and underwent cesarean section at 33 weeks in view of eclampsia. Second case presented with history of vasculotoxic snake bite in her third trimester (29 weeks) with a deranged WBCT of >20 minutes. She too was treated with ASV and antibiotics following which her coagulation parameters normalized and she underwent spontaneous preterm labor at 36 weeks and delivered a healthy baby.

Cardiac effects of snake envenomations: Sunil Kumar et al.[7] in study of 96 cases of snake envenomations reported a cardiac toxicity of 42.7%, with majority of them as ECG changes

(34.3%—documented as bradycardia, early repolarization, ST elevation, T wave inversion, Brugada pattern, premature atrial complexes, and ST depression), rise in troponin-I levels (21.9%), hypertension (15.6%), hypotension (13.5%), 2D echo changes (4.2%) and takotsubo cardiomyopathy (1%). It should be noted that the above cohort had both neurotoxic and vasculotoxic snake bite patients. Cardiac toxicity is not a well-documented finding in snake envenomations, above study highlights the need for cardiac monitoring in all snake bite patients.

Case 3

A 16-year-old boy without any previous underlying illness presented to a rural peripheral center following history of a scorpion sting on his right hand while he was collecting wood in a local forest. He had excruciating pain at the sting site and was anxious and restless. He was administered injection Tetanus toxoid along with local 2% lignocaine injection and was referred to a tertiary care hospital. On arriving at our emergency department 2 hours later, he complained of abdominal pain, vomiting and increased salivation. He also had profuse sweating and visual blurring. There was no bleeding from any site, chest pain or breathing difficulty.

On examination, the patient had cold, clammy extremities with a pulse rate of 102 beats/min, blood pressure of 160/100 mm Hg and respiratory rate of 16 breaths/min. Local examination revealed no oozing/redness/edema or tenderness at the sting site.

On systemic examination, respiratory system had bilateral rhonchi on auscultation, per abdomen examination demonstrated epigastric tenderness. Central nervous system (CNS) and cardiovascular system showed no obvious abnormality.

Q1. What is your diagnosis?
It is a case of scorpion sting with autonomic storm.

Q2. How will you manage a case of scorpion sting?
- Reassure the patient, give tetanus toxoid injection to prevent tetanus. Local lignocaine infiltration (2%) should be given promptly for pain relief.
- Use of analgesics or oral diazepam also alleviates the pain.
- Ice fomentation reduces localized edema.
- All patients need pulse and blood pressure monitoring with urine output charting.

What not to do: Application of tight tourniquets proximal to sting site, incision around sting site, local use of $KMnO_4$ (potassium permanganate) or herbal remedies can worsen the localized tissue damage and can lead to infection and gangrene.

Patients with systemic manifestations (hypertensive crisis and pulmonary edema) are ideally managed in ICU with central line insertion for IV fluid management and monitoring for cardiac arrhythmias.

In patients with hypertensive crises, IV labetalol or oral prazosin (alpha blockers) is preferred. For patients with hypotension, IV noradrenaline and dobutamine may be used. Patients with pulmonary edema require parenteral diuretics (IV frusemide) and mechanical ventilation. Antihypertensive medications should be titrated cautiously in order to avoid precipitous hypotension.

Q3. What complications can develop in scorpion sting?
Autonomic features (storm) set in rapidly within 15–30 minutes and are characterized by features of parasympathetic nervous system (PNS) stimulation. These include diaphoresis, vomiting, bradycardia or ventricular premature complexes, and low blood pressure and could be attributed to acetylcholine excess. Priapism, ropy salivation, and ventricular premature complexes may also be seen. Occasionally, patient may present with tachycardia and high blood pressure as part of sympathetic nervous system (SNS) stimulation. Often, systolic blood pressure exceeds over 200 mm Hg even in young patients which can lead to flash pulmonary edema.

Cardiovascular features include myocarditis which can be fatal and usually leads to hypotension, arrhythmias including ventricular arrhythmias and cardiogenic shock. Ventricular arrhythmias can lead to death even within the first half hour following the sting.

Central nervous system features include dilated or non-reactive pupils due to excitation of alpha receptors of the dilator pupillary muscle as a result of overt catecholamine levels in the blood. Hemiparesis due to hemorrhagic or thrombotic stroke can be seen in red scorpion sting patients secondary to DIC. Coma, cerebral edema, constricted or dilated pupils and convulsions are associated with poor prognosis.

Some stings can lead to renal failure within 48 hours. The causes may be pre-renal due to hypovolemic shock or renal due to toxin or hemolysis-induced kidney damage.

Rarely, DIC can lead to intermittent thrombosis, thrombocytopenia and fatal bleeding (reported by stings from *Hemiscorpius lepturus*).

Q4. How do you grade scorpion stings?
Based on the clinical features at the time of presentation to the hospital and their severity, there are four grades:
- *Grade 1:* Localized excruciating and severe pain at the sting site along with radiation to the concerned

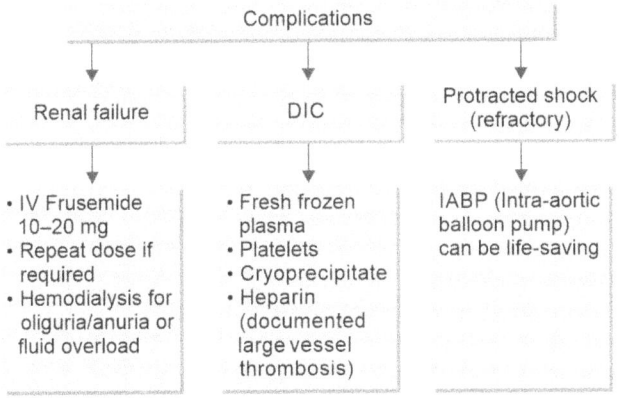

Flowchart 2: Management of complications of scorpion sting.

(DIC: disseminated intravascular coagulation)

TABLE 4: Investigations chart on admission.			
Hemoglobin	12.9 g%	Total protein	6.5 g%
Leukocyte count	7,100 /mm³	Serum albumin	3.9 g%
Platelet count	262,000/mm³	Serum Na⁺/K⁺	139/4.1 mEq/L
Prothrombin time	12.7 (control 11.7 seconds)	Serum Calcium	9.1 mg%
INR	1.1	Serum Magnesium	2.1 mg%
Chest X-ray	Normal	Total bilirubin	0.6 mg%
WBCT	<20 minutes	SGOT/SGPT	14/17 U/L
		BUN/creatinine	18/0.9 mg%
ECG	Sinus tachycardia, heart rate 106 beats/min, T-wave inversion in II, III, and aVF	2 D Echo	Normal study

(BUN: blood urea nitrogen; ECG: electrocardiogram; INR: international normalized ratio; SGPT: serum glutamic pyruvic transaminase; SGOT: serum glutamic oxaloacetic transaminase ; WBCT: whole blood clotting time)

dermatomes, localized swelling (mild) and without any systemic features
- *Grade 2:* Clinical features of autonomic storm due to excess of acetylcholine or due to PNS stimulation and SNS stimulation
- *Grade 3*: Tachycardia, cool peripheries, low or high blood pressure along with pulmonary edema
- *Grade 4:* Low blood pressure, tachycardia, and warm peripheries with or without pulmonary edema (warm shock).

Q5. How do you manage the complications of scorpion sting?
Management of complications of scorpion sting is shown in **Flowchart 2**.

Case 3 continued…

A provisional diagnosis of scorpion sting with autonomic storm was made and patient was shifted to Medical ICU for further management. Patient initially received stat doses of injection prazosin (1 mg), injection chlorpheniramine maleate, injection hydrocortisone (100 mg), injection frusemide (20 mg) along with other supportive measures and vitals monitoring.

After 4 hours of the bite, there was a sudden fall in SpO₂ level to 92% and the patient became tachypneic with respiratory rate of 30 breaths/min, pulse rate of 110 beats/min and blood pressure of 122/96 mm Hg with his peripheries now turning warm. On auscultation of respiratory system, patient had bilateral scattered crepitations with no changes in clinical findings of other systems. Patient had to be intubated and put on ventilatory support. He was extubated 48 hours after, following which he was shifted to general ward on day 5 of admission and discharged on day 7.

*Investigations are summarized in **Table 4**.*

Q6. What are the rare complications of scorpion sting which are reported in literature?
Rare complications of scorpion sting which are reported in literature are as follows: Multiple IC hemorrhages[8] or cerebral infarction,[9] pancreatitis, defibrination syndrome, and bilateral cerebellar infarction.[10]

Q7. What is the role of scorpion antivenom and how is it administered?
Scorpion anti-venom (SAV): It is a lyophilized, monovalent, enzyme-refined immunoglobulin (equine) available as a freeze-dried powder which can be stored at room temperature. Each mL of reconstituted serum (in 10 mL of sterile water) neutralizes 1 mg of red scorpion venom. Each vial costs around Rs 1,500/- and is usually in short supply. Initially a test dose of 0.1 mL is administered subcutaneously and monitored for any reactions for 30 minutes. If no adverse reactions are seen/documented, immediate treatment dose of one vial (total 10 mL reconstituted) is given intravenously. Further doses depend on persistence of clinical signs. A cumulative dose of around 30–100 mL of SAV is usually required. Use of SAV along with prazosin has also demonstrated a faster recovery than oral prazosin administered alone.[11]

Caution: Some scorpion sting patients may directly present to the emergency with hypertensive crises and pulmonary edema along with pink frothy sputum. Attempts to reduce the blood pressure with prazosin or labetalol may be followed by "precipitous hypotension" within 30–60 minutes which may require inotrope support. Hence, utmost care with strict monitoring of vitals in an ICU setting is advisable along with a careful titration of prazosin or labetalol.

REFERENCES

1. Saini RK, Singh S, Sharma S, Rampal V, Manhas AS, Gupta VK. Snake bite poisoning presenting as early morning neuroparalytic syndrome in jhuggi dwellers. J Assoc Physicians India. 1986;34(6):415-7.
2. WHO. (2013). Guidelines for the production, control and regulation of snake antivenom immunoglobulins Replacement, Annex 5, TRS No 1004— Replacement of Annex 2 of WHO Technical Report Series, No. 964. , No. 964. [online] Available from: https://www.who.int/publications/m/item/snake-antivenom-immunoglobulins-annex-5-trs-no-1004 [Last accessed August, 2023].
3. Wium L. Neurotoxic snake bite in pregnancy. Obstet Med. 2021;14(3):187-9.
4. Gupta A, Bhandari S, Anand A, Sharma SK, Gautam A, Priyanka KC, et al. Management of snake bite during third trimester of pregnancy with coagulopathy and delivery of live baby in resource-limited setting in Nepal: A case report. Oxf Med Case Reports. 2022;2022(10):omac105.
5. Bolliger D, Görlinger K, Tanaka KA. Pathophysiology and treatment of coagulopathy in massive hemorrhage and hemodilution. Anesthesiology. 2010;113:1205-19.
6. Singh S, Mohanty RR. Vasculotoxic snakebite envenomation: Management challenges in pregnancy. Obstet Med. 2021; 14(3):190-2.
7. Kumar S, Joseph K, Joseph S, Varghese AM, Jose MP. Cardiac involvement in vasculotoxic and neurotoxic snakebite—A not so uncommon complication. J Assoc Physicians India. 2020;68(11):39-41.
8. Kishore D, Misra S. Atypical systemic manifestation of scorpion envenomation. J Assoc Physicians India. 2009;57: 344.
9. Jain MK, Indurkar M, Kastwar V, Malviya S. Myocarditis and multiple cerebral and cerebellar infarction following scorpion sting. J Assoc Physicians India. 2006;54:491-2.
10. Gadwalkar SR, Bushan S, Pramod K, Gouda C, Kumar PM. Bilateral Cerebellar Infarction: A Rare Complication of Scorpion Sting. J Assoc Physicians India. 2006;54:581-3.
11. Bawaskar HS, Bawaskar PH. Efficacy and safety of scorpion anti-venom plus prazosin compared with prazosin alone for venomous scorpion (Mesobuthus tamulus) sting: randomised open label trial. BMJ. 2011;342:c7136.

CHAPTER 19

Infective Endocarditis

Sachin Gupta, Deeksha Singh Tomar

CASE STUDIES

Case 1

A 36-year-old male presents to the emergency department with fever of 6 days duration, easy fatigability, and vomiting of 3 days duration. His attendants also informed that he has become drowsy over last 3 days and now only responds to loud verbal commands. His vital parameters on arrival are heart rate 135 beats/min, blood pressure 108/66 mm Hg, respiratory rate 26 breaths/min, and temperature 102.5°F. He is drowsy but responding to loud verbal commands. Pupils are 3 mm, sluggishly reacting to light. There is history of recent hospitalization for 10 days for severe community-acquired pneumonia (CAP) where he received intravenous medications. Patient had taken intramuscular penicillin G injections for rheumatic heart disease in his childhood. On examination, he also has small punctate hemorrhages at the shin of tibia.

Q1. What is the differential diagnosis that should be considered in this scenario?

This patient is having sepsis as he is having high-grade fever, altered sensorium, tachycardia, and history of recent hospitalization. The probable differential diagnosis for this scenario can be:
- *Consolidation:* As patient had been recently treated for severe CAP, there could be relapse of pneumonia for another multidrug-resistant organism.
- *Meningoencephalitis:* The patient has presented with altered sensorium with high-grade fever.
- *Infective endocarditis (IE):* As the patient presented with high-grade fever, altered sensorium, and previous history of prolonged injectable drug therapy, mostly through a central venous access, should raise the suspicion. Rheumatic heart disease is a risk factor for IE.[1] More than 25% cases of IE present with features of embolic phenomena.[2]
- *Pulmonary embolism:* Fever, tachycardia, and fatigability are nonspecific symptoms of pulmonary embolism. Patient also has recent history of hospitalization, which increases the risk of pulmonary embolism.

Q2. How will you confirm the diagnosis in this patient?

All patients should undergo routine blood investigations including blood and other appropriate cultures (according to suspected site/s of infection) and radiological tests such as chest X-ray, computed tomography (CT) scan, and 2-dimensional echocardiography. The routine blood tests should include complete blood count, renal function test, liver function test, D-dimer, and coagulation profile.

On physical examination at presentation and the clinical features, the most probable diagnosis looks to be IE, although every investigation will be done to rule out other diagnosis as well.

Q3. What are the risk factors for IE?

Structural heart disease, especially valvular heart disease, is a significant risk factor for IE. Patients with long-term central venous catheters are also at increased risk. Cardiac surgery for structural heart disease also increases the chances of IE.[3] Any residual cardiac defect after cardiac surgery increases the risk for IE.

In pediatric population, presence of central venous catheter without any structural heart disease is a risk factor for IE. Prolonged intravenous drug usage can cause IE of the tricuspid valve in adolescent individuals. **Box 1** enumerates the various risk factors.

Q4. What are the clinical presentations of IE?

A very high index of suspicion should be kept while interpreting the symptoms of the patients. The infective

---

BOX 1: Risk factors for infective endocarditis.
- Structural heart disease
- Valvular heart disease
- Rheumatic heart disease
- Prosthetic valve
- Recent cardiac surgery
- Prolonged intravenous drug therapy
- Drug addicts
- Prolonged central venous line
- Dental extraction
- Coronavirus disease-2019

foci can present as embolic phenomenon at various body parts. The severity of clinical symptoms will vary according to cardiac dysfunction that the vegetation has created and the embolic or metastatic spread of the infection.[4] The initial symptoms are very vague with fever and chills being the most common presentation. Anorexia, malaise, weight loss, headache, and restlessness are the most symptoms, which the patients complain. Joint pain or inability to bear weight is a sign of metastatic spread of infection at the knee joint and presenting as osteomyelitis.[5]

Congestive heart failure (CHF) can be a finding in patients with prior structural heart disease. Patients can have altered sensorium due to embolic stroke or even brain abscess due to metastatic spread of infection[6] (just like in our patient who is in altered sensorium).

Drug abusers generally present with cough and dyspnea as they are more prone to tricuspid valve vegetation and the symptoms are due to embolic showers to pulmonary vasculature.

The peripheral manifestations of IE are nonsuppurative lesions, which are irregular, nontender, erythematous papules which are generally located on the palm of hands or soles. These are called Janeway lesions[7] and are signs of subacute IE as these lesions last for days and weeks. Osler nodes[7] are defined as red-colored tender lumps and represent embolic manifestation of IE. Roth's spots[8] can be found in many medical conditions but are most associated with IE and they are defined as white-centered retinal hemorrhages. Patients also develop bleeding under the nailbed, which is called subungual hemorrhages. All the clinical features are represented in **Table 1**.

TABLE 1: Clinical presentation.	
Nonspecific symptoms	• Fever • Myalgia • Weakness • Easy fatigability • Anorexia • Weight loss • Cough
Cardiac manifestations	• Pleuritic chest pain • Irregular heart rhythm • Tachycardia • Breathlessness • Syncope • Myocarditis
Noncardiac manifestations	• Altered sensorium • Stroke • Janeway lesions • Osler nodes • Roth's spots • Subungual hemorrhages • Osteomyelitis • Petechiae at various body areas • Clubbing

Q5. How to classify IE?
Infective endocarditis can be classified as acute or subacute presentation.[9] Acute IE is a fulminant disease with poor outcome if not recognized in a timely manner. Subacute IE can present as vague and slow progressive symptoms such as fever, anorexia, weakness, and fatigability.[10] The development of cerebral events is less in subacute IE. The differentiation between acute and subacute IE is important as the treatment aggressiveness depends on the course of symptoms.

Case 2

Looking at the symptoms and rapid onset, the preliminary diagnosis of the patient was established as acute IE. Cultures and certain radiological test and echocardiogram were ordered.

Q1. What should be the protocol for blood cultures if there is high index of suspicion of IE?
Blood culture positivity is a sign of bacteremia, and it is essential to the diagnosis of IE. For all infective etiologies, blood culture is sent as paired sets to culture for aerobic and anaerobic organisms from different venipuncture sites at the same time. But for IE, at least three sets of blood cultures are sent 30 minutes apart. Each set consists of two bottles, one aerobic and another anaerobic, at least 10 mL of blood in each bottle (total 60 mL of blood for three sets). All the samples should be taken from different venipuncture sites.[5] If all the cultures turn out to be positive, then it confirms continued bacteremia, which is diagnostic of IE. But on 10–20% occasions the blood culture will be false negative due to previous antibiotic use or improper volume of blood sample in the culture bottle.[11]

Q1a. What findings are expected in echocardiogram?
Transthoracic echocardiography (TTE) is the first imaging modality that should be performed for all patients with suspected IE. **Box 2** highlights the various findings in echocardiogram. TTE has good sensitivity (almost 60%)[12] in detecting vegetations in native valves but transesophageal echocardiography (TEE) has almost 90%[13] sensitivity in detecting prosthetic valve endocarditis (PVE). Presence of vegetation on any valve is diagnostic of IE. TEE should also be done when the suspicion of IE is high but TTE is negative. Three-dimensional TEE complements the findings

BOX 2: Echocardiography findings in infective endocarditis.
• Vegetation • Annular abscess • Dehiscence of prosthetic valve • New valvular regurgitation • Oscillating intracardiac mass

of conventional TEE and helps in describing the entire architecture of the vegetation and also helps in surgical planning for that patient.[14]

Q1b. What are the other imaging modalities that can be done to diagnose IE?

There are couple of imaging techniques that can be done to confirm the diagnosis and also help in diagnosing certain complications that have occurred due to IE.

Cardiac computed tomography

This imaging modality should be done to detect perivalvular abscess and to detect any vegetations around the aortic root.[15] Recently Wang et al. proposed that cardiac CT has prognostic value in surgery planning and in predicting mortality.[16]

Chest radiograph

Features of pulmonary embolism and infarcts can be seen. Other features like lung abscess can also be identified.

Case 3

On echocardiogram, mitral valve vegetation was detected. Moderate mitral regurgitation was present. Broad-spectrum antibiotics were initiated as the culture reports were still awaited.

Q1. What are the most common organisms causing IE?

The most common organisms are *Staphylococcus aureus*, *Streptococcus viridans,* and *Enterococcus* species.[2] *S. aureus* can cause IE even in structurally normal heart and can cause fulminant presentation. The other organism causing endocarditis is coagulase-negative staphylococci (CoNS).

Most of the studies have detected *S. viridans* as the most common organism causing IE.[17] These organisms are present in oral cavity and gastrointestinal tract and do not affect normal heart valves. But patients with valvular pathology are prone to microbial seeding even after minor procedures like dental extraction or mucosal damage during toothbrushing.

Other less common organisms causing IE belong to HACEK group of gram-negative organisms.[18] HACEK stands for *Haemophilus* species, *Aggregatibacter* species, *Cardiobacterium hominis*, *Eikenella corrodens*, and *Kingella* species. These organisms also colonize the oral cavity and are responsible for small number of pediatric IE. Catheter-related blood stream infection leading to IE is generally caused by enteric gram-negative rods-like *Escherichia coli* and *Klebsiella* species. Around 5% cases may be caused by candida species.

Case 4

The blood culture report reported no growth, although the patient has vegetations on echocardiogram. The patient was already initiated on cefepime and vancomycin.

Q1a. What is the significance of culture-negative IE?

If the patient is having culture-negative endocarditis, it is generally due to the following reasons:
- Recent antibiotic exposure that has suppressed the growth of offending organism
- Infection due to fastidious organism or slow organism
- Intracellular organism such as *Bartonella* species, *Coxiella burnetii*, and *Chlamydia* species causing endocarditis[2,19]
- Noncandida fungi endocarditis or
- Noninfectious endocarditis

These patients should be identified promptly as delay in appropriate treatment may affect the overall outcome of the patient.

Case 5

On eliciting the history again, it was found that our patient had received cefoperazone and sulbactam during the previous hospitalization for CAP.

Q1b. What factors should be considered while prescribing antibiotics?

The prime objective of antibiotic therapy in IE is to eradicate vegetations and reduce the incidence of complications due to infection. The antibiotic therapy should be selected based on the pharmacokinetic and pharmacodynamic properties of the drug and the penetration properties of the antibiotic into the vegetation.[20] All antibiotics should be given parenterally for prolonged periods till the time desired results are obtained. Bactericidal antibiotics should be chosen over bacteriostatic ones.

Q1c. What are the antibiotic choices for IE?

High-dose β-lactam with antistaphylococcal properties or addition of a glycopeptide is recommended for most of the patients with IE. The antibiotic can be modified once the culture reports are available.

Streptococci

As streptococci are mostly sensitive to penicillin, the treatment depends on the minimum inhibitory concentration of penicillin to the isolate.[21] Sensitive organisms can be treated with monotherapy with either high-dose penicillin or ceftriaxone. Ampicillin can be used as an alternative to penicillin when it is not available or there is allergy to penicillin. Combination of β-lactam with aminoglycoside has shown excellent cure rates and has reduced the duration of treatment to almost 2 weeks.[22] This treatment regimen is effective in treating native valve endocarditis (NVE). Gentamicin is not recommended nowadays due to increased incidence of ototoxicity and nephrotoxicity.

For PVE, the same treatment can be given, except the duration which has to be at least 4 weeks.

Staphylococci

The treatment depends whether the isolate is coagulase positive (*S. aureus*) or coagulase negative (*S. epidermidis*). This differentiation is important as *S. aureus* generally causes NVE, whereas CONS generally causes PVE. As there is overlap in infection, one should consider both the organisms while prescribing antibiotics.

Staphylococcus aureus which is methicillin-sensitive can be easily treated with β-lactam antibiotic like cefazolin or nafcillin. Vancomycin needs to be added only if the isolated organism is *methicillin-resistant S. aureus* (MRSA). Daptomycin has also been found to be an effective alternative to vancomycin and does not require therapeutic drug monitoring for its trough levels in the blood.[23] Addition of aminoglycoside or rifampicin is not recommended for treatment of NVE as it can create resistance among organisms.[24,25] Aminoglycoside is associated with increased incidence of nephrotoxicity with any major clinical benefit when it is added to β-lactam antibiotic.[26]

Drug combination with rifampicin or aminoglycoside has been found useful in antibiotics therapy of PVE.

Enterococci

There is increasing resistance to penicillin and aminoglycosides among the enterococci species; hence, combination therapy has been used for bactericidal synergy. Enterococci can only be killed by an antibiotic combination, which is cell wall active and achieves high serum concentration (penicillin, ampicillin, and vancomycin) along with an aminoglycoside, which is not resistant.[27] If there is documented resistance to aminoglycoside, then high-dose ampicillin along with ceftriaxone can be used.

Table 2 lists the recommended antibiotics for common organisms causing endocarditis.

Case 6

The patient continued to have fever despite initiating antibiotics. Repeat blood culture was sent, which cultured as E. coli along with Candida.

Q1. What should be the antibiotic prescription for this situation?

This patient has growing nosocomial infection as he had history of previous hospitalization. The incidence of non-HACEK gram-negative infection is around 1.8% as per 1 large multinational database, which included 2,761 patients affected with IE.[28] The most common risk factor for this kind IE is prolonged antibiotic exposure and cardiac surgery. The following factors should be kept in mind while deciding the antibiotic choice: chances of multidrug resistance as it is a nosocomial infection, chances of increased nephrotoxicity due to combined usage of aminoglycoside and colistin, knowledge of drug–drug interaction, and high chances of mortality in these patients.

The patient should receive combination therapy with β-lactam–β-lactamase inhibitor (penicillin, cephalosporin, and carbapenems) along with antipseudomonal aminoglycoside or fluoroquinolone.[28] The antibiotics can be modified as per the local antibiogram.

Q1a. Which antifungal therapy should be initiated for candida?

Prolonged central venous catheters, pacemakers, or implantable cardiac devices are the common risk factors for fungal IE, although the incidence is very low.[29,30] Fungal IE mostly causes PVE. *Candida* and *Aspergillus* species are the most common culprit species.[30] *Aspergillus* can be a cause of culture negative IE. With fungal IE, the incidence of metastatic complications is high and one should look for endophthalmitis. Combination of medical-surgical treatment is required with liposomal amphotericin B or echinocandins as the antifungal agents.

Q1b. What are the antibiotic choices for HACEK group of organisms?

Ceftriaxone should be considered as the drug of choice due to rise in β-lactamase-producing strains, hence causing ampicillin resistance.[31] Fluoroquinolone can also be used to treat HACEK group of organisms due to in vitro susceptibility, although there is limited data on this.[32]

Q1c. What should be the duration of antibiotic therapy?

Microbiological relapse is a possibility even in antibiotic susceptible organisms; hence, the duration has to be long enough to achieve complete sterilization of vegetation. The standard duration for NVE is 4 weeks, whereas for PVE the duration has to be extended for 6 weeks. The literature also mentions a short 2-week therapy for right-sided endocarditis and when the combination of β-lactam and aminoglycoside is used for penicillin-susceptible streptococci *viridans*.[33,34]

If the patient undergoes surgical intervention during the active phase of medical management, then the exact duration will be decided by the culture report of the valve. It is recommended to give the antibiotic therapy for 2 weeks postsurgery if the valve culture is negative, whereas to restart the 6-week therapy if the valve culture is positive as it represents absence of sterilization of vegetation at the time of surgery.[35]

The appropriate duration of antifungal therapy for fungal IE is not clear and generally involves surgical management as well.[36] The duration should be at least 6 weeks and the antifungal agent should be continued at least for 14 days

TABLE 2: Antimicrobial therapy for organisms causing infective endocarditis.

Organism	Native valve endocarditis	Prosthetic valve endocarditis
Methicillin-sensitive *Staphylococcus aureus*	*Nafcillin/oxacillin:* 12 g/24 h in six divided doses or *Cefazolin:* 6 g/24 h in three divided doses Duration: 4 weeks	*Nafcillin/oxacillin:* 12 g/24 h in six divided doses or *Cefazolin:* 6 g/24 h in three divided doses Duration: 6 weeks
Methicillin-resistant *S. aureus*	*Cefepime:* 2 g 8th hourly plus *Vancomycin:* 15 mg/kg twice daily or *Daptomycin:* 6 mg/kg once daily Duration: 4 weeks	*Cefepime:* 2 g 8th hourly plus *Vancomycin:* 15 mg/kg twice daily or *Daptomycin:* 6 mg/kg once daily plus Rifampicin 300 mg thrice daily Duration: 6 weeks
Streptococcus viridans	*Ceftriaxone sodium:* 2 g once daily Duration: 4 weeks *Ceftriaxone sodium:* 2 g once daily plus *Gentamicin:* 3 mg/kg once daily Duration: 2 weeks	*Ceftriaxone sodium:* 2 g once daily Duration: 6 weeks *Ceftriaxone sodium:* 2 g once daily plus *Gentamicin:* 3 mg/kg once daily Duration: 2 weeks of combination followed by 4 weeks of ceftriaxone
Enterococci species	*Ampicillin sodium:* 2 g 4th hourly plus (optional) *Gentamicin:* 3 mg/kg three divided doses or *Ampicillin:* 2 g 4th hourly plus *Ceftriaxone:* 2 g 12th hourly Duration: 6 weeks	*Ampicillin sodium:* 2 g 4th hourly plus (optional) *Gentamicin:* 3 mg/kg three divided doses or *Ampicillin:* 2 g 4th hourly plus *Ceftriaxone:* 2 g 12th hourly Duration: 6 weeks
Enterococcus species resistant to penicillin, aminoglycoside, or vancomycin	*Linezolid:* 600 mg twice daily or *Daptomycin:* 10–12 mg/kg once daily Duration: 6 weeks	*Linezolid:* 600 mg twice daily or *Daptomycin:* 10–12 mg/kg once daily Duration: 6 weeks
HACEK organism	*Ceftriaxone sodium:* 2 g once daily or *Ampicillin sodium:* 2 g 4th hourly or *Ciprofloxacin:* 800 mg in two divided doses Duration: 4 weeks	*Ceftriaxone sodium:* 2 g once daily or Ampicillin sodium 2 g 4th hourly or *Ciprofloxacin:* 800 mg in two divided doses Duration: 6 weeks
Culture-negative endocarditis including Bartonella endocarditis	*Ampicillin sulbactam:* 3 g 6th hourly plus Gentamicin sulfate 3 mg/kg in three divided doses plus *Ciprofloxacin:* 800 mg in two divided doses Duration: 4–6 weeks	Cefepime 2 g thrice daily plus Gentamicin sulfate 3 mg/kg in three divided doses plus Vancomycin 15 mg/kg twice daily plus Rifampicin 300 mg thrice daily Duration: 6 weeks

(HACEK: *Haemophilus* species, *Aggregatibacter* species, *Cardiobacterium hominis*, *Eikenella corrodens*, and *Kingella*)

after a negative blood culture report. Similarly for culture-negative IE, the exact duration is not mentioned, but the decision should be based on clinical presentation of the patient, presence or absence of prosthetic valve, and other risk factors. Combination of antibiotics can be given for at least 4 weeks for NVE and 6 weeks for PVE.

Case 7

The appropriate antibiotic and antifungal therapy were initiated for the patient. At the end of second week of medical therapy, the patient started to have breathing difficulty and episodes of pulmonary edema. Despite diuretic therapy and application of noninvasive ventilation, his distress increased.

It was also noticed that there is tenderness at left knee joint and swelling over the patella.

Q1. What is the reason for the above finding, and what intervention should be done to stabilize the patient?

The patient is developing complications of IE and warrants surgical intervention in the form of valve replacement. The accepted indication for surgery is uncontrolled infection despite medical management, episodes of heart failure, and appearance of embolic events. The exact timing of surgical intervention is not clear. The American[24] and European[1] guidelines have suggested that early valve surgery which is defined as surgery during the medical treatment phase of IE needs to be performed in significant proportion of patients. **Table 3** lists the indications for surgery as per the timing.

The data about timing of surgery is controversial as there are no randomized trials. Most of the data is derived from observational studies, and most of the studies have found that the benefit of early valve surgery is mostly seen in NVE.[37]

Q1a. What investigations should be done to investigate for embolic complications of IE?

The emboli can be deposited in any body site and the patients can present with symptoms only pertaining to these embolic manifestations. The risk of systemic embolization has been estimated to be around 50% and includes brain, lungs, spleen, or extremities. Most of the embolic symptoms happen from mitral valve IE.[38] More than 65% patients with systemic embolization manifest as neurological symptoms and should undergo CT brain to diagnose embolic stroke or brain abscess. One should always look for hemorrhagic conversion in the infarcted area.

Similarly, for osteomyelitis, CT scan of the affected joint or magnetic resonance imaging can be performed. In unstable patients, bedside ultrasound can be utilized to detect collection in the synovial joints.

Computed tomography of abdomen should be done to look for hepatic or splenic infarcts due to embolic shower.

Case 8

The patient underwent mitral valve replacement with drainage of synovial collection from left knee. The culture also grew E. coli and Candida, and the antibiotics were continued as per previous prescription. Noncontrast CT scan of brain revealed small embolic strokes. The intensive care unit (ICU) team wanted to initiate anticoagulation for this patient.

Q1. What should be the protocol for initiating anticoagulation in this patient?

Anticoagulation is controversial in patients with IE. There is no consensus on initiation of anticoagulation in NVE, and similarly it is advisable to stop all anticoagulation for at least 2 weeks in PVE due to risk of neurological deterioration and hemorrhagic conversion of stroke.[39] Deep vein thrombosis prophylaxis should be initiated first with mechanical compression devices. If anticoagulation is deemed necessary, then unfractionated heparin should be started and activated partial thromboplastin time (aPTT) should be monitored and maintained at 50–70 seconds.

Case 9

The patient was initially managed with compression devices and later on initiated with unfractionated heparin therapy. He improved with combined medical surgical treatment for mitral valve endocarditis. The therapy continued for 6 weeks, and all the repeat cultures were negative. The patient was eventually discharged in healthy condition.

Q1. What precautions should be advised for the patient on discharge?

Presence of prosthetic heart valve is a risk factor for developing IE; hence, these patients should be advised long-term prevention strategies. These patients should receive prophylactic antibiotics before undergoing dental procedures. Oral amoxicillin 2 g 1 hour prior to the procedure should be administered.

Q2. What are Duke's criteria?

Durack and colleagues in 1994 at Duke university defined criteria which can help in diagnosing IE with good sensitivity.[40] These criteria stratified patients into three categories: *definite,* where IE was diagnosed clinically or microbiologically; *possible,* where patients did not meet

TABLE 3: Indications for surgery.

Timing	Indications
Emergent (within 24 hours of presentation)	• Cardiogenic shock • Pulmonary edema • Acute aortic regurgitation
Urgent (within 24–48 hours)	• Valve obstruction by vegetation • Prosthetic valve dehiscence • Septal perforation • Uncontrolled infection • Perivalvular abscess • Extension of vegetation despite antibiotic • Effective antibiotic not available • Vegetation >10 mm plus embolic episodes • Vegetation >30 mm
Elective	• Fungal endocarditis • Progressive valvular regurgitation despite medical management • Prosthetic valve endocarditis due to *Staphylococcus aureus*

the criteria for definite IE; and *rejected,* where patients improved with short-term treatment with antibiotics and did not have any clinical or microbiological confirmation of IE. **Tables 4 and 5** depict the Modified Duke's Criteria for defining terminologies and diagnosing IE, respectively.

Q3. What are the complications of IE?

The following complications can happen during medical treatment of IE, and most of these complications are then managed surgically.

Congestive heart failure

Congestive heart failure has the greatest impact on overall prognosis of these patients and affects 6-month mortality.[41] In patients with NVE, aortic valve followed by mitral valve IE can cause CHF.[42] CHF presentation can be varied with patients being most distressed with aortic regurgitation than with mitral regurgitation. CHF can happen due to valve dehiscence, rupture of chordae, valve obstruction, or massive intracardiac shunts. Severity of CHF guides the decision to operate on these patients.

Embolization

Almost half of the patients affected with IE will have some systemic embolization during the medical management. The emboli can be dislodged in almost all vital organs with central nervous system embolization being the most common. The highest incidence is associated with aortic valve followed by mitral valve endocarditis. The most common time frame of embolization is between 2 and 4 weeks after initiation of medical management.[43] Prediction of embolization is difficult in patients with IE. Roughly, echocardiography finding of >1 cm left-sided vegetation is a risk factor for embolization.[44] If there are more than two major embolic events due to IE, then it warrants surgical intervention.[45]

Periannular extension of vegetation

This is associated with very high mortality and can lead to destruction of nearby structures.[45] In aortic valve IE, the infection may spread to atrioventricular node and cause heart block.[46] These abscesses may create fistula tracts and cause pericardial shunts.

Splenic abscess

Bacteremic seeding causing a localized infraction of spleen can lead to splenic abscess formation. It is a rare complication of IE. In roughly 40% of left-sided IE, splenic infarction occurs, but splenic abscess is not a common

TABLE 4: Definition of various criteria as per Modified Duke's criteria.

Criteria severity	Criteria	Description
Major criteria	Positive blood culture consistent with IE	• Bacteremia with *Staphylococcus aureus, Streptococcus viridans,* enterococci species or HACEK group of organisms • At least two positive blood cultures taken >12 hours apart or all three cultures positive taken 30 minutes apart • Single blood culture positive for *Coxiella burnetii*
	Evidence of endocardial involvement	• Echocardiography confirmation of intracardiac valvular mass, which is oscillating • New valvular regurgitation • Prosthetic valve dehiscence • Perivalvular abscess
Minor criteria	Predisposing heart condition or intravenous drug user	
	Fever >38°C	
	Vascular phenomenon	• Janeway lesions • Arterial emboli • Intracranial hemorrhage • Pulmonary infarcts
	Immunological phenomenon	• Osler's nodes • Roth's spots • Glomerulonephritis • Rheumatoid factor
	Microbiological evidence	Positive blood culture but not meeting major criteria

(HACEK: *Haemophilus* species, *Aggregatibacter* species, *Cardiobacterium hominis, Eikenella corrodens,* and *Kingella;* IE: infective endocarditis)

TABLE 5: Modified Duke's criteria definition of infective endocarditis (IE).

Definite IE	• Pathological criteria • Microbiology detected by culture or histological examination of vegetation, or culture positive found in embolized vegetation or in intracardiac abscess specimen • Vegetation or intracardiac abscess specimen showing active endocarditis pathologically *Clinical criteria:* • Two major criteria or • One major and three minor criteria or • Five minor criteria
Possible IE	• One major criterion and one minor criterion or • Three minor criteria
Rejected	• Confirmed alternative diagnosis against IE • Rapid symptom resolution with antibiotic therapy of <4 days • No pathological evidence of IE at histological examination

finding.[47] Patients may complain of vague symptoms such as back pain, persistent fever, and other signs of sepsis unrelated to cardiac symptoms should raise the suspicion of splenic abscess. Abdominal CT scan can diagnose these abscesses. Splenectomy with appropriate antibiotic cover should be given to all patients.

Prognosis

The prognosis of these patients depends on the long-term follow-up advice that the patient is following. Good oral hygiene is an important factor to be kept in mind. Any episode of fever should not go unnoticed, and they should consult a physician and if required an echocardiogram should be performed.

REFERENCES

1. Habib G, Lancellotti P, Antunes MJ, Bongiorni MG, Casalta JP, Del Zotti F, et al.; ESC Scientific Document Group. 2015 ESC Guidelines for the management of infective endocarditis: The Task Force for the Management of Infective Endocarditis of the European Society of Cardiology (ESC). Endorsed by: European Association for Cardio-Thoracic Surgery (EACTS), the European Association of Nuclear Medicine (EANM). Eur Heart J. 2015;36(44):3075-128.
2. Murdoch DR, Corey GR, Hoen B, Miró JM, Fowler VG Jr, Bayer AS, et al.; International Collaboration on Endocarditis-Prospective Cohort Study (ICE-PCS) Investigators. Clinical presentation, etiology, and outcome of infective endocarditis in the 21st century: the International Collaboration on Endocarditis-Prospective Cohort Study. Arch Intern Med. 2009;169(5):463-73.
3. Baltimore RS, Gewitz M, Baddour LM, Beerman LB, Jackson MA, Lockhart PB, et al.; American Heart Association Rheumatic Fever, Endocarditis, and Kawasaki Disease Committee of the Council on Cardiovascular Disease in the Young and the Council on Cardiovascular and Stroke Nursing. Infective Endocarditis in Childhood: 2015 Update: A Scientific Statement From the American Heart Association. Circulation. 2015;132(15):1487-515.
4. Starke JR, Endocarditis I. In: Cherry JD, Harrison GJ, Kaplan SL, Steinbach WJ, Hotez PJ (Eds). Feigin and Cherry's Textbook of Pediatric Infectious Diseases, 7th edition. Philadelphia, PA: Elsevier; 2014.
5. Snygg-Martin U, Gustafsson L, Rosengren L, Rosengren L, Alsiö A, Ackerholm P, et al. Cerebrovascular complications in patients with left-sided infective endocarditis are common: a prospective study using magnetic resonance imaging and neurochemical brain damage markers. Clin Infect Dis. 2008;47(1):23-30.
6. Pruitt AA, Rubin RH, Karchmer AW, Duncan GW. Neurologic complications of bacterial endocarditis. Medicine (Baltimore). 1978;57(4):329-43.
7. Farrior JB, Silverman ME. A consideration of the differences between a Janeway's lesion and an Osler's node in infectious endocarditis. Chest. 1976;70(2):239-43.
8. Arora N, Dhibar DP, Bashyal B, Agarwal A. Roth's Spots, a clinical diagnostic clue for Infective Endocarditis. Perm J. 2020;24:20.038.
9. Bansal RC. Infective endocarditis. Med Clin North Am. 1995;79(5):1205-40.
10. Cunha BA, Gill MV, Lazar JM. Acute infective endocarditis. Diagnostic and therapeutic approach. Infect Dis Clin North Am. 1996;10(4):811-34.
11. Bragg L, Alvarez A. Endocarditis. Pediatr Rev. 2014;35(4):162-7; quiz 168.
12. Li JS, Sexton DJ, Mick N, Nettles R, Fowler VG Jr, Ryan T, et al. Proposed modifications to the Duke criteria for the diagnosis of infective endocarditis. Clin Infect Dis. 2000;30(4):633-8.
13. Doherty JU, Kort S, Mehran R, Schoenhagen P, Soman P. ACC/AATS/AHA/ASE/ASNC/HRS/SCAI/SCCT/SCMR/STS 2017 Appropriate Use Criteria for Multimodality Imaging in Valvular Heart Disease: A Report of the American College of Cardiology Appropriate Use Criteria Task Force, American Association for Thoracic Surgery. J Am Coll Cardiol. 2017;70:1647-72.
14. Singh P, Inamdar V, Hage FG, Kodali V, Karakus G, Suwanjutah T, et al. Usefulness of live/real time three-dimensional transthoracic echocardiography in evaluation of prosthetic valve function. Echocardiography. 2009;26(10):1236-49.
15. Sifaoui I, Oliver L, Tacher V, Fiore A, Lepeule R, Moussafeur A, et al. Diagnostic performance of transesophageal echocardiography and cardiac computed tomography in infective endocarditis. J Am Soc Echocardiogr. 2020;33(12):1442-53.
16. Wang TKM, Bin Saeedan M, Chan N, Obuchowski NA, Shrestha N, Xu B, et al. Complementary diagnostic and prognostic contributions of cardiac computed tomography for infective endocarditis surgery. Circ Cardiovasc Imaging. 2020;13:e011126.
17. Gupta S, Sakhuja A, McGrath E, Asmar B. Trends, microbiology, and outcomes of infective endocarditis in children during 2000-2010 in the United States. Congenit Heart Dis. 2017;12(2):196-201.
18. Feder HM Jr, Roberts JC, Salazar J, Leopold HB, Toro-Salazar O. HACEK endocarditis in infants and children: two cases and a literature review. Pediatr Infect Dis J. 2003;22(6):557-62.
19. Habib G, Erba PA, Iung B, Donal E, Cosyns B, Laroche C, et al.; EURO-ENDO Investigators. Clinical presentation, aetiology and outcome of infective endocarditis. Results of the ESC-EORP EURO-ENDO (European infective endocarditis) registry: a prospective cohort study. Eur Heart J. 2019;40(39):3222-32.
20. Durack DT, Beeson PB. Experimental bacterial endocarditis. II. Survival of a bacteria in endocardial vegetations. Br J Exp Pathol. 1972;53(1):50-3.
21. Francioli P, Etienne J, Hoigné R, Thys JP, Gerber A. Treatment of streptococcal endocarditis with a single daily dose of ceftriaxone sodium for 4 weeks. Efficacy and outpatient treatment feasibility. JAMA. 1992;267(2):264-7.
22. Sexton DJ, Tenenbaum MJ, Wilson WR, Steckelberg JM, Tice AD, Gilbert D, et al. Ceftriaxone once daily for four weeks compared with ceftriaxone plus gentamicin once daily for

two weeks for treatment of endocarditis due to penicillin-susceptible streptococci. Endocarditis Treatment Consortium Group. Clin Infect Dis. 1998;27(6):1470-4.
23. Fowler VG Jr, Boucher HW, Corey GR, Abrutyn E, Karchmer AW, Rupp ME, et al.; S. aureus Endocarditis and Bacteremia Study Group. Daptomycin versus standard therapy for bacteremia and endocarditis caused by Staphylococcus aureus. N Engl J Med. 2006;355(7):653-65.
24. Baddour LM, Wilson WR, Bayer AS, Fowler VG Jr, Tleyjeh IM, Rybak MJ, et al.; American Heart Association Committee on Rheumatic Fever, Endocarditis, and Kawasaki Disease of the Council on Cardiovascular Disease in the Young, Council on Clinical Cardiology, Council on Cardiovascular Surgery and Anesthesia, and Stroke Council. Infective Endocarditis in Adults: Diagnosis, Antimicrobial Therapy, and Management of Complications: A Scientific Statement for Healthcare Professionals From the American Heart Association. Circulation. 2015;132(15):1435-86.
25. Riedel DJ, Weekes E, Forrest GN. Addition of rifampin to standard therapy for treatment of native valve infective endocarditis caused by Staphylococcus aureus. Antimicrob Agents Chemother. 2008;52(7):2463-7.
26. Cosgrove SE, Vigliani GA, Fowler VG Jr, Abrutyn E, Corey GR, Levine DP, et al. Initial low-dose gentamicin for Staphylococcus aureus bacteremia and endocarditis is nephrotoxic. Clin Infect Dis. 2009;48(6):713-21.
27. Wilson WR, Wilkowske CJ, Wright AJ, Sande MA, Geraci JE. Treatment of streptomycin-susceptible and streptomycin-resistant enterococcal endocarditis. Ann Intern Med. 1984;100(6):816-23.
28. Morpeth S, Murdoch D, Cabell CH, Karchmer AW, Pappas P, Levine D, et al.; International Collaboration on Endocarditis Prospective Cohort Study (ICE-PCS) Investigators. Non-HACEK gram-negative bacillus endocarditis. Ann Intern Med. 2007;147(12):829-35.
29. Pierrotti LC, Baddour LM. Fungal endocarditis, 1995-2000. Chest. 2002;122(1):302-10.
30. Boland JM, Chung HH, Robberts FJ, Wilson WR, Steckelberg JM, Baddour LM, et al. Fungal prosthetic valve endocarditis: Mayo Clinic experience with a clinicopathological analysis. Mycoses. 2011;54(4):354-60.
31. Coburn B, Toye B, Rawte P, Jamieson FB, Farrell DJ, Patel SN. Antimicrobial susceptibilities of clinical isolates of HACEK organisms. Antimicrob Agents Chemother. 2013;57(4):1989-91.
32. Tsigrelis C, Singh KV, Coutinho TD, Murray BE, Baddour LM. Vancomycin-resistant Enterococcus faecalis endocarditis: linezolid failure and strain characterization of virulence factors. J Clin Microbiol. 2007;45(2):631-5.
33. Ribera E, Gómez-Jimenez J, Cortes E, del Valle O, Planes A, Gonzalez-Alujas T, et al. Effectiveness of cloxacillin with and without gentamicin in short-term therapy for right-sided Staphylococcus aureus endocarditis. A randomized, controlled trial. Ann Intern Med. 1996;125(12):969-74.
34. Francioli P, Ruch W, Stamboulian D. Treatment of streptococcal endocarditis with a single daily dose of ceftriaxone and netilmicin for 14 days: a prospective multicenter study. Clin Infect Dis. 1995;21(6):1406-10.
35. Morris AJ, Drinković D, Pottumarthy S, MacCulloch D, Kerr AR, West T. Bacteriological outcome after valve surgery for active infective endocarditis: implications for duration of treatment after surgery. Clin Infect Dis. 2005;41(2):187-94.
36. Arnold CJ, Johnson M, Bayer AS, Bradley S, Giannitsioti E, Miró JM, et al. Candida infective endocarditis: an observational cohort study with a focus on therapy. Antimicrob Agents Chemother. 2015;59(4):2365-73.
37. Lalani T, Cabell CH, Benjamin DK, Lasca O, Naber C, Fowler VG Jr, et al.; International Collaboration on Endocarditis-Prospective Cohort Study (ICE-PCS) Investigators. Analysis of the impact of early surgery on in-hospital mortality of native valve endocarditis: use of propensity score and instrumental variable methods to adjust for treatment-selection bias. Circulation. 2010;121(8):1005-13.
38. García-Cabrera E, Fernández-Hidalgo N, Almirante B, Ivanova-Georgieva R, Noureddine M, Plata A, et al.; Group for the Study of Cardiovascular Infections of the Andalusian Society of Infectious Diseases; Spanish Network for Research in Infectious Diseases. Neurological complications of infective endocarditis: risk factors, outcome, and impact of cardiac surgery: a multicenter observational study. Circulation. 2013;127(23):2272-84.
39. Tornos P, Almirante B, Mirabet S, Permanyer G, Pahissa A, Soler-Soler J. Infective endocarditis due to Staphylococcus aureus: deleterious effect of anticoagulant therapy. Arch Intern Med. 1999;159(5):473-5.
40. Durack DT, Lukes AS, Bright DK. New criteria for diagnosis of infective endocarditis: utilization of specific echocardiographic findings. Duke Endocarditis Service. Am J Med. 1994;96(3):200-9.
41. Hasbun R, Vikram HR, Barakat LA, Buenconsejo J, Quagliarello VJ. Complicated left-sided native valve endocarditis in adults: risk classification for mortality. JAMA. 2003;289(15):1933-40.
42. Sexton DJ, Spelman D. Current best practices and guidelines. Assessment and management of complications in infective endocarditis. Cardiol Clin. 2003;21(2):273-82, vii-viii.
43. Vilacosta I, Graupner C, San Román JA, Sarriá C, Ronderos R, Fernández C, et al. Risk of embolization after institution of antibiotic therapy for infective endocarditis. J Am Coll Cardiol. 2002;39(9):1489-95.
44. Sanfilippo AJ, Picard MH, Newell JB, Rosas E, Davidoff R, Thomas JD, et al. Echocardiographic assessment of patients with infectious endocarditis: prediction of risk for complications. J Am Coll Cardiol. 1991;18(5):1191-9.
45. Alsip SG, Blackstone EH, Kirklin JW, Cobbs CG. Indications for cardiac surgery in patients with active infective endocarditis. Am J Med. 1985;78(6B):138-48.
46. Omari B, Shapiro S, Ginzton L, Robertson JM, Ward J, Nelson RJ, et al. Predictive risk factors for periannular extension of native valve endocarditis. Clinical and echocardiographic analyses. Chest. 1989;96(6):1273-9.
47. Ting W, Silverman NA, Arzouman DA, Levitsky S. Splenic septic emboli in endocarditis. Circulation. 1990;82(5 Suppl):IV105-9.

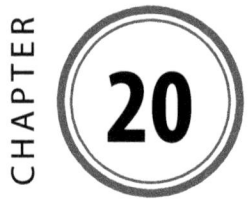

Acute Aortic Emergencies

Khalid Ismail Khatib

CASE STUDY

A 35-year-old male presented to emergency department with history of severe chest pain for the last 6 hours. Chest pain was retrosternal with a tearing feeling. There was no breathlessness, diaphoresis, or palpitation. On examination, pulse rate was 94 beats/min, regular and there was inequality in the bilateral radial pulses. Blood pressure (BP) was 190/116 mm Hg. However, there were no abnormal cardiac sounds or murmurs and respiratory system examination was normal. Electrocardiogram (ECG) done was normal. Chest X-ray (CXR) was done, and it demonstrated widened mediastinum with abnormal aortic contour.

Q1. What are the various conditions which comprise acute aortic emergencies (AAE)? How common are these?

The conditions which majorly comprise AAE are: (1) Aortic dissection (AD), (2) abdominal aortic aneurysm (AAA), and (3) thoracic aortic aneurysm (accounts for only a small fraction of AAEs).[1]

The term "acute aortic syndrome" encompasses AD (almost 90–95%), penetrating aortic ulcer (approximately 5%), and intramural hematoma (0–25%).[2] The term was coined initially by Vilacosta and Roman in 2001.

Incidence of various entities comprising AAS/AAEs: The reported incidence of AD is 2–3.5 patients/100,000 patients/year, though it is impossible to accurately report these patients due to occurrence of sudden deaths in these patients.[3-5]

Incidence of AAAs varies according to the methods used to detect it. Screening in elderly (>65 years) will lead to its detection in 7% of patients. AAA presenting with symptoms are seen in 25 per 1 lakh in patients aged 50 years and increasing almost three times in patients aged over 70 years.

Q2. What are the causes and risk factors for developing AD?

Aortic dissection develops when micro tears develop in the intimal lining of the aorta due to atherosclerotic disease (most common) or from other conditions affecting the aortic walls, such as medial degeneration, trauma or infection. Presence of risk factors **(Table 1)** leads to increasing of these microtears both proximally and distally. Sometimes some of the branches of the aorta may be involved in the dissection. Patients may then present with typical signs and symptoms related to that branch in addition to general symptoms and signs of AD. The already weakened wall along with the increasing microtears leads the blood to enter the wall of the aorta separating an intimal flap to form a false lumen as opposed to the true lumen of the blood vessel. The false lumen may or may not reconnect with the true lumen.

Q3. What are the various symptoms and signs of AD?

Symptoms and signs of AD are given in **Table 2**.

Q4. How are ADs classified?

Aortic dissections are classified as per the anatomical, DeBakey, and Stanford classifications **(Table 3)**.

Q5. What are the CXR findings in AD?

The CXR may show (1) widened mediastinum (>80 mm is a cause of concern), (2) calcium sign (due to separation of the layers of the aorta), (3) pleural effusion (left > right), and (4) downward shift of left main bronchus (due to pressure from the widened aorta). The CXR is the most common investigation done in patients presenting with AD and will

TABLE 1: Risk factors for aortic dissection.

Sr. No.	Risk factors
1.	Hypertension
2.	Trauma
3.	Genetic causes (Ehlers–Danlos syndrome, Marfan syndrome)
4.	Vasculitides (Takayasu arteritis, giant cell arteritis, Behçet's disease)
5.	Presence of thoracic aortic aneurysm
6.	Family history of aortic abnormalities

TABLE 2: Clinical features of aortic dissection.

Sr. No.	Symptoms	Signs
1.	Chest pain/back pain (most common presenting symptom, sudden onset, tearing in character, and severe)	Inequality of bilateral pulses (more commonly upper limb pulses)
2.	Abdominal pain	Focal neurological deficit including transient ischemic attacks and stroke
3.	Flank pain	Diastolic murmur of aortic regurgitation
4.	Migrating pain	Hypertension

TABLE 3: Classification of aortic dissection (AD).

Classification	Types	Remarks
Anatomical	A. AD of ascending aorta B. AD of descending aorta	AD of ascending aorta >2 times as common as AD of descending aorta
DeBakey	*Type I:* Intimal tear originates in ascending aorta and involves the whole length of the aorta (both ascending and descending) *Type II:* Intimal tear originates in ascending aorta and the dissection is limited to the ascending aorta *Type III:* Intimal tear originates in descending aorta and the dissection is limited to the descending aorta	
Stanford	*Type A:* Involving the ascending aorta with/without affecting descending aorta *Type B:* Restricted only to descending aorta	• Type A also called proximal type and requires surgical treatment • Type B also called distal and requires medical management

be abnormal in more than three-fourths of the patients.[6] The CXR should be looked at carefully in patients who present with chest pain and have normal ECG.

Q6. How will you manage the hemodynamics of the patient on presentation?

Patients with AD need aggressive control of their BP and heart rate (HR). The target BP is 100–120 mm Hg systolic and target HR is 60 beats/min.

Beta-blockers are the drug of choice in the medical management of AD due to their negative inotropic and negative chronotropic effects.

Intravenous esmolol can be used due to its short duration of action. It is used as an IV infusion.

Dose: 500 µg/kg as bolus and then 50 µg/kg/min as infusion. Dose may be titrated to achieve target HR and BP. Labetalol is an equally excellent choice. For those with contraindications to beta-blocker use, calcium channel blockers such as verapamil or diltiazem may be tried.

For patients who continue to have high systolic BP despite adequate rate control, sodium nitroprusside infusion (0.5–3 mg/kg/min) is the drug of choice. However, it should be given after beta blockade or it may result in reflex tachycardia.

Case continued: The patient continued to have chest pain. He was given esmolol infusion following which his symptoms reduced. His HR was 64 beats/min and BP was 100/62 mm Hg on infusion of esmolol. However, he continued to be restless.

Q7. How will you further investigate the patient?

Computed tomography (CT) angiography is the gold standard investigation in patients with AD. It can depict the extent of the dissection along with its characteristics and also help in planning operative treatment. It will help to differentiate AD from penetrating aortic ulcer and intramural hematoma. The patient needs to be hemodynamically stable to be shifted for the study and this may be a disadvantage of this modality. Moreover, the administration of contrast may not be ideal in patients with elevated creatinine.

For hemodynamically unstable patients, other modalities such as transesophageal echocardiography (TEE) and/or transthoracic echocardiography (TTE) can be done to secure the diagnosis.

Transesophageal echocardiography is the modality of choice in hemodynamically instable patients who cannot be moved for CT angiography. Bedside TEE has advantages like being highly sensitive and specific for detection of AD, besides also being able to evaluate the aortic root and aortic valve for any regurgitation. However, expertise in TEE is not always available and is operator dependent.

Transthoracic echocardiography should not be used by itself to rule out the presence of AD. The dissecting flap may not be visible and TTE is not sensitive enough to detect AD. It may be used alongside TEE as the proximal most portion of aortic arch may not be visible clearly on TEE.

Magnetic resonance imaging (MRI) when available can easily identify in detail the presence and extent of AD. Another advantage of MRI is the absence of radiation.

However, patient needs to be stable enough to be shifted to the MRI department.

Q8. What is the definitive treatment for patients with AD?

Surgery: AD involving the ascending aorta (Type A) requires surgical management and such patients should be referred to centers where it is available. Medical management must be continued aggressively till such time that surgery is performed. Surgery may be required in those patients with descending aorta AD (Type B) who have complications such as visceral or limb ischemia. Unstable patients with shock and elderly patients have higher perioperative mortality.[7]

Endovascular interventions: These are indicated in patients with Type B ADs with limb or vital organ ischemia who are poor candidates for surgery (patients with refractory hypertension and pain). Endovascular interventions are especially superior in patients with ruptured descended aorta aneurysm as compared to surgery.[8]

REFERENCES

1. Wittels K. Aortic emergencies. Emerg Med Clin North Am. 2011;29(4):789-800, vii.
2. Voitle E, Hofmann W, Cejna M. Aortic emergencies-diagnosis and treatment: a pictorial review. Insights Imaging. 2015;6(1):17-32.
3. Baliyan V, Parakh A, Prabhakar AM, Hedgire S. Acute aortic syndromes and aortic emergencies. Cardiovasc Diagn Ther. 2018;8(Suppl 1):S82-S96.
4. Fattori R, Cao P, De Rango P, Czerny M, Evangelista A, Nienaber C, et al. Interdisciplinary expert consensus document on management of type B aortic dissection. J Am Coll Cardiol. 2013;61(16):1661-78.
5. Moll FL, Powell JT, Fraedrich G, Verzini F, Haulon S, Waltham M, et al.; European Society for Vascular Surgery. Management of abdominal aortic aneurysms clinical practice guidelines of the European society for vascular surgery. Eur J Vasc Endovasc Surg. 2011;41(Suppl 1):S1-S58.
6. Braverman AC. Acute aortic dissection: clinician update. Circulation. 2010;122(2):184-8.
7. Trimarchi S, Nienaber CA, Rampoldi V, Myrmel T, Suzuki T, Bossone E, et al.; IRAD Investigators. Role and results of surgery in acute type B aortic dissection: insights from the International Registry of Acute Aortic Dissection (IRAD). Circulation. 2006;114(1 Suppl):I357-64.
8. Jonker FH, Trimarchi S, Verhagen HJ, Moll FL, Sumpio BE, Muhs BE. Meta-analysis of open versus endovascular repair for ruptured descending thoracic aortic aneurysm. J Vasc Surg. 2010;51(4):1026-32, 1032.e1-1032.e2.

CHAPTER 21: Hyponatremia

Harish Mallapura Maheshwarappa, Richa Narang

INTRODUCTION

Hyponatremia, defined as a serum sodium concentration <135 mmol/L, is the most common disorder of body fluid and electrolyte balance encountered in clinical practice occurring in up to 30% of hospitalized patients causing a wide spectrum of clinical symptoms. Hyponatremia is more of a pathophysiologic process rather than a disease, indicating disturbed water homeostasis. Commonly seen causes of hyponatremia are the syndrome of inappropriate antidiuresis (SIAD), diuretics use, polydipsia, adrenal insufficiency, hypovolemia, heart failure, and liver cirrhosis.

CLINICAL FEATURES

Symptoms can vary from mild, nonspecific to severe and life-threatening symptoms **(Table 1)**. This variation seen in symptomatology is because when hyponatremia develops rapidly, and the brain has had too little time to adapt to its hypotonic environment, the brain cells start to swell due to the movement of water from the extracellular to

TABLE 1: Comparison of the United States and European Guidelines.

Subject	United States Guideline	European Guideline
Acute or symptomatic hyponatremia	• *Severe symptoms:* Bolus 3% NaCl (100 mL over 10 min × 3 as needed) • *Moderate symptoms:* Continuous infusion 3% NaCl (0.5-2 mL/kg/h)	• *Severe symptoms:* Bolus 3% NaCl (150 mL over 20 min two to three times as needed) • *Moderate symptoms:* Bolus 3% NaCl (150 mL 3% over 20 minutes once)
Chronic hyponatremia		
SIAD	• Fluid restriction (first line) • Demeclocycline, urea, or vaptan (second line)	• Fluid restriction (first line) • Urea or loop diuretics + oral • NaCl (second line) • Do not recommend or recommend against vaptan[a] • Recommend against lithium or demeclocycline
Hypovolemic hyponatremia	Isotonic saline	Isotonic saline or balanced crystalloid solution
Hypervolemic hyponatremia	• Fluid restriction • Vaptans[b]	• Fluid restriction • Recommend against vaptan
Correction rates	• *Minimum:* 4–8 mmol/L/day, • 4–6 mmol/L/day (high risk of ODS) • *Limits:* 10–12 mmol/L/day, 8 mmol/L/day (high risk of ODS)	• No minimum • *Limit:* 10 mmol/L per day
Management of overcorrection	• Baseline SNa ≥120 mmol/L: Probably unnecessary • Baseline SNa <120 mmol/L: Start relowering with electrolyte-free water or desmopressin after correction exceeds 6–8 mmol/L/day	• Start once limit is exceeded • Consult an expert to discuss infusion containing electrolyte-free water (10 mL/kg) with or without 2 μg desmopressin IV

[a]"Do not recommend" when SNa <130 mmol/L, "recommend against" when SNa <125 mmol/L.
[b]In liver cirrhosis, restrict to patients where potential benefit outweighs risk of worsened liver function.
(SNa: serum sodium concentration; ODS: osmotic demyelination syndrome)

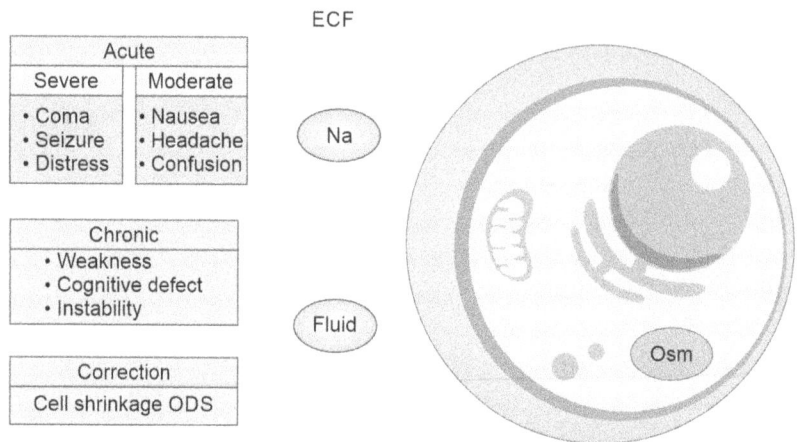

Fig. 1: Rate of fall in sodium levels is holds more importance than absolute levels. (ECF: extracellular fluid; ODS: osmotic demyelination syndrome)

the intracellular compartment caused by the difference in effective osmolality created by the sodium deficit (**Fig. 1**).

CLINICAL SPECTRUM (FIG. 2)

Overtime, the brain reduces the number of osmotically active particles within its cells (mostly potassium and organic solutes) by extruding them in extracellular space in an attempt to restore the brain volume. This process takes 24–48 hours, hence the reason for using the 48-hour threshold to distinguish acute (<48 hours) from chronic (>48 hours) hyponatremia.

PATHOLOGY UNDERLYING SEIZURES IN SEVERE HYPONATREMIA

Hyponatremia is considered significant in terms of severity when the level is below 125 mEq/L. The clinical presentation is more severe when the decrease in serum sodium concentrations is severe or when it occurs rapidly (within hours). Swelling of brain cells and herniation of the brain tissue are the main pathologic finding along with neurologic symptoms being evident when sodium level approaches 120 mEq/L.

This risk of cerebral edema and neurologic manifestations are less if the drop in serum sodium occurs slowly and gradually (≥48 hours), even in case of a marked overall reduction of serum sodium values.

The neurological symptoms of low sodium go hand-in-hand with the severity of cerebral edema (which indirectly depends on rapidity of decrease in level), approximately half of the patients with chronic hyponatremia are asymptomatic, even with serum sodium concentration <125 mEq/L.

Symptoms in these patients rarely occur until the serum sodium is <120 mEq/L and are more usually associated with values around 110 mEq/L or lower. Severe and rapidly

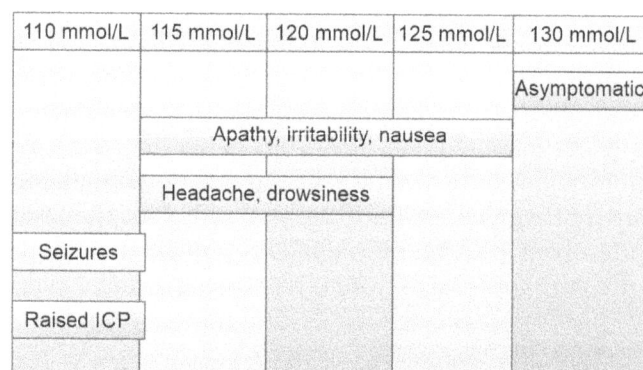

Fig. 2: Clinical features at various sodium levels. (ICP: intracranial pressure)

decreasing sodium level may cause seizures, which are usually generalized tonic-clonic, and generally occur if the plasma sodium concentration rapidly decreases to <115 mEq/L.

PATHOPHYSIOLOGY OF HYPONATREMIA (FIG. 3)

Hyponatremia is primarily a disorder of water balance, with a relative excess of body water compared to total body sodium and potassium content. It is usually associated with a disturbance in the hormone that governs water balance, vasopressin (also called antidiuretic hormone). Even in disorders associated with (renal) sodium loss, vasopressin activity is generally required for hyponatremia to develop (**Fig. 3**).

Changes in serum osmolality are primarily determined by changes in the serum concentration of sodium and its associated anions.

It is important to differentiate the concepts of total osmolality and effective osmolality.

Total osmolality is defined as the concentration of all solutes in a given weight of water (mOsm/kg), regardless of

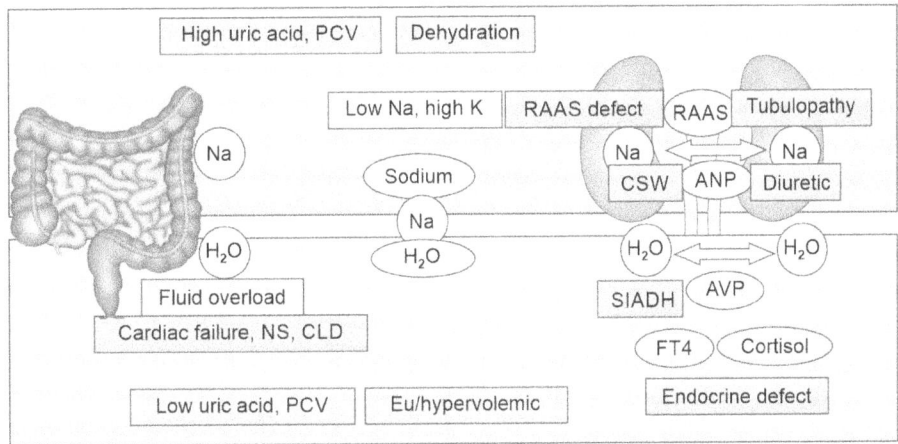

Fig. 3: Pathophysiology of hyponatremia: Hyponatremia can be due to free water excess or sodium deficit. (ANP: atrial natriuretic peptide; AVP: arginine vasopressin; CLD: chronic liver disease; CSW: cerebral salt wasting; PCV: packed cell volume; SIADH: syndrome of inappropriate secretion of antidiuretic hormone; RAAS: rennin-angiotensin-aldosterone system)

whether or not the osmoles can move across the biological membranes.

Effective osmolality or tonicity refers to the number of osmoles that contribute to the water movement between the intracellular and extracellular compartment. It is a function of the relative solute permeability properties of the membrane separating the intracellular and extracellular fluid (ECF) compartments. Only effective solutes create osmotic pressure gradients across cell membranes leading to osmotic movement of water between the intracellular and ECF compartment.

Regulation of Water Intake and Homeostasis

As the serum sodium concentration is determined by the amount of extracellular water relative to the amount of sodium, it can be regulated by changing intake or output of water.

Osmoregulation of Vasopressin Release

The major mechanisms responsible for regulating water metabolism are thirst, and the pituitary secretion and renal effects of vasopressin. A decrease in cell stretch due to changes in systemic effective osmolality increases the firing rate of osmoreceptive neurons located in the anterior hypothalamus which leads to both increased thirst and increased release of vasopressin from the posterior pituitary gland. Vasopressin in turn causes excretion of a concentrated urine by increasing the reabsorption of water from the urine in the distal tubules of the nephron.

Baroregulation of Vasopressin Release

Stretch-sensitive receptors in the left atrium, carotid sinus, and aortic arch sense circulating volume. When the circulating volume is increased, afferent neural impulses inhibit the secretion of vasopressin. Conversely, when the volume is decreased, the discharge rate of the stretch receptors slows and vasopressin secretion increases.

Unregulated Vasopressin Release

Under pathological conditions, vasopressin is secreted independent of serum osmolality or circulating volume from both pituitary and other cells.

Renal Actions of Vasopressin

Reabsorption of water from the collecting duct for the concentration of urine requires the collecting duct to become permeable to water. The basolateral membrane is always permeable to water because of aquaporin-3 and aquaporin-4 water channels. Vasopressin regulates the permeability of the apical membrane by insertion of aquaporin-2 water channels through vasopressin-2 receptor activation. The counter current mechanism of the loops of Henle creates solute gradients from the cortex to the inner medulla and results in high osmolality of the medulla, which provides the driving force needed for reabsorption of water from the collecting duct. Because of the reabsorption of both sodium and urea from the lumen, the osmolality of the tip of the medulla may reach 1,200 mOsm/L in case of water depletion. The medullary osmolality determines maximum urine osmolality and is influenced by the actions of vasopressin.

To capture the current approach to hyponatremia, two sets of guidelines have been developed, one is "United States Guideline" and the other one from within Europe, the "European Guideline" (*see* **Table 1**).

TABLE 2: Classification of hyponatremia.

Classification	Criteria	Limitations of clinical utility
Moderate (125–129 mmol/L) versus severe/profound[a] (<125 mmol/L)	Absolute SNa concentration	Symptoms do not always correlate with degree of hyponatremia
Acute versus chronic	Time of development (cut-off 46 hours)	Time of development not always known
Symptomatic versus asymptomatic	Presence of symptoms	Many symptoms aspecific; chronic hyponatremia may be symptomatic
Hypotonic, isotonic, or hypertonic	Measured serum osmolality	Ineffective osmoles (e.g., urea and ethanol) are also measured
Hypovolemic, euvolemic, and hypervolemic	Clinical assessment of volume status	Clinical assessment of volume status has low sensitivity and specificity

[a]SNa < 125 mmol/L is defined as "severe hyponatremia" by the United States guideline, and as "profound hyponatremia" by the European guideline. (SNa: serum sodium concentration)

CLASSIFICATION OF HYPONATREMIA

Classification of hyponatremia is given in **Table 2**.

CASE STUDY

A 46-year-old female 60 kg in weight, known case of cancer of breast was started on chemotherapy with carboplatin. The next day, she presented to the casualty with disorientation and drowsiness. In the casualty while awaiting investigations, she had an episode of seizure.

Arterial blood gas (ABG) taken at that time showed a serum sodium (S. Na) of 117 mEq/mL. Levetiracetam was started and the patient was shifted to intensive care unit (ICU). In ICU, her GCS remained low—E3M5V3.

Q1. How will you evaluate this case? What will be your diagnostic approach for this patient?

The above patient had severe symptomatic hyponatremia (**Flowchart 1**).

Is it because of free water excess or sodium loss? Differentiation of the two is essential as while fluid restriction is required in free water excess states, saline bolus is indicated in sodium loss states.

Stepwise approach:
- *Serum osmolality:* The initial step in evaluation is exclusion of pseudohyponatremia, therefore identify and rule out high protein, lipid, and glucose concentration for confirmation of hyponatremia.
  Because hyperglycemia is by far the most common cause of nonhypotonic hyponatremia, excluding hyperglycemic hyponatremia is the first step in the diagnostic algorithm.
- *Urine osmolality to assess vasopressin activity:* To confirm excess of fluid intake relative to solute intake, we recommend it as the second step in the diagnostic strategy.
- *Urine sodium concentration in a spot urine sample:* A urine sodium concentration threshold of 30 mmol/L is used for distinguishing hypovolemia from euvolemia or hypervolemia. This means that a urine sodium concentration ≤30 mmol/L suggests low effective arterial blood volume, even in patients on diuretics while increased levels suggest salt loss.
- *ECF volume status:* Clinicians often misclassify hyponatremia when using algorithms that start with a clinical assessment of volume status. Therefore, using an algorithm in which urine osmolality and urine sodium concentration are prioritized over assessment of volume status. Assessment of hydration status is vital with hypovolemia indicating sodium loss and euvolemia/hypervolemia suggesting free water excess.
  Laboratory pointers of hydration include uric acid and hematocrit (high with dehydration). Uric acid excretion is directly proportional to plasma volume. Hypervolemic states have increased urinary excretion and low serum uric acid levels while levels are high in hypovolemia.

Diagnostic difficulty with diuretics: Patients on diuretics may have increased, normal, or decreased extracellular circulating volume and can have increased or decreased urine sodium concentration.

The natriuresis induced by diuretics may cause "appropriate" vasopressin release and subsequently hyponatremia because of a decrease in circulating volume.

In patients using diuretics, a fractional excretion of uric acid >12% may be better than urine sodium concentration to differentiate reduced effective circulating volume from SIAD as the underlying cause of hyponatremia.

Although all types of diuretics have been associated with hyponatremia, thiazide diuretics are most commonly the culprit.

Q2. What are the common causes of hyponatremia in intensive care unit (ICU)?

The most common causes of hyponatremia in adults are patient on diuretics, the excessive fluid given in postoperative

Flowchart 1: The diagnosis of hyponatremia.

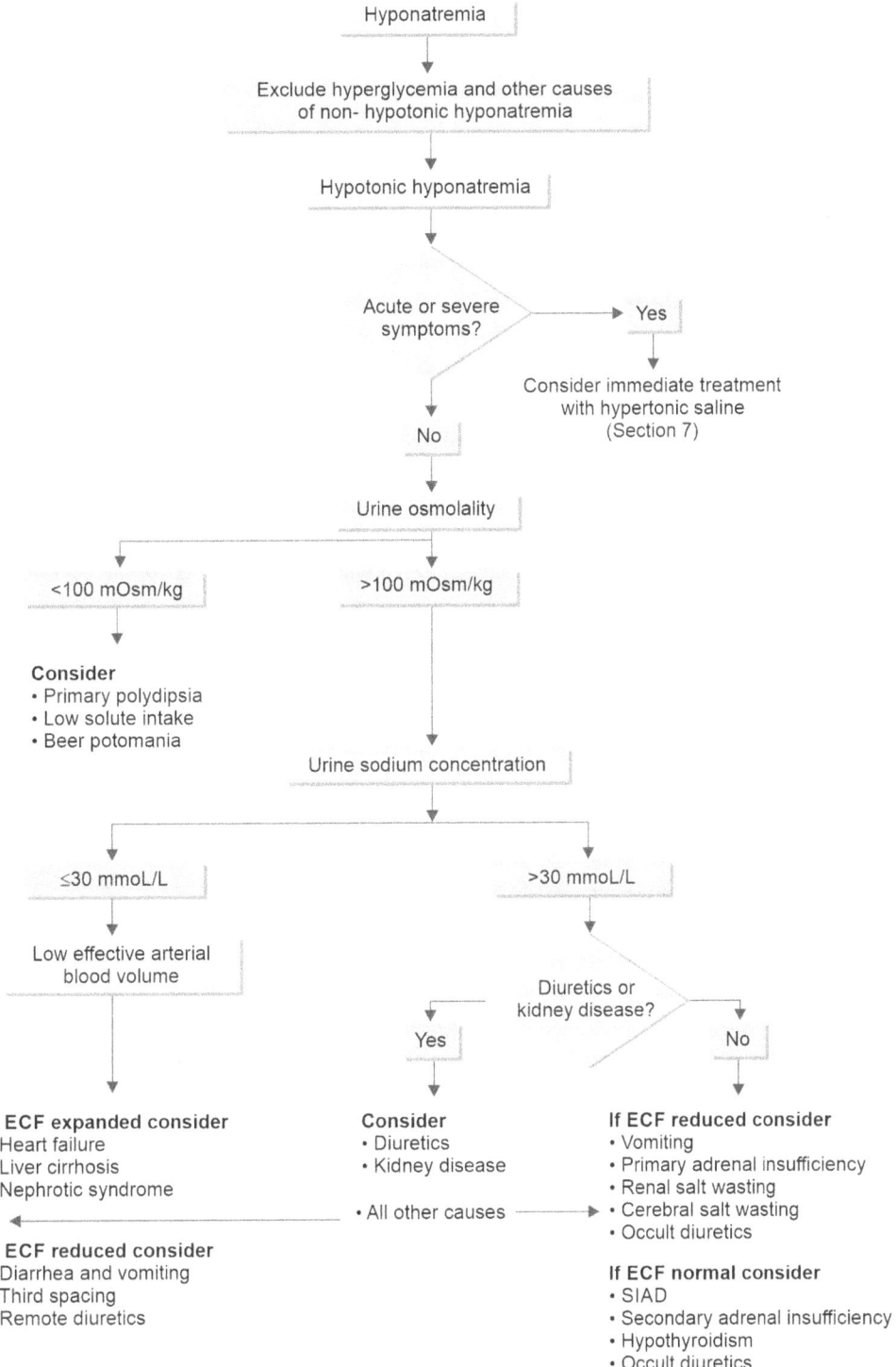

(ECF: extracellular fluid; SIAD: syndrome of inappropriate antidiuresis)

state and various causes of the syndrome of inappropriate secretion of antidiuretic hormone (SIADH), primary polydipsia in psychiatric patients, and after transurethral prostatectomy. Gastrointestinal fluid loss, ingestion of dilute formulas, and receipt of multiple tap-water enemas are the main causes of severe hyponatremia in infants and children.

Following is the overall etiology/differential diagnosis of hyponatremia in ICU patients:

Hyponatremia can be broadly classified as:
- Hypotonic hyponatremia
- *Nonhypotonic hyponatremia:* It does not cause brain edema and is managed differently from hypotonic hyponatremia.

Normal serum osmolality is 280–295 mOsm/kg. The serum osmolality can be calculated by the concentration in millimoles per liter of the major serum solutes according to the following equation:

Serum osmolality (mmol/kg) = (2 × serum [Na]) + (serum [glucose]/18) + (blood urea nitrogen/2.8)

Nonhypotonic hyponatremia:
There are further three categories of nonhypotonic hyponatremia (**Table 3**)
- Isotonic known as pseudohyponatremia
- Hypertonic known as translocational hyponatremia, hyponatremia in the presence of a surplus of "effective" osmoles
- Hyponatremia in the presence of a surplus of "ineffective" osmoles

1. *Pseudohyponatremia (normo-osmolal) or isotonic hyponatremia* is a laboratory artifact seen in the presence of abnormally high concentrations of lipids (hypertriglyceridemia) or plasma proteins (multiple myeloma) in the blood which interfere with the accurate measurement of sodium.

   In normal subjects, the plasma water is 93% of the plasma volume, fats, and proteins account for the remaining 7%.

   Plasma water fraction falls below 80% in cases with marked hyperlipidemia (triglycerides >1,500 mg/dL) or hyperproteinemia (protein > 10 g/dL).

   Here, the plasma water sodium concentration and plasma osmolality are unchanged, but the measured sodium concentration in the total plasma volume is reduced since the specimen contains less plasma water. In pseudohyponatremia, serum osmolality is normal and no shifts of water occur.

2. *Translocational (hyperosmolal)/hypertonic or redistributive hyponatremia:* It is due to the presence of significant amounts of osmotically active unmeasured solutes in the serum to which cell membranes are impermeable, and are restricted to the ECF compartment and are effective osmoles because they create osmotic pressure gradients across cell membranes leading to osmotic movement of water from the intracellular to the extracellular compartment.

   Because dilutional hyponatremia results from the water shift from the intracellular to the extracellular compartment, there is no risk of brain edema.

   It is important to make the distinction between measured osmolality and effective osmolality. Effective osmolality may be calculated with the following equations:

Effective osmolality (mmol/kg H_2O)
 = 2 × (serum sodium (mmol/L)
 + serum K (mmol/L) + serum glycemia (mg/dL)/18

Depending on the serum concentration of effective osmoles, the resulting nonhypotonic hyponatremia can be isotonic or hypertonic. The prime example is hyperglycemia. Others include infusion of mannitol or perioperative absorption of irrigation fluids such as glycine, which most frequently occurs during transurethral resection of the prostate (TURP) and is therefore also referred to as "TURP syndrome".

When glucose, mannitol, and glycine are metabolized or excreted, serum osmolality decreases. This reduces the osmotic gradient, resulting in less water being pulled from the cells and spontaneously limiting the degree of hyponatremia. It explains why during treatment of diabetic ketoacidosis or the hyperosmolar hyperglycemic state a decrease in serum glycemia leads to a "spontaneous" rise in the serum sodium concentration.

TABLE 3: Three categories of nonhypotonic hyponatremia.

Setting	Serum osmolality	Examples
Presence of "effective" osmoles that raise serum osmolality and can cause hyponatremia	Isotonic or hypertonic	• Glucose • Mannitol • Glycine • Histidine-tryptophan-ketoglutarate • Hyperosmolar radiocontrast media • Maltose
Presence of "ineffective" osmoles that raise serum osmolality but do not cause hyponatremia	Isotonic or hyperosmolar	• Urea • Alcohols • Ethylene glycol
Presence of endogenous solutes that cause pseudohyponatremia (laboratory artifact)	Isotonic	• Triglycerides, cholesterol, and protein • Intravenous immunoglobulins • Monoclonal gammapathies

Estimates of the serum sodium concentration corrected for the presence of hyperglycemia can be obtained from the following equations:

Corrected serum sodium = measured Na + 2.4 × [glucose (mg/dL) − 100 mg/dL/100 mg/dL]

This translates into adding 2.4 mmol/L to the measured serum sodium concentration for every 100 mg/dL incremental rise in serum glucose concentration above a standard serum glucose concentration of 100 mg/dL.

3. *Hyponatremia due to Ineffective osmoles:* Seen with high urea concentrations in kidney disease, ethanol, and methanol

Solutes which readily pass across the cellular membrane are ineffective solutes because they do not create osmotic pressure gradients across cell membranes and therefore cause no water shifts, to the ECF compartment increase the measured osmolality. It does not change effective osmolality. Consequently, they do not cause hyponatremia.

Hypotonic hyponatremia—True (hypoosmolal) hyponatremia: In the majority of patients that present with hyponatremia, the serum is hypotonic, i.e., both the sodium concentration and the effective osmolality are low.

From physiology basics, we know sodium is the major extracellular cation. Changes in serum sodium is always accompanied by changes in water and thus the volume status. Since sodium is mainly extracellular cation, by volume status we mean mainly extracellular volume and when we encounter hyponatremia, fundamentally there is greater retention of water relative to sodium and the resultant serum osmolality will be low.

Change in Na^+ = change in water = change in ECF volume
Hyponatremia H_2O > Na → low serum osmolality

Causes of hyponatremia are further characterized as per three possible ECF volume statuses into:
1. Euvolemic
2. Hypervolemic and
3. Hypovolemic.

Determining volume status will help us narrow down the differentials of hypotonic hyponatremia.
1. If the patient is hypovolemic, there is depletion of Na and water, but sodium deficit exceeds the water deficit, causing hypovolemia and hyponatremia ↓ Na^+ ↓ H_2O ↓
2. The second situation is if the patient is in volume overload (hypervolemic), excessive water retention secondary to sodium retention, and there is volume expansion ↑ Na ↑ H_2O ↑ T
3. Thirdly the volume status is normal, there are no major disturbances of body sodium content and the patient is euvolemic Na ↔ H_2O

Hypotonic hyponatremia with decreased ECF volume: Depletion of circulating volume, with or without deficit of total body sodium, can markedly increase the secretion of vasopressin leading to water retention despite hypotonicity (in order to preserve intravascular volume) causing hyponatremia.

For further understanding of the causes, we check urine sodium loss **(Flowchart 2)**.

Renal sodium loss when urine sodium is > 20 mEq/dL:
- *Diuretic agents/osmotic diuresis (glucose, urea, and mannitol):* Diuretics especially thiazides are frequently implicated as a cause of hyponatremia. The renal sodium loss leads to volume contraction with subsequent release of vasopressin. Despite the potential for causing more urinary sodium loss, loop diuretics rarely cause hyponatremia because they reduce osmolality in the

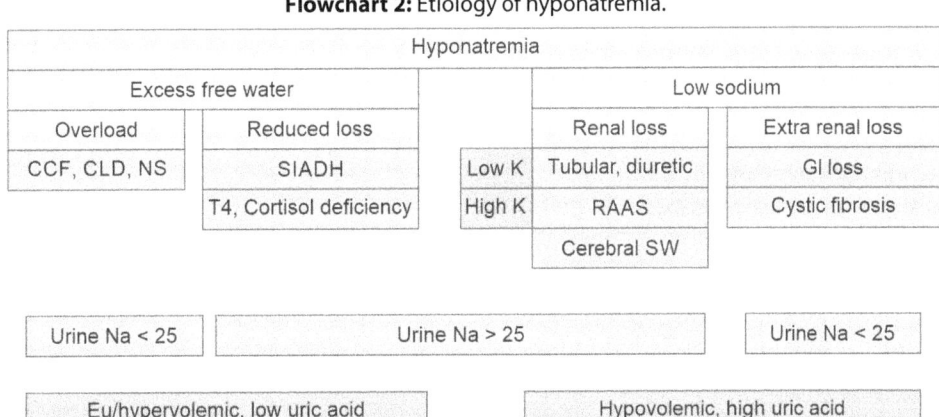

Flowchart 2: Etiology of hyponatremia.

(CCF: congestive cardiac failure; CLD: chronic liver disease; GI: gastrointestinal; RAAS: renin-angiotensin-aldosterone system; SIADH: syndrome of inappropriate antidiuretic hormone; SW: salt wasting)

renal medulla and thus limit the kidney's ability to concentrate urine.

- *Adrenal insufficiency:* In primary adrenal insufficiency, hypoaldosteronism causes renal sodium loss, contracted ECF volume and hyponatremia. Here, hyponatremia can be its first and only sign.
- *Cerebral salt wasting:* Cerebral salt wasting is characterized by urinary sodium loss due to release of increased levels of brain natriuretic peptide in the setting of neurological insults such as infection, surgery, or subarachnoid bleeding. The condition presents with orthostatic hypotension, low central venous pressure (dehydration), hyponatremia and markedly elevated urinary sodium levels, and a high serum urea. It is often confused with SIADH and can be differentiated from it by the demonstration of high uric acid, dehydration, and very high sodium loss. Cerebral salt wasting is important because its treatment requires volume resuscitation rather than water restriction, and fludrocortisone.
- *Salt-wasting nephropathy kidney disease:* Renal salt wasting can also occur in salt-losing nephropathies, such as tubulopathy after chemotherapy or in analgesic nephropathy, medullary cystic kidney disease and certain pharmacological compounds can inhibit the kidney's ability to reabsorb appropriate amounts of sodium.

Extrarenal sodium loss: When urine sodium is <20 mEq/dL:
- *Diarrhea:* In case of severe diarrhea, the kidneys respond by preserving sodium and so urine sodium concentrations are very low.
- *Transdermal sodium loss:* Excessive sweating (e.g., in marathon runners) impaired reabsorption of sodium in the sweat duct as in cystic fibrosis or by an impaired natural barrier function due to extensive skin burns.
- *Third spacing:* Fluid sequestration in "third space" as seen in bowel obstruction peritonitis, pancreatitis, muscle trauma, and burns may markedly reduce effective circulating blood volume through fluid leakage from blood vessels. This causes baroreceptor activation and vasopressin release, which may result in hyponatremia.

Hypotonic hyponatremia with increased ECF volume:
- *Congestive heart failure:* Approximately 20-30% of patients with chronic heart failure [New York Heart Association (NYHA)] classes III and IV have hyponatremia. Baroreceptor-mediated neurohumoral activation commonly results in increased secretion of vasopressin by the pituitary. Simultaneous activation of the renin–angiotensin system and increased release of vasopressin reduces urinary sodium excretion and increases urine osmolality.
- *Cirrhosis:* Systemic vasodilation and arteriovenous shunting of blood may reduce the effective arterial blood volume. As in heart failure, this reduction can lead to neurohumoral activation and water retention due to baroreceptor mediated vasopressin release.
- *Nephrotic syndrome:* In nephrotic syndrome, blood volume may be decreased due to the lower serum oncotic pressure. If this happens, stimulation of vasopressin secretion can cause patients to develop hyponatremia.
- *Renal failure (acute or chronic):* When glomerular filtration rate deteriorates, or when there is tubular injury or scarring, the ability to reabsorb sodium and excrete free water decreases. Consequently, hyponatremia can readily develop if patients do not adhere to fluid restriction.
- *Reset osmostat:* In reset osmostat, there is a change in the set point of osmoregulation. The response to changes in osmolality remains intact. This phenomenon is seen in pregnancy where the serum sodium concentration may mildly decrease by 4–5 mmol/L.

Hypotonic hyponatremia with normal ECF volume: Euvolemic hyponatremia is caused by an absolute increase in body water, which results from an excessive fluid intake in the presence of an impaired free water excretion, either due to inappropriate release of vasopressin or due to a low intake of solutes.

- *Hypothyroidism* very rarely causes hyponatremia. Only severe cases of clinically manifest hypothyroidism resulted in clinically important hyponatremia.
- *Secondary adrenal insufficiency:* The production of aldosterone is less impaired in secondary than in primary adrenal insufficiency. Under normal circumstances, cortisol suppresses both production of corticotrophin-releasing hormone and vasopressin in the hypothalamus. In secondary adrenal insufficiency, persistently low concentrations of cortisol fail to suppress vasopressin and hyponatremia results from impaired free water excretion, as it does in SIAD.
- *SIADH:* It represents inappropriately increased arginine vasopressin (AVP) secretion in the absence of an osmotic stimuli. It is characterized by euvolemic hyponatremia, reduced urine output with high urinary sodium (>25 mmol/L) and osmolality (>100 mOsm/kg). Uric acid levels are low suggesting fluid excess.

Syndrome of inappropriate secretion of antidiuretic hormone should be diagnosed only after exclusion of diuretic use, renal, thyroid, and adrenal diseases. Because of the vasopressin activity, urine osmolality will be inappropriately high (usually >100 mOsm/L) and this is one of the criteria required for a diagnosis of SIAD. Treatment includes fluid restriction and V2 receptor antagonists.

- *Excessive water intake:* Seen in primary polydipsia patients, sodium-free irrigant solutions (used in hysteroscopy and laparoscopy). Multiple tap-water enemas under conditions of high water and low solute intake, the excess water intake is primarily responsible for hyponatremia. Vasopressin release is suppressed/activity is absent, which is reflected by an appropriately low urine osmolality, usually <100 mOsm/kg. A urine osmolality <100 mOsm/kg on a spot urine sample always indicates maximally dilute urine.

Q3. How will you manage symptomatic hyponatremia in this patient?

Principles of treatment of hyponatremia: The plasma sodium concentration can be increased by either salt administration (hypertonic saline/normal saline/salt capsules) or by restricting their water intake to less than the level of excretion.

Choice of treatment depends on:
- Duration of hyponatremia (whether acute or >48 hours)
- Presence or absence of symptoms
- Volume status
- Etiology of hyponatremia

During treatment of hyponatremia, we set a target and a limit. Target is the change in serum sodium concentration that we expect to achieve with a particular treatment. By contrast, a limit is a change in serum sodium concentration which we do not want to exceed and if surpassed, requires prompt counter-regulating intervention.

As it is usually not possible to determine the duration of hyponatremia, clinical symptoms are used as a surrogate with neurological symptoms indicating acute hyponatremia.

Treatment of acute hypotonic hyponatremia:
- With severe symptoms
- With moderately severe symptoms
- Without severe or moderately severe symptoms.

Treatment of acute hypotonic hyponatremia with severe or moderately severe symptoms is reflected by seizures, encephalopathy, and focal deficits. These patients have not had time for the brain adaptations to occur. Severe symptoms result from brain edema (a dangerous condition, which may lead to permanent brain damage or death if left untreated) caused by an acute drop in effective osmolality or by rapid further decrease in preexisting chronic hyponatremia. Given the immediate risk of severe neurological damage (the risk of brain herniation is high), reducing brain edema should be prioritized in severely symptomatic hyponatremia as the risk of brain edema outweighs the risk of possibly inducing osmotic demyelination or fluid overload. So, a rapid correction is needed irrespective of biochemical degree or timing (acute vs. chronic) of hyponatremia (**Flowchart 3**).

First-hour management: Regardless of whether hyponatremia is acute or chronic:

- Treatment recommended is giving a bolus of 150 mL (3-5 ml/kg) 3% NaCl (1 liter = 513 mEq Na$^+$) intravenous (IV) over 20 minutes, repeated up to three doses till acute symptoms subside with 3% NaCl. The aim of this treatment is to correct the symptoms and not to raise sodium levels to the normal range.
- The goal is to provide an urgent correction by 4-6 mmol/L to prevent brain herniation.
- This approach allows monitoring of the change in serum sodium concentration in relationship to the clinical response and aims to manage the risk of overly rapid correction. We suggest repeating the 150 mL infusions of 3% hypertonic saline until the serum sodium concentration has increased 5 mmol/L, or until the symptoms improve, whichever comes first. This treatment can provide rapid but controlled correction of hyponatremia. Hypertonic saline is usually combined with furosemide to limit treatment-induced volume expansion.

Follow-up management: In case of improvement of symptoms after a 5 mmol/L increase in serum sodium concentration in

Flowchart 3: Management of hyponatremia.

Symptoms		
Acute severe	Acute moderate	Chronic
3–5 mL/kg 3% NaCl in 20 min	Avoid bolus	No acute treatment
Only till symptomatic	Rise <6–9 mmol/L/day	Rise <6 mmol/L/day
<12 mmol/L/day		

3% NaCl infusion in severe cases

the first hour, regardless of whether hyponatremia is acute or chronic:

- It is recommended to stop the infusion and start cause-specific treatment to maintain the achieved serum sodium concentration.
- Limit the increase in serum sodium concentration to a total of 10 mmol/L during the first 24 hours and an additional 8 mmol/L during every 24 hours thereafter until the serum sodium concentration reaches 130 mmol/L. It is very difficult, to set "safe" rate limits for correcting hyponatremia. A correction rate of 10 mmol/L during the first 24 hours and 18 mmol/L during the first 48 hours is probably a safe limit.
- Serum sodium concentration should be closely monitored after 1, 6, and 12 hours during the first 24 hours of treatment and daily afterward until the serum sodium concentration has stabilized under stable treatment.

Follow-up management: In case of no improvement of symptoms after a 5 mmol/L increase in serum sodium concentration in the first hour, regardless of whether hyponatremia is acute or chronic (*see* **Flowchart 3**).

- If the symptoms do not improve after a 5 mmol/L increase in serum sodium concentration during the first hour, causes other than hyponatremia for the symptoms should be explored. Depending on the clinical history, additional neurological investigations such as imaging may be helpful.
- It is advised attempting a further increase in serum sodium concentration of 1 mmol/L by infusing 3% hypertonic saline.
- If symptoms do not improve after a 10 mmol/L increase in sodium concentration, it is (even more) likely they are caused by something other than hyponatremia.
- Hence, we believe that serum sodium concentration should not increase 10 mmol/L during the first 24 hours (the first 5 mmol included), even if symptoms do not improve.
- It is also recommended stopping hypertonic saline if the serum sodium concentration reaches 130 mmol/L, because it is unlikely that symptoms are caused by hyponatremia if they persist after the serum sodium concentration has reached 130 mmol/L.

Equation to estimate achievement of 1 mmol/L/h increase in sodium:

- The degree to which one liter of a given solution initially raises the serum sodium concentration in a hyponatremic patient is estimated from the Adrogué-Madias formula described in the **Table 4**.

TABLE 4: Formulas for use in managing hyponatremia and characteristics of infusates.

Formula*	Clinical use
1. Change in serum $Na^+ = \dfrac{\text{Infusate } Na^+ - \text{Serum } Na^+}{\text{Total body water} + 1}$	Estimate the effect of 1 liter of any infusate on serum Na^+
2. Change in serum $Na^+ = \dfrac{(\text{Infusate } Na^+ + \text{infusate } K^+) - \text{serum } Na^+}{\text{Total body water} + 1}$	Estimate the effect of 1 liter of any infusate containing Na^+ and K^+ on serum Na^+

Infusate	Infusate Na^+ mmol/L	Extracellular fluid Distribution %
5% sodium chloride in water	855	100†
3% sodium chloride in water	513	100†
0.9% sodium chloride in water	154	100
Ringer's lactate solution	130	97
0.45% sodium chloride in water	77	73
0.2% sodium chloride in 5% dextrose in water	34	55
5% dextrose in water	0	40

*The numerator in formula 1 is a simplification of the expression (infusate Na^+ —serum Na^+) × 1 liter, with the value yielded by the equation in millimoles per liter. The estimated total body water (in liters) is calculated as a fraction of body weight. The fraction is 0.6 in children; 0.6 and 0.5 in nonelderly men and women, respectively; and 0.5 and 0.45 in elderly men and women, respectively. Normally, extracellular and intracellular fluids account for 40 and 60% of total body water, respectively.
†In addition to its complete distribution in the extracellular compartment, this infusate induces osmotic removal of water from the intracellular compartment.

However, these formulae have limitations and cannot be used to accurately predict the magnitude of change in serum sodium and frequent measurements are necessary.

- In the current guidelines, these formulae are not used. Instead 1 mL/kg of 3% NaCl is estimated to raise the serum sodium by 1 mEq/L.

Acute hyponatremia with moderately severe symptoms: The immediate threat from hyponatremia and for osmotic demyelination syndrome (ODS) (which may occur due to rapid correction of sodium) is less pronounced than that for hyponatremia with severe symptoms. Consequently, the reduced immediate threat shifts the priority, from inducing a rapid increase in sodium to preventing a further decrease in serum sodium concentration. Thus, a prompt diagnostic assessment for hyponatremia is to be done.

If possible stop medications and other factors that can contribute to or provoke hyponatremia. Start immediate treatment with a single IV infusion of 150 mL 3% hypertonic saline or equivalent over 20 minutes. Limit the increase in serum sodium concentration to 10 mmol/L in the first 24 hours and 8 mmol/L during every 24 hours thereafter, until a serum sodium concentration of 130 mmol/L is reached. If the symptoms do not improve with an increase in serum sodium concentration, additional diagnostic workup for other causes of the symptoms should be done.

Acute hyponatremia with mild symptoms: In the absence of severe or moderately severe symptoms, there is time for diagnostic assessment and cause-specific treatment is the most reasonable approach. For mild-to-moderate symptoms, consider using weight-based (2 mL/kg) rather than the fixed 150 mL infusion volumes of 3% hypertonic saline. Aim for a 5 mmol/L per 24-hour increase in serum sodium concentration. Stop nonessential fluids, medications, and other factors that can contribute to or provoke hyponatremia. Do not treat with the sole aim of increasing the serum sodium concentration.

Infusion of 0.9% NaCl should not be used to acutely increase $P^-(Na^+)$ as in the case story such an infusion does not cause an immediate, controllable increase in $P^-(Na^+)$, and 0.9% NaCl might worsen the hyponatremia in SIADH.

Most reported cases of osmotic demyelination occurred after rates of correction that exceeded 12 mmol/L/day were used, commended indications for stopping the rapid correction of symptomatic hyponatremia (regardless of the method used) are the cessation of life-threatening manifestations, moderation of other symptoms, or the achievement of a serum sodium concentration of 125–130 mmol/L (or even lower if the base-line serum sodium concentration is below 100 mmol/L). Long-term management of hyponatremia (described below) should then be initiated. Another formula was proposed to estimate both the sodium deficit and the direct effect of a given fluid (3% NaCl) on the serum sodium concentration:

For example:

Sodium deficit = Total body water (TBW) × (desired serum sodium concentration – actual serum sodium concentration)

Q4. Innumerate the causes of SIADH.

The various causes are mentioned in **Table 5**.

The most frequent causes of increased inappropriate secretion of vasopressin include cancers (e.g., small cell carcinoma of the lung) and diseases of the lung (e.g., pneumonia) or central nervous system (e.g., subarachnoid hemorrhage).

Q5. What are the diagnostic criteria for SIADH?

Diagnostic criteria for the SIADH are given in **Box 1**.

Q6. Enumerate the differences between SIADH and cerebral salt wasting.

Differences between SIADH and cerebral salt wasting are given in **Table 6**.

The patients' symptoms improved with the initial bolus of hypertonic saline. She became conscious, oriented, and did not have further episodes of seizures. Sodium level increased to 126 mmol/L after 6 hours. She was monitored in the ICU for 48 hours and discharged.

Q7. What is ODS? Who are the patients at high risk of ODS?

The ODS is a central nervous system disorder caused by rapid changes in serum osmolality resulting in neuronal damage. Patients at high risk of developing the ODS include those with alcohol abuse, concomitant hypokalemia, liver diseases, use of diuretics, malnutrition, and patients on psychoactive agents.

Chronicity of hyponatremia, severity of symptoms, and susceptibility to ODS should be kept in mind while treating hyponatremia and overcorrection should always be avoided. Whenever possible, in these cases, the conservative measures such as water restriction and stopping the offending drug should be given the chance before implementation of more active measures, especially in absence of severe symptoms. In cases of concomitant hypokalemia, the administration of potassium may raise the serum sodium and osmolality in the hyponatremic patient. Therefore, the impact of the given potassium on hyponatremia correction should be taken into account. Additionally, whenever hypokalemia and severe hyponatremia present simultaneously, slow correction is necessary. Generally, in all high-risk patients, slower rates

TABLE 5: Various causes of syndrome of inappropriate antidiuresis hormone.

Malignant diseases	Pulmonary disorders	Disorders of the nervous system	Drugs	Other causes
Carcinoma	Infections	Infection	Vasopressin release or action stimulants	Hereditary
Lung	Bacterial pneumonia	Encephalitis	Antidepressants	Gain-of-function mutation of the vasopressin V2 receptor
Oropharynx	Viral pneumonia	Meningitis	SSRIs	Idiopathic
Gastrointestinal tract	Pulmonary abscess	Brain abscess	Tricyclic	Transient
	Tuberculosis	Rocky Mountain spotted fever	MAOI	Exercise-associated hyponatremia
Stomach				
Duodenum	Aspergillosis	AIDS	Venlafaxine	General anesthesia
Pancreas	Asthma	Malaria	Anticonvulsants	Nausea
Genitourinary tract	Cystic fibrosis	Vascular and masses	Carbamazepine	Pain
Ureter	Respiratory failure associated with positive pressure breeding	Subdural hematoma	Oxcarbazepine	Stress
Bladder		Subarachnoid hemorrhage	Sodium valproate	
Prostate		Stroke	Lamotrigine	
Endometrium		Brain tumors	Antipsychotics	
Endocrine thymoma		Head trauma	Phenothiazines	
Lymphomas		Other	Butyrophenones	
Sarcomas		Hydrocephalus	Anticancer drugs	
Ewing's sarcoma		Cavernous sinus thrombosis	Vinca alkaloids	
Olfactory neuroblastoma		Multiple sclerosis	Platinum compounds	
		Guillain–Barré syndrome	Ifosfamide	
		Shy–Drager syndrome	Melphalan	
		Delirium tremens	Cyclophosphamide	
		Acute intermittent porphyria	Methotrexate	
			Pentostatin	
			Antidiabetic drugs	
			Chlorpropamide	
			Tolbutamide	
			Miscellaneous	
			Opiates	
			MDMA (XTC)	
			Levamisole	
			Interferon	
			NSAIDs	
			Clofibrate	
			Nicotine	
			Amiodarone	
			Proton pump inhibitors	
			MABs	
			Vasopressin analogs	
			Desmopressin	
			Oxytocin	
			Terlipressin	
			Vasopressin	

(AIDS: acquired immunodeficiency syndrome; MOAI: monoamine oxidase inhibitors; MDMA: 3,4-methylenedioxymethamphetamine; NSAID: nonsteroidal anti-inflammatory drug; SSRIs: selective serotonin reuptake inhibitors)

of correction and lower targets of serum sodium should be considered along with vigilant monitoring. Weighing the risk of developing the ODS versus the benefit of correcting the severe hyponatremia is always crucial.

Q8. What is the mechanism of injury in ODS and how will you prevent it?
Osmotic demyelination syndrome is characterized by the development of demyelinating brain lesions that classically

BOX 1: Diagnostic criteria for the syndrome of inappropriate antidiuresis hormone.

Essential criteria:
- Effective serum osmolality <275 mOsm/kg
- Urine osmolality >100 mOsm/kg at some level of decreased effective osmolality
- Clinical euvolemia
- Urine sodium concentration >30 mmol/L with normal dietary salt and water intake
- Absence of adrenal, thyroid, pituitary, or renal insufficiency
- No recent use of diuretic agents

Supplemental criteria:
- Serum uric acid <0.24 mmol/L (<4 mg/dL)
- Serum urea <3.6 mmol/L (<21.6 mg/dL)
- Failure to correct hyponatremia after 0.9% saline infusion
- Fractional sodium excretion >0.5%
- Fractional urea excretion >55%
- Fractional uric acid excretion >12%
- Correction of hyponatremia through fluid restriction

TABLE 6: Differences between syndrome of inappropriate antidiuresis hormone (SIADH) and cerebral salt wasting.

	SIADH	Cerebral salt wasting
Serum urea concentration	Normal—low	Normal—high
Serum uric acid concentration	Low	Low
Urine volume	Normal-low	High
Urine sodium concentration	>30 mmol/L	>30 mmol/L
Blood pressure	Normal	Normal—orthostatic hypotension
Central venous pressure	Normal	Low

occur in the basis pontis (central pontine myelinolysis); and sometimes at few extrapontine sites including the cerebellum, basal ganglia, lateral geniculate bodies, thalamus, and cerebral cortex (extrapontine myelinolysis). Histopathologic findings include noninflammatory injury or death of oligodendrocytes as well as astrocytes; and loss of myelin with relative axonal sparing.

Rapid correction of chronic (≥48 hours or unknown duration) hyponatremia is the main pathologic reason for the ODS. The brain adapts to hyponatremia by losing extracellular water into the cerebrospinal fluid and by extruding sodium, potassium, and certain organic solutes (osmolytes) out of the brain cells to maintain extracellular osmolality. This preventive mechanism results in keeping the brain volume toward normal, thus avoiding brain edema. Accumulation of organic osmolytes occurs slow as compared to inorganic ions.

In the setting of chronic hyponatremia, the overly rapid correction or of serum sodium concentration without giving sufficient time for osmolytes to reaccumulate back into the brain cells may cause fluid shifts into extracellular space resulting in an undesired brain cell shrinkage injury (osmotic demyelination).

Thus, overcorrection of severe hyponatremia may result in brain edema with its symptoms in the form of headache, vomiting, disturbed level of sensorium, and convulsions. The increase in intracranial pressure carries the risk of brain herniation and death. However, the detrimental consequences of brain edema are more likely to occur with the acute severe hyponatremia rather than with the chronic one. Previously, it was believed that oligodendrocytes that constitute the sheaths are particularly sensitive to osmotic changes and that the distribution of ODS lesions parallels that of oligodendroglial cells injury as also supported by the pathologic findings of loss of myelin sheaths with relative axonal preservation. Researchers are recently shedding the light on the role of astrocytes in the process of osmotic demyelination. The foot processes of astrocytes, which encircle both brain capillaries and neurons, express aquaporins (such as aquaporin-4) that allow water to cross the blood–brain barrier. Astrocytes protect neurons from osmotic stress; in response to hypotonicity allowing neurons to lose water and maintain their volume while astrocytes swell.[7] Within 24-48 hours after this transfer, astrocytes restore their volume through loss of organic osmolytes, but this makes them vulnerable to injury from rapid normalization of the plasma sodium concentration. Recapture of lost brain osmolytes may take a week or longer. Therefore, rapid correction of hyponatremia is a hypertonic stress to astrocytes that are depleted of osmolytes, triggering astrocyte apoptosis, and, eventually, brain demyelination.

Prevention of ODMS:
- *Differentiation of acute from chronic hyponatremia:* First step in prevention is to differentiate chronic from acute hyponatremia. Patients with severe hyponatremia of <48 hours duration (acute hyponatremia) usually present with neurological symptoms due to brain edema and they tolerate the controlled rapid rises of serum sodium and their risk of developing ODS is significantly low.

  On the other hand, patients with chronic hyponatremia (hyponatremia of ≥48 hours or uncertain duration) are presumed to have already developed the process of adaptation with extrusion of water, electrolytes as well as organic osmolytes out of the brain cells. Therefore they are at significant risk to develop the post-therapeutic neurological deterioration in terms of ODS. Whenever uncertainty exists about the duration of hyponatremia, it is prudent to consider it chronic.

- *The method used to raise serum sodium:* Stopping the drug which caused the low sodium may be the first step (such as a diuretic or a drug that may produce inappropriate antidiuretic hormone release) in chronic hyponatremia. Hypertonic saline is usually reserved for patients with severe chronic hyponatremia with severe neurological symptoms; particularly convulsions and coma. Isotonic saline (0.9% saline) infusion is usually indicated for the treatment of hypovolemic hyponatremia. Isotonic saline infusion may indeed cause an overly rapid correction of plasma sodium with ODS as a possible consequence. Treating chronic hyponatremia patients with isotonic saline should be associated with as much caution as with hypertonic saline.

- *Target and rate of serum sodium rise:* The risk of developing the ODS seems to depend not only on the rate of increase in serum sodium concentration but also on associated underlying risk factors. In patients with chronic hyponatremia and severe neurological symptoms (active convulsions or coma), a rapid correction of hyponatremia is required to control the severe symptoms. An increase in serum sodium of 2-4 mmol/L in 2-4 hours may be beneficial with low risk of ODS; provided it is followed by caution not to exceed the total of 6-8 mmol/L in 24 hours. This rapid controlled rise is usually achieved with a bolus or two of 100 mL of 3% saline.
- *Extra caution with high-risk patients:* Conservative measures should be the first option in high-risk patients in the absence of symptoms, it may be by simply stopping the offending drug. Generally, in all high-risk patients, slower rates of correction and lower targets of serum sodium should be considered in the presence of vigilant monitoring. Risk-benefit assessment of developing the ODS versus the benefit of correcting the severe hyponatremia is always crucial.
- *Monitoring:* It is difficult to precisely predict the rise in serum sodium in response to a given rate of infusion of isotonic or hypertonic saline. Many times, treatment with salt tablets was ended in overshoot of serum sodium. Hence, monitoring is of very important. Monitoring helps to predict or early detect the inadvertent rise in serum sodium. Initial monitoring of serum sodium should be carried out every 2-4 hours, whenever the rate of sodium rise exceeds 0.5 mmol/L/h while others prefer to record it in terms of increments for a specified period (12 hours or 24 hours).

Monitoring of urine output and urine osmolality is also as important as monitoring of serum sodium; however, it is not always feasible. The water diuresis phase is characterized by a remarkably rapid excretion of dilute urine and is observed in a significant proportion of sodium overcorrections. An increase in urine output of 100 mL/h or more in the background of hyponatremia active treatment indicates increased risk of overly rapid rise in serum sodium concentration and requires measuring urine osmolality.

- *Prophylaxis against overcorrection:* Prophylaxis against inadvertent serum sodium rise may be indicated in patients with high risk of developing the ODS, or in hypovolemic patients who are liable to overcorrection after volume resuscitation. Desmopressin (DDAVP) administration in conjunction with the hypertonic saline might result in a more controlled rate of correction of hyponatremia and helps in avoiding the unanticipated emergence of water diuresis in patients at high risk for overcorrection (e.g., patients with inappropriate antidiuretic hormone secretion as a result of antidepressants; hyponatremia caused by hypovolemia, low dietary solute intake, cortisol deficiency, or thiazide diuretics).

Data suggested that patients admitted with sodium <120 mmol/L treated with a combination of DDAVP and hypertonic saline infusion achieved expected sodium level without overcorrection. This helps to achieve a rise of sodium within the first 24 hours in an expected way. DDAVP is also not so effective in hypervolemic hyponatremia patients. DDAVP is typically prescribed for central diabetes insipidus, von Willebrand disease, and for enuresis.

It has been observed that patients with azotemia have lower risk to develop ODS on rapid correction of hyponatremia by renal replacement therapy. The reasons why ODS is uncommon in patients treated with hemodialysis are not completely understood; however, one mechanism which helps in maintaining the sodium level is that a rise in serum osmolality induced by the rise in serum sodium during dialysis may be counterbalanced by a fall in serum osmolality induced by the removal of urea.

Q9. Describe the management of chronic hyponatremia.

Chronic hyponatremia without severe or moderately severe symptom: In chronic hyponatremia, the brain undergoes adaptation and hence the risk of cerebral herniation is very low unlike the risk in acute hyponatremia. Since a very rapid correction can lead to ODS, hence chronic hyponatremia generally needs gradual correction. High risk of ODS is seen especially if serum sodium is 120 mEq/L or less or if comorbidities such as alcoholism, liver disease, malnutrition, or severe hypokalemia are present.

In case of chronic hyponatremia without severe symptoms, it is advocated to adopt a cautious approach and limit the correction to 6-8 mmol/L in the first 24 hours, 12-14 mmol/L in the first 48 hours.

In patients with low risk of ODS, a rise of 8 mmol/day (maximum of 10 mmol/day) sodium concentration in 24 hours is sufficient to reverse most severe manifestations of chronic hyponatremia.

In patients with high risk of ODS, the serum sodium concentration be raised by a goal of 4 to 6 mEq/L per 24 h and by <9 mEq/L in any 24-h period.

In moderate or profound hyponatremia, we suggest restricting fluid intake as first-line treatment.

Increasing salt intake with combination of low-dose loop diuretics and oral sodium chloride capsules or 0.25–0.50 g/kg per day of urea

Lithium or demeclocycline and vasopressin receptor antagonists are not strongly recommended.

Patients with expanded ECF: Increasing serum sodium concentration here has not resulted in improved patient outcomes in moderate hyponatremia with expanded ECF volume, such as seen in liver cirrhosis or heart failure.

Given treatments directed solely at increasing serum sodium concentration have risks of overcorrection.

Thus, it is recommended not treating in case of mild or moderate hyponatremia in patients with expanded extracellular volume. For patients with profound hyponatremia, it is reasonable to avoid further decreases in serum sodium.

Fluid restriction here can be used as a means to reduce further fluid overload.

Patients with reduced circulating volume: Patients with hyponatremia and a contracted ECF volume have a combination of a true sodium and water deficit (lack water as well as sodium). They require a different approach than other causes of hyponatremia. Consequently, replenishing both deficits with isotonic saline seems logical. It is strongly recommended to restore extracellular volume with IV infusion of 0.9% saline or a balanced crystalloid solution at 0.5–1.0 mL/kg/h.

In case of hemodynamic instability, the need for rapid fluid resuscitation overrides the risk of an overly rapid increase in serum sodium concentration.

The vasopressin activity is suddenly suppressed, when intravascular volume is restored in hypovolemia, free water clearance can than dramatically increase, resulting in serum sodium concentrations rising more rapidly. Therefore, these patients are at high risk of an overly rapid increase in serum sodium concentration. A sudden increase in urine output to >100 mL/h signals increased risk of overly rapid rise in serum sodium concentration. If urine output suddenly increases, we would advise measuring the serum sodium.

In patients who are hemodynamically unstable, the immediate risk of decreased organ perfusion is more important than the potential risk of overly rapid increases in serum sodium concentration. Hence, the need for volume resuscitation overrides any concerns for overly rapid correction of hyponatremia.

V2 receptor antagonists are contraindicated in acute hypernatremia as they induce rapid fall in serum sodium levels **(Table 7)**.

TABLE 7: Specific management of hyponatremia.

Disorder	Management
Fluid overload	Correct cause, fluid restriction
SIADH	Fluid restriction, V2 receptor antagonists
Adrenal insufficiency	Hydrocortisone, fludrocortisone
PHA	NaCl, frusemide
Bartter syndrome	Indomethacin and amiloride

Q10. How will you manage a case of SIADH?

Specific treatment for euvolemic hyponatremia SIADH:
SIAD: Hyponatremia in SIADH is usually chronic, hence slow correction is needed and fluid restriction is the main cornerstone of treatment. Several days of restriction are usually necessary before a significant increase in plasma osmolality occurs; and only fluid, not sodium, should be restricted. Thirst can be ameliorated by substituting hard candy or ice chips for drinking fluids.

As a second-line treatment, increased intake of osmotic solutes to enhance clearance of water can be done. Oral urea might be the most practical method to achieve increased solute intake. The problem of bitter taste of urea, can be solved by combining urea with sweet-tasting substances.

In some severe, symptomatic, or acute cases, 3% NaCl is needed. 0.9% NaCl has a limited role in correction of the hyponatremia in SIADH and 3% NaCl is the fluid of choice. The amount of 3% NaCl needed can be calculated as the per formulae given for sodium correction. Approximately, 1 mL/kg of 3% NS increases the serum sodium by 1 mEq/L.

Some causes of SIADH can be corrected, e.g., self-limited disease (e.g., nausea, pain, and surgery), cessation of drugs that cause SIADH and treatment of tuberculosis or meningitis. Diuretics and vaptans are the other drugs used.

Diuretics: Concurrent use of a loop diuretic is beneficial in patients with SIADH who have a high urine to serum electrolyte (>1). Furosemide inhibits the sodium chloride reabsorption in the thick ascending limb of the loop of Henle and cause more of water loss than sodium loss.

Other drugs used for chronic SIADH are urea, demeclocycline, and the vaptans.

Demeclocycline: Causes a nephrogenic form of diabetes insipidus, thereby decreasing urine concentration even in the presence of high plasma AVP levels. Appropriate doses of demeclocycline range from 600 to 1,200 mg/day administered in divided doses. Demeclocycline can cause reversible azotemia and sometimes nephrotoxicity, especially in patients with cirrhosis and should be discontinued if increasing azotemia occurs.

Cause specific management of hyponatremia:
- *Primary polydipsia:* Fluid restriction is warranted in hyponatremic patients with primary polydipsia.
- *Adrenal insufficiency:* Glucocorticoid deficiency can be ruled out with a random or early morning cortisol level >18 mg/dL, or a cosyntropin stimulation test for a definitive diagnosis. Initial management of salt wasting crisis includes fluid resuscitation with sodium chloride, correction of hyperkalemia and stress dose of hydrocortisone (50 mg/m stat followed by 100 mg/m/day in four divided doses). The dose is tapered over the next 48 hours to 10-15 mg/m/day. Fludrocortisone is added when hydrocortisone dose is below 50 mg/m/day.
- *Hypothyroidism:* Unless hypothyroidism is severe (i.e., symptoms and signs of myxedema or thyroid-stimulating hormone >50 mIU/mL), other causes of hyponatremia should be sought rather than ascribing the hyponatremia to hypothyroidism. Treatment should consist of thyroid hormone replacement.

FURTHER READING

1. Abbott R, Silber E, Felber J, Ekpo E. Osmotic demyelination syndrome: BMJ. 2005;331:829-30.
2. Adrogué HJ, Madias NE. Aiding fluid prescription for the dysnatremias. Intensive Care Med 1997;23:309-16.
3. Adrogué HJ, Madias NE. Hyponatremia. N Engl J Med. 2000;342:1581-9.
4. Berl T. Treating hyponatremia: damned if we do and damned if we don't. Kidney Int. 1990;37:1006-18.
5. Bhardwaj A. Neurological impact of vasopressin dysregulation and hyponatremia. Ann Neurol. 2006;59:229-36.
6. Burg MB, Ferraris JD. Intracellular organic osmolytes: function and regulation. J Biol Chem. 2008;283:7309-13.
7. Castilla-Guerra L, del Carmen Fernández-Moreno M, López-Chozas JM, Fernández-Bolaños R. Electrolytes disturbances and seizures. Epilepsia. 2006;47:1990-8.
8. Clinical practice guideline on diagnosis and treatment of hyponatraemia European Journal of Endocrinology (2014) 170, G1-G47
9. Decaux G, Andres C, Gankam Kengne F, Soupart A. Treatment of euvolemic hyponatremia in the intensive care unit by urea. Crit Care. 2010;14:R184.
10. Dhrolia MF, Akhtar SF, Ahmed E, Naqvi A, Rizvi A. Azotemia protects the brain from osmotic demyelination on rapid correction of hyponatremia. Saudi J Kidney Dis Transpl. 2014;25: 558-66.
11. Gankam Kengne F, Nicaise C, Soupart A, Boom A, Schiettecatte J, Pochet R, et al. Astrocytes are an early target in osmotic demyelination syndrome. J Am Soc Nephrol. 2011;22: 1834-45.
12. Hegazi MO, Nawara A. Prevention and treatment of the osmotic demyelination syndrome: a review. JSM Brain Sci. 2016;1(1):1004.
13. Kerns E, Patel S, Cohen DM. Hourly oral sodium chloride for the rapid and predictable treatment of hyponatremia. Clin Nephrol. 2014;82:397-401.
14. Martin RJ. Central pontine and extrapontine myelinolysis: the osmotic demyelination syndromes. J Neurol Neurosurg Psychiatry. 2004;75:22-8.
15. Oh MS, Carroll HJ. Regulation of intracellular and extracellular volume. In: Arieff AI, DeFronzo RA, eds. Fluid, electrolyte, and acid-base disorders. 2nd ed. New York: Churchill Livingstone, 1995:1-28.
16. Overgaard-Steensen C, Ring T. Clinical review: practical approach to hyponatremia and hypernatraemia in critically ill patients. Crit Care. 2013;17:206.
17. Overgaard-Steensen C, Stodkilde-Jorgensen H, Larsson A, Broch-Lips M, Tonnesen E, Frokiaer J, et al. Regional differences in osmotic behavior in brain during acute hyponatremia: an in vivo MRI-study of brain and skeletal muscle in pigs. Am J Physiol Regul Integr Comp Physiol. 2010;299:R521-32.
18. Sarnaik AP, Meert K, Hackbarth R, Fleischmann L. Management of hyponatremic seizures in children with hypertonic saline: a safe and effective strategy. Crit Care Med. 1991;19: 758-62.
19. Sood L, Sterns RH, Hix JK, Silver SM, Chen L. Hypertonic saline and desmopressin: a simple strategy for safe correction of severe hyponatremia. Am J Kidney Dis. 2013;61:571-8.
20. Soupart A, Penninckx R, Stenuit A, Decaux G. Azotemia (48 h) decreases the risk of brain damage in rats after correction of chronic hyponatremia. Brain Res. 2000;852:167-72.
21. Spasovski G, Vanholder R, Allolio B, Annane D, Ball S, Bichet D, et al. Clinical practice guideline on diagnosis and treatment of hyponatremia. Eur J Endocrinol. 2014;170:1-47.
22. Sterns RH, Hix JK, Silver S. Treating profound hyponatremia: a strategy for controlled correction. Am J Kidney Dis. 2010;56:774-9.
23. Sterns RH, Hix JK, Silver SM. Management of hyponatremia in the ICU. Chest. 2013;144:672-9.
24. Sterns RH, Riggs JE, Schochet SS Jr. Osmotic demyelination syndrome following correction of hyponatremia. N Engl J Med. 1986;314:1535-42.
25. Sterns RH. Disorders of plasma sodium—causes, consequences, and correction. N Engl J Med. 2015;372:55-65.
26. Verbalis JG, Goldsmith SR, Greenberg A, Korzelius C, Schrier RW, Sterns RH, et al. Diagnosis, evaluation, and treatment of hyponatremia: expert panel recommendations. Am J Med. 2013;126:1-42.

CHAPTER 22

Guillain–Barré Syndrome

Jitendra Choudhary, Rahul Anil Pandit

CASE STUDY

A 25-year-old male was brought to the intensive care unit (ICU) with complaints of acute-onset weakness of both lower limb for 4 hours. There was history of diarrhea 1 week prior that subsided with treatment. After admission to ICU, clinical examination revealed diffuse weakness in all the four extremities with three-fifths power in upper limb and two-fifths power in lower limb. Muscle tone was decreased. Deep tendon reflexes were absent. Other neurological examination including higher mental function, speech, memory, and cranial nerve examination was normal. Spine was nontender to deep palpation.

Q1. What is the likely diagnosis in this patient? What are the differential diagnoses?[1]

Acute neuromuscular weakness is most commonly caused by Guillain-Barré syndrome (GBS) or myasthenia gravis. Less commonly, it may be due to motor neuron disease, myotonic dystrophy, polymyositis, muscular dystrophy, or acute brainstem/upper cervical spinal cord disease. Always consider botulism and tetanus, particularly if there is a history of intravenous drug abuse. Poisoning with organophosphates, lead, arsenic, and certain shellfish can also cause neuromuscular weakness **(Table 1)**.

Guillain-Barré syndrome is acute-onset polyneuropathy which is characterized by progressive symmetrical weakness and areflexia. Sometimes, sensory involvement and autonomic dysfunction may also be present. It is presumed that patients with GBS have good prognosis but up to 20% patients may have severe disability despite immunotherapy.

Guillain-Barré syndrome mainly presents in various variants.

Two main pathological types are:
1. Acute motor axonal neuropathy
2. Acute inflammatory demyelinating polyneuropathy (AIDP)

Classification:
There are axonal and demyelinating forms:
- *Sensory and motor:*
  - Classic or AIDP or acute motor and sensory axonal neuropathy (AMSAN)
- *Motor:*
  - Acute motor demyelinating neuropathy (ADMN) or acute motor axonal neuropathy (AMAN)
- *Sensory:*
  - Acute sensory loss, areflexia but no motor involvement

TABLE 1: Conditions that mimic GBS.

Disorder	Major features
Myasthenia gravis	• Reflexes are spared • Ocular weakness predominates • Positive response to edrophonium • *EMG:* Decremental motor response
Porphyria neuropathy	• Mental disturbance • Abdominal pain
Botulism	• Predominant bulbar involvement • Autonomic abnormalities (pupils) • *EMG:* Normal velocities, low amplitudes, incremental response (with high-frequency repetitive nerve stimulation)
Organophosphorus poisoning	Acute cholinergic reaction toxicity
Poliomyelitis	• Weakness, pain, and tenderness • Preserved sensation • *Cerebrospinal fluid:* Protein and cell count elevated
Periodic paralysis	• Reflexes normal • Cranial nerves and respiration spared • Abnormal serum potassium concentration
Shellfish poisoning	• Rapid onset (face, finger, and toe numbness) • Follows consumption of mussels/clams
Tick paralysis	• Rapid progression (1–2 days) • Tick present
West Nile virus neuroinvasive disease	• Associated fever, meningitis, or encephalitis • Asymmetric weakness • *Cerebrospinal fluid:* Protein and cell count elevated
Critical illness neuropathy	• Sepsis and multiorgan failure >2 weeks • *EMG:* Axon loss

(EMG: electromyography; GBS: Guillain–Barré syndrome)

- *Miller Fisher variant (~5%):*
  - Classic triad of ophthalmoplegia, ataxia, and areflexia
  - May present as isolated oculomotor palsy
  - May progress to weakness of the limbs (Miller Fisher-Guillain-Barré overlap syndrome)
- *Bickerstaff's brainstem encephalitis (BBE):*
  - Similar to the Miller Fisher variant but with altered level of consciousness and long tract signs
- Pharyngeal-cervical-brachial
  - Arm weakness, dysphagia, and facial weakness
- *Pandysautonomia:*
  - Diarrhea, vomiting, dizziness, abdominal pain, ileus, orthostatic hypotension, urinary retention, bilateral tonic pupils, fluctuating heart rate and dysrhythmias, decreased sweating, salivation, and lacrimation.

It is not always possible to classify disease in one particular category.

Q2. What is pathophysiology of GBS?

Guillain-Barré syndrome (GBS) is an autoimmune response to an immune activating event, such as:
- *Campylobacter jejuni* enteritis (25–50%)
- Viral [e.g., Cytomegalovirus (CMV), Epstein-Barr virus (EBV), hepatitis A-E viruses, HIV, influenza, arboviruses (e.g., Zika and Chikungunya)]
- *Mycoplasma* infection
- Vaccination (e.g., influenza and rabies).

Precise interplay of host and infectious factor remains unclear but one of the above-mentioned events leads to autoantibody production. Autoantibodies affect peripheral nerves. Autonomic nerves are also sometimes affected.

In the case of GBS associated with *Campylobacter jejuni* infection, autoantibodies result from molecular mimicry [e.g., glycans expressed on bacterial lipooligosaccharides (LOS)].

There are two major distinct pathologies of immune injury:
1. The myelin sheath and related Schwann cell components are targeted in acute inflammatory demyelinating polyneuropathy.
2. Membranes on the nerve axon (the axolemma) are targeted in acute motor axonal neuropathy.

Guillain-Barré syndrome is mainly humorally mediated, rather than T-cell-mediated disorder, at least in progressive stage of nerve injury.

Immunobiology:
- *Antiganglioside antibodies:* It has been proposed that antiganglioside antibodies contribute to the immunopathogenesis of GBS and certain other inflammatory neuropathies. The mechanism by which antiganglioside antibodies production is triggered is not very well known. Antiganglioside antibodies bind to the nodal axolemma or the paranodal myelin, thus leading to axonal degeneration or demyelination. Four gangliosides—GM1, GD1a, GT1a, and GQ1b—described in GBS differ with regard to the number and position of their sialic acids, in which M, D, T, and Q represent mono-, di-, tri-, and quadri-sialosyl groups, respectively. IgG antiganglioside antibodies to GM1 and GD1a are more commonly associated with AMAN, AMSAN, and acute motor conduction block neuropathy, but not with AIDP[2,3] **(Table 2)**.

Molecular mimicry and cross-reactivity:
Campylobacter jejuni isolates from patients express lipo-oligosaccharides (LOS) that mimic the carbohydrates of gangliosides. The type of ganglioside mimicry in *C. jejuni* seems to determine the specificity of the antiganglioside antibodies and the associated variant of GBS. *C. jejuni* isolates from patients with pure motor or axonal GBS frequently express a GM1-like and GD1a-like LOS, whereas isolates from patients with ophthalmoplegia or Miller Fisher syndrome (MFS) usually express a GD3-like, GT1a-like, or GD1c-like LOS.

Complement activation:
Some antiganglioside antibodies are highly toxic for peripheral nerves. These antibodies cause complement activation and formation of membrane attack complex, which is characterized by a dramatic release of acetylcholine, resulting in a depletion of this neurotransmitter at the nerve terminals, and final blockade of nerve transmission and paralysis of the nerve-muscle preparation. The nerve

TABLE 2: Association of IgG antiganglioside antibodies with GBS subtypes.

Subtypes/variants	IgG antibodies against
Acute inflammatory demyelinating polyradiculoneuropathy (AIDP)	None
Acute motor axonal neuropathy (AMAN)	GM1 and GD1a
Acute motor and sensory axonal neuropathy (AMSAN)	GM1 and GD1a
• Acute motor conduction block neuropathy • Pharyngeal–cervical–brachial (PCB) variant	• GM1 and GD1a • GT1a (less frequently with GQ1b and GD1a)
Miller Fisher syndrome (MFS)[4]	GQ1b and GT1a
Acute ataxic neuropathy (without ophthalmoplegia)	GQ1b and GT1a
Pure sensory ataxic variant	GD1b (less frequently with GQ1b and GT1a)
Bickerstaff brainstem encephalitis (BBE)	GQ1b and GT1a

(GBS: Guillain–Barré syndrome; Ig: immunoglobulin)

terminal and perisynaptic Schwann cell are also destroyed. Antibodies to GM1 affect the sodium channels at the nodes of Ranvier of rabbit peripheral nerves.

In an excellent review, Yuki and colleagues have described the possible immunogenetic mechanism for development of GBS. They suggest that the GBS progresses through four phases—binding of autoantibodies to the myelin sheath antigens, leading to activation of complement system. This leads to the formation of membrane attack complex (MAC) on the surface of Schwann cells injuring the nerves. At the same time, there is initiation of vesicular vesicles. Macrophages then enter and remove the myelin debris. The axon is attacked simultaneously and injured through formation of MAC due to interaction between IgG anti-GM1 or anti-GD1a autoantibodies and the axolemma. This results in detachment of myelin in the paranodal regions resulting in failure of nerve conduction and muscle weakness. Macrophages later scavenge the axonal debris.

Q3. What is the clinical course of GBS and what are the clinical features?

Guillain–Barré syndrome (GBS) often occurs 2-4 weeks after a flu-like or diarrheal illness caused by a variety of infectious agents (e.g., *Campylobacter*, viral, or *Mycoplasma*). The illness is heralded by the presence of dysesthesias of the feet or hands, or both. The major feature is weakness that evolves rapidly (usually over days) and classically has been described as ascending from legs to arms and, in severe cases, to respiratory and bulbar muscles. Weakness may, however, start in the cranial nerves or arms and descend to the legs or start simultaneously in the arms and legs. Clinical deficit reaches peak at 2-4 weeks (usually 2 weeks). Progression of symptoms beyond 4 weeks but arresting within 8 weeks has been termed subacute inflammatory demyelinating polyneuropathy (SIDP), while progression beyond 2 months is designated chronic inflammatory demyelinating polyradiculoneuropathy (CIDP), a disorder with a natural history different from GBS. A small percentage of patients (2-5%) have recurrent GBS. The extent and distribution of weakness in GBS are variable. Within a few days, a patient may become quadriparetic and respirator dependent, or the illness may take a benign course and after progression for 3 weeks produce only mild weakness of the face and limbs.

Motor-sensory features:
- Bilateral, symmetrical limb weakness, typically ascending:
  - May initially only affect lower limbs
  - Usually starts distally, but can start more proximally
  - May have facial, oculomotor, or bulbar weakness, which might then extend to involve the limbs (Miller Fisher syndrome)
- *Areflexia:*
  - May initially be normal or even hyperreflexic.
- *Paresthesia:*
  - Sensory symptoms and signs are common
  - Usually milder than motor
  - 15% of GBS patients have no sensory symptoms (pure motor)
- *Muscular or radicular pain*:
  - Commonly back pain, but not always
  - May precede weakness in one-third cases

Other features:
- *Autonomic dysfunction:*
  - Diarrhea, vomiting, dizziness, abdominal pain, ileus, orthostatic hypotension, urinary retention, bilateral tonic pupils, fluctuating heart rate and dysrhythmias, decreased sweating, salivation, and lacrimation
- Respiratory failure (affects 20–30% of cases)
- Corneal ulceration (poor lid closure)

Q4. How do you investigate this case?

The diagnosis is largely based on clinical patterns. There are no diagnostic biomarkers available for most variants of the syndrome.

Cerebrospinal fluid (CSF) examination:

A lumbar puncture is performed primarily to rule out infectious processes. CSF examination shows cytoalbumino dissociation (increased CSF protein in the absence of increased WBCs) in approximately 50% of patients if done in 1st week of illness. Absence of cytoalbumino dissociation does not rule out GBS. 5% of GBS patients have a mild increase in CSF cell count (5–50 cells per μL).

Blood tests:
- High IgG
- Antiganglioside GM1 and GD1a antibodies (axonal forms)
- GQ1b antibodies (Miller Fisher variant)

Nerve conduction studies:

They are helpful in clinical practice, but are generally not essential for diagnosis of GBS. They are required for GBS classification. At least four motor nerves, three sensory nerves, F-waves, and H-reflexes should be assessed.
- *Acute inflammatory demyelinating polyneuropathy:*
  - Decreased motor nerve conduction velocity
  - Prolonged distal motor latency
  - Increased F-wave latency
  - Multifocal conduction blocks
  - Abnormal temporal dispersion of compound muscle action potentials (CMAPs)

- *Acute motor axonal neuropathy*
  - No features of demyelination
  - Decreased motor, sensory amplitudes, or both
  - One demyelinating feature in one nerve, if distal CMAP amplitude is <10% lower limit of normal, can be found
  - Distal CMAP amplitude <80% lower limit of normal in at least two nerves
  - Transient motor nerve conduction block might be present
- Abnormalities are most pronounced 2 weeks after start of weakness.

MRI spine:
Performed to exclude a high-cervical lesion.

Lung function tests:
- If forced vital capacity (FVC) <20 mL/kg transfer to ICU
- Intubate if FVC <15 mL/kg or negative inspiratory pressure < −25 cmH$_2$O

Screen for infection:
- Viral polymerase chain reaction (PCR)/antibodies
- Stool culture for *Campylobacter*
- *Mycoplasma* antibodies and chest X-ray (CXR).

Q5. How will you manage a patient with GBS?
Patients with GBS are in particular need of excellent multidisciplinary care to prevent and manage potentially fatal complications. Thus, patients need careful and regular monitoring of pulmonary function (at least vital capacity and respiratory frequency) and possible autonomic dysfunction (reflected in heart rate and blood pressure). The infections that can occur during the course of illness need to be prevented.

Q6. After 2 weeks in ICU, patient is still not generating enough tidal volume and has a very poor cough reflex. How will you continue to manage the ventilation now?
The development of respiratory compromise requiring mechanical ventilation is the most common fatal complication of GBS and occurs in up to 30% of patients.[5,6] Early identification of respiratory deterioration and transfer to critical care usually leads to a positive outcome. There are several prediction tools that are used to recognize the development of respiratory dysfunction. The Erasmus GBS Respiratory Insufficiency Score (EGRIS) is a point-based tool that can accurately predict the probability of development of respiratory failure in 90% of patients **(Table 3)**.

Pulmonary function tests are used by many studies as predictor for need for intubation. Most commonly used rule is 20-30-40 rule.[7]
- Forced vital capacity (FVC) <20 mL/kg
- Maximum inspiratory pressure <30 cmH$_2$O

TABLE 3: Erasmus GBS Respiratory Insufficiency Score (EGRIS).

Measure	Categories	Score
Days between onset of weakness and hospital admission	>7 days	0
	4–7 days	1
	≤3 days	2
Facial and/or bulbar weakness at hospital admission	Absence	0
	Presence	1
Medical Research Council (MRC) sum score at hospital admission	60–51	0
	50–41	1
	40–31	2
	30–21	3
	≤20	4
EGRIS		0–7

(GBS: Guillain–Barré syndrome)

- Maximum expiratory pressure <40 cmH$_2$O

The only bedside pulmonary function test which is useful is the FVC. Patients with an FVC <20 mL/kg are at risk for respiratory failure and should receive ICU-level monitoring. Intubation is typically required when the FVC falls below 10–15 mL/kg. However, the decision to intubate is a *clinical decision* based primarily on ability to protect the airway, work of breathing, vital signs, and overall appearance. For patients who are dyspneic but do not require intubation, consider giving a trial of bilevel positive airway pressure (BiPAP) or high-flow nasal cannula to see if this improves the patient's comfort and reduce the work of breathing.

Possible approach to ventilatory support in GBS:
Evaluate patient's work of breathing, ability to protect airway:
- No respiratory distress at rest, not tachypneic >> no ventilatory support needed
- Severe distress or other indication for intubation >> intubate
- Mild–moderate distress and no indication for intubation >> potential candidate for BiPAP or high-flow nasal cannula.

Tracheostomy:
Tracheostomy improves patient's comfort, resulting in minimal sedation; it reduces the risk of laryngeal and vocal cord damage; it enhances airway toilet; and it facilitates liberation from mechanical ventilation. The timing of tracheostomy is unclear and should be considered if mechanical ventilation is likely to exceed 2 weeks. Clinical clues that would suggest the need for tracheostomy include persisting neck and proximal arm weakness, severe autonomic instability, development of ventilator-associated pneumonia, or advanced age. Percutaneous dilatational

tracheostomy is preferred over the conventional surgical approach.[8]

Q7. What are specific therapy options available for GBS?

Immunotherapy: First studies which showed benefits of immunotherapy in Guillain-Barré syndrome (GBS) studied plasma exchange for immunotherapy. Plasma exchange was beneficial when applied within the first 4 weeks of onset, but the largest effect was seen when started early (within the first 2 weeks). Later, intravenous immunoglobulin (IVIg) was studied for treatment of GBS. Studies showed that IVIg was equally effective as plasma exchange.[2,9,10]

Immunotherapy, either plasma exchange or IV immunoglobulin, is first-line option:
- Plasma exchange:
  - Within the first 4 (preferably 2) weeks from onset in GBS patients who are unable to walk unaided
  - GBS patients who are still able to walk might improve more rapidly after 2 plasma exchange sessions
  - 5 plasma exchanges of 2–3 L (50 mL/kg) over 2 weeks
  - Use albumin as replacement fluid
- Intravenous immunoglobulin:
  - Start within the first 2 weeks after onset of weakness in patients unable to walk unaided
  - 0.4 g/kg/day for 5 doses over 5 days
  - Alternative is (2 g/kg bodyweight) given in 2 days (1 g/kg per day) but may have more side effects and children with this regimen have higher rates of treatment-related fluctuations (TRFs)
  - More convenient, less side effects, but more expensive than plasma exchange
- *Treatment-related fluctuations:*[3,9]
  - TRFs refer to deteriorations after initial improvement or stabilization.
  - TRFs affect 10% patients and usually occur within the first 8 weeks after start of treatment.
  - Repeated treatment with IVIg is indicated (2 g IVIg/kg in 2–5 days)
  - Repeat treatment of TRFs with IVIg, it is not proven in RCTs but supported by observational studies.[3,9]

There is no evidence of additional benefit for both IVIg and plasma exchange as co-therapy.[9] There is no role of steroids for treatment of GBS.[11,12]

Q8. What are other adjuvant and emerging therapies for treatment of GBS?

Despite plasmapheresis and immunoglobulin therapy, many patients with Guillain-Barré syndrome (GBS) still have an incomplete recovery, thus various potential therapeutic targets for immune therapy have been considered such as anti-B-cell therapy, anticomplement therapy, and anticytokine therapy. These therapies are being tested in diverse animal and human models.[13-16]

Newly developed biological medications like eculizumab have displayed considerable potency.[13]

Severity and progression of GBS correlate with nutritional factors such as vitamin deficiencies and folate levels. Therefore, neurotrophic therapies, including vitamin supplementation, might benefit GBS outcomes.[14,15]

Despite some promising results in animal and human models, there is not much evidence to support use of interferon beta-1a (IFN-β1a), brain-derived neurotrophic factor (BDNF), CSF filtration with PE, *Tripterygium* polyglycoside, and eculizumab in treating GBS.[17]

Supportive care:
- Assess for signs of autonomic dysfunction, e.g., tachycardia, urinary retention, postural hypotension, sweating, or ileus. Management of cardiovascular instability may require anticholinergics (for bradycardia), beta-blockers (for tachycardia and hypertension), or vasopressors (for hypotension). There have been reports of patient requiring temporary or permanent pacemaker for severe bradycardia or asystole.[18]
- Assessment for ability to swallow and nasogastric feeding if bulbar function is poor.
- *Venous thromboembolism (VTE) prophylaxis:* Sequential compression devices or low-molecular weight heparin.
- Eye care if inadequate eye closure due to bulbar weakness.
- Patients may develop severe neuropathic pain. Consider amitriptyline or gabapentin.
- Cognitive behavior therapies, and psychological support for GBS-related mental status alteration, such as vivid dreams, hallucinations, and psychosis.[19]
- Guillain-Barré syndrome is associated with long-term disability. Early rehabilitative intervention ensures medical stability and prevents long-term complications. Rehabilitative efforts can be started since acute phase of illness.

Q9. How do you prognosticate in a patient with GBS?

The prognosis of GBS is difficult to predict in individual patients because of the substantial variation in outcome. Advanced age, however, is generally reported to be indicative of a worse prognosis. Peroneal nerve conduction block and age above 40 years were independent predictors of disability at 6 months. Typical course of illness in patients who recover to walk unassisted is 3 months and full recovery in 6 months; however, there is permanent disability in many cases.[20]

The EGOS score (Erasmus GBS outcome scale)[5,6] can be used 2 weeks after admission to predict the ability of the patient to walk at 6 months, and is based on:
- Age >40 years

- Preceding *Campylobacter* infection or diarrheal illness (in the past 4 weeks) high disability at nadir.

The mEGOS score (Modified Erasmus GBS Outcome Scale)[21,22] can be used at 1 week and replaces disability with the Medical Research Council (MRC) Scale for Muscle Strength score.

3–7% mortality in GBS is from medical complications that occur in the hospital. Death is usually due to respiratory failure or complications and autonomic complications. Though many patients recover from GBS, up to 20% of patients are still significantly disabled at 6 months and 15% still have significant functional disability at 1 year. Most patients have residual pain and fatigue due to persistent axonal loss.[2,3,6,23,24]

After 2 weeks, the patient was not generating enough tidal volume, and his cough reflex was weak, so elective tracheostomy was done. The patient was initiated on home BiPAP with tracheostomy and discharged to home. Gradually after 4 months, the cough reflex improved. Physiotherapy continued, and power also improved gradually.

REFERENCES

1. Fokke C, van den Berg B, Drenthen J. Diagnosis of Guillain-Barré syndrome and validation of Brighton criteria. Brain. 2014;137(Pt 1):33-43.
2. Yuki N, Hartung HP. Guillain-Barré syndrome. New Engl J Med. 2012;366(24):2294-304.
3. van Doorn PA, Ruts L, Jacobs BC. Clinical features, pathogenesis, and treatment of Guillain-Barré syndrome. Lancet Neurol. 2008;7:939-50.
4. Wakerley BR, Uncini A, Yuki N. GBS Classification Group. Guillain-Barré and Miller Fisher syndromes—new diagnostic classification. Nat Rev Neurol. 2014;10:537-44.
5. Rajabally YA, Uncini A. Outcome and its predictors in Guillain-Barre syndrome. J Neurol Neurosurg Psychiatry. 2012;83:711-8.
6. Walgaard C, Lingsma HF, Ruts L. Prediction of respiratory insufficiency in Guillain-Barré syndrome. Ann Neurol. 2010;67:781-7.
7. Lawn ND, Fletcher DD, Henderson RD. Anticipating mechanical ventilation in Guillain-Barre syndrome. Arch Neurol. 2001;58:893-8.
8. Higgins KM, Punthakee X. Meta-analysis comparison of open versus percutaneous tracheostomy. Laryngoscope. 2007;117:447-54.
9. Hughes RA, Swan AV, van Doorn PA. Intravenous immunoglobulin for Guillain-Barré syndrome. Cochrane Database Syst Rev. 2004;(1):CD002063.
10. Raphaël JC, Chevret S, Hughes RA. Plasma exchange for Guillain-Barré syndrome. Cochrane Database Syst Rev. 2017;(2):CD001798.
11. Hughes RA, Swan AV, van Koningsveld R, van Doorn PA. Corticosteroids for Guillain-Barré syndrome. Cochrane Database Syst Rev. 2016;(10):CD001446.
12. Lehmann HC, Hartung HP, Hetzel GR, Stüve O, Kieseier BC. Plasma exchange in neuroimmunological disorders: part 2. Treatment of neuromuscular disorders. Arch Neurol. 2006;63:1066-71.
13. Misawa S, Kuwabara S, Sato Y, Yamaguchi N, Nagashima K, Katayama K, et al. Safety and efficacy of eculizumab in Guillain-Barre syndrome: a multicentre, double-blind, randomised phase 2 trial. Lancet Neurol. 2018;17:519-29.
14. Staff NP, Windebank AJ. Peripheral neuropathy due to vitamin deficiency, toxins, and medications. Continuum. 2014;20:1293-306.
15. Gao Y, Zhang HL, Xin M, Wang D, Zheng N, Wang S, et al. Serum folate correlates with severity of Guillain-Barre syndrome and predicts disease progression. Biomed Res Int. 2018;2018:5703279.
16. Soltani ZE, Rahman F, Rezaei N. Autoimmunity and cytokines in Guillain-Barre syndrome revisited: review of pathomechanisms with an eye on therapeutic options. Eur Cytokine Netw. 2019;30:1-14.
17. Doets AY, Hughes RAC, Brassington R, Hadden RDM, Pritchard J. Pharmacological treatment other than corticosteroids, intravenous immunoglobulin and plasma exchange for Guillain-Barre syndrome. Cochr Database Syst Rev. 2020;2020(1):CD008630.
18. Patel MB, Goyal SK, Punnam SR, Pandya K, Khetarpal V, Thakur RK. Guillain-Barre syndrome with asystole requiring permanent pacemaker: a case report. J Med Case Reports. 2009;3:5.
19. Cochen V, Arnulf I, Demeret S, Neulat ML, Gourlet V, Drouot X, et al. Vivid dreams, hallucinations, psychosis and REM sleep in Guillain-Barré syndrome. Brain. Brain. 2005;128(Pt 11):2535-45.
20. Walgaard C, Lingsma HF, Ruts L, van Doorn PA. Early recognition of poor prognosis in Guillain-Barré syndrome. Neurology. 2011;76:968-75.
21. González-Suárez I, Sanz-Gallego I, Rodríguez de Rivera FJ, Arpa J. Guillain Barre Syndrome: Natural history and prognostic factors: a retrospective review of 106 cases. BMC Neurol. 2013;13:95.
22. Bella I, Chad D. Guillain-Barré Syndrome. In: Richard I, James R (Eds). Irwin and Rippe's Intensive Care Medicine, 7th edition. Philadelphia: Lippincott Williams & Wilkins; 2011. pp. 1798-805.
23. Willison HJ, Jacobs BC, van Doorn PA. Guillain-Barré syndrome. Lancet. 2016;388(10045):717-27.
24. Joy V, Yuki N. How Should Guillain Barre Syndrome be managed in the ICU? In: Deutschman CS, Neligan JP (Eds). Evidence-Based Practice of Critical Care, 2nd edition. Canada: Elsevier; 2016. Chapter 66: p. 475.

CHAPTER 23

Approach to a Patient with Unknown Poisoning

Bindu M, Rahul Anil Pandit

CASE STUDY

A 63-year-old male, known case of depression on treatment, was found unconscious on the bathroom floor. He was recently complaining that he was feeling low and was also talking of futility of living further. He was prescribed Escitalopram and Amitriptyline; however, he was not taking medications for the last few days. On arrival to the intensive care unit (ICU), he was unconscious, hyperthermic, and had a history of an episode of vomiting. In the ICU, the patient was looking dehydrated, was febrile (103°C), tachycardic (heart rate 130/minute), and hypertensive (BP 170/110 mm Hg). His both pupils were dilated and sluggishly reacting to light, and the bowel sounds were sluggish.

Q1. How do we approach this patient?

Patients with exposure to poison may present with a spectrum of various clinical signs, symptoms, and problems. There are, however, general principles that may be employed as a framework on which approach to most poisonings. These should be employed when managing adverse effects from poisoning by unknown substances. Thorough general supportive care is the most important approach in caring for most poisoned patients. Critical step is recognition that poison exposure occurred. "Airway, breathing, circulation, disability, dextrose, exposure, and ECG" comprise the general "A, B, C, D, D, E, E" mantra of poison management.[1]

Six steps in the management in critical care management of unknown poisoning:
1. Initial assessment and stabilization
2. History and physical examination
3. Laboratory and ECG
4. Decontamination
5. Antidote administration
6. Enhanced elimination.[1]

Initial assessment and stabilization:
According to the patient's condition, resuscitation using basic life support (BLS) or advanced cardiac life support (ACLS) should be given. "Airway, Breathing, Circulation, Disability, Dextrose, Exposure, ECG" comprise the general "A, B, C, D, D, E, E" mantra of poison management.

Patients who have consumed poison can deteriorate rapidly. Frequent assessment of their ability to protect their airway and breathing is necessary. Rapid-sequence intubation or drug-assisted intubation (DAI) should be used on comatose or obtunded patients.

Fluid resuscitation of the poisoned patient must be individualized. Initial resuscitation includes the administration of intravenous crystalloid fluid, whenever indicated; vasopressor infusion should be started as early as possible in the course of the resuscitation. In a distributive shock or cardiogenic shock, administration of vasopressors or inotropes (noradrenaline) is more appropriate than simply administering fluids. Bedside sonography is a useful tool to determine volume responsiveness and to estimate cardiac contractility to further guide resuscitation. Hence, the choice of vasopressor must be made on patient profile and clinical grounds. Nonadrenergic vasoactive drugs are an effective therapy for shock caused by β-adrenergic blocking agents and calcium channel antagonists.[2]

When standard therapy fails to relieve the symptoms of poisoned individuals in refractory shock, extracorporeal membrane oxygenation (ECMO) is recommended. When a patient is poisoned, ECMO acts as a stopgap measure until the poisons are broken down or cleared, at which point the patient should resume normal circulatory function. Although ECMO is more expensive and has side effects, new technological advancements have made it a more viable option for patients with refractory shock.

Prolonged cardiopulmonary resuscitation (CPR), heroic treatments such as cardiopulmonary bypass and ECMO, and antidotes (such as a digoxin fragment antibody, bicarbonate, and high-dose insulin) should all be taken into consideration because patients are frequently young and have the ability to fully recover if they are maintained through this time.[3]

History and physical examination:
Patient may be an unreliable source of information about the event. Relatives, friends and roommates, and previous medical records may be able to provide useful information of all ailments, medical history, medication history, and other medications or substances the patient had access to.

A good approach will include:
- Identify the reason of exposure (i.e., intentional, unintentional, and misadventure)
- The type of substance involved (i.e., prescription, over-the-counter, herbal, and illicit drug), the formulation (i.e., immediate *vs.* sustained release)
- The dose of the substance
- The amount of substance involved
- The route of exposure (i.e., ingestion, inhalation, intravenous, and dermal)
- The time of exposure (hours since exposure, acute *vs.* chronic)
- Any potential coingestion
- The severity of exposure.

Examining vital signs including temperature, abnormal pupil size, abnormal eye movements, the condition and color of the skin and mucous membranes, the presence or absence of bowel noises, and deep tendon reflexes is integral part of a physical examination.[1]

The constellation of symptoms and indications will aid the clinician in identifying potential toxidromes; therefore, abnormalities of each system should be documented. A toxidrome is a collection of warning signs and symptoms that herald toxicity **(Table 1)**.

There are five well-described toxidromes (Table 2):
1. *Adrenergic (sympathomimetic):* Sympathomimetic agents capable of alpha- and/or beta-adrenergic agonism, for example, cocaine, amphetamines, theophylline, caffeine, pseudoephedrine, ephedrine, epinephrine, norepinephrine, and methylenedioxymethamphetamine (ecstasy).
2. *Anticholinergic:* Cholinergic receptor blockers, for example, atropine, scopolamine, antihistamines, phenothiazines, cyclic antidepressants, and cyclobenzaprine.
3. *Cholinergic:* Substances that affect cholinergic receptors, for example, organophosphate pesticides and nerve agents, physostigmine, rivastigmine, and nicotine.
4. *Opioid:* Substances that afflict opioid receptors, for example, heroin, morphine, hydromorphone, methadone, diphenoxylate, clonidine, and tramadol.
5. *Sedative–hypnotic:* Substances that increase gamma-aminobutyric acid (GABA) activity, for example, benzodiazepines, barbiturates, alcohols, gamma-hydroxybutyrate (GHB), and zolpidem.[4]

TABLE 1: Vital signs and symptoms.

Vital signs	Symptoms
Pulse	Tachycardia, bradycardia, and normal
Blood pressure	Hypertension and hypotension
Temperature	Hypothermia/hyperthermia
Reflexes	Hyperreflexia/hyporeflexia/normal
Eyes	Icterus and nystagmus
Pupils	Miosis and mydriasis
Lungs	Bradypnea, tachypnea, rhonchi, and crepitations
Skin and mucous membrane	Hot, moist, red, pale, and dry
Bowel sounds	Present/absent/increased/decreased

Q2. What is the role of ECG in poisoning?
The ECG is important in the assessment and management of poisoned patients for screening, diagnosis, prognosis, monitoring progression to guide management and disposition.
- Rate and rhythm
- PR interval—is there any degree of heart block?
- Determine QRS duration in lead II. The studies examining QRS duration in tricyclic antidepressant intoxication use manual measurements to measure QRS in limb lead II.
- *Right axis deviation of the QRS:* A large terminal R wave in AVR or increased R/S ratio indicates slow rightward conduction and is characteristic of fast sodium channel blockade. If not pathological, it remains static in appearance and severity throughout the course of the poisoning. Comparison with prepoisoning ECGs is useful.
- *Determine QT interval:* Prolonged QT interval predisposes to the development of Torsade de pointe, a polymorphic ventricular tachycardia. Torsade des pointes is more likely to occur where there is coexisting bradycardia. The arrhythmogenic risk for drug-induced QT prolongation is accurately predicted by the "QT nomogram" which plots QT versus heart rate.
- Evidence of increased cardiac ectopy or automaticity
- Evidence of myocardial ischemia.[2]

Laboratory tests:
History may be inaccurate and hence the following laboratory tests should usually be obtained: complete blood count, renal function tests, liver function test, serum lactate, arterial blood gas, urine pregnancy test in all women of childbearing age, and a urine toxin screen (to support a history of cocaine, opiate, or benzodiazepine use).

The following lethal ingestions with specific therapies should always be ruled out: acetaminophen (serum level),

TABLE 2: Vital signs in various toxidromes.

Group	BP	P	R	T	Mental status	Pupil size	Peristalsis	Diaphoresis	Other
						Vital signs			
Anticholinergics	—/↑	↑	±	↑	Delirium	↑	↓	↓	Dry mucous membranes, flush, urinary retention
Cholinergic	±	±	—/↑	—	Normal to depressed	±	↑	↑	Salivation, lacrimation, urination, diarrhea, bronchorrhea, fasciculations, paralysis
Ethanol or sedative hypnotics	↓	↓	↓	—/↓	Depressed	±	↓	—	Hyporeflexia, ataxia
Opioids	↓	↓	↓	↓	Depressed	↓	↓	—	Hyporeflexia
Sympathomimetics	↑	↑	↑	↑	Agitated	↑	—/↑	↑	Tremor, seizures
Withdrawal from ethanol or sedative hypnotics	↑	↑	↑	↑	Agitated, disoriented, hallucinations	↑	↑	↑	Tremor, seizures
Withdrawal from opioids	↑	↑	—	—	Normal, anxious	↑	↑	↑	Vomiting, rhinorrhea, piloerection, diarrhea, and yawning

tricyclic antidepressants (EKG), and salicylates (serum level). Serum level of digoxin, lithium, theophylline, phenytoin, and iron should be obtained if the patient is known to take or have immediate access to these medicines. Management should be guided by a careful history, clinical findings, and identification of a toxidrome. It should not be guided by drug toxicology screening results.

The three gaps to look for are (1) the anion gap, (2) the osmolal gap, and (3) the oxygen saturation gap.

1. Anion gap elevations may indicate the ingestion of toxins such as ethylene glycol, methanol, or salicylates (**Box 1**).

   Anion gap = $[Na^+] - ([Cl^-] + [HCO_3^-])$

2. Osmolal gap elevations may be present following toxic ingestions of alcohols. The serum osmolal gap is the difference between the measured and calculated serum osmolality (**Table 3**).

   Osm calculated = $2[Na^+] + [Urea]/2.8 + [Glucose]/18 + [Ethanol]/4.6$

   Where $[Na^+]$ is in mmol/L and [Urea], [Glucose], and [Ethanol] are in mg/dL.

3. The term "oxygen saturation gap" refers to disparities between the oxyhemoglobin percentage (SaO_2) as measured by co-oximetry and the oxyhemoglobin percentage (SpO_2) as measured by pulse oximetry or inferred from arterial oxygen tension (PaO_2). An oxygen saturation gap may be a sign of methemoglobinemia, acquired hemoglobinopathy, or poisoning from carbon monoxide (CO), cyanide, or hydrogen sulfide. A co-oximeter, which can measure the quantities of oxyhemoglobin, deoxyhemoglobin, methemoglobin, and carboxyhemoglobin in the specimen, must analyze arterial blood if these toxins are suspected.[5]

BOX 1: Toxicological causes of elevated anion gap.

- Salicylates
- Ethylene glycol
- Methanol
- Paraldehyde
- Isoniazid
- Iron

Toxicological cause of low anion gap:
- Lithium

TABLE 3: Osmolal and anion gap.

Elevated osmolal gap + normal anion gap	Elevated osmolal gap + elevated anion gap
Isopropanol	Methanol
Acetone	Ethylene glycol
Mannitol	Formaldehyde
Diethyl ether	Paraldehyde

*Specific treatment strategies (**Table 4**):*
Special therapies:
Intravenous lipid emulsion (e.g., lipid parenteral nutrition, 20% lipid) in overdoses with lipophilic drugs (e.g., bupivacaine, verapamil, chlorpromazine, and clomipramine). It is theorized that the intravenous lipid sequesters toxins from physiologic binding sites.

Dose: 1.5 mL/kg bolus of 20% lipid followed by a 0.25 mL/kg/min infusion until hemodynamic stability is achieved.

TABLE 4: Specific treatment strategies.

Toxin	Antidotes
Paracetamol	N-acetylcysteine
Beta-blockers	Atropine
Calcium blockers	Glucagon/high-dose insulin euglycemia/intralipid/ECMO
Carbon monoxide	Oxygen hyperbaric/100%
Organophosphorus poisoning	Atropine/pralidoxime
Cyanide	Sodium nitroprusside
Digoxin	Digoxin specific antibodies
Ethylene glycol	Fomepizole and ethanol
Methanol	Fomepizole, ethanol
Iron	Desferrioxamine
Methemoglobinemia	Methylene blue
Opioids	Naloxone
Sulfonylureas	Octreotide/dextrose
Tricyclic antidepressants	Sodium bicarbonate/intralipid

(ECMO: extracorporeal membrane oxygenation)

The American Society of Anesthesiology and the American Heart Association now recommend lipid infusion as a therapy in local anesthetic toxicity. There are multiple reports of lipid emulsion therapy (LET) reversing the toxicity of calcium channel antagonists, tricyclic antidepressants, benzodiazepines, anticonvulsants, and β-adrenergic blocking agents.[2,5]

Glucagon, the peptide hormone that is produced by alpha cells of the pancreas, stimulates adenyl cyclase, which in turn increases intracellular cyclic adenosine monophosphate (cAMP) through a nonadrenergic mechanism. This increase in cAMP causes an increase in intracellular calcium, which leads to positive chronotropic and inotropic actions.

High-dose insulin euglycemia (HIE) therapy is used to treat β-adrenergic blocking agents and calcium channel antagonists toxicity. The pathophysiology of calcium channel antagonist toxicity is decrease in insulin release from pancreatic β-cells causing insulin resistance in the myocardium and changes in myocyte metabolism from fatty acids to carbohydrates. High-dose insulin euglycemia therapy improves myocyte use of carbohydrates as an energy source and, therefore, increases cardiac contractility and improves perfusion.[2]

Gastric decontamination:
There are two ways to prevent medications from being absorbed in the gastrointestinal (GI) tract, activated charcoal, and whole-bowel irrigation (WBI). Due to their lack of efficacy and interference with enterally administered antidotes, induced emesis and cathartics are not advised. Only use gastric lavage if patient has taken substantial amount of sustained release drugs.

BOX 2: Indications for activated charcoal.
- Carbamazepine
- Dapsone
- Phenobarbital
- Quinine
- Theophylline

BOX 3: Indications whole-bowel irrigation.
- Iron poisoning
- Retained illicit drug packets
- Lithium poisoning
- Sustained release/enteric-coated medication toxicity

Activated charcoal:
The efficacy of activated charcoal is greatest when given within 1 hour of ingestion and is generally ineffective by 4 hours postingestion. Alcohols, iron, and lithium are examples of substances that activated charcoal cannot effectively adsorb. For adults and adolescents, a single dose of 1 g/kg of activated charcoal is advised. Unprotected airways and ingestion of a hydrocarbon are contraindications. In the case of substantial GI pathology or recent GI surgery, caution should be exercised. Repeated enteral administration of activated charcoal is known as multiple-dose activated charcoal (MDAC), which may aid in the removal of some toxins. However, there is little proof of effectiveness. There are many different dosage plans, but a common plan would start with a 1 g/kg loading dose and then provide 0.5 g/kg every 2–4 hours for at least three doses. MDAC should not be administered alongside cathartics (**Box 2**).

Whole-bowel irrigation:
Enterally delivering large amounts of an osmotically balanced polyethylene glycol electrolyte solution to induce diarrhea and hasten the outflow of unabsorbed toxins from the GI tract is known as WBI. The optimum way to deliver fluid during WBI is by a nasogastric tube, and the suggested dosage is 1,500–2,000 mL/h of enterally supplied fluid, sustained until the rectal effluent is clear. Unprotected airways, intestinal obstruction or perforation, ileus, substantial GI hemorrhage, toxic colitis, uncontrollable vomiting, and hemodynamic instability are examples of contraindications (**Box 3**).

Enhancing drug elimination can be done by urine alkalinization, hemodialysis, and hemoperfusion.

Urine alkalinization is a method of enhancing the renal elimination of certain poisons by increasing urine pH to levels ≥7.5 (e.g., pH = 8.0) through the administration of

BOX 4: Potential indications for urine alkalinization.
- Salicylates
- 2,4-D herbicide
- Fluoride
- Diflunisal

BOX 5: Toxins removed by hemodialysis.
- Salicylates
- Lithium
- Methanol
- Ethylene glycol
- Isopropanol
- Calcium-channel blockers
- Beta-blockers

BOX 6: Indication for hemoperfusion.
- Barbiturates
- Carbamazepine
- Theophylline
- Valproic acid

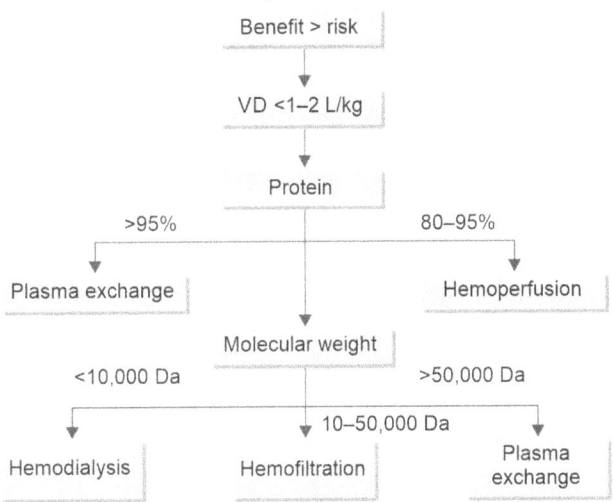

Flowchart 1: Criteria to go in for extracorporeal support.

intravenous (IV) sodium bicarbonate (e.g., 1-2 mEq/kg IV during 3-4 hours) **(Box 4)**.

To treat toxicity that poses a life-threatening risk, extracorporeal toxin removal techniques such as hemoperfusion and hemodialysis may be necessary. Clinical worsening despite rigorous alternative therapy, impairment of normal toxin elimination capacity (such as liver or renal failure), and severe medication toxicity are all general criteria for use. Extracorporeal procedures can also eliminate toxins from the body more quickly than conventional methods. When hemodialysis or hemoperfusion is being considered, a prompt consultation with a nephrologist and a medical toxicologist should be obtained **(Boxes 5 and 6)**.[5]

Risk benefit of extracorporeal support should be assessed **(Flowchart 1)**. If risk is more than benefit or if other alternative therapy is available or volume of distribution of the drug is more than 1-2 L/kg then extracorporeal therapy should not be considered.[2]

Ancillary support:
Patients who are poisoned and are critically unwell have a higher risk of GI hemorrhage. By 18 hours after being admitted to the ICU, 75% of poisoned patients exhibit endoscopic signs of stomach mucosal injury, with 5% of patients experiencing overt bleeding. Proton-pump inhibitors or histamine-2 receptor antagonists are the best medications to utilize to prevent gastrointestinal bleeding after ICU admission.

If a poisoning has a protracted duration that necessitates bed rest, poisoned ICU patients are at risk for venous thromboembolic illness. Despite receiving prophylaxis, deep vein thrombosis (DVT) is detected by ultrasonography in about 33% of ICU patients. According to meta-analyses, the incidence of DVT is reduced by at least 50% when heparin or pneumatic compression stockings are used. If a longer stay is anticipated, DVT prophylaxis should start as soon as the patient is brought to the ICU. This can be done by using compression devices, unfractionated heparin, or low-molecular weight heparin.

Meeting the patient's dietary needs without overfeeding is the aim of nutritional support. Overfeeding should be avoided since too many carbohydrates can increase the generation of carbon dioxide. Parenteral feedings are preferred to enteral feedings because they assist preserve the integrity of the gut's mucosal barrier.[4,6]

REFERENCES

1. Hoffman RJ, Punja M. Chapter 40. Approach to Poisoning. In: Farcy DA, Chiu WC, Flaxman A, Marshall JP (Eds). Critical Care Emergency Medicine. New York: McGraw Hill; 2012.
2. Panchal AR, Bartos JA, Cabañas JG, Donnino MW, Drennan IR, Hirsch KG, et al. Part 3: Adult Basic and Advanced Life Support: 2020 American Heart Association Guidelines for Cardiopulmonary Resuscitation and Emergency Cardiovascular Care. Circulation. 2020;142:S366-468.
3. Little M. Emergency management and resuscitation of poisoned patients: perspectives from "down under". Scand J Trauma Resusc Emerg Med. 2009;17:36.
4. Chandran J, Krishna B. Initial Management of Poisoned Patient. Indian J Crit Care Med. 2019;23(Suppl 4):S234-40.
5. Kollef MH. Toxicology. In: Mecham JL, Brody SL (Eds). Washington Manual, 3rd edition. Gurgaon: Wolters Kluwer India; 2018.
6. Bersten AD, Handy JM. Poisoning and drug intoxication. In: Murfin BR, Barrett NA (Eds). Oh's Intensive Care Manual, 8th edition. Amsterdam: Elsevier; 2018.

CHAPTER 24

Organophosphorus Poisoning

JV Peter, Binila Chacko

CASE STUDY

A 32-year-old female is brought to the emergency department (ED) by relatives after being found unconscious at home. On examination, she is unconscious with saliva drooling from the angle of the mouth. On examination, heart rate is 62/min, systolic blood pressure (BP) is 60 mm Hg, and respiratory rate is 32/min with shallow breathing; bilateral crepitations are heard over both lung fields. Pupils are constricted, equal, and reacting to light. The Glasgow Coma Scale (GCS) is 4/15. There is a strong pungent garlic odor. Relatives found an empty bottle of chlorpyrifos in the bedroom.

Q1. How will you approach this case? What are the initial management strategies? Should we use atropine or glycopyrrolate?

Initial management

This patient has been brought to the ED with cholinergic toxidrome[1] in a cholinergic crisis. The classical presentation of the cholinergic toxidrome is described in the acronym SLUDGE, which includes salivation, lacrimation, urination, defecation, gastrointestinal dysfunction, and emesis.[1,2] The presence of an empty bottle of chlorpyrifos in the bedroom corroborates with the clinical picture of acute organophosphorus poisoning, although at times relatives bring the first bottle of pesticide that they find, a common phenomenon in India. It is important to send a blood sample for butyrylcholinesterase, pseudocholinesterase, or red cell cholinesterase activity. Suppression of cholinesterase activity to <25% is taken as supportive evidence of significant poisoning with an organophosphorus or carbamate compound.[3]

Immediate management involves the general approach to the management of any critically ill patient, namely airway, breathing, circulation, disability, exposure (ABCDE) approach.[4] Three aspects of the respiratory component warrant discussion in acute organophosphorus poisoning—airway issues, pacemaker problems, and problems with the gas exchange.[5] The airway issues in acute organophosphorus poisoning include the inability to protect the airway and airway obstruction. Inability to protect the airway may be due to a reduced conscious state as a result of the toxin per se, coingestion of other neurodepressive agents such as alcohol, or secondary injury to the brain as a result of fall, hypoxia, hypotension, or metabolic effects of the toxin on the central nervous system (CNS). Intrinsic airway obstruction can be direct, due to intraluminal contents such as vomitus, secretions, or foreign body,[6] oral structures (tongue falling back), laryngeal edema (traumatic intubation), or laryngeal muscle dysfunction.[7] Extrinsic airway obstruction can be direct as a result of trauma to the neck as a result of fall (uncommon) or indirect (iatrogenic) as in insertion of central venous access (uncommon). Airway obstruction may be suspected if there is stridor or hoarseness of voice, gurgling respirations, reduced consciousness level, or neck swelling or trauma **(Table 1)**.

TABLE 1: Reasons for airway obstruction in the setting of organophosphorus poisoning.

Inability to protect the airway due to reduced consciousness	Airway obstruction	
	Intrinsic causes	*Extrinsic causes*
Direct CNS depression due to OP	Excessive oral secretions	Direct (trauma)
Coingestion of CNS depressants (alcohol, hypnotics)	Vomiting, oral bleeding	Indirect (subcutaneous emphysema)*
Seizures	Tongue falling back (due to low GCS)	
Cortical dysfunction (secondary to hypoxia, hypotension)	Laryngeal edema and dysfunction	
Head injury (secondary to fall)		

*Post insertion of a central line.
(CNS: central nervous system; GCS: Glasgow Coma Scale; OP: organophosphorus compound)

Respiratory failure, both type I and type II, may be observed in acute organophosphorus poisoning. Type I respiratory failure is contributed by ventilation–perfusion (V/Q) mismatch as a result of shunting or dead space, while type II respiratory failure, which is more often seen in clinical practice in organophosphorus poisoning, is contributed by central hypoventilation due to central effects of the poison, neuromuscular weakness, and increased work of breathing with resultant fatigue due to increase in airway resistance and reduction in lung compliance.

In this patient who presented with a low GCS, the airway is likely to be compromised and hence it is important to take control of the airway. Respiratory support is also required since the patient has manifested rapid, shallow breathing suggesting respiratory failure. An arterial blood gas (ABG) estimation should be performed to ascertain the nature and severity of respiratory failure while the patient is being stabilized. Supplemental oxygen should be started if there is evidence of hypoxia.

The airway can be kept open by clearing the secretions by suctioning and with the triple maneuver[8] that involves jaw thrust, head tilt, and chin lift. While this is being done, the patient should be atropinized (see below). Recent evidence suggests that administration of atropine need not be withheld till hypoxia is corrected.[9] Delay in administering atropine may further deteriorate respiratory status. Atropine may help by drying up respiratory secretions, clearing the airway, improving the GCS by its central effects on the brain, and improving the respiratory function by partially reversing neuromuscular blockade.[10] If the airway is still compromised despite these measures, an oral or nasopharyngeal airway may be introduced while preparing the patient for intubation and ventilation. The patient is preoxygenated with bag and mask ventilation and an assessment of the anticipated difficulty of the airway is undertaken simultaneously.[11] If a difficult airway is anticipated, having an anesthetist standing by is recommended along with the availability of a difficult airway cart. Succinylcholine should be avoided for neuromuscular blockade for intubation since clearance of this drug may be delayed due to acetylcholinesterase inhibition by the organophosphorus compound.[12]

The circulatory component of resuscitation is managed by fluid resuscitation, rapid atropinization, preferably within 30 minutes,[13] and judicious use of vasoactive agents if the patient has persistent hypotension. It is recommended that atropine is started at an initial dose of 2 mg bolus with a doubling of atropine doses every 2-5 minutes till atropinization.[13] Mandatory atropine targets that should be achieved are heart rate >100/min, systolic BP >90 mm Hg, and clear lung fields.[14] The heart rate targets may be lowered on subsequent days. Since a low heart rate, low blood pressure, and flooded lungs are potentially life-threatening, rapid atropinization is recommended. Other targets of atropinization that are monitored in clinical practice include pupil size (midposition pupils) and bowel sounds (which should just be present). Once atropinization is achieved, the target heart rate and BP may be maintained with atropine infusion. There is some evidence that atropine administration as an infusion may be preferred over bolus doses.[15]

The choice of the anticholinergic agent is based on several factors. Since atropine crosses the blood-brain barrier, it may be preferred in patients who manifest CNS effects (e.g., drowsiness, coma) of the organophosphorus compound;[2] however, some patients may develop atropine psychoses.[16] In these patients, glycopyrrolate may be used instead of atropine. In the one study that compared atropine with glycopyrrolate, there was no distinct advantage of one over the other.[17] In one anecdotal case report, scopolamine, an anticholinergic with high blood-brain penetration, reversed the central neurological effects of organophosphorus.[18]

Q2. What is the role of gastric lavage and activated charcoal?

The role of gastric lavage and activated charcoal warrant discussion. Studies on gastric lavage are limited. The position paper on gastric lavage suggests that the risk and harm may outweigh the benefits.[19] In particular, in organophosphorus poisoning where gastric emptying may be accentuated by the poison, the expected return of the poison on lavage is likely to be small, particularly if the time interval elapsed between ingestion and lavage exceeds 2 hours. Gastric lavage should also not be attempted in patients with reduced GCS whose airway is not protected. Although there are a few studies in Chinese that suggest potential benefit, there are methodological weaknesses that limit its clinical applicability.[19] Many centers practice gastric lavage even in delayed presentations. However, since the evidence is weak, gastric lavage should only be attempted in patients who present very early, particularly with megadose ingestions in whom the airway is protected and the likelihood of benefit outweighs the risk.

The role of activated charcoal in organophosphorus poisoning was assessed in a large, randomized trial from Sri Lanka.[20] This study did not show the benefit of multidose activated charcoal administration in acute poisoning. However, the authors concluded that studies on the early administration of charcoal are required to answer the question.[20] In countries such as India where patients present late, often beyond 6 hours,[2] gastric lavage and activated charcoal may have a limited role in acute organophosphorus poisoning.

Q3. What is the role of oxime therapy in patients with organophosphorus poisoning?

Oximes have been the subject of debate for several decades. Individual studies[21-28] and meta-analyses[29-31] have failed to consistently show the benefit of administration of oximes in acute poisoning. Barring the one study from Pune[32] which showed the benefit of pralidoxime in acute poisoning of moderate severity who presented to the hospital within 2 hours of poisoning, the remaining studies and meta-analyses[29-31] have not shown benefit. In fact, there was evidence of potential harm with the use of oximes. Several reasons may explain the lack of benefit in acute organophosphorus poisoning. They include megadose intoxications where the rate of binding of the organophosphorus compound far exceeds the rate of reactivation of acetylcholinesterase by the antidote (oximes), late administration of the antidote due to delayed presentation, aging characteristics of the compound, and potential toxicity of the antidote.[29] In the absence of evidence, the use of oximes may be restricted to very early presenters (<2 hours) with diethyl organophosphorus poisoning of moderate toxicity; even in this group, the evidence is not strong and consistent.

The patient was intubated, stabilized, and transferred to the intensive care unit (ICU). In the ICU, the patient has a heart rate of 64/min on 50 mg of atropine/hour and a systolic BP of 90 mm Hg. She is ventilated and oxygenation is adequate; lung fields are clear. GCS has improved to 9T/15. The patient is commenced on small doses of morphine and midazolam for analgosedation in view of restlessness.

Q4. How would you manage the hemodynamic parameters?

Inadequate heart rate response to atropine

Some patients fail to respond to standard doses of atropine and require escalating doses to achieve atropine targets. These patients manifest with a persistently low (<70/min) heart rate and/or low systolic blood pressure (<90 mm Hg), despite the reversal of other cholinergic signs of bronchorrhea and increased salivation.[33] This phenomenon is seen in megadose intoxications, particularly with monocrotophos. This should be suspected in any individual who requires >30 mg/h of atropine infusion for at least 3 hours or >100 mg of atropine over 6 hours. This phenomenon is probably due to the blockade of preganglionic sympathetic neurons with reduced sympathetic outflow. Administration of a small dose of adrenaline as an *infusion* (1–2 μg/min) improves hemodynamics with rapid reduction of atropine requirement.[33]

Q5. When would you start nutritional support?

Enteral nutritional support in acute organophosphorus poisoning is generally not commenced in the first 24 hours since high-dose atropine therapy used to counter the effects of the poison reduces gastric motility. Preliminary evidence suggests that enteral feeds may be safely commenced after 24–48 hours of poisoning at 500 mL/day and gradually increased based on tolerability.[34]

The patient's hemodynamics improves with the treatments initiated. On day 3, the patient develops severe neck muscle weakness and proximal muscle weakness. The GCS remains at 9–10T.

Q6. What are we dealing with? How will you manage the patient? What are the complications that you can expect?

Intermediate syndrome

This patient has developed the classical symptoms of intermediate syndrome. First described by Wadia et al. in 1974[10] and observed in 8–49% of patients,[2] intermediate syndrome or type II paralysis is characterized by acute onset of muscle paralysis following the cholinergic crisis or persistence of muscle paralysis after the initial muscle weakness during the cholinergic phase.[2] It typically occurs after 24–96 hours following acute poisoning,[2] although delayed-onset intermediate syndrome on day 5 has also been reported.[35] The clinical picture is characterized by proximal muscle, neck muscle, respiratory muscle weakness, and cranial nerve palsies.[2] Patients either require mechanical ventilation after initial stabilization of the cholinergic phase or need ongoing ventilation if it was required initially. Muscle weakness typically lasts 5–7 days but sometimes it may last longer, even up to 1–2 weeks.

Electromyography (EMG) is characterized typically by neuromuscular transmission defects.[36,37] Patients with moderate muscle weakness have an initial decrement-increment pattern at high rates of stimulation which progresses to decrement-increment patterns at intermediate and low frequencies.[37] Further progression of muscle weakness results in decrement-increment response and repetitive fade patterns.[37]

Prolonged mechanical ventilation can lead to problems such as ventilator-associated pneumonia and other mechanical complications of ventilation, which need to be dealt with. If patients do not improve muscle function within 5–7 days of poisoning, it is our practice to do an early tracheostomy. Although there are no studies to show the benefit of early tracheostomy in organophosphorus poisoning, in our experience, early tracheostomy facilitates weaning from analgosedation and enables ease of tracheal toileting and increased patient cooperation with the weaning process.

On day 5, you notice that the patient becomes progressively drowsier, and the GCS drops rapidly from 9T to 2T. There is no cough or gag reflex and no response to deep painful stimuli. The oculocephalic and pupillary light reflexes are absent.

Q7. What is happening to the patient? Is the patient brain-dead? How will you manage the patient? What is the prognosis?

Delayed organophosphorus coma

Delayed organophosphate encephalopathy and coma occur in some patients with severe organophosphorus poisoning usually between 4 and 7 days after poisoning.[38,39] In some patients, there is a reduced conscious state following a period of normal or near-normal consciousness, while in others, the clinical picture mimics brain death with bedside tests consistent with a clinical picture of brain death. The clinical clue to this brain death mimic is *pinpoint pupils* in delayed organophosphate coma as opposed to fixed dilated pupils in brain death. Although a computed tomography (CT) scan or magnetic resonance imaging (MRI) may be done to rule out structural changes in the brain, these are often negative. An electroencephalography (EEG) may be done, although not necessary, which would show bihemispheric slowing.[38] This phenomenon lasts 3–5 days and spontaneously resolves. The coma is thought to be due to the saturation of central receptors by the organophosphorus compound over time and the delay is attributed to the redistribution of the compound from the lipid tissue.[38,39] Clinicians should be aware of this problem and manage it appropriately and counsel the patient's family that this is generally a transient phenomenon.

Q8. What are the adjunct therapies in organophosphorus poisoning?

Several other therapies and adjuncts have been tried in acute organophosphorus poisoning. Some have shown some promise and may be considered for further trials in humans. Others have not shown promise or consistent benefit in human poisoning. These therapies are summarized in **Table 2**. These include bioscavenger therapy,[40,41]

TABLE 2: Adjunct and alternative therapies in acute organophosphate poisoning.

Therapy	Physiological basis	Human studies	Recommendations
Bioscavenger therapy	BuChE can bind to free OP and decrease its binding to neuronal sites	Two studies[40,41] showed improvement in BuChE levels with FFP therapy; one study[40] suggested clinical improvement; one[41] did not	Small numbers and methodological limitations limit its use; trials on purified BuChE and modified BuChE which has a prolonged half-life underway
Magnesium	Potential for reversing neuromuscular junction effects; improve skeletal muscle CMAP; cardioprotective effect[42]	Eight comparative studies summarized in a meta-analysis;[43] reasonably well tolerated; some studies showed clinical benefit, some no benefit; pooled odds ratio benefit for mortality, ventilation	Methodological weakness and risk of bias are limitations; magnesium could be considered as an adjunct; more trials required
Calcium channel blocker	Blocking calcium channels thereby reducing acetylcholine release[43]	No human studies; studies on rats[43] reduced lethality (nimodipine) and protection against muscle fasciculation and convulsions (verapamil)	Need more animal studies before human studies are planned; the potential to reduce blood pressure may be a limitation
Diazepam	Used for control of seizures and beneficial when given early[44]	No human studies; pretreatment with diazepam in animal models decreases toxicity[42]	Use diazepam or other newer benzodiazepines (e.g., midazolam) for control of seizures
Clonidine	Dose-related inhibition of soman induced cardiovascular channels[42]	One phase II trial of 48 patients;[45] drop in blood pressure after the third dose in 42%; no difference in mortality	Side effects preclude use
N-acetyl cysteine	Attenuation of generation of free radicals and alterations in antioxidant status[42]	One trial in humans involving 46 patients; less atropine requirements; no other outcome benefits; no major adverse effects[46]	Need further trials before routine use in humans OP poisoning
Alkalinization	Enhanced pesticide clearance, volume expansion, improved tissue perfusion, effect on neuromuscular function[42]	Five studies summarized in a meta-analysis; marked heterogeneity;[47] trend toward lower dose of atropine required	Insufficient evidence for routine use in humans
Hemoperfusion	Extracorporeal removal of toxins	Several series; three recent trials;[48-50] less use of atropine; shorter time to improve GCS; some studies mortality improvement	Cost and availability of resources may limit its use; more randomized trials required as well as comparisons with standard therapy

(BuChE: butyrylcholinesterase; CMAP: compound muscle action potential; FFP: fresh frozen plasma; GCS: Glasgow Coma Scale; OP: organophosphorus compound)

Note: In addition to the above agents, adenosine agonists[41] have been tried in animal models; however, there are no studies on humans.

TABLE 3: Differences between organophosphorus and organocarbamate compounds.

Feature	Organophosphate	Organocarbamate
Compound type	Phosphoric or thiophosphoric acid esters	Esters of N-methyl carbamic acid
Some examples	Malathion, parathion, monocrotophos, chlorpyrifos	Aldicarb, carbaryl, propoxur
Absorption	Well absorbed from skin, lung, gastrointestinal tract	Well absorbed from skin, lung, gastrointestinal tract
Mechanism of action	Cholinesterase inhibitor	Cholinesterase inhibitor
Effect on enzyme/receptor	Permanent, irreversible*	Temporary (<48 hours), reversible
Fate of compound in humans	Undergoes "aging" by dealkylation of alkoxyl group	Spontaneous hydrolysis from cholinesterase enzymatic site
Duration of toxicity	5–15 days	2–3 days
Diagnosis	Clinical features of cholinergic toxidrome	Clinical features of cholinergic toxidrome
Laboratory diagnosis	Suppression of cholinesterase activity	Suppression of cholinesterase activity
Intermediate syndrome	Common	Rare, reported in massive overdose[50]
Outcome	5–15%	Limited information; 12.8% in one study[51]

*If oximes are used early before aging occurs, the effect of the compound can be reversed.

intravenous magnesium,[42,43] calcium channel blockers,[43] diazepam,[44] clonidine,[45] N-acetyl cysteine,[46] alkalinization,[47] and hemoperfusion.[48-50] Of these, intravenous magnesium, a commonly available and cheap drug, should be evaluated further in randomized clinical trials. Diazepam and other benzodiazepines are recommended for seizure control. Hemoperfusion may be beneficial if initiated early. However, the high cost of hemoperfusion and the lack of availability of dialysis in all centers limit its routine use. There is no evidence for the benefit of calcium channel blockers, clonidine, N-acetyl cysteine, and alkalinization in human organophosphorus poisoning.

On day 10, the GCS of the patient improves to 10T and the patient is down to minimal ventilatory support, is hemodynamically stable, and has a good forced vital capacity (FVC) and a positive leak test. He is extubated. However, he fails extubation and needs to be reintubated.

Q9. What are the reasons for extubation failure?
Extubation failure in organophosphorus poisoning
The reasons for extubation failure are often due to factors that are seen in any mechanically ventilated patient that are related to the airway or nonairway causes.[51] However, extubation failure in organophosphorus poisoning can be contributed by neuromuscular weakness affecting the respiratory muscles, neck and proximal muscles, or laryngeal muscle dysfunction per se.[52] In the setting of organophosphorus poisoning, it is prudent to assess for "readiness for extubation" on at least two occasions, 6 hours apart, since neuromuscular weakness can be fluctuant, particularly in the setting of patients who are recovering from the intermediate syndrome.

Q10. What are the differences between organophosphorus and organocarbamate poisoning?
Although both organophosphorus and organocarbamate compounds present with the same toxidrome, organocarbamates have a shorter period of toxicity as their binding to the receptors is reversible. Intermediate syndrome is frequently seen with organophosphorus poisoning but rarely reported with organocarbamate poisoning.[53] Mortality is similar with both poisonings.[54] The similarities and differences between organophosphorus and organocarbamate poisoning are summarized in **Table 3**.

CONCLUSION
The outcome of patients admitted with acute organophosphorus poisoning has improved considerably over the last two decades. This has been possible not because of newer therapies, but because of a better understanding of the pathophysiology of the disease, avoidance of potentially harmful therapies, and improvement in intensive care and supportive therapy.[55] Except in severe poisoning, where the need for prolonged mechanical ventilation may result in ventilator-related events and nosocomial infections, which may increase morbidity and contribute to mortality, most patients are expected to survive to hospital discharge. The key to reducing the burden of organophosphorus poisoning would be through suicide prevention, strict legislation regarding the sale of the more harmful pesticide formulations, prompt treatment of a patient with deliberate self-harm, and appropriate supportive and intensive care therapy in severely poisoned patients.

REFERENCES

1. Holstege CP, Borek HA. Toxidromes. Crit Care Clin. 2012;28:479-98.
2. Peter JV, Sudarsan TI, Moran JL. Clinical features of organophosphate poisoning: a review of different classification systems and approaches. Indian J Crit Care Med. 2014;18:735-45.
3. Peter JV, Cherian AM. Organic insecticides. Anaesth Intensive Care. 2000;28:11-21.
4. Thim T, Krarup NH, Grove EL, Rohde CV, Løfgren B. Initial assessment and treatment with the airway, breathing, circulation, disability, exposure (ABCDE) approach. Int J Gen Med. 2015;5:117-21.
5. Peter JV. Acute respiratory failure. In: David S (Ed.). Clinical Pathways in Emergency Medicine, Vol. I. New York: Springer; 2016. pp. 161-78.
6. Jose R, Chacko B, Iyyadurai R, Peter JV. Polythene predicament. J Emerg Med. 2012;43:e31-33.
7. Jin YH, Jeong TO, Lee JB. Isolated bilateral vocal cord paralysis with intermediate syndrome after organophosphate poisoning. Clin Toxicol (Phila). 2008;46:482-4.
8. Matten EC, Shear T, Vender JS. Nonintubation management of the airway: airway maneuvers and mask ventilation. In: Benumof and Hagberg's Airway Management, 3rd edition. Philadelphia, PA: Elsevier Saunders; 2013. pp. 324-39.
9. Konickx, LA, Bingham K, Eddleston M. Is oxygen required before atropine administration in organophosphorus or carbamate pesticide poisoning?—a cohort study. Clin Toxicol (Phila). 2014;52:531-7.
10. Wadia RS, Sadagopan C, Amin RB, Sardesai HV. Neurological manifestations of organophosphorous insecticide poisoning. J Neurol Neurosurg Psychiatry. 1974;37:841-7.
11. El-Ganzouri AR, McCarthy RJ, Tuman KJ, Tank EN, Invankovich AD. Preoperative airway assessment: predictive value of a multivariate risk index. Anesth Analg. 1996;82:1197-204.
12. Sener EB, Ustun E, Kocamanoglu S, Tur A. Prolonged apnea following succinylcholine administration in undiagnosed acute organophosphate poisoning. Acta Anaesthesiol Scand. 2002;46:1046-8.
13. Eddleston M, Buckley NA, Checketts H, Senarathna L, Mohamed F, Sheriff MH, et al. Speed of initial atropinisation in significant organophosphorus pesticide poisoning—a systematic comparison of recommended regimens. J Toxicol Clin Toxicol. 2004;42:865-75.
14. Peter JV, Jerobin J, Nair A, Bennett A, Samuel P, Chrispal A, et al. Clinical profile and outcome of patients hospitalized with dimethyl and diethyl organophosphate poisoning. Clin Toxicol (Phila). 2010;48:916-23.
15. Abedin MJ, Sayeed AA, Basher A, Maude RJ, Hoque G, Faiz MA. Open-label randomized clinical trial of atropine bolus injection versus incremental boluses plus infusion for organophosphate poisoning in Bangladesh. J Med Toxicol. 2012;8:108-17.
16. Deo A, Mehta HG, Pathare S, Biniyala R, Mehta PJ, Mehtalia SD. Spontaneous reversal of atropine induced delirium in organophosphorus compound poisoning: an early sign of re-excretion. J Assoc Physicians India. 1993;41:611.
17. Bardin PG, Van Eeden SF. Organophosphate poisoning: grading the severity and comparing treatment between atropine and glycopyrrolate. Crit Care Med. 1990;18:956-60.
18. Kventsel I, Berkovitch M, Reiss A, Bulkowstein M, Kozer E. Scopolamine treatment for severe extra-pyramidal signs following organophosphate (chlorpyrifos) ingestion. Clin Toxicol (Phila). 2005;43:877-9.
19. Benson BE, Hoppu K, Troutman WG, Bedry R, Erdman A, Jer JHO, et al. Position paper update: gastric lavage for gastrointestinal decontamination. Clin Toxicol (Phila). 2013;51:140-6.
20. Eddleston M, Juszczak E, Buckley NA, Senarathna L, Mohamed F, Dissanayake W, et al. Multiple-dose activated charcoal in acute self-poisoning: a randomised controlled trial. Lancet. 2008;371:579-87.
21. Cherian AM, Peter JV, Samuel J, Jaydevan R, Peter S, Joel S, et al. Effectiveness of P2AM (PAM—pralidoxime) in the treatment of organophosphate poisoning (OPP). A randomized, double-blind placebo-controlled clinical trial. J Assoc Physicians India. 1997;45:22-4.
22. Johnson S, Peter JV, Thomas K, Jeyaseelan L, Cherian AM. Evaluation of two treatment regimens of pralidoxime (1 gm single bolus dose vs. 12 gm infusion) in the management of organophosphorous poisoning. J Assoc Physicians India. 1996;44:529-31.
23. Cherian MA, Roshini C, Visalakshi J, Jeyaseelan L, Cherian AM. Biochemical and clinical profile after organophosphate poisoning—a placebo-controlled trial using pralidoxime. J Assoc Physicians India. 2005;53:427-31.
24. de Silva HJ, Wijewickrema R, Senanayake N. Does pralidoxime affect outcome of management in acute organophosphorus poisoning? Lancet. 1992;339:1136-8.
25. Abdollahi M, Jafaria A, Jalali N, Balali-Mood M, Kebriaeezadeh A, Nifkar S. A new approach to the efficacy of oximes in the management of acute organophosphorus poisoning. Ir J Med Sci. 1995;20:105-9.
26. Chugh SN, Aggarwal N, Dabla S, Chhabra B. Comparative evaluation of "atropine alone" and "atropine with pralidoxime (PAM)" in the management of organophosphorus poisoning. JIACM. 2005;6:33-7.
27. Balali-Mood M, Shariat M. Treatment of organophosphate poisoning. Experience of nerve agents and acute pesticide poisoning on the effects of oximes. J Physiol Paris. 1998;92:375-8.
28. Eddleston M, Eyer P, Worek F, Juszczak E, Alder N, Mohamed F, et al. Pralidoxime in acute organophosphorus insecticide poisoning—a randomized controlled trial. PLoS Med. 2009;6:e1000104.
29. Peter JV, Moran JL, Graham PL. Advances in the management of organophosphate poisoning. Expert Opin Pharmacother. 2007;8:1451-64.
30. Peter JV, Moran JL, Graham P. Oxime therapy and outcomes in human organophosphate poisoning: an evaluation using meta-analytic techniques. Crit Care Med. 2006;34:502-10.
31. Buckley NA, Eddleston M, Li Y, Bevan M, Robertson J. Oximes for acute organophosphate pesticide poisoning. Cochrane Database Syst Rev. 2011;16:CD005085.

32. Pawar KS, Bhoite RR, Pillay CP, Chavan SC, Malshikare DS, Garad SG. Continuous pralidoxime infusion versus repeated bolus injection to treat organophosphorus insecticide poisoning: a randomized controlled trial. Lancet. 2006;368:2136-41.
33. Samprathi A, Chacko B, D'sa SR, Rebekah G, Kumar CV, Sadiq M, et al. Adrenaline is effective in reversing the inadequate heart rate response in atropine treated organophosphorus and carbamate poisoning. Clin Toxicol. 2021;59:604-10.
34. Moses V, Mahendri NV, John G, Peter JV, Ganesh A. Early hypocaloric enteral nutritional supplementation in acute organophosphate poisoning—a prospective randomized trial. Clin Toxicol (Phila). 2009;47:419-24.
35. Yardan T, Baydin A, Aygun D, Karatas AD, Deniz T, Doganay Z. Late-onset intermediate syndrome due to organophosphate poisoning. Clin Toxicol (Phila). 2007;45:733-4.
36. Jayawardane P, Senanayake N, Buckley NA, Dawson AH. Electrophysiological correlates of respiratory failure in acute organophosphate poisoning: evidence for differential roles of muscarinic and nicotinic stimulation. Clin Toxicol (Phila). 2012;50:250-3.
37. Jayawardane P, Senanayake N, Dawson A. Electrophysiological correlates of intermediate syndrome following acute organophosphate poisoning. Clin Toxicol (Phila). 2009;47:193-205.
38. Peter JV, Prabhakar AT, Pichamuthu K. Delayed-onset encephalopathy and coma in acute organophosphate poisoning in humans. Neurotoxicology. 2008;29:35-342.
39. Peter JV, Prabhakar AT, Pichamuthu K. In-laws, insecticide—and a mimic of brain death. Lancet. 2008;371(9612):622.
40. Güven M, Sungur M, Eser B, Sari I, Altuntaş F. The effects of fresh frozen plasma on cholinesterase levels and outcomes in patients with organophosphate poisoning. J Toxicol Clin Toxicol. 2004;42:617-23.
41. Pichamuthu K, Jerobin J, Nair A, John G, Kamalesh J, Thomas K, et al. Bioscavenger therapy for organophosphate poisoning—an open-labeled pilot randomized trial comparing fresh frozen plasma or albumin with saline in acute organophosphate poisoning in humans. Clin Toxicol (Phila). 2018;56:725-36.
42. Peter JV, Moran JL, Pichamuthu K, Chacko B. Adjuncts and alternatives to oxime therapy in organophosphate poisoning—is there evidence of benefit in human poisoning? A review. Anaesth Intensive Care. 2008;36:339-50.
43. Brvar M, Chan MY, Dawson AH, Ribchester RR, Eddleston M. Magnesium sulfate and calcium channel blocking drugs as antidotes for acute organophosphorus insecticide poisoning—a systematic review and meta-analysis. Clin Toxicol (Phila). 2018;56:725-36.
44. Reddy DS. Neurosteroids for the potential protection of humans against organophosphate toxicity. Ann N Y Acad Sci. 2016;1378:25-32.
45. Perera PM, Jayamanna SF, Hettiarachchi R, Abeyshinghe C, Karunatilake H, Dawson AH, et al. A phase II clinical trial to assess the safety of clonidine in acute organophosphorus pesticide poisoning. Trials. 2009;10:73.
46. El-Ebiary AA, Elsharkawy RE, Soliman NA, Soliman MA, Hashem AA. N-acetylcysteine in acute organophosphorus pesticide poisoning: a randomized, clinical trial. Basic Clin Pharmacol Toxicol. 2016;119:222-7.
47. Roberts D, Buckley NA. Alkalinisation for organophosphorus pesticide poisoning. Cochrane Database Syst Rev. 2005;1:CD004897.
48. Liang MJ, Zhang Y. Clinical analysis of penehyclidine hydrochloride combined with hemoperfusion in the treatment of acute severe organophosphorus pesticide poisoning. Genet Mol Res. 2015;14:4914-9.
49. Dong H, Weng YB, Zhen GS, Li FJ, Jin AC, Liu J. Clinical emergency treatment of 68 critical patients with severe organophosphorus poisoning and prognosis analysis after rescue. Medicine (Baltimore). 2017;96:e7237.
50. Bo L. Therapeutic efficacies of different hemoperfusion frequencies in patients with organophosphate poisoning. Eur Rev Med Pharmacol Sci. 2014;18:3521-3.
51. Jaber S, Qunitard H, Cinotti R, Asehnoune K, Arnal JM, Guitton C, et al. Risk factors and outcomes for airway failure versus non-airway failure in the intensive care unit: a multicenter observational study of 1514 extubation procedures. Crit Care. 2018;22:236.
52. Mani GS, Mathews SS, Victor P, Peter JV, Yadav B, Albert RR. Laryngeal dysfunction in acute organophosphorus and carbamate poisoning. Ind J Crit Care Med. 2022;26:167-73.
53. Paul N, Mannathukkaran TJ. Intermediate syndrome following carbamate poisoning. Clin Toxicol. 2005;43:867-8.
54. Arulmurugan C, Ahmed S, Gani M. A retrospective study of paradigm and outcome of acute poisoning cases in a tertiary care teaching hospital in Southern India. Int J Res Med Sci. 2015;3:2654-7.
55. Peter JV, John G. Management of acute organophosphorus pesticide poisoning. Lancet. 2008;371:2170.

Acute Kidney Injury

Srinivas Samavedam

CASE STUDY

A 45-year-old gentleman, known diabetic on OHAs, is brought to the emergency room with pain abdomen of 4 days duration and vomiting of 1 day duration. There is no history of alcohol consumption. The pain is epigastric in location and radiates to the back. There is no history of hematemesis or melena. On evaluation, he seems to be in distress and has sinus tachycardia of 140 beats/min. His extremities are cool and his blood pressure is recorded at 90/50 mm Hg. An ultrasonographic assessment excludes a hemoperitoneum and cardiac dysfunction. Wide-bore cannulae are secured and fluid resuscitation is commenced. Catheterization of his urinary bladder yielded 150 mL of concentrated urine. His creatinine is reported to be 1.8 mg/dL and he has a high anion gap metabolic acidosis. The treating specialist ordered a contrast-enhanced CT of his abdomen, which revealed necrotizing pancreatitis.

Q1. How will you approach a patient with acute kidney injury (AKI)?

Approach to AKI has to take into account the etiology, the risk factors, the severity, and the assessment of the outcome. All these have to be prioritized for an early diagnosis and stratification of risk. It is also important to understand if this AKI is occurring on a background of preexisting chronic kidney disease (CKD).

Q2. How is AKI diagnosed?

Acute kidney injury is diagnosed if any one of the following are present:
- Increase in serum creatinine by ≥0.3 mg/dL within 48 hours, or
- Increase in serum creatinine to ≥1.5 times baseline, which is known or presumed to have occurred within the prior 7 days, or
- Urine volume < 0.5 mL/kg/h for 6 hours.

Several systems of classification of AKI are available, starting from the RIFLE (risk, injury, failure, loss, end-stage kidney disease),[1] AKIN (Acute Kidney Injury Network),[2] and the KDIGO (Kidney Disease: Improving Global Outcomes)[3] systems. The criteria for diagnosis of AKI as described by each of these systems are shown in **Table 1** (RIFLE), **Table 2** (AKIN), and **Table 3** (KDIGO).

Q3. How do you approach an oliguric patient?

Approach to a patient with AKI usually begins with stratifying the presentation into oliguric and nonoliguric. Patients with

TABLE 1: RIFLE criteria.

Class	Glomerular filtration rate (GFR)	Urine output
Risk	↑ SCr × 1.5 or ↓ GFR >25%	<0.5 mL/kg/h × 6 h
Injury	↑ SCr × 2 or ↓ GFR >50%	<0.5 mL/kg/h × 12 h
Failure	↑ SCr × 3 or ↓ GFR >75% or if baseline SCr ≥353.6 µmol/L (≥4 mg/dL) ↑ SCr >44.2 µmol/L (>0.5 mg/dL)	<0.3 mL/kg/h × 24 h or anuria × 12 h
Loss of kidney function	Complete loss of kidney function >4 weeks	
End-stage kidney disease	Complete loss of kidney function >3 months	

(RIFLE: risk, injury, failure, loss, end-stage kidney disease; SCr: serum creatinine)

TABLE 2: AKIN criteria.

Stage	Serum creatinine	Urine output
1	↑ SCr ≥26.5 µmol/L (≥0.3 mg/dL) or ↑ SCr ≥150–200% (1.5–2×)	<0.5 mL/kg/h (>6 h)
2	↑ SCr >200–300% (>2–3×)	<0.5 mL/kg/h (>12 h)
3	↑ SCr >300% (>3×) or if baseline SCr ≥353.6 µmol/L (≥4 mg/dL) ↑ SCr ≥44.2 µmol/L (≥0.5 mg/dL)	<0.3 mL/kg/h (24 h) or anuria (12 h)

(AKIN: Acute Kidney Injury Network; SCr: serum creatinine)

TABLE 3: KDIGO criteria.

Stage	Description
I	• Cr 1.5–1.9 times baseline • Cr increase >0.3 mg/dL • Urine output (UO) <0.5 mL/kg/h for 6–12 hours
II	• Cr 2–2.9 times baseline. • UO <0.5 mL/kg/h for 12–24 hours
III	• Cr >three times baseline • Cr >4 mg/dL • Initiation of dialysis • UO <0.3 mL/kg/h for >24 hours • Anuria >12 hours

(KDIGO: Kidney Disease: Improving Global Outcomes; Cr: creatinine)

TABLE 4: Stepwise approach to oliguria.

Step	Description
1.	Exclude obstruction
2.	Assess and optimize
3.	Consider volume challenge
4.	Consider vasopressor challenge
5.	Consider inotrope challenge
6.	Perform a frusemide stress test

AKI who have a urine output <0.3–0.5 mL/kg/h for 12–24 hours are deemed to be oliguric.[4] Patients with oliguria seem to require renal replacement therapy (RRT) more often than patients who develop AKI but are not oliguric. Although hypovolemia is the most common cause of oliguria among critically ill patients, other caused such as obstruction and low cardiac output could also present with oliguric AKI.

The approach to oliguria should be structured and sequential. While obstruction is a less common cause of oliguria among ICU patients, it is essential to exclude this etiology first since all other interventions aim to increase the urine output. The steps of approach to oliguria are listed in **Table 4**.

Q4. What is a Frusemide stress test (FST) and its significance?
An FST is performed to assess the renal reserve. It entails administering a diuretic (frusemide) and assessing the renal response.[5] For patients who have previously been exposed to diuretic a higher dose (1.5 mg/kg) is administered. For patients who have not been exposed to frusemide, a dose of 1 mg/kg is used. The urine output after the dose is measured and an hourly output of 200 mL is considered as optimum response. An inadequate response to the FST indicates a diminished renal reserve and also a probable need for RRT. Such patients are also less likely to respond to attempts at optimizing volume status and hemodynamics.

Q5. How do you decide on the optimum timing of initiation of RRT among patients with AKI?
Initiation of RRT among critically ill patients is a complex decision. Life-threatening indications such as hyperkalemia and metabolic acidosis warrant immediate initiation of therapy. However, initiating the RRT for nonconventional indications at earlier time points might not be beneficial and could expose the critically ill patient to procedure and therapy related morbidity.[6] On the contrary, delaying the initiation could result in irreversible metabolic and hemodynamic consequences. Several studies have tried to answer this query of optimum timing over the past 10 years. Two studies, ELAIN[7] and AKIKI[8] were published in the same year (2016). The single center ELAIN study included patients with KDIGO II AKI and compared early initiation (8 hours) of RRT with late initiation (>12 hours) after reaching KDIGO III stage. They reported a decrease in all-cause mortality at 90 days and 1 year in the early initiation group. On the contrary, the AKIKI study, a larger multicenter study, did not report any advantage with early initiation of RRT among patients with KDIGO stage III AKI. Subsequently, several studies have followed the Artificial Kidney Initiation in Kidney Injury (AKIKI) study design and evaluated the benefit of early initiation of RRT. The Initiation of Dialysis Early versus Late in the Intensive Care Unit (IDEAL-ICU) study published in 2018[9] and the Standard versus Accelerated Initiation of RRT in AKI (STARRT-AKI) trial published in 2020[10] also did not show any benefit in initiating RRT early. Holding the dialysis off for longer than 72 hours after the onset of KDIGO III AKI was found to be detrimental in the multi center AKIKI 2 trial.[11] As a summary, initiation of RRT too early (within 12 hours of onset of AKI) or too late (>72 hours after the onset of AKI) seems to be associated with adverse outcomes.

Q6. Which modality of RRT is ideal for ICU patients?
Patients in the ICU, who develop AKI and become eligible for RRT can be offered three forms of RRT—(1) intermittent hemodialysis (IHD), continuous RRT (CRRT), and (3) hybrid form [sustained low-efficiency daily dialysis (SLEDD)]. The three modalities are compared in **Table 5**.

The obvious advantage of CRRT being a continuous form of RRT and operating blood flow being low makes it an appealing option for hemodynamically unstable ICU patients. However, data available so far does not establish the superiority of CRRT over SLEDD.

Q7. How do you prescribe RRT in the ICU?
Initiation of RRT and modality to choose from have been already discussed. Once the decision to initiate RRT has been taken, a methodical prescription is needed for efficient execution of this decision. The prescription has to be

TABLE 5: Comparison of different modalities of renal replacement therapy.

Parameter	Intermittent hemodialysis	Sustained low-efficiency daily dialysis	Continuous renal replacement therapy
Molecules removed	Mostly low molecular weight	Small + middle molecules	Small + middle molecules
Blood flow	300–400 mL/min	100–150 mL/min	150–200 mL/min
Dialysate flow	500 mL/min; 30L/h	100–200 mL/min; 6–12 L/h	1 L/h
Urea clearance	150 mL/min	80 mL/min	30 mL/min
Duration	4 h × 3 times a week	6–12 h/day	Continuous
Anticoagulation	Not needed	Can be avoided	Mostly needed

structured to answer the main queries related to the need for AKI for each patient:[12]

- Fluid management
- Acidosis correction
- Hyperkalemia correction
- Uremia
- Toxin removal

The prescription has to take into account the:

- Mode—IHD, SLEDD, or CRRT
- Duration (for IHD and SLEDD)
- Blood flow rate
- Dialysate flow rate
- Ultrafiltrate rate
- Replacement fluid
- Net fluid removal
- Anticoagulation strategy

Q8. What is the role of sodium bicarbonate in AKI?

Patients in the ICU who develop AKI quite often have a high anion gap metabolic acidosis. The metabolic acidosis could worsen the hemodynamic status further. Correction of this acidosis have long been thought to be in the domain of RRT. However, there has been some interest in the use of sodium bicarbonate infusion for the correction of metabolic acidosis. Jaber et al.[13] randomized 389 critically ill patients with severe metabolic acidemia (i.e., pH, ≤7.20; bicarbonate, ≤20 mmol/L; partial pressure of carbon dioxide, ≤45 mm Hg) to receive 4.2% $NaHCO_3$ aiming for Ph >7.30 and observe for mortality. The authors could not show a difference in mortality but incidence of AKI was less in the group receiving the infusion.

Q9. What are the indications of renal biopsy in a case of AKI?

In situations of AKI, renal biopsy is indicated in following settings:

- Acute kidney injury of unknown etiology
- Suspected vasculitis or significant proteinuria
- Transplant rejection

SUMMARY

- AKI is a common problem among ICU patients.
- Oliguric AKI has a worse course.
- Early RRT has no advantages.
- CRRT does not confer additional advantage over conventional modes.
- Infusion of bicarbonate can be tried in selected patients.

REFERENCES

1. Bellomo R, Ronco C, Kellum JA, Mehta RL, Palevsky P; Acute Dialysis Quality Initiative workgroup. Acute renal failure — definition, outcome measures, animal models, fluid therapy and information technology needs: the Second International Consensus Conference of the Acute Dialysis Quality Initiative (ADQI) Group. Crit Care. 2004;8:R204-12.
2. Mehta RL, Kellum JA, Shah SV, Molitoris BA, Ronco C, Warnock DG, et al. Acute Kidney Injury Network: Report of an initiative to improve outcomes in acute kidney injury. Crit Care. 2007;11:R31.
3. Kellum JA, Lameire N, Aspelin P, Barsoum RS, Burdmann EA, Goldstein SL, et al. Kidney Disease: Improving Global Outcomes (KDIGO) Acute Kidney Injury Work Group. KDIGO clinical practice guideline for acute kidney injury. Kidney Int Suppl. 2012;2:1-138.
4. Kunst G, Ostermann M. Intraoperative permissive oliguria—how much is too much? Br J Anaesth. 2017;119(6): 1075-7.
5. McMahon BA, Chawla LS. The furosemide stress test: current use and future potential. Ren Fail. 2021;43(1):830-9.
6. Cove ME, MacLaren G, Brodie D, Kellum JA. Optimising the timing of renal replacement therapy in acute kidney injury. Crit Care. 2021;25:184.
7. Zarbock A, Kellum JA, Schmidt C, Aken HV, Wempe C, Pavenstädt H, et al. Effect of early vs delayed initiation of renal replacement therapy on mortality in critically Ill patients with acute kidney injury: the ELAIN randomized clinical trial. JAMA. 2016; 315:2190-9.
8. Gaudry S, Hajage D, Schortgen F, Martin-Lefevre L, Pons B, Boulet E, et al. Initiation strategies for renal-replacement therapy in the intensive care unit. N Engl J Med. 2016;375:122-33

9. Barbar SD, Clere-Jehl R, Bourredjem A, Hernu R, Montini F, Bruyère R, et al. Timing of renal-replacement therapy in patients with acute kidney injury and sepsis. N Engl J Med. 2018;379:1431-42
10. The STARRT-AKI Investigators. Timing of initiation of renal-replacement therapy in acute kidney injury. N Engl J Med. 2020;383:240-51.
11. Gaudry S, Hajage D, Martin-Lefevre L, Lebbah S, Louis G, Moschietto S, et al. Comparison of two delayed strategies for renal replacement therapy initiation for severe acute kidney injury (AKIKI 2): a multicentre, openlabel, randomised, controlled trial. Lancet. 2021;397:1293-300.
12. See EJ, Bellomo R. How I prescribe continuous renal replacement therapy. Crit Care. 2021;25:1.
13. Jaber S, Paugam C, Futier E, Lefrant JY, Lasocki S, Lescot T, et al. Sodium bicarbonate therapy for patients with severe metabolic acidaemia in the intensive care unit (BICAR-ICU): A multicentre, open-label, randomised controlled, phase 3 trial. Lancet. 2018; 392:31.

CHAPTER 26

Upper Gastrointestinal Bleeding

Lalita Gouri Mitra, Jagdeep Sharma, Atul Prabhakar Kulkarni

CASE STUDY

A 56-year-old male, a known case of liver cirrhosis due to chronic alcohol intake, presents with acute-onset hematemesis followed by loss of consciousness. The relatives reveal that he had bouts of blood-stained vomiting overnight and might have lost some blood in the vomitus.

He was previously admitted 2 weeks ago for massive ascites, which required tapping and was detected to have grade II esophageal varices for which endoscopic variceal ligation (EVL) was done. In the intensive care unit (ICU), he is unconscious with Glasgow Coma Scale (GCS) of 8 (E2M3V3). Pupils are equal in size and reacting to light, pallor is present. He is tachycardic [heart rate (HR) 115/min, regular], hypotensive [blood pressure (BP) 70/36 mm Hg], tachypneic [respiratory rate (RR) 28/min], and hypoxic [oxygen saturation (SpO$_2$) 85% on room air]. Auscultation of the chest reveals decreased air entry at both bases. His abdomen is warm, tense, and distended.

Laboratory investigations reveal a total leukocyte count of 13,000/mm^3 (predominantly polymorphs 88%), international normalized ratio (INR) 3.5, prothrombin time (PT) 22 seconds, activated partial thromboplastin time (aPTT) 40 seconds, and platelets 40,000/mm^3. His liver function [total bilirubin is 6.2 mg%, alkaline phosphatase (ALP) 208 IU/L, serum glutamic-pyruvic transaminase (SGPT) 78 IU/L, serum glutamic-oxaloacetic transaminase (SGOT) 88 IU/L, serum albumin 1.4 g/dL, globulin 4.2 g/dL, random blood sugar 40 mg/dL, and renal function (serum urea 52 mg/dL and creatinine 2.0 mg/dL)] appear deranged.

Baseline creatinine during past admission was 1.3. Serum ammonia was 88 µg/dL (units).

Q1. How will you manage this patient immediately after admission?

General management

In case of active bleed, secure two large-bore (18G or larger) peripheral cannulas. Secure a central venous line when feasible, but this is not a priority unless peripheral venous access is difficult. Supplemental oxygen can be given by nasal cannula and the patient should be kept nil by mouth. The European Society of Gastrointestinal Endoscopy (ESGE) suggests intubation prior to upper gastrointestinal (UGI) endoscopy in patients with suspected variceal hemorrhage with ongoing hematemesis and encephalopathy.[1] If there is worsening in mentation or respiration, consider elective intubation to prevent aspiration. However, chances of developing pneumonia within 48 hours are higher in patients who require intubation (14.0 vs. 2.0) and are more likely to have cardiopulmonary complications (20.0 vs. 6.0) as seen in a study by Hayat et al.[2] Hypotension and active bleed should be treated as per established transfusion guidelines. Vigorous resuscitation with saline or overtransfusion should be avoided in patients of variceal bleed as it can precipitate recurrent variceal hemorrhage and worsen/precipitate ascites or extravascular fluid collection. The National Institute for Health and Care Excellence (NICE) guidelines recommend giving fresh frozen plasma (FFP) for coagulopathy and platelets for thrombocytopenia (platelets <50,000) or platelet dysfunction. The ESGE guidelines do not recommend the transfusion of FFP as the initial management of esophageal gastric variceal hemorrhage (EGVH).[1]

Risk stratification and triage: Patients who are hemodynamically unstable and actively bleeding patients will present with shock and orthostatic hypotension or may require vasopressors to maintain their hemodynamics, and they should be admitted to an ICU for close monitoring with at least electrocardiography (ECG), pulse oximetry, and automated or invasive BP measurement and resuscitation should be done aggressively. The ESGE recommends that patients with suspected acute variceal bleed must be risk-stratified according to Child–Pugh score and Model for End-Stage Liver Disease (MELD) score. It must be documented if the bleeding is active/inactive at the time of UGI endoscopy.[1]

The NICE and Scottish Intercollegiate Guidelines Network (SIGN) advocate a two-step risk assessment strategy: Variceal assessment and severity assessment. The variceal assessment is based on the presence of confirmed varices, or if the patient has risk factors for developing portal hypertension, like proven cirrhosis chronic liver disease along with relevant radiological and biochemical findings.[3] The severity assessment is commonly done based on two scores: The Blatchford score **(Table 1)** and the Rockall score **(Table 2)**, which predict endoscopic and clinical outcomes. Endoscopy should be done within 24 hours of admission in patients with higher risk scores.

The modified Glasgow-Blatchford score is a simpler score, calculated using only the blood urea nitrogen, hemoglobin, systolic BP, and pulse. The score ranges from 0 to 16. It outperformed the Rockall score with regard to predicting rebleeding requiring clinical intervention, and mortality in a prospective study.[5]

AIMS65 uses pre-endoscopy data which has high accuracy for predicting inpatient mortality among patients with UGI bleeding, and five factors are associated with increased inpatient mortality:[7]
1. Albumin < 3.0 g/dL (30 g/L)
2. INR > 1.5
3. Altered mental status (GCS < 14, disorientation, lethargy, stupor, or coma)
4. Systolic BP of 90 mm Hg or less
5. Age older than 65 years

The mortality rate increases significantly as the number of risk factors present increases as shown by Hyett et al. in their validation cohort:[8]
- *Zero risk factors:* 0.3%
- *One risk factor:* 1%
- *Two risk factors:* 3%
- *Three risk factors:* 9%
- *Four risk factors:* 15%
- *Five risk factors:* 25%

Q2. Describe the initial evaluation and management of UGI bleed.

Bleeding from a source proximal to the ligament of Treitz is defined as UGI bleeding and can be defined as variceal or nonvariceal bleed. Variceal hemorrhage is a complication of end-stage liver disease and nonvariceal bleed can be due to peptic ulcer disease and various other causes **(Table 3)**.

With the aim of assessing the severity of the bleeding, a complete medical history, physical examination, nasogastric lavage, and laboratory assessment should be done when the patient presents in the emergency.

The ESGE recommends the following risk stratification definitions:
- Patients with Child–Pugh A/Child–Pugh B without active bleeding at UGI endoscopy or MELD score <11 have a low risk of poor outcomes.

TABLE 1: Blatchford score.[4]

Criteria (on admission)		Score
Hemoglobin (g/L)		
Hb—Male	Hb—Female	
120–139	100–120	1
100–120	–	3
<100	<100	6
Urea (mmol/L)		
6.5–8		2
8–10		3
10–25		4
≥25		6
Systolic blood pressure (mm Hg)		
100–109		1
90–99		2
<90		3
Others		
Pulse ≥ 100		1
Melena		1
Syncope		2
Hepatic disease		2
Cardiac failure		2

TABLE 2: Rockall score.[6]

Criteria (on admission)	Score
Age (years)	
<60	0
60–79	1
≥80	2
Shock	
Pulse >100	1
Systolic blood pressure (BP) <100 mm Hg	2
Comorbidity	
Cardiac, other major	2
Renal/liver failure, cancer	3
Endoscopic diagnosis	
Normal, Mallory–Weiss	0
Ulcer, erosion, esophagitis	1
Cancer	2
Endoscopic stigmata of recent hemorrhage (ESRH)	
Clean base ulcer, flat pigmented spot	0
Active bleeding, clot, vessel, blood	2

TABLE 3: Disorders that cause upper GI bleeding in adults.

Cause	Associated risk factors and conditions	Associated signs and symptoms	Bleeding manifestations
Complications of portal hypertension			
• Esophagogastric varices • Ectopic varices • Portal hypertensive gastropathy	Portal hypertension from: • Cirrhosis • Portal vein thrombosis • Noncirrhotic portal hypertension	Stigmata of chronic liver disease,^Δ signs of portal hypertension (splenomegaly, ascites, thrombocytopenia)	• Hematemesis • Melena • Hematochezia (indicates brisk bleeding)
Ulcerative or erosive			

Duodenal and/or gastric ulcer	• Infections:
	  – *Helicobacter pylori*
	  – CMV
	  – HSV
	• NSAIDs
	• Stress ulcer (e.g., in patients who are critically ill)
	• Excess gastric acid production (ZES)
	• Idiopathic
		• Upper abdominal pain
		• Pain associated with eating (worse when eating suggests gastric ulcer, improvement with eating suggests duodenal ulcer)
		• Dyspepsia*
			• Hematemesis
			• Melena
			• Hematochezia (indicates brisk bleeding)
			• Occult blood loss

Esophagitis	• Gastroesophageal reflux disease
	• *Medications that may cause "pill esophagitis"*:
	  – Erythromycin
	  – Tetracycline
	  – Doxycycline
	  – Clindamycin
	  – Trimethoprim-sulfamethoxazole
	  – NSAIDs
	  – Oral bisphosphonates
	  – Potassium chloride
	  – Quinidine
	  – Iron supplements
	• Infections:
	  – HSV
	  – CMV
	  – *Candida albicans*
	  – HIV
		• Dysphagia/odynophagia
		• Retrosternal pain
		• Food impaction
			• Hematemesis
			• Melena
			• Occult blood loss

Gastritis/gastropathy Duodenitis/duodenopathy	*Risk factors:* • *H. pylori* • NSAIDs • Excessive alcohol consumption • Radiation injury • Physiologic stress • Weight loss surgery • Bile reflux *Risk factors for bleeding:* • Anticoagulant use	Dyspepsia*	
Vascular lesions			
Angiodysplasia	• End-stage kidney disease • Aortic stenosis • Left ventricular assist device • Hereditary hemorrhagic telangiectasia • von Willebrand disease • Radiation therapy • Idiopathic	Cutaneous angiodysplasia in patients with hereditary hemorrhagic telangiectasia (Osler-Weber-Rendu syndrome)	• Hematemesis • Melena • Hematochezia • Occult blood loss • May have brisk bleeding

Contd...

Contd...

Cause	Associated risk factors and conditions	Associated signs and symptoms	Bleeding manifestations
Dieulafoy's lesion	• Etiology unknown • Bleeding may be associated with NSAIDs, cardiovascular disease, hypertension, chronic kidney disease, diabetes, or alcohol abuse		
Gastric antral vascular ectasia (GAVE)	• Idiopathic • Cirrhosis with portal hypertension • Kidney disease/transplantation • Diabetes mellitus • Systemic sclerosis (scleroderma) • Bone marrow transplantation	In patients with cirrhosis, there may be stigmata of chronic liver disease,$^\Delta$ signs of portal hypertension (splenomegaly, ascites, thrombocytopenia)	
Blue rubber bleb nevus syndrome (Bean syndrome)		*Venous malformations and hemangiomas of any organ, including:* • Skin • Central nervous system • Liver • Muscles • Lymphatics Intussusception	
Traumatic or iatrogenic			
Mallory-Weiss syndrome	• Vomiting/retching (often related to alcohol consumption) • Straining at stool or lifting • Coughing • Seizures • Blunt abdominal trauma • Hiatal hernia may increase the risk of developing a tear	• Epigastric pain • Back pain	• Hematemesis following an increase in intra-abdominal pressure • Melena • Hematochezia (indicates brisk bleeding)
Foreign body ingestion	• Psychiatric disorders • Altered mental status (toxin induced, dementia, etc.) • Loose dentures	• Dysphagia • Odynophagia • Neck or abdominal pain • Choking • Hypersalivation • Retrosternal fullness	• Hematemesis • Melena • Hematochezia (indicates brisk bleeding) • Occult blood loss
Postsurgical anastomotic bleeding ("marginal ulcers")	• Billroth II surgery • Gastric bypass surgery • NSAID use • *H. pylori* infection • Smoking	• Epigastric pain • Nausea	
Postpolypectomy/ endoscopic resection/ endoscopic sphincterotomy	Large lesions	Past history of instrumentation (may be as long as three weeks prior to presentation)	
Cameron lesions	• Hiatal hernia • Reflux esophagitis		
Aortoenteric fistula	• Infectious aortitis (syphilis, tuberculosis) • Prosthetic aortic graft • Atherosclerotic aortic aneurysm • Penetrating ulcers • Tumor invasion • Trauma • Radiation injury • Foreign body perforation	• Back pain • Fever • Signs of sepsis • Pulsatile abdominal mass • Abdominal bruit	• Hematemesis • Melena • Hematochezia (indicates brisk bleeding) • May have a "herald" bleed followed by massive bleeding

Contd...

Contd...

Cause	Associated risk factors and conditions	Associated signs and symptoms	Bleeding manifestations
Tumors			

Upper GI tumors	• Virtually any tumor type may bleed
	• *Benign tumors:*
	  – Leiomyoma
	  – Lipoma
	  – Polyp (hyperplastic, adenomatous, hamartomatous, inflammatory)
	• *Malignant tumors:*
	  – Adenocarcinoma
	  – GI stromal tumors
	  – Lymphoma
	  – Kaposi sarcoma
	  – Carcinoid
	  – Melanoma
	  – Metastatic tumors
		• Weight loss
		• Anorexia
		• Nausea/vomiting
		• Early satiety
		• Epigastric pain
		• Dysphagia (for tumors in the esophagus or proximal stomach)
		• Gastric outlet obstruction
		• Palpable mass
		• *Paraneoplastic manifestations:*
		  – Diffuse seborrheic keratoses
		  – Acanthosis nigricans
		  – Membranous nephropathy
		  – Coagulopathy
			• Hematemesis
			• Melena
			• Hematochezia (indicates brisk bleeding)
			• Occult blood loss

Miscellaneous			
Hemobilia	*Past history of liver or biliary tract instrumentation and/or injury, including the following:* • Liver biopsy • Cholecystectomy • Endoscopic biliary biopsies or stenting • TIPS placement • Angioembolization • Blunt or penetrating abdominal trauma • Gallstones • Cholecystitis • Hepatic or bile duct tumors • Intrahepatic stents • Hepatic artery aneurysms • Hepatic abscesses	• Biliary colic • Jaundice (obstructive) • Sepsis (biliary)	• Hematemesis • Melena • Hematochezia (indicates brisk bleeding)

Hemosuccus pancreaticus	• Chronic pancreatitis
	• Pancreatic pseudocysts
	• Pancreatic tumors
	• Pancreatic pseudoaneurysm
	• Therapeutic endoscopy of the pancreas or pancreatic duct:
	  – Pancreatic stone removal
	  – Pancreatic duct sphincterotomy
	  – Pseudocyst drainage
	  – Pancreatic duct stenting
		• Abdominal pain
		• Past evidence of symptoms/signs of pancreatitis
		• Imaging evidence of pancreatitis (current or in the past)
		• Elevated amylase and lipase (current or in the past)	

*Postprandial fullness, early satiety, epigastric pain, or burning.
ΔEvidence of chronic liver disease includes jaundice, splenomegaly, ascites, thrombocytopenia, palmar erythema, spider angiomata, gynecomastia, testicular atrophy, and Dupuytren's contracture.
(CMV: cytomegalovirus; HSV: herpes simplex virus; ZES: Zollinger-Ellison syndrome; NSAID: nonsteroidal anti-inflammatory drug; HIV: human immunodeficiency virus; GI: gastrointestinal).

- Patients with Child-Pugh B with active bleeding at UGI endoscopy despite vasoactive medications, Child-Pugh C, or MELD score > 19 are at a high risk for poor outcomes.[1]

High-risk patients should be identified, and timely intervention is essential to reduce mortality and morbidity. Red flags for severe bleeding include tachycardia, frank blood detected during nasogastric lavage, and a significant and rapid fall in hemoglobin level or a value < 8 g/dL at presentation.

Hematemesis which is frankly bloody suggests moderate-to-severe bleeding. It suggests ongoing active bleed. Limited bleeding is suggested by coffee-ground emesis. If a patient has hematemesis and black tarry melena, the source is likely to be proximal to the ligament of Treitz **(Table 4)**.[9]

History
Rule out past medical history of varices or portal hypertensive gastropathy, angiodysplasia, peptic ulcer disease, nonsteroidal anti-inflammatory drug (NSAID) use, smoking, malignancy, and history of comorbid conditions such as coronary artery disease (CAD), pulmonary disease (to prevent adverse effects of anemia), any condition that may cause volume overload (e.g., renal disease or heart failure), or difficult to control bleeding (coagulopathies or patients on antiplatelet therapy), risk of aspiration such as hepatic encephalopathy or associated severe ascites, history of medication like NSAIDs, aspirin, clopidogrel, bismuth or iron **(Table 5)**.[9]

Signs and symptoms
Severe bleeding is indicated by orthostatic hypotension, confusion, angina, cold and clammy peripheries, and palpitations. Less than 15% of blood volume lost will cause mild-to-moderate hypovolemia and resting tachycardia. If the blood volume loss is at least 15%, there will be orthostatic hypotension. Supine hypotension occurs with a blood volume loss of at least 40% **(Table 6)**.[9]

Laboratory investigations
On presentation, it is essential to get a complete blood count, liver function tests, renal function tests, serum electrolytes, arterial blood gases (to acid–base status and lactate levels), and coagulation profile done. Monitor ECG and cardiac enzymes in the elderly or in patients with CAD and history of dyspnea. Depending on the severity of the bleeding, measure hemoglobin every 2–8 hours, keeping in mind that the hemoglobin could be falsely low because of hemodilution following fluid resuscitation. In chronic bleeding, peripheral smear will show microcytic red blood cells (RBCs), and in acute bleeding, normocytic RBCs. The blood urea nitrogen to creatinine ratio and urea to creatinine ratio is elevated (values >36:1 or >100:1) in acute UGI bleed due to decreased renal perfusion, and the bleed is likely to be from the UGI tract if the ratio is high.[10] A rapid hemoglobin estimate along with acid–base disturbances and hyperlactatemia associated with tissue hypoperfusion can be obtained from an arterial blood gas.

TABLE 4: Probable source of gastrointestinal (GI) bleeding within the gut.

Clinical indicator	Probability of upper GI source	Probability of lower GI source
Hematemesis	Almost certain	Rare
Melena	Probable	Possible
Hematochezia	Possible	Probable
Blood-streaked stool	Rare	Almost certain
Occult blood in stool	Possible	Possible

TABLE 5: Clinical features.

History:
- *Medication:* Nonsteroidal anti-inflammatory drugs (NSAIDs), aspirin, anticoagulants, antiplatelet agents
- Alcohol abuse/intake; previous gastrointestinal (GI) bleed; liver disease; coagulopathy

Symptoms and signs:
- Abdominal pain
- Hematemesis or "coffee ground" emesis
- Melena/tarry stool

Examination:
- Tachycardia
- Orthostatic blood pressure (changes suggest moderate-to-severe blood loss)
- Hypotension (life-threatening blood loss)
- Rectal examination—examine stool color

TABLE 6: Estimated fluid and blood loss in shock.[8]

	Class 1	Class 2	Class 3	Class 4
Blood loss, mL	Up to 750	750–1,500	1,500–2,000	>2,000
Blood loss, % blood volume	Up to 15%	15–30%	30–40%	>40%
Pulse rate, bpm	<100	>100	>120	>140
Blood pressure	Normal	Normal	Decreased	Decreased
Respiratory rate	Normal or increased	Decreased	Decreased	Decreased
Urine output, mL/h	>35	30–40	20–30	14–20
Central nervous system (CNS)/mental status	Slightly anxious	Mildly anxious	Anxious, confused	Confused, lethargic
Fluid replacement, 3-for-1 rule	Crystalloid	Crystalloid	Crystalloid and blood	Crystalloid and blood

Q3. How will you manage blood loss in this patient?

The dynamic definitions, which identify rapid blood transfusions, are better suited for use in day-to-day practice, hence in acute variceal bleed. Transfusion of more than four units of packed red blood cells (PRBCs) in 1 hour when the ongoing need is foreseeable or replacement of 50% of total blood volume (TBV) within 3 hours, would be considered as massive blood transfusion.[11]

The principles of management of massive blood loss are as follows:

Critical hypoperfusion occurs once the body has lost 30% TBV and the physiological hemodynamic compensatory mechanisms begin to fail. The patient will develop shock if resuscitation is inadequate at this stage. It is important to remember that overzealous resuscitation leads to high arterial and venous pressures, which may dislodge hemostatic clots, cause more bleeding, and hence can be deleterious.

Management of loss of blood components

Since laboratory turnaround time can be long, coagulation factors can be empirically replaced as per protocol in massive blood losses. The aim is to break the lethal triad of acidosis, hypothermia, and coagulopathy that invariably follows a massive transfusion, thereby improving outcome. Patients without active bleeding who become hemodynamically stable with fluid resuscitation should receive a blood transfusion if the hemoglobin is <8 g/dL (90 g/L) for high-risk patients and if it is <7 g/dL (70 g/L) in low-risk patients. The desired hemoglobin post transfusion is 8–9 g/dL.[1] Transfusion of platelets may be required if the platelet count is <50,000/μL and prothrombin complex concentrate is indicated if the INR is >2. After transfusion of 4–10 units, a massive blood transfusion protocol is initiated and it has a predefined ratio of RBCs, FFP/cryoprecipitate, and platelet units (random donor platelets) in each pack (e.g., 1:1:1 or 2:1:1 ratio) for transfusion.[12] These ratios were suggested by the PROPPR trial in which more patients in the 1:1:1 group achieved hemostasis and fewer experienced death due to exsanguination by 24 hours.[13] There were only two large randomized controlled trials (RCTs) studying massive blood transfusion with focus on patients with acute UGI hemorrhage.[14,15] In both studies, the restrictive group had significantly lower 45-day mortality and rebleeding. Patients with chronic liver disease and portal hypertension showed more positive and pronounced effects of restriction. All patients received urgent endoscopy within 6 hours from presentation, which may have impacted outcomes, and patients with exsanguinating hemorrhage were excluded.

The reason why transfusion worsens outcomes in some UGI bleed with parathyroid hormone (PTH) also remains unclear. It has been proposed that transfusion increases portal and/or systemic pressures, thereby promoting further bleeding. These patients also have impairment of coagulation, and the transfused RBCs are transiently unable to effectively deliver oxygen to end organs (due to depleted 2,3-diphosphoglycerate). Stored RBCs have stiff membranes and blood transfusion in portal hypertension decreases functional capillary density, antigen-mediated immune reactions, and paradoxical dampening of the immune response.[14]

Complications of massive blood transfusion

An immediate complication seen during massive blood transfusion is inadequate resuscitation, which leads to hypoperfusion that causes lactic acidosis and systemic inflammatory response syndrome (SIRS). Disseminated intravascular coagulation ensues and multiorgan dysfunction sets in.

It is prudent to keep in mind that overzealous resuscitation leads to transfusion-associated circulatory overload and interstitial edema due to increased hydrostatic pressure, which may lead to abdominal compartment syndrome.[11] It also causes dilutional coagulopathy and low colloid oncotic pressure that gives rise to interstitial edema. 80 mL of citrate phosphate dextrose adenine solution present in each blood bag contains approximately 3 g citrate and hypoperfusion or hypothermia associated with massive blood loss can decrease this rate of metabolism leading to citrate toxicity, which causes hypocalcemia and hypomagnesemia and worsens the acidosis.

Stored PRBCs have high potassium content (7–77 mEq/L depending on the age of stored blood), hence causing hyperkalemia.

Infusion of cold fluids and blood and blood products, opening of gut/abdomen cavities (surgical cases), and decreased heat production all cause hypothermia which not only reduces citrate metabolism and drug clearance but also contributes to the development of coagulopathy.

Hypomagnesemia occurs as citrate also binds to magnesium. Each unit has an acid load of approximately 6 mEq/L; hence acidosis is caused by the lower pH of stored PRBCs, and it directly reduces the activity of both extrinsic and intrinsic coagulation pathways.[11]

Late complications seen are respiratory failure due to transfusion-related acute lung injury (TRALI), SIRS, sepsis, and thrombotic complications.[11]

Q4. What are the options available to stop the UGI bleed?

Medical management

Patients with acute UGI bleeding should be started empirically on an intravenous (IV) proton-pump inhibitor (PPI) (both intermittent boluses and continuous infusion are equally effective) as it reduces the rate of rebleeding even though in the setting of active UGI bleed, H_2 receptor antagonists have not been shown to significantly lower the rate of ulcer rebleeding.[15] Stabilization of blood clots occurs with neutralization of gastric acid. The ESGE recommends in the absence of contraindications, administration of IV erythromycin 250 mg, 30-120 minutes prior to UGI endoscopy.[1] Prokinetic agents such as erythromycin at a dose of 3 mg/kg intravenously over 20-30 minutes, 30-90 minutes prior to endoscopy, clear the stomach of blood, clots, and food residue, thereby improving visualization, and decrease the need for second-look endoscopy.[16] Vasoactive medications such as somatostatin (250 μg/h continuous infusion can be increased to 500 μg/h), its analog octreotide (50 μg bolus followed by 50 μg/h infusion), and terlipressin (2 mg/4 h during the first 4 hours followed by 1 mg/4 h) reduce the risk of bleeding due to both variceal and nonvariceal causes.[17] These vasoactive agents terlipressin, octreotide and somatostatin should be initiated at the time of presentation, in patients with suspected variceal bleed and continued for a duration of up to 5 days. Following successful endoscopic management, these agents might be stopped 24-48 hours post procedure in select group of patients.[1]

The ESGE recommends antibiotic prophylaxis with ceftriaxone 1 g/day for all patients with advanced chronic liver disease presenting with acute variceal hemorrhage.[1] Prophylactic antibiotics (ceftriaxone 1 g/24 h in those who are already on quinolones such as norfloxacin 400 mg BID) should be given to patients with cirrhosis who present with acute UGI bleeding (from varices or other causes). Up to 20% of patients with cirrhosis who are hospitalized with GI bleeding have bacterial infections and hence should be given antibiotics before endoscopy. Multiple trials suggest that prophylactic antibiotics reduce infectious complications and possibly decrease mortality, reducing the risk of recurrent esophageal variceal bleeding in hospitalized patients.[18]

Withhold anticoagulants and antiplatelet agents in patients with UGI bleeding whenever possible, and the decision to discontinue medications or administer reversal agents or resume after hemostasis needs to be individualized.[19] There is no role for tranexamic acid or recombinant factor VIIa in the treatment of UGI bleeding. Cochrane reviews of various trials found that tranexamic acid appears to have a beneficial effect on mortality; however, a few trials had a dropout rate. Hence, one cannot be sure of these findings until further studies are published. Tranexamic acid did not reduce mortality in the trials that included antiulcer drugs or endoscopic therapy. The results of TXA TAUGIB trials are awaited and HALT-IT trial suggests that tranexamic acid did not reduce death from GI bleeding. It also suggests that it should not be used for the treatment of GI bleeding. It also suggests that the use of tranexamic acid increases the risk of venous thromboembolism.[20] At least two RCTs and a meta-analysis of those trials failed to demonstrate a clear benefit of recombinant factor VIIa in active variceal bleeding. Thus, the role of recombinant factor VIIa in the management of bleeding awaits further clarification, and it cannot yet be recommended for routine clinical use in patients with variceal hemorrhage as most patients will be acidotic.[21] The ESGE guidelines do not recommend the transfusion recombinant factor VIIa as the initial management of EGVH.[1]

Endoscopic management

The management of bleeding lesions varies for variceal and nonvariceal sources. Endoscopy evaluation should be carried out within 12 hours from the time the patient presents to the emergency, provided the patient has been hemodynamically resuscitated to determine the cause and initiate early therapeutic interventions.[1]

Portal hypertension causes the formation of portosystemic shunts and varices causing variceal bleed. The ESGE recommends that variceal bleeds be managed with endoscopic band ligation.

The ESGE recommends the use of hemostatic powders/spray only as a bridge before definitive endoscopic treatment.[1] Mechanical tamponade can be applied with Sengstaken-Blakemore (SB) tube or Minnesota tube or Linton-Nachlas tube insertion and self-expanding metal stent for the esophagus **(Figs. 1 and 2)**.

Nonvariceal UGI bleed (NVUGIB) presents in one of the following three ways:
1. Active bleeding
2. A nonbleeding visible vessel
3. Adherent clot

Endoscopic therapies for NVUGIB comprise injection therapy (injection of adrenaline into and around the point

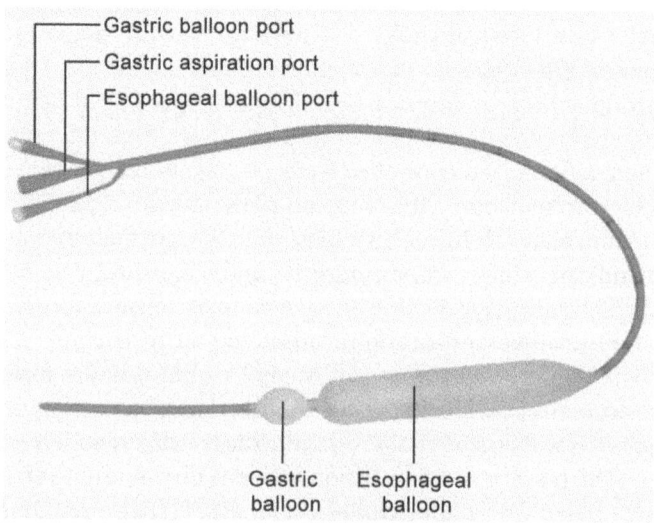

Fig. 1: Sengstaken-Blakemore tube.[26]

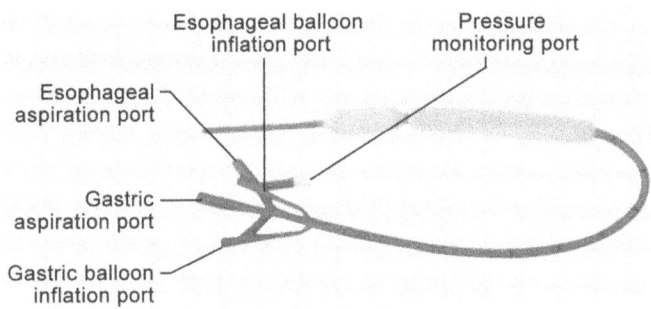

Fig. 2: Minnesota tube.

of bleeding), thermal treatments (contact-monopolar diathermy compresses and seals a bleeding lesion and noncontact-argon plasma coagulation), mechanical adjuncts (endoclip or hemoclip), and hemospray therapy. The ESGE recommends early endoscopy <24 hours, rather than urgent endoscopy. The ESGE recommends high-dose PPI for patients who undergo endoscopic hemostasis. It should be given as a bolus dose of 80 mg followed by 8 mg/h for the next 72 hours.[22]

Q5. How will you manage this patient after endoscopy has been performed?
Terlipressin: It is a synthetic analog of vasopressin that has a longer biological activity and significantly fewer side effects and NICE recommends continuing until the certainty of hemostasis or up to 5 days at a dose of 1–2 mg IV every 4 hours.[23]

Nonselective beta-blockers: Within 6 weeks, the risk of rebleeding is 15–30%. Recent British Society of Gastroenterology (BSG) guidelines recommend the use of propranolol or nadolol for secondary prevention of variceal bleeding, with carvedilol as an alternative.[24] The ESGE recommends the use of nonselective beta-blockers (propranolol/carvedilol) in combination with endoscopic therapy for secondary prophylaxis.[1]

Variceal band ligation (VBL): Elective repeat endoscopy should be scheduled every 1–4 weeks after variceal hemorrhage until varices have been eradicated.[1]

Transfusion thresholds: The BSG recommends a transfusion threshold of 7–8 g/dL in hemodynamically stable patients with variceal hemorrhage.[1]

The ESGE suggests against the routine use of PPIs in the postendoscopic management of acute variceal bleed.[1]

Q6. What is the role of mechanical tamponade? Describe Minnesota and Sengstaken–Blakemore (SB) tubes and discuss their use. How is SB tube inserted? Which balloon is inflated first and how? How is the SB tube fixed? Which balloon is inflated next and how? Which cuff is deflated and when? What if bleeding persists?
Sengstaken–Blakemore (SB) tube has three components: (1) A gastric balloon, (2) an esophageal balloon, and (3) a gastric suction port. The balloons are for tamponade, while the gastric port is for aspiration of blood from the stomach.

Procedure for insertion: Most patients will need to be intubated as it is a large tube and very uncomfortable for the patient; however, local anesthesia may be used. The patient is put in 45% head elevation. Alternatively, a left lateral decubitus position can be used. The balloons are checked by inflating and submerging under water for leaks; then ports are clamped after removing all air. Sometimes, a nasogastric tube is tied about 4 cm above the esophageal balloon and used for aspiration of blood from the esophagus. The tube (and balloons) is lubricated and then it is passed (either nasally or orally) in the stomach up to the 50 cm mark. First, the gastric balloon is inflated with 100 mL increments and the pressure is measured. If the pressure is >15 mm Hg, the balloon may be in the esophagus and it needs to be deflated, and the tube is advanced further, till it is correctly positioned. Then the gastric balloon is inflated with 450–500 mL of air, and the ports are clamped. Proper placement can be confirmed by irrigating the gastric aspiration port with water while auscultating over the stomach. The tube is pulled back gently until resistance is felt. The tube is put on a traction device (0.45–0.91 kg, generally a 0.5 L saline bottle) using a pulley.

The gastric port is aspirated to check for bleeding. If bleeding continues, the esophageal balloon is inflated to the lowest pressure needed to stop bleeding (30–45 mm Hg) and then the port is clamped. A periodic watch is kept on the balloon pressure. If bleeding still continues, the traction is increased further to a maximum of 1.1 kg. Once bleeding is controlled, esophageal balloon pressure is decreased by 5 mm Hg every 3 hours to 25 mm Hg. This pressure is maintained for 12–24 hours. The esophageal balloon should be deflated for 5 minutes every 6 hours to help prevent esophageal necrosis. If bleeding recurs, the gastric balloon and, if necessary, the esophageal balloon may be reinflated for an additional 24 hours.

The SB tube and Minnesota tube are devices which provide a balloon tamponade and can be temporarily used in uncontrollable hemorrhage. The *SB tube* is 85 cm long, and comes in various sizes, from 14 to 21 Fr. Air is filled in increments of 100 mL and up to 250–300 mL for an SB tube and 400 mL for a Minnesota tube once 50 cm of the tube has been inserted. Check pressures at each step. Withdraw till resistance is felt (30–35 cm). Appropriate esophageal pressures are 25–30 mm Hg up to a maximum of 40 mm Hg. Traction is usually 1–2 kg, which is equivalent to a 500-mL fluid bag. Always get an X-ray chest with upper abdomen done after insertion to rule out esophageal placement of the gastric balloon. If the bleeding has stopped, then it should be deflated by 10 mm Hg every 2 hours. Tracheal intubation will then be needed and to avoid esophageal rupture, ensure proper device placement prior to inflation. To avoid necrosis, it should be removed within 24–36 hours and pressures kept at 15 mm Hg.[25] The ESGE suggests that for persistent esophageal variceal bleeding despite vasoactive pharmacological and endoscopic hemostasis therapy, self-expandable metal stents are preferred over balloon tamponade for bridging to definitive hemostasis therapy.[1]

Contraindications for the use of the SB tube:
- Unprotected airway
- Esophageal rupture (e.g., Boerhaave syndrome)
- Esophageal stricture
- Uncertainty regarding the source of bleeding, i.e., duodenal bleed
- Well-controlled variceal bleeding

Q7. What is the role of interventional radiology?

Transjugular intrahepatic portosystemic shunt (TIPS)
A portosystemic shunt is created across the liver parenchyma with the target to rapidly reduce portal pressures. The ESGE recommends that in patients at high risk of recurrent acute variceal bleeding following successful endoscopic management [Child–Pugh C ≤13, Child–Pugh B >7 with active EVH at the time of endoscopy despite vasoactive agents, or hepatic venous pressure gradient (HVPG) >20 mm Hg], pre-emptive TIPS within 72 hours (preferably within 24 hours) must be considered.[1] TIPS is contraindicated in primary prevention, severe pulmonary hypertension (pulmonary arterial pressure >45 mm Hg), polycystic liver disease, uncontrolled systemic infection, unrelieved biliary obstruction, moderate pulmonary hypertension, severe congestive cardiac failure, and advanced cirrhosis (Child C).[23]

Balloon-occluded retrograde transvenous obliteration (BRTO) is a relatively newer radiologic technique used for the management of gastric varices with large gastrosystemic shunts, mainly gastrorenal shunts. The goal of treatment is to obliterate the varices and their feeding shunts.[27] The ESGE suggests BRTO for gastric variceal bleeding when there is a failure of endoscopic hemostasis or early recurrent bleeding.[1]

Q8. What is the role of nonselective beta-blockers in the presence of varices and variceal bleed? Discuss the grades of varices and the indications for the use of beta-blockers.

At all sites where the portal and systemic circulations communicate, collaterals develop as sequelae of portal hypertension, and this is accompanied by splanchnic vasodilatation. The portal sinusoidal pressure can be determined by the HVPG. This can be obtained by passing a balloon catheter under radiologic guidance into the hepatic vein via the femoral or the internal jugular vein. HVPG predicts the risk of developing varices and the overall prognosis **(Table 7)**.[28]

TABLE 7: Prognostic value of hepatic venous pressure gradient (HVPG) in patients with chronic liver disease.[29]

Value (mm Hg)	Significance
1–5	Normal
6–10	Preclinical sinusoidal portal hypertension
≥10	Clinically significant portal hypertension
≥12	Increased risk of rupture of varices
≥16	Increased risk of mortality
≥20	Treatment failure and increased risk of mortality in acute variceal bleed

The following is the summary of the terminology used to describe prophylaxis of variceal bleeding.[27]

Preprimary prophylaxis: It is the prevention of the development of varices in patients with portal hypertension. In a large, multicenter, placebo-controlled, double-blinded trial that enrolled participants with compensated cirrhosis (i.e., those patients who did not have ascites, encephalopathy, jaundice, or varices), investigators showed that nonselective beta-blockers do not prevent the development of varices and are associated with unwanted side effects **(Table 8)**.

Primary prophylaxis: It is the prevention of variceal hemorrhage in patients with known esophageal varices but no history of variceal hemorrhage.

Small esophageal varices: Nonselective beta-blockers (NSBBs) may slow down variceal formation in patients with small esophageal varices that have not bled but have not been shown any survival advantage.[30] Since they has potential for side effects, they are recommended only for those at higher risk of hemorrhage, small varices that have red marks or red spots, or those with Child–Turcotte–Pugh (CTP) class C cirrhosis with annual follow-up.

Medium and large esophageal varices: For patients with medium/large varices, the use of a nonselective beta-blocker or treatment with EVL has been shown to significantly reduce the risk of variceal bleeding. For patients with medium/large varices, the 2016 American Association for the Study of Liver Diseases (AASLD) prevention guidance recommends primary prophylaxis with either (1) a NSBBs-propranolol or nadolol or carvedilol, or (2) endoscopic variceal ligation. The use of combination therapy with a NSBBs or carvedilol and endoscopic variceal ligation are not recommended.[29]

Gastric varices: The data for primary prophylaxis for typical fundo-varicael varices or isolated fundic varices is more

TABLE 8: Recommended beta-blockers for primary prophylaxis against variceal bleeding.[29]

Drug	Initial dose		Titration of the dose	Maximum dose	Goal
	No ascites	With ascites			
Carvedilol	6.25–12.5 mg OD	NA	↑ 6.25 mg BD after 3 days	12.5 mg/day [not in persistent hypertension (HTN)]	Systolic pressure ≥90 mm Hg
Nadolol (nonselective beta-blocker)	10–20 mg OD	10–20 mg OD	↑ every 2–3 days till either maximum dose or treatment goal achieved	• 160 mg (without ascites) • 80 mg (with ascites)	• Systolic pressure ≥90 mm Hg • Resting heart rate (HR) 55–60/min
Propranolol (nonselective beta-blocker)	20–40 mg OD	10–20 mg OD	↑ every 2–3 days till either maximum dose or treatment goal achieved	• 320 mg (without ascites) • 160 mg (with ascites)	• Systolic pressure ≥90 mm Hg • Resting HR 55–60/min

limited, but the 2016 AASLD guideline recommends using the same NSBBs dosing goals used for esophageal varices.[29]

NSBBs should be used with caution in patients with refractory ascites because it is in these patients that NSBBs can lead to a decrease in renal perfusion pressure and acute kidney injury. It is important that mean arterial pressure is maintained at greater than 65 mm Hg in patients with ascites because this will not only prevent kidney injury, but it is the threshold pressure that has been associated with improved survival. In addition, it should be noted that the maximal recommended doses of NSBBs are lower compared with patients without ascites.

Q9. How will you approach a patient with recurrent bleed, after it was treated and stopped once?

Secondary prophylaxis: Untreated cirrhotic patients with a history of variceal bleeding have a 60% risk of rebleeding within 1 year. The risk of dying with each rebleeding episode is approximately 20%. Modalities used to prevent rebleeding are considered secondary prophylaxis of variceal bleeding.

Pharmacologic therapy
NSBBs can reduce the risk of rebleeding by about 40% and improve overall survival by 20%. Side effects of adding isosorbide mononitrate to a NSBBs are more, hence its recommended to use NSBBs without isosorbide mononitrate. ESGE recommends the use of NSBBs propranolol or carvedilol in combination with endoscopic therapy for secondary prophylaxis.[1]

Endoscopic variceal ligation therapy
Endoscopic variceal ligation therapy is superior to sclerotherapy for secondary prophylaxis. It decreases the rebleeding rate to around 32%. Endoscopic sessions should be repeated every 7–28 days until the varices are eradicated and then surveillance endoscopy should be repeated every 3–6 months.[29]

Combination therapy
Combination therapy of a nonselective beta-blocker and EVL therapy is superior to either modality alone for secondary prophylaxis of variceal bleeding as it decreases the rebleeding rate to about 14–23%. There is no statistical difference in mortality but combination therapy is considered the standard first-line therapy for secondary prophylaxis of variceal bleeding.[31]

Transjugular intrahepatic portosystemic shunt
Placement of TIPS has been shown to be superior to EVL therapy and pharmacologic therapy in reducing the risk of rebleeding. TIPS does not improves mortality nor does it decrease the incidence of hepatic encephalopathy. If a patient had placement of a TIPS during an acute bleeding episode, they do not need additional therapy for portal hypertension or varices, but they should be referred for liver transplantation evaluation.[32] If a patient has rebleeding after combination therapy with nonselective beta-blockers and EVL therapy, placement of a TIPS is the recommended rescue therapy.

Portacaval shunt surgery
Surgical placement of a portacaval shunt is effective in preventing rebleeding; this procedure, however, does not improve survival, increases the risk of developing hepatic encephalopathy, and has largely been replaced by TIPS. Portacaval shunt surgery is primarily reserved for patients with CTP class A liver disease.

Gastric varices
The combination of nonselective beta-blocker and endoscopic therapy can be used for secondary variceal hemorrhage prophylaxis for gastroesophageal varices but for fundal varices, TIPS and/or BRTO (transvenous occlusion of gastro- or splenorenal collateral via the left renal vein using sclerosants or embolic agents) can be performed.[29]

Q10. What is the role of thromboelastography (TEG) in the presence of bleeding?

Coagulation abnormalities seen in patients with liver disease include INR, aPTT, PT, thrombocytopenia, and elevated D-dimer. These values worsen as liver failure progresses.[33] Since they only reflect changes in procoagulant factors, these tests are very poor at predicting the risk of bleeding in individuals with liver disease. Therefore, viscoelastic testing such as TEG or thromboelastometry (ROTEM) is being studied in patients with liver disease and used during liver transplantation.[34] Dynamic changes in clot formation and lysis can be assessed from the changes in torque between a pin and a cup that occur as blood clots from the trace produced in both. In TEG, the cup rotates, and the pin is stationary; in ROTEM, the pin rotates, and the cup is stationary **(Flowchart 1)**.

Studies of TEG and ROTEM in patients with liver disease confirm relatively preserved hemostatic function despite a prolonged INR; hence, blood products are used judiciously. The drawback is that they may not pick up subtle changes. Parameters most likely to be abnormal in cirrhosis are the clot formation time and the maximum clot firmness with a normal coagulation time as seen in a small study comparing ROTEM parameters in blood samples from 51 patients with cirrhosis.[35] Viscoelastic testing may be able to predict hypercoagulability in liver disease.[35] **Table 9** compares the values of TEG and ROTEM, and how one can use these values to guide the management.

Multiple choice questions:

1. Intravenous erythromycin must be administered how much time before an endoscopy procedure?
   a. 10 minutes
   b. 15 minutes
   c. 20 minutes
   d. 40 minutes
2. In nonvariceal UGI bleed, infusion of PPI should be continued for how long after bolus dose?
   a. 6 hours
   b. 24 hours
   c. 72 hours
   d. 12 hours

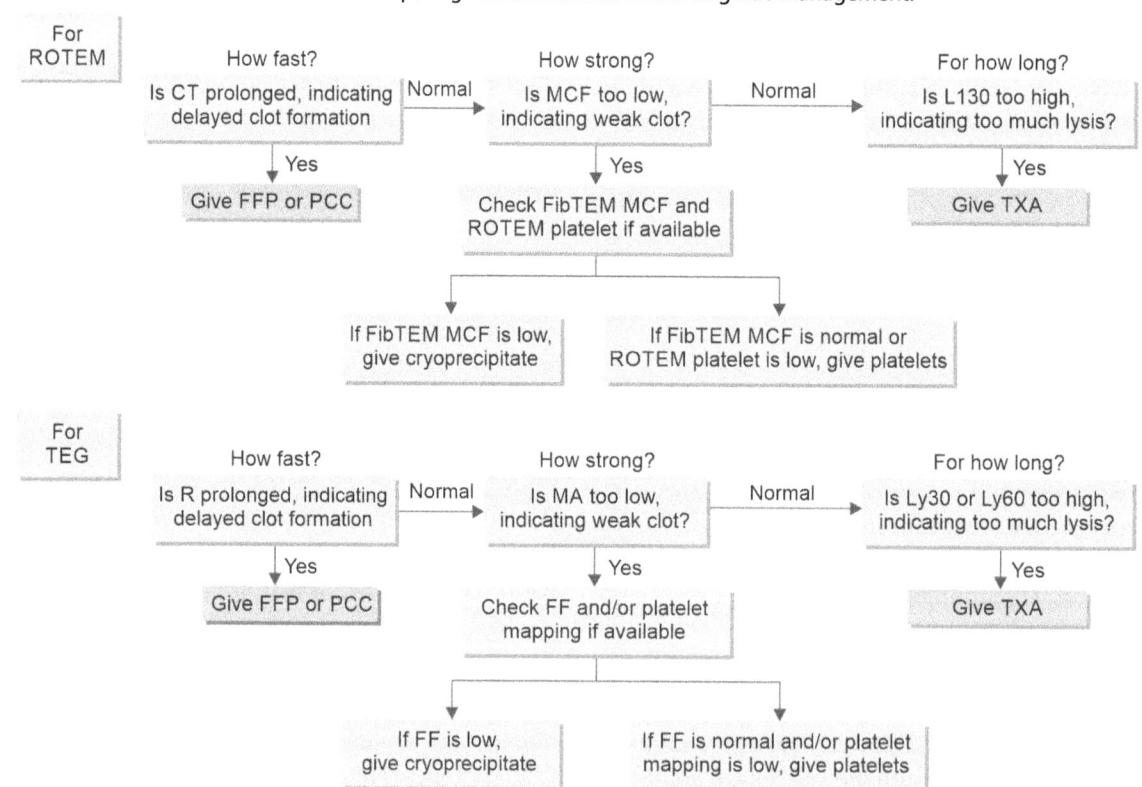

Flowchart 1: Comparing TEG and ROTEM values to guide management.[37]

(CT: computed tomography; FF: functional fibrinogen; FFP: fresh frozen plasma; MA: maximum amplitude; MCF: maximum clot firmness; PCC: prothrombin complex concentrate; ROTEM: thromboelastometry; TEG: thromboelastography; TXA: tranexamic acid)

TABLE 9: Comparing TEG and ROTEM values and treatment options.[36]

ROTEM	TEG	Coagulopathy	Treatment options
ExTEM CT 80–100 seconds InTEM CT 200–240 seconds	R 10–14 minutes	↓ Coagulation factors	FFP 20 mL/kg
ExTEM CT >100 seconds InTEM CT >240 seconds	R >14 minutes	↓↓ Coagulation factors	FFP 30 mL/kg
FibTEM MCF 6–9 mm	FF_{MA} 7–14 mm	↓ Fibrinogen	FFP 20 mL/kg or cryoprecipitate 3 mL/kg or fibrinogen concentrate 20 mg/kg
FibTEM MCF 0–6 mm	FF_{MA} 0–7 mm	↓↓ Fibrinogen	FFP 30 mL/kg or cryoprecipitate 5 mL/kg or fibrinogen concentrate 30 mg/kg
ExTEM A_{10} 35–42 mm or ExTEM MCF <50 mm and FibTEM >10 mm	MA 45–49 mm and FF_{MA} >14 mm	↓ Platelets	Platelet 5 mL/kg
ExTEM A_{10} <35 mm and FibTEM >10 mm	MA <45 mm and FF_{MA} >14 mm	↓↓ Platelets	Platelet 10 mL/kg
ExTEM Li30 <94%	Ly30 >8%	Hyperfibrinolysis	TXA 1–2 g IV or 10–20 mg/kg
InTEM CT/HepTEM CT >1.25	Difference in R HepTEG R >2 minutes	Heparinization	• Protamine 50–100 mg or • FFP 10–20 mL/kg

[A_{10}: amplitude after 10 minutes (normal range ExTEM A10 43–65 mm, InTEM A10 7–3 mm); CT: clotting time (normal range ExTEM CT 38–79 seconds, InTEM CT 100–240 seconds); FF_{MA}: functional fibrinogen maximum amplitude (normal range 14–24 mm); FFP: fresh frozen plasma; Ly30: hyperfibrinolysis after 30 minutes (normal range < 8%); MA: maximum amplitude (normal range 51–69 mm); MCF: maximum clot firmness (normal range ExTEM MCF 50–72 mm); R: reaction time (normal range 3–8 minutes); ROTEM: thromboelastometry; TEG: thromboelastography; TXA: tranexamic acid]

REFERENCES

1. Gralnek IM, Camus Duboc M, Garcia-Pagan JC, Fuccio L, Karstensen JG, Hucl T, et al. Endoscopic diagnosis and management of esophagogastric variceal hemorrhage: European Society of Gastrointestinal Endoscopy (ESGE) Guideline. Endoscopy. 2022;54(11):1094-120.
2. Hayat U, Lee PJ, Ullah H, Sarvepalli S, Lopez R, Vargo JJ. Association of prophylactic endotracheal intubation in critically ill patients with upper GI bleeding and cardiopulmonary unplanned events. Gastrointest Endosc. 2017;86:500-9.e1.
3. Kim J. Management and prevention of upper GI bleed. PSAP VII Gasterentol Nutr. 2012;7-26.
4. Blatchford O, Murray WR, Blatchford M. A risk score to predict need for treatment for upper-gastrointestinal haemorrhage. Lancet. 2000;356:1318-21.
5. Lahiff C, Shields W, Cretu I, Mahmud N, McKiernan S, Norris S, et al. Upper gastrointestinal bleeding: predictors of risk in a mixed patient group including variceal and nonvariceal haemorrhage. Eur J Gastroenterol Hepatol. 2012;24:149-54.
6. Rockall TA, Logan RF, Devlin HB, Northfield TC. Risk assessment after acute upper gastrointestinal haemorrhage. Gut. 1996;38:316-21.
7. Saltzman JR, Tabak YP, Hyett BH, Sun X, Travis AC, Johannes RS. A simple risk score accurately predicts in-hospital mortality, length of stay, and cost in acute upper GI bleeding. Gastrointest Endosc. 2011;74:1215-24.
8. Cappell MS, Friedel D. Initial management of acute upper gastrointestinal bleeding: from initial evaluation up to gastrointestinal endoscopy. Med Clin North Am. 2008;92:491-509.
9. Richards RJ, Donica MB, Grayer D. Can the blood urea nitrogen/creatinine ratio distinguish upper from lower gastrointestinal bleeding? J Clin Gastroenterol. 1990;12:500-4.
10. Patil V, Shetmahajan M. Massive transfusion and massive transfusion protocol. Indian J Anaesth. 2014;58:590-5.
11. Villanueva C, Colomo A, Bosch A, Concepción M, Hernandez-Gea V, Aracil C, et al. Transfusion strategies for acute upper gastrointestinal bleeding. N Engl J Med. 2013;368:11-21.
12. Holcomb JB, Tilley BC, Baraniuk S, Fox EE, Wade CE, Podbielski JM, et al. Transfusion of plasma, platelets, and red blood cells in a 1:1:1 vs a 1:1:2 ratio and mortality in patients with severe trauma: the PROPPR randomized clinical trial. JAMA. 2015;313(5):471-82.
13. Yen AW. Blood transfusion strategies for acute upper gastrointestinal bleeding: are we back where we started? Clin Transl Gastroenterol. 2018;9:150.
14. Hyett BH, Abougergi MS, Charpentier JP, Kumar NL, Brozovic S, Claggett BL, et al. The AIMS65 score compared with the Glasgow-Blatchford score in predicting outcomes in upper GI bleeding. Gastrointest Endosc. 2013;77:551-7.
15. Dorward S, Sreedharan A, Leontiadis GI, Howden CW, Moayyedi P, Forman D. Proton pump inhibitor treatment initiated prior to endoscopic diagnosis in upper gastrointestinal bleeding. Cochrane Database Syst Rev. 2006; CD005415.
16. Barkun AN, Bardou M, Martel M, Gralnek IM, Sung JJY. Prokinetics in acute upper GI bleeding: a meta-analysis. Gastrointest Endosc. 2010;72:1138-45.

17. Seo YS, Park SY, Kim MY, Kim JH, Park JY, Yim HJ, et al. Lack of difference among terlipressin, somatostatin, and octreotide in the control of acute gastroesophageal variceal hemorrhage. Hepatology. 2014;60:954-63.
18. Chavez-Tapia NC, Barrientos-Gutierrez T, Tellez-Avila F, Soares-Weiser K, Mendez-Sanchez N, Gluud C, et al. Meta-analysis: antibiotic prophylaxis for cirrhotic patients with upper gastrointestinal bleeding—an updated Cochrane review. Aliment Pharmacol Ther. 2011;34:509-18.
19. Bennett C, Klingenberg SL, Langholz E, Gluud LL. Tranexamic acid for upper gastrointestinal bleeding. Cochrane Database Syst Rev. 2014;2014:CD006640.
20. Roberts I, Still HS, Afolabi A, Akere A, Arribas M, Brenner A, et al. Effects of a high-dose 24-h infusion of tranexamic acid on death and thromboembolic events in patients with acute gastrointestinal bleeding (HALT-IT): an international randomised, double-blind, placebo-controlled trial. Lancet. 2020;1927-36.
21. Martí-Carvajal AJ, Karakitsiou DE, Salanti G. Human recombinant activated factor VII for upper gastrointestinal bleeding in patients with liver diseases. Cochrane Database Syst Rev. 2012:CD004887.
22. Gralnek IM, Stanley AJ, Morris AJ, Camus M, Lau J, Lanas A, et al. Endoscopic diagnosis and management of nonvariceal upper gastrointestinal haemorrhage (NVUGIH): European Society of Gastrointestinal Endoscopy (ESGE) Guideline—Update 2021. Endoscopy. 2021;53(3):300-32.
23. Wolf AT, Wasan SK, Saltzman JR. Impact of anticoagulation on rebleeding following endoscopic therapy for nonvariceal upper gastrointestinal hemorrhage. Am J Gastroenterol. 2007;102:290-6.
24. Barkun A, Bardou M, Kuipers E, Sung J, Hunt RH, Martel M, et al. International consensus recommendations on the management of patients with nonvariceal upper gastrointestinal bleeding. Ann Intern Med. 2010;152:101-13.
25. National Institute for Health and Care Excellence (NICE). (2012). Acute upper gastrointestinal bleeding in over 16s: management. [online] Available from: https://www.nice.org.uk/guidance/cg141. [Last accessed July, 2023].
26. Nadler J, Stankovic N, Uber A, Holmberg MJ, Sanchez LD, Wolfe RE, et al. Outcomes in variceal hemorrhage following the use of a balloon tamponade device. Am J Emerg Med. 2017;35:1500-2.
27. MA Saad WE, Sabri SS. Balloon-occluded Retrograde Transvenous Obliteration (BRTO): Technical results and outcomes. Semin Intervent Radiol. 2011;28(3):333-8.
28. Tripathi D, Stanley AJ, Hayes P, Patch D, Millson C, Mehrzad H, et al. U.K. guidelines on the management of variceal haemorrhage in cirrhotic patients. Gut. 2015;64:1680-704.
29. Garcia-Tsao G, Bosch J. Varices and variceal hemorrhage in cirrhosis: a new view of an old problem. Clin Gastroenterol Hepatol. 2015;13:2109-17.
30. Garcia-Tsao G, Abraldes JG, Berzigotti A, Bosch J. Portal hypertensive bleeding in cirrhosis: risk stratification, diagnosis, and management: 2016 practice guidance by the American Association for the study of liver diseases. Hepatology. 2017;65:310-35.
31. Merkel C, Marin R, Angeli P, Zanella P, Felder M, Bernardinello E, et al. A placebo-controlled clinical trial of nadolol in the prophylaxis of growth of small esophageal varices in cirrhosis. Gastroenterology. 2004;127:476-84.
32. Sarin SK, Wadhawan M, Agarwal SR, Tyagi P, Sharma BC. Endoscopic variceal ligation plus propranolol versus endoscopic variceal ligation alone in primary prophylaxis of variceal bleeding. Am J Gastroenterol. 2005;100:797-800.
33. Rudler M, Cluzel P, Corvec TL, Benosman H, Rousseau G, Poynard T, et al. Early-TIPSS placement prevents rebleeding in high-risk patients with variceal bleeding, without improving survival. Aliment Pharmacol Ther. 2014;40:1074-80.
34. Weeder PD, Porte RJ, Lisman T. Hemostasis in liver disease: implications of new concepts for perioperative management. Transfus Med Rev. 2014;28:107-13.
35. Davis JPE, Northup PG, Caldwell SH, Intagliata NM. Viscoelastic testing in liver disease. Ann Hepatol. 2018;17:205-13.
36. Tripodi A, Primignani M, Chantarangkul V, Viscardi Y, Dell'Era A, Fabris FM, et al. The coagulopathy of cirrhosis assessed by thromboelastometry and its correlation with conventional coagulation parameters. Thrombin Res. 2009;124:132-6.
37. Whiting D, DiNardo JA. TEG and ROTEM: technology and clinical applications. Am J Hematology. 2014;89:228-32.

Oncologic Emergencies

Suhail Sarwar Siddiqui, Syed Nabeel Muzaffar, Atul Prabhakar Kulkarni

CASE STUDY

A 36-year-old male, recently diagnosed with acute myeloid leukemia (AML) presented to the casualty with respiratory distress. On arrival to intensive care unit (ICU), he is tachycardic [heart rate (HR)—120 beats/min], and tachypneic [respiratory rate (RR)—30 breaths/min], but normotensive [systolic blood pressure (SBP) 130 mm Hg].

His oxygen saturation is 99% on room air. The investigations are hemoglobin (Hb)—6.6 g/dL, white blood cell (WBC)—100,000/mm^3, platelets—86,000/cubic mm (cumm). The urea is 66 mg/dL, uric acid (UA) 16 mg/dL, and serum creatinine (Cr) 2.1 mg/dL. The electrolyte values are Na$^+$ 146 mEq/L, K$^+$ 6.1 mEq/L, Cl$^-$ 110 milliequivalent/liter (mEq/L) and HCO$_3^-$ 18 mEq/L. The arterial blood gas (ABG) reveals partial pressure of arterial oxygen (PaO$_2$) 46 mm Hg, partial pressure of carbon dioxide (PCO$_2$) 46 mm Hg and O$_2$ saturation to be 86%.

Echocardiography revealed normal right ventricle (RV) and left ventricle (LV) function. There were scattered B lines in both lung bases. The urine output was 15 mL/h for the past 2 hours.

Q1. What are the current issues in this patient? How will you manage the patient?

Specific problems that need to be addressed in this patient are:
- Acute respiratory failure (ARF)
- Acute kidney injury (AKI)
- Dyselectrolytemia
- Hyperleukocytosis and hyperuricemia
- Hematologic dysfunction

These problems may be malignancy-related, treatment-related, or an infective complication secondary to immunosuppression. We need to employ a systematic and comprehensive organ-wise evaluation approach.

In immunocompromised patients, hypoxemic ARF is the leading cause of ICU admission.[1]

Etiology of ARF[2,3]

The ARF may be of either infectious or noninfectious origin:
- *Infectious etiology:* Pulmonary infections (bacteria, viruses, fungi, mycobacteria, *Nocardia*, *Pneumocystis*, etc.)
- *Noninfectious etiology:* Comorbidities [e.g., chronic obstructive pulmonary disease (COPD), interstitial lung disease, etc.], malignancy-related direct pulmonary involvement, cancer-related medical disorders, chemotherapy-induced respiratory failure, pulmonary edema, pulmonary thromboembolism, and pleural effusion.

Management of acute respiratory failure

As invasive mechanical ventilation (IMV) in these patients is associated with high mortality, therefore, strategies, which improve oxygenation noninvasively (without delaying IMV when required), should be tried first.[4]

Factors such as undetermined ARF etiology, delayed ICU admission, noninvasive ventilation (NIV) failure, and invasive fungal infection (IFI) have been shown to increase mortality to 60% in these patients.[5-8]

Noninvasive ventilation in immunocompromised patients with acute respiratory failure[9]

The BRICNet (Brazilian Research in Intensive Care Network) study to evaluate clinical characteristics and outcome of patients with cancer requiring ventilation showed that IMV as initial ventilatory strategy, NIV followed by IMV, and sequential organ failure assessment (SOFA) score were associated with increased hospital mortality.[10] The recent Efraim multinational prospective cohort study in critically ill immunocompromised patients with ARF concluded that patients with unknown ARF etiology and IMV [first-line IMV or after standard oxygen/NIV/high-flow nasal cannula (HFNC)/NIV + HFNC failure] had high hospital mortality rates.[4]

Thus, avoiding IMV and an appropriate diagnostic approach for determining the etiology of ARF are essential.

Moreover, the selected oxygenation device should be able to facilitate the required diagnostic workup.

The evidence for benefit of NIV in immunocompromised patients with ARF is based upon many observational studies and only two small randomized controlled trials (RCTs) with heterogeneous population.[11,12]

However, recent RCTs have failed to show benefit of early NIV in ARF. Still, the utility of NIV cannot be negated as these studies had limitations like being underpowered, allowing crossover between the arms, and use of HFNC in both NIV and control groups.[13,14]

Table 1 summarizes the RCTs comparing NIV and conventional oxygen therapy in immunocompromised patients with hypoxemic ARF.

According to a recent systematic review and meta-analysis, early use of NIV could reduce intubation rates and short-term mortality in selected patients. Although further studies are needed to identify for which patients NIV could be beneficial.[15] A retrospective study showed that factors such as acute respiratory distress syndrome (ARDS), delay between admission and first NIV use, RR when on NIV, ARDS, need for vasopressors, or renal replacement therapy (RRT) were independently associated with NIV failure **(Table 2)**.[5,8,16]

As suggested by Peñuelas and Esteban, "selecting patients for NIV, closely monitoring the response, identifying failure of NIV, stopping NIV, and proceeding to IMV" are crucial steps for ensuring success of NIV.[17]

The criteria for terminating NIV and endotracheal intubation (ETI) and invasive ventilation in immunocompromised patients are:
- Inability to tolerate interface
- Agitation under sedation
- Coma or seizures (for airway protection)
- Copious tracheal secretions
- *Persistent dyspnea:* Tachypnea or use of accessory respiratory muscles
- *Hypoxemia:* PaO_2 ≤65 at fraction of inspired oxygen (FiO_2) 0.6 or PaO_2/FiO_2 <85 or PaO_2/FiO_2 <150 (after 1 hour of NIV)[5-8]
- *Respiratory acidemia:* Increase in PCO_2 with pH ≤7.3
- Severe hemodynamic instability

TABLE 1: Randomized controlled trials (RCTs) of noninvasive ventilation (NIV) in immunocompromised patients with acute respiratory failure (ARF).

	Antonelli et al.[11]	*Hilbert et al.*[12]	*Wermke et al.*[13]	*Lemiale et al.*[14]
Setting	Single-center ICU n = 40	Single-center ICU n = 52	Single-center, hematology ward n = 86	Multicenter, 28 ICUs France and Belgium n = 374
Study population	Solid organ transplant recipients	Hematologic cancer with neutropenia (postchemotherapy or bone marrow transplant), solid organ transplant recipients, steroid or cytotoxic therapy for nonmalignant disease, and AIDS	Allogeneic, hematopoietic stem cell transplant	Hematologic cancer, solid tumor, solid organ transplant recipients, steroids >1 mg/kg/day or >30 days, immunosuppressive drugs in high dose for or >30 days
Intervention arm	NIV (by facemask) PS set to obtain: • Vt 8–10 mL/kg • RR <25 • Patient comfort	NIV (by facemask) PS set to obtain: • Vt 7–10 mL/kg • RR <25 • FiO_2 for SpO_2 >90% PEEP 2–10	NIV (by facemask) PS 15 and PEEP 7 cm initially; titrated as per patient comfort and blood gases	NIV (by facemask) PS set to obtain: • Vt 7–10 mL/kg • PEEP 2–10 cm • FiO_2 and PEEP for SpO_2 ≥92%
Control arm	Oxygen by Venturi mask	Oxygen by Venturi mask	Oxygen by nasal insufflation or Venturi mask	Oxygenation methods and HFNC at clinician's discretion
Primary outcome	Need for ETI and IMV	Need for ETI and IMV	100-day mortality	28-day mortality
Results	Reduction in patients requiring ETI in NIV group	Reduction in patients requiring ETI in NIV group	No difference	No difference
Remark	Patients with cardiogenic pulmonary edema included		Crossover from control to NIV group	Underpowered, HFNC used in control group

(AIDS: acquired immune deficiency syndrome; ETI: endotracheal intubation; FiO_2: fraction of inspired oxygen; HFNC: high-flow nasal cannula; IMV: invasive mechanical ventilation; n: number of patients; PEEP: positive end-expiratory pressure; PS: pressure support; RR: respiratory rate; SpO_2: peripheral oxygen saturation; Vt: tidal volume)

TABLE 2: Risk factors for noninvasive ventilation (NIV) failure in patients with acute respiratory failure (ARF).	
Prior to NIV	• Airway involvement by malignancy • Delay between admission and first NIV use, unknown etiology of ARF • ARDS • Need for vasopressors or RRT, multiple organ failure
During NIV	• Unknown ARF etiology, tachypnea >30/min • No improvement of ABG within 6 hours, not tolerating NIV • Clinical deterioration NIV dependency ≥3 days

(ARDS: acute respiratory distress syndrome; ABG: arterial blood gas; RRT: renal replacement therapy)

High-flow nasal cannula in immunocompromised patients with acute respiratory failure

The HFNC improves oxygenation by delivering a mixture of air and oxygen (constant FiO_2 0.21–1.0) through nasal cannulae (better tolerance) at high flows (up to 40–60 L/min) at normal body temperature and with 100% humidification. It was initially developed for use in neonates and is recently gaining popularity for use in adults. There is still much debate regarding its role in critically ill population but as of now, HFNC may be used as an intermediate therapy between standard oxygen therapy and NIV.[18-22] HFNC has shown conflicting and poor quality data in immunocompromised patients with ARF.[23]

In this case, the patient is tachypneic but is maintaining good oxygenation [peripheral oxygen saturation (SpO_2): 99%] 99% on room air. The discrepancy between pulse oximetry and ABG vis-à-vis oxygenation may be attributed to "leukocyte larceny" (see below) secondary to hyperleukocytosis.[24] There are scattered bibasal B lines at lung bases which may be attributed to septal edema (pulmonary edema) due to either cardiogenic (unlikely as 2D echocardiography reveals normal biventricular function) or noncardiogenic causes (inflammation either due to infectious or noninfectious causes).[25] As this patient is hypercapnic, despite being tachypneic, indicating respiratory muscle fatigue. Since the patient is conscious and has protective airway reflexes, NIV can be used to start with. The positive end-expiratory pressure (PEEP) during NIV can decrease the extravascular lung water.[9]

Early diagnosis and prompt initiation of antimicrobial coverage help to reduce morbidity and mortality. Advanced diagnostic modalities [i.e., such as polymerase chain reaction (PCR)-based methods] facilitate early and effective therapy. Invasive procedures [including fiberoptic bronchoscopy, biopsy, video-assisted thoracoscopic surgery (VATS)] are essential in view of the possibility of varied pulmonary pathogens, and the need to establish a specific diagnosis.[3]

NIV is of great help in performing diagnostic and therapeutic fiberoptic bronchoscopy [e.g., for obtaining bronchoalveolar lavage (BAL) samples, removing mucous plugs, etc.] by preventing procedure-related gas exchange deterioration.

Besides ARF, this patient also has AKI and dyselectrolytemia as manifested by oliguria, acidemia (metabolic and respiratory components), hyperkalemia, hypernatremia, and hyperuricemia.

The AKI is common in patients like this, due to either cancer or therapy-related injuries or other causes (see below) and is associated with increased morbidity and mortality in patients.[26,27]

- *Cancer-related injury:*
  - Obstructive nephropathy (due to retroperitoneal lymphadenopathy)
  - Tumor infiltration of kidneys
  - Direct tubular injury (associated with lysozymuria)
  - Hemophagocytic lymphohistiocytosis with acute interstitial disease
  - Vascular occlusion [associated with disseminated intravascular coagulation (DIC) and hyperleukocytosis]
  - Glomerular diseases
  - Hypercalcemia
- *Therapy-related injury:*
  - Tumor lysis syndrome (TLS) with acute UA nephropathy
  - Nephrotoxicity
  - Intratubular obstruction from medications (e.g., methotrexate)
- *Other causes:*
  - Renal hypoperfusion
    - Hypovolemia (diarrhea, vomiting, and third spacing)
    - Cardiomyopathy, cirrhosis, nephrotic syndrome
    - Shock of various etiologies
  - Sepsis

As AKI can be secondary to diverse etiologies and the management should focus the cause of AKI. In this patient, acute UA nephropathy needs to be specifically tackled.

If the patient is hypovolemic (as might be expected from tachycardia and oliguria), hemodynamic monitoring including indices of fluid responsiveness and tissue perfusion monitoring and lung ultrasound (monitoring B lines) can help in guiding fluid therapy.[28] The fluid infused should be a balanced crystalloid solution (e.g., Ringer's lactate and plasmalyte, sterofundin) because the electrolyte composition is similar to plasma (therefore not normal saline).[29] Hyperkalemia needs urgent treatment, decision to offer RRT is complex and needs to take into the account likelihood of reversibility of AKI, likely long-term prognosis of cancer and the input from the family.

Thrombotic microangiopathies, thrombotic, or bleeding diathesis may be seen in patients with hematological malignancies. Anemia and thrombocytopenia in AML patients are due to bone marrow infiltration by leukemic cells and bone marrow suppression due to chemotherapy. Thrombocytopenia spectrum may extend from being asymptomatic or patient having life-threatening bleeding. Bleeding complications are seen more often in patients with acute promyelocytic leukemias (AML M3). Major bleeding is defined by International Society on Thrombosis and Haemostasis (ISTH) in nonsurgical patients as fatal bleeding and/or bleeding at critical sites (intracranial, intraspinal, intraocular, pericardial, retroperitoneal, intra-articular, and intramuscular bleed with compartment syndrome) and/or any bleeding event associated with ≥2 g/dL drop in Hb or requiring at least two units of packed red blood cells (PRBCs) transfusion.[30]

Strict vigilance is required to detect intracranial and retroperitoneal bleeding, which if unnoticed can end in mortality. Blood component therapy may be urgently needed at any time during the course of illness. Due to presence of coagulopathy, all invasive procedures should be performed under ultrasound guidance by a skilled person.

Venous thromboembolism (VTE) is not uncommon in hematological malignancies with an incidence between 2 and 12% and a significant impact on morbidity and mortality.[31] Pharmacological treatment and prophylaxis of VTE are challenging owing to the thrombocytopenia. Nonpharmacological methods such as sequential compression devices, for VTE prophylaxis may be safer.[30]

Adequate nutrition is an essential part of the management. Infection control practices need to be strictly adhered to.

A multidisciplinary approach with appropriate organ support is the optimum management plan in this patient.[32]

Q2. Why do you observe a discrepancy between SpO_2 and partial pressure of arterial oxygen from the ABG sample?
This patient has AML with high WBC count (100,000/mm^3). Here, the SpO_2 is 99% and the PaO_2 is 46 mm Hg; this discrepancy is known as "leukocyte larceny", which was first reported by Fox et al. (1979).[33] This phenomenon occurs due to high number of metabolically active cells (leukocytosis of >50,000/mm^3 or severe thrombocytosis) leading to consumption of oxygen, thereby giving spuriously low level of PaO_2 in ABG in patients with normal SpO_2. It is imperative for the intensivists to interpret the low PaO_2 with caution especially if SpO_2 is normal. This helps in avoiding unnecessary investigations and interventions.[34]

Objectively, this is confirmed by increased PaO_2 after leukocyte reduction due to chemotherapy[34] or leukapheresis.[35] It has been suggested that putting ABG sample on ice will slow down the metabolic rate, resulting in an increase in PaO_2.[33,36] Alternatively, use of potassium cyanide or sodium fluoride in ABG samples arrests the ex vivo metabolism by cells and results in increased PaO_2.[33,37]

Q3. What are the causes of AKI in this patient? How will you manage TLS?
Likely, causes of AKI in this patient are enumerated in **Table 3**.

Tumor lysis syndrome is an oncological emergency caused by efflux of intracellular contents of the tumor cells. This can occur either spontaneously or due to cancer therapy (chemotherapy, radiotherapy, interventional radiology, or immunotherapy). It presents with changes in biochemical parameters such as hyperuricemia, hyperphosphatemia, hyperkalemia, and hypocalcemia.[38-40] It can be a laboratory diagnosis or clinical TLS. It is classified using the Cairo-Bishop classification **(Table 4)**.

The risk factors for development of TLS are enumerated in **Table 5**.[42]

Prophylactic measures to reduce the concentration effects of metabolic abnormalities or the extent of kidney injury.

The concentration effects of biochemical abnormalities are myocardial irritability causing fatal cardiac arrhythmias either due to hyperkalemia or hypocalcemia (secondary to hyperphosphatemia-induced precipitation of calcium),

TABLE 3: Causes of acute kidney injury (AKI).

Category	Etiology
Prerenal causes	• Poor oral intake due to anorexia • Fluid loss due to fever, vomiting and diarrhea • *Bleeding due to coagulopathy:* GI bleed and retroperitoneal bleed • *Third spacing of fluid:* Malignant pleural effusion and ascites
Renal causes	• Malignant infiltration of kidney • Crystal induced nephropathy • *Nephrotoxic drugs:* Nonsteroidal anti-inflammatory drugs, radiocontrast agent, antibiotics, nephrotoxic chemotherapeutic agents, e.g., cisplatin and cyclophosphamide
Postrenal causes	Retroperitoneal lymphadenopathy, retroperitoneal hematoma or tumor infiltration causing outflow obstruction
Miscellaneous	Tumor lysis syndrome, sepsis, rhabdomyolysis, raised intra-abdominal pressure due to bowel edema or ascites or enterocolitis

(GI: gastrointestinal)

neuromuscular excitability causing seizures, or laryngospasm or bronchospasm due to hypocalcemia.

The AKI due to crystallization of phosphate or UA crystals. Phosphate crystallizes also with calcium causing further hypocalcemia.

Principles of management of TLS: Prevention of TLS is of prime importance. Prevention of AKI, cardiac arrhythmias, seizures, and management of established renal failure are the basic tenets of management of TLS. Patient at "intermediate" or "high" risk of developing TLS should be transferred to the ICU for continuous hemodynamic and input and output monitoring.[42] Also monitoring of serum levels of sodium, potassium, phosphate, UA, calcium, urea, and Cr should be done 6–8 hourly.

Prevention of acute kidney injury: Intravascular volume repletion: Intravascular volume expansion using intravenous (IV) fluids is done using 2,500–3,000 mL/m² in 24 hours with a target of maintaining 2 mL/kg/h of urine output.[42] Volume expansion dilutes the concentration of biochemicals and reduces their propensity of crystallization. It also improves renal blood flow and excretion of UA, potassium, and phosphate thus lowering their blood levels. It also treats hypotension and decreases in lactic acidosis.[43] If the patient develops fluid overload; a low dose of loop diuretic may be used; however, routine use of diuretic is not recommended.

TABLE 4: Cairo and Bishop classification of tumor lysis syndrome (TLS) adapted from Cairo et al.[41]

Types of TLS	Laboratory TLS	Clinical TLS
Prerequisite	Two or more of the following laboratory abnormalities occurring simultaneously 3 days before or within a week of initiation of tumor-directed therapy	Laboratory TLS with additional one or more of the following findings
Parameters	• *Serum uric acid level:* An absolute value of >8 mg/dL or a rise of 25% or more from baseline • *Serum phosphate level:* An absolute value of >6.5 mg/dL (adults) or >4.5 mg/dL (children) or a rise of 25% or more from baseline • *Serum calcium level:* An absolute value of <7 mg/dL (adults) or a fall of 25% or more from baseline • *Serum potassium level:* >6 mEq/L or 25% rise from baseline	• Cardiac arrhythmia or sudden death • Raised level of serum creatinine to 1.5 times the upper limit of normal value for that age • Seizures or signs of neuromuscular irritability (tetany, paresthesia and laryngospasm)

TABLE 5: Risk factors for tumor lysis syndrome (TLS).[42]

Types	Risk factors	Comments
Tumor-related risk factors	High tumor burden, organ involvement, extensive metastasis extrinsic compression of renal outflow system	• High tumor burden is related to high number of tumor cells in circulation or bulky tumor • Tumor infiltration to other organs such as kidney, spleen, liver, or bone marrow • Extensive and distant spread of tumor • This particular problem is caused by enlarged lymph node or spleen causing postrenal type of acute kidney injury by obstructing the flow of urine
Tumor-related risk factors	• Highly sensitive tumor to anticancer therapy • Short doubling time of tumor • Intensity of tumor-directed therapy	• If the tumor is highly sensitive to cancer-directed therapy, more chances of release of intracellular content of tumor cells • Highly proliferative tumors are highly prone cause TLS • If high intensity tumor-directed therapy is given for a tumor, then there may be rapid lysis of tumor cell beyond the homeostatic capacity of human body
Patient-related risk factors	• Preexisting nephropathy • Dehydration or reduced intravascular volume • Hypotension • Acidic urinary pH • Nephrotoxic drug or agent exposure	• Patients with preexisting nephropathy due to systemic diseases will not be able to handle high intravascular biochemical excess and will rapidly show features of TLS • As a consequence of reduced intravascular volume, the concentration of biochemicals released due to TLS is increased and has high chances of causing symptoms due to crystal formation in renal tubules • Hypotension by causing poor renal perfusion complicates TLS by inability to excrete the biochemicals • As a result of acidic urinary pH, there is decreased solubility of uric acid, thus causing crystallization and renal failure • Exposure to nephrotoxic drugs (vancomycin and aminoglycosides) or agents (radiocontrast dye) lead to accelerated worsening of kidney functions

Management of hyperuricemia: Hypouricemic agents such as allopurinol, febuxostat, or rasburicase can be used to reduce the UA concentrations in blood.

- *Allopurinol:* Allopurinol is a xanthine oxidase inhibitor. Xanthine oxidase is the enzyme that catalyzes the production of UA from xanthine and hypoxanthine.[44,45] Efflux of deoxyribonucleic acid (DNA) from the cells caused its degradation into purines **(Flowchart 1)**.

  Exogenously supplemented UA oxidase (rasburicase) enzyme acts on UA and converts it to allantoin which is more water soluble than UA.

  Allopurinol by inhibiting xanthine oxidase enzyme reduces the formation of UA. However, it increases the concentration of hypoxanthine and xanthine, which can crystallize and can injure the kidney, also allopurinol does not cause any effect on already produced UA.[44] Over and above allopurinol can cause serious hypersensitivity reactions[46] and its metabolite oxypurinol is renally excreted, thus it requires dose reduction in cases of established renal failure.

- *Febuxostat:* Febuxostat is a newer generation oral hypouricemic agent, which inhibits xanthine oxidase enzyme but unlike allopurinol, it does not need dose modification in AKI. It is costly and hence not used much.[47]

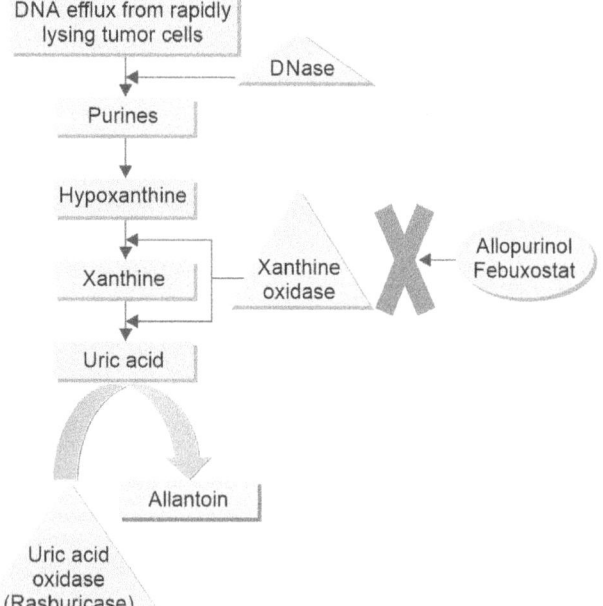

Flowchart 1: Schematic diagram showing deoxyribonucleic acid (DNA) metabolism.

Key: Substrates and products: rectangular shape; gray cross: enzyme inhibition; enzyme inhibitors: oval shape; enzymes: triangular shape; curved arrow shows the step that normally does not occur in humans as they lack uric acid (UA) oxidase enzyme.

- *Rasburicase:* It is United States Food and Drug Administration (US FDA) approved recombinant urate oxidase, which converts UA to allantoin, which is more water soluble[48] and thus reduces UA levels. It is costly, and can cause methemoglobinemia and in severe cases, hemolytic anemia in patients with glucose-6-phosphate dehydrogenase (G6PD) deficiency.[49,50] The patients should be screened for G6PD deficiency before administering rasburicase. It is given as 0.2 mg/kg in 50 mL normal saline over 30 minutes. Duration of treatment once daily for 5 days, however, one dose usually serves the purpose, failing which it can be administered again.

  Rasburicase has ex vivo effect, hence when a patient is on rasburicase, the blood sample should be stored and transported in ice to avoid getting spuriously low levels of serum UA.[47]

Urinary alkalinization: Urinary alkalinization was previously recommended to increase the solubility of UA. However, the alkalinization of urine can lead to phosphate crystallization formation in renal tubules[42] and decreased ionic calcium, worsening hypocalcemia.[47] Our patient has isolated hyperuricemia and phosphate is normal, so urinary alkalinization can be tried with careful monitoring of serum phosphate and ionic calcium levels.

Management of hyperphosphatemia

Hyperphosphatemia is treated with phosphate binders. Continuous renal replacement therapy (CRRT) or extended duration sustained low-efficiency dialysis (SLED) can be offered in the following situations:

- Hyperphosphatemia refractory to phosphate binders
- Established renal failure
- The product of serum calcium and phosphate concentration >60 mg^2/dL.

Prevention of life-threatening cardiac arrhythmias

Life-threatening cardiac arrhythmias can occur in presence of hyperkalemia and/or hypocalcemia. Hyperkalemia should be managed by reducing exogenous potassium supplementation, β_2 agonist inhalation, glucose insulin drip, and potassium binders. IV soda bicarbonate should be used only if acidosis is deemed to be the cause of hyperkalemia and should be used cautiously as it can precipitate arrhythmias by decreasing ionic calcium.

Calcium gluconate in prevention of hyperkalemia should be used cautiously. Calcium supplementation can cause phosphate crystal deposition in renal tubules and can also cause ectopic calcification.[42]

Management of established renal failure

The RRT is needed apart from monitoring of urine output and serum electrolytes, urea, Cr, calcium, and phosphate levels. Patient's prognosis should be explained to the family. Patients with TLS-induced AKI have higher rates of mortality as compared to those without AKI.[51]

Q4. Describe TLS risk stratification classification for various tumors?

Tumor lysis syndrome is a life-threatening but preventable oncologic emergency, the occurrence of which may have negative impact on outcome including increased hospital length of stay and treatment cost.[39] Various risk stratification models have been developed for its early identification in order to manage better but these models lacked uniformity and versatility or were for specific set of patients.[44,52] The search for an apt risk stratification system for TLS continued and an expert panel of TLS published a more elaborate and versatile stratification model taking into account laboratory TLS features, malignancy-related traits (tumor type, stage and bulk), and evidence of renal dysfunction or renal involvement. These factors were considered in classifying the risk of TLS as low-risk disease with a TLS likelihood of <1%, intermediate-risk disease with a TLS likelihood of <1–5%, and high-risk disease with a TLS likelihood of >5%. The intent to develop such classification is to better work on its prevention and plan management. **Table 6** shows TLS risk stratification model and its prophylaxis recommendations.[39,53]

Q5. What hyperviscosity syndromes (HVS) are common in patients with hematologic malignancies? How are they managed?

Hyperviscosity syndromes are the cluster of disorders with varied underlying mechanisms presenting with constellation of signs and symptoms of increased blood or serum viscosity causing change in blood rheologic characteristics. Viscosity is one of the principal factors defining fluid dynamics and it defines the thickness or ability of a liquid to flow.[54,55] The thicker is the fluid, the slower it will flow. Centipoise (Cp) is used for measuring viscosity. Viscosity of water is 1 Cp; normal blood viscosity varies from 1.4 to 1.8 Cp. Increase in blood viscosity can result from increase in cellular or acellular components. Cellular components include WBCs, RBCs, and platelets and acellular components are plasma proteins. Increase in acellular components in blood causes HVS more commonly. HVS can also occur due to one of the following reasons:

- Increased cellular components (leukemia, polycythemia, and thrombocytosis)
- Increased acellular components (plasma cell dyscrasias, e.g., Waldenstrom's macroglobulinemia and multiple myeloma)
- Decreased cellular deformability (e.g., spherocytosis)
- Due to pathogenic complexes as in collagen vascular diseases (e.g., systemic lupus erythematosus, rheumatoid arthritis, and Sjögren's syndrome).

Conventionally, disorders of paraproteinemias as in plasma cell dyscrasias is called HVS and that due to excess of leukocytes is called leukostasis.

Pathophysiology: Increase in blood viscosity leads to poor flow and adversely affects tissue perfusion. In case of Waldenstrom's macroglobulinemia, there is excess production of immunoglobulin (Ig) M, which is a large pentameric molecule of around 1,000 kDA, which has predominantly intravascular distribution (80%).[56] However, in cases of multiple myeloma, there is excess production of IgA or IgG, which are not as large as IgM and have relatively less intravascular distribution.[57,58] Pathologic elevations of Igs not only increase the viscosity of blood but also cause rouleaux formation of RBCs and resultant hindrance to the microvascular flow.[59-64] Also, these proteins coat the platelet surface thus creating a functional platelet deficit and contribute to bleeding diathesis.[56] Increase in serum proteins also causes increase in total intravascular volume and consequent high-output cardiac failure.[65]

On the other hand, pathophysiology of leukostasis is related to the symptoms due to sludging of leukocytes and clogging of pulmonary and neurologic vasculature. Leukostasis is more common with acute leukemias; however, it may occur with chronic leukemias in blast crisis. Leukostasis is associated with WBC count of >1 lakh/mm^3 in AML and >4 lakh/mm^3 in acute lymphocytic leukemia (ALL).[66-68] It is more common with AML as compared to ALL as the blast cells of AML are larger than those of ALL.[69]

Clinical features: The HVS, apart from general features of anorexia, weight loss, presents with a classic triad of bleeding tendency, and ophthalmological and neurological manifestations.[57] Bleeding usually presents from skin or mucous membrane. Easy bruisability, epistaxis, menorrhagia, and gastrointestinal tract bleeding are common. Ophthalmological symptoms include blurred vision, nystagmus which may progress to retinal detachment, and blindness if appropriate measures to treat HVS are not taken immediately. On ophthalmoscopy, one can find exudates, flame hemorrhages, and characteristic boxcar or sausage-link appearance due to dilated retinal veins.[59,70]

Neurologic manifestation may range from headache, confusion, deafness, seizures, dementia, peripheral neuropathy, and stroke to coma. Anemia is often present but it is dilutional and should not be corrected, as its correction will further increase the viscosity. Hypercalcemia and hyponatremia are also common. In these cases, hyponatremia should be interpreted with caution, as it is spurious due to excess of paraproteins.

Pulmonary leukostasis may present with symptoms of dyspnea, hypoxemia, respiratory distress syndrome,

TABLE 6: Risk stratification of malignancies for tumor lysis syndrome (TLS).

TLS category[a]	Solid malignancies	Hematolymphoid malignancies	Prophylaxis recommendations
Low-risk disease (LRD)	MM solid tumors except those classified as IRD	*Chronic:* • CML • CLL except if classified as IRD or WBC count ≥50 × 10^9/L *Acute:* *Lymphomas:* • Hodgkin's lymphoma • Small lymphocytic lymphoma • Follicular lymphoma *Marginal zone B-cell lymphoma:* • MALT lymphoma • Mantle cell lymphoma (non-blastoid) • Mantle cell lymphoma (blastoid, normal LDH) cutaneous T-cell lymphoma *Anaplastic large cell lymphoma:* • ATL with normal LDH • Diffuse large B-cell lymphoma with normal LDH • Peripheral T-cell lymphoma with normal LDH *Leukemia:* AML with WBC count <25 × 10^9/L and LDH <2 × ULN	• Monitoring • Hydration ± Allopurinol
Intermediate-risk disease (IRD)	Neuroblastoma germ cell tumors SCLC	*Chronic:* CLL receiving targeted or biological therapies *Acute:* Any LRD with renal dysfunction/involvement *Lymphomas:* • Non-bulky ATL with LDH >ULN • Non-bulky diffuse large B-cell lymphoma with LDH >ULN • Non-bulky peripheral T-cell lymphoma with LDH >ULN • Non-bulky mantle cell lymphoma (blastoid, LDH >ULN) *Leukemia:* • AML with WBC count <25 × 10^9/L and LDH ≥2 × ULN • AML with WBC count 25–99×10^9/L • ALL with WBC count <100 × 10^9/L and LDH <2 × ULN • Burkitt's lymphoma with LDH <2 × ULN	• Monitoring • Hydration • Allopurinol
High-risk disease (HRD)	NA	*Chronic:* NA *Acute:* Any IRD with renal dysfunction and/or renal involvement or where uric acid, phosphate or potassium levels are elevated with uric acid and potassium/phosphate levels >ULN *Lymphomas:* • Bulky ATL with LDH >ULN • Bulky diffuse large B-cell lymphoma with LDH >ULN Bulky peripheral T-cell lymphoma with LDH >ULN • Bulky mantle cell lymphoma (blastoid, LDH >ULN) *Leukemia:* • AML with WBC count ≥100 × 10^9/L • ALL with WBC count <100 × 10^9/L and LDH ≥2 × ULN ALL with WBC count ≥100 × 10^9/L • Burkitt's lymphoma with LDH ≥2 × ULN	• Monitoring • Hydration • Rasburicase[$]

[a]Risk categories were defined as low-risk disease (LRD) with an approximate risk <1% of developing TLS, intermediate-risk disease (IRD) approximately 1–5% risk of developing TLS, and high-risk disease (HRD) with a risk of >5% of developing TLS.
[$]In suspected or documented glucose-6-phosphatase deficiency patients, rasburicase is contraindicated and should be substituted with allopurinol.
(ALL: acute lymphoblastic leukemia; AML: acute myeloid leukemia; ATL: adult T-cell lymphoma; CML: chronic myeloid leukemia; CLL: chronic lymphoid leukemia; LDH: lactate dehydrogenase; MALT: mucosa-associated lymphoid tissue; MM: multiple myeloma; SCLC: small cell lung cancer; ULN: upper limit of normal; WBC: white blood cell)
Source: Adapted from Cairo et al.[39] and Sury et al.[53]

or respiratory arrest with or without overt chest X-ray abnormality. Even if chest X-ray abnormality is present, it does not have any specific pattern and resembles the usual causes of respiratory distress such as pneumonia, pleural effusion, or lung infiltrate.

Neurologic leukostasis symptomatology may include headaches altered mental status, intracranial hemorrhage, or thrombosis of intracranial vasculature.[71-73]

Diagnosis: High index of suspicion is required for diagnosis and it is based on patient's history and examination. Patients undergo hematological screening tests such as complete blood count, general blood picture, platelet counts, and coagulogram. Blood biochemistry, electrolyte panel, and serum electrophoresis with bone marrow examination are done to ascertain the cause. Suspicion of HVS should mandate prompt hematology or oncology referral.

Treatment: Treatment of HVS starts with basic supportive management, targeted management for reduction of serum viscosity, treatment of complications, and for control of underlying disorder.

Basic supportive management includes support of airway, breathing, and circulation, and if the need arises patient should be intubated.

For reduction of serum viscosity plasmapheresis is recommended. Plasmapheresis will give immediate relief of symptoms in case of IgM-related hypergammaglobulinemia due to its predominant intravascular distribution.[56] However, in cases of IgA- or IgG-related disorders multiple sessions of plasmapheresis are required to obtain observable effect as these Igs have high volume of distribution.

Definitive treatment: Definitive management of underlying disorder includes chemotherapy with hematology or oncology referral.

Leukostasis treatment: Pharmacologic or leukapheresis is the emergency treatment, pharmacologic leukocytoreduction can be done using hydroxyurea while arranging for central venous line and leukapheresis. For therapy, WBC count target should be $<50,000/mm^3$.[74]

Specific therapy for treatment of underlying malignancy should be as per hematologist or oncologist.

The patient continued to have oliguria and with hyperkalemia not getting controlled, dialysis was initiated. Chemotherapy was initiated, and the WBC counts started to fall. By day 8 of chemotherapy, he had a WBC count of $100/cc^3$, with absolute neutrophil count (ANC) of 80.

He remained oliguric requiring dialysis. By day 12 in the ICU, he started to have fever. A paired blood culture was sent, and broad-spectrum antibiotics were added. Even after starting broad-spectrum antibiotics, he continued to have fever spikes. He started to have associated loose stools also for which IV metronidazole was added.

Despite adequate fluid resuscitation and antibiotics, he continued to have fever spikes and also had an episode of hypotension. With a decision to start antifungal therapy, pending blood culture is made. Justify addition of antifungal in this scenario.

Several terminologies are relevant to know in this context which are mentioned below:[75,76]

Neutropenia: Neutropenia is defined as ANC $<1,500/mm^3$. ANC includes both the mature and immature neutrophils and can be calculated by multiplying the percentage of polymorphonuclear cells by total WBC count.

- *Severe neutropenia:* ANC $<500/mm^3$
- *Profound neutropenia:* ANC $<100/mm^3$
- *Protracted neutropenia:* Neutropenia persisting for >7 days.

Febrile neutropenia: Febrile neutropenia (FN) is defined as oral temperature $>38.3°C$ ($101°F$) or two successive readings of $>38°C$ for 2 hours with ANC $<500/mm^3$ or ANC $>1,000/mm^3$ with a predicted decline to $<500/mm^3$ over next 48 hours.[77]

The FN is an oncological emergency and has substantial morbidity and mortality.[78] Incidence is higher in hematological malignancies as compared to solid tumors.[79]

Risk stratification: Multinational Association of Supportive Care in Cancer (MASCC) risk index scoring is widely used for assessing risk of complications in FN and it classifies the patients into low and high-risk categories.[80]

- *Low-risk patients:* MASCC ≥ 21
- *High-risk patients:* MASCC <21.

Factors associated with good prognosis (high score) in MASCC risk index have been summarized in **Table 7**.

TABLE 7: Factors associated with good prognosis (high score) in Multinational Association of Supportive Care in Cancer (MASCC) risk index.

Patient characteristics	Points
Burden of febrile neutropenia with no or mild symptoms	5
Absence of hypotension (systolic blood pressure >90 mm Hg)	5
Absence of chronic obstructive pulmonary disease	4
Solid organ or hematological malignancies with no previous fungal infection	4
No dehydration requiring intravenous volume expansion	3
Outpatient status	3
Burden of febrile neutropenia with moderate symptoms	3
Age <60 years	2

> **BOX 1:** Initial assessment and workup of patients with febrile neutropenia (FN).
>
> *Initial assessment and workup of patients with FN*
> - Detailed history and examination and stabilization of cardiorespiratory status
> - Symptoms and signs of infective focus
>   - Central nervous system (CNS), respiratory system, oropharynx and gastrointestinal tract (GIT), skin and perineal or genitourinary discharges
>   - Examine all the indwelling catheters
>   - Complete blood count (CBC)
>   - Renal and liver function tests
>   - Coagulation screen
>   - C-reactive protein or procalcitonin
>   - Blood cultures (at least two sets) including samples from indwelling venous and arterial catheters
>   - Sputum microscopy and culture*
>   - Urinalysis and culture*
>   - Stool microscopy and culture*
>   - Skin lesion (swab/aspirate/biopsy)*
>   - Chest X-ray (even in absence of pulmonary signs/symptoms)
> - Further investigations (profound/prolonged neutropenia/after allografts)
>   - High-resolution CT chest (HRCT) if fever despite 72 hours of appropriate antibiotics to look for invasive pulmonary aspergillosis
>   - CT sinuses for fungal infections, e.g., mucormycosis
>   - CT abdomen for hepatosplenic candidiasis
>   - *Bronchoalveolar lavage (BAL):* Stains, cultures, and biomarkers
>   - Look for noninfectious causes of fever, e.g., venous thromboembolism (VTE)
>
> *Only if focus of infection is suspected at these sites.
> (CT: computed tomography)

Low-risk patients can be managed on outpatient department (OPD) basis with oral antibiotics while high-risk patients need to be hospitalized and managed with IV broad-spectrum antibiotics. Moreover, mortality related to bacteremia is higher in patients with high-risk FN. Fungal pathogens are also more common in high-risk patients.[75]

Initial assessment and workup of febrile neutropenia[78]
Box 1 summarizes the workup required in patients with FN.

Prompt empirical IV antibiotic therapy: Prompt diagnosis and treatment of infection is essential.[78] In all febrile neutropenic patients, empiric broad-spectrum antibiotic therapy should be initiated immediately after obtaining blood cultures within 60 minutes of presentation.[81] For high-risk patients, European Society for Medical Oncology (ESMO) guidelines recommend initiating monotherapy with a beta-lactam having anti-*Pseudomonas aeruginosa* activity.[82]

In a meta-analysis comparing different beta-lactams–beta-lactamase inhibitors (BL-BLI) combinations (piperacillin-tazobactam, ceftazidime, cefepime, meropenem, and imipenem–cilastatin) mortality was found to be significantly less with piperacillin-tazobactam.[83] Initial empirical antibiotic coverage should take into account local microbiological data and resistance patterns are available.

Indications for including alternative initial empirical therapies have been mentioned below:
- Resistant gram-negative organisms
- Methicillin-resistant *Staphylococcus aureus* (MRSA) infections
- Suspected central nervous system (CNS) infection (meningitis or encephalitis)
- *Central venous catheters:* Central line-associated bloodstream infections (CLABSI)
- Pneumonia
- Lung infiltrates
- Intra-abdominal or pelvic sepsis
- Diarrhea or *Clostridium difficile*
- Cellulitis
- Vesicular lesions or suspected viral infections **(Flowchart 2)**

Antifungal therapy in febrile neutropenia
Invasive FIs have significant morbidity and mortality in hematologic and transplant patients.[79,80] Numerous risk factors predispose these patients to IFIs-like advanced underlying disease, prior history of corticosteroid usage, use of broad-spectrum antibiotics, presence of indwelling central venous catheters, intensive chemotherapy, and severe and protracted neutropenia (ANC ≤500/mm^3 >7–10 days).[77] The presence of a colonized environment along with a breach in physiological barriers by indwelling catheters potentiates the risk of these infections.

In an autopsy study in cancer patients, incidence of IFIs was as high as 25% in patients with leukemia, 12% in those with lymphoma and 5% in those with solid organ tumors. Most of these infections had *Candida* as the causative pathogen (58%) followed by *Aspergillus* (30%).[84]

Incidence of IFIs in hematopoietic stem cell transplant (HSCT) recipients is around 3.4% with *Aspergillus* being the most common (43%) followed by *Candida* (28%), fusariosis (15%), scedosporiosis (16%), and zygomycosis (8%).[85,86]

Prophylactic antifungal therapy
Antifungal prophylaxis against *Candida* is used for allogeneic HSCT and in those undergoing intensive remission-induction or salvage-induction chemotherapy for acute leukemias.[73]

Antifungal prophylaxis against *Aspergillus* is considered for selected patients undergoing intensive chemotherapy for AML or myelodysplastic syndrome (MDS) and during pre-engraftment phase of allogeneic HSCT.

Empiric antifungal therapy
The guidelines recommend adding an empiric antifungal agent after 4–7 days in high-risk neutropenic patients who are expected to have a total duration of neutropenia

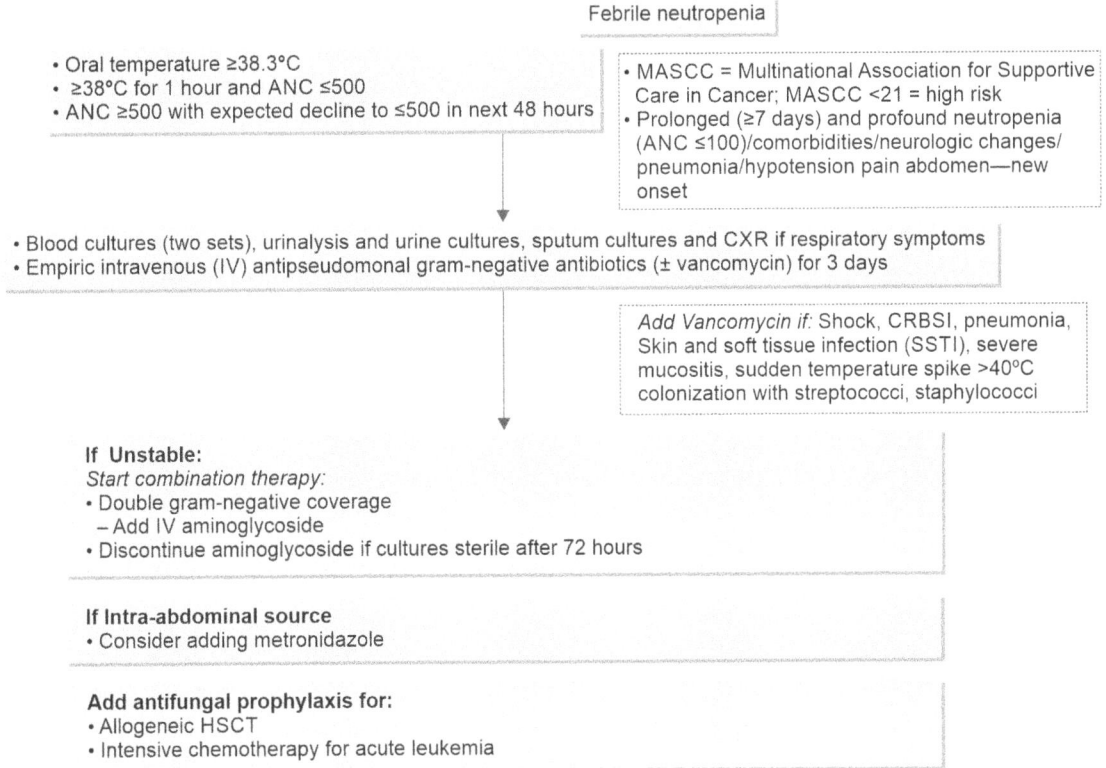

Flowchart 2: Initial management of patients with febrile neutropenia (FN).

(ANC: absolute neutrophil count; CRBSI: catheter-related bloodstream infection; CXR: chest X-ray; HSCT: hematopoietic stem cell transplant)

>7 days who have persistent or recurrent fever and in whom reassessment does not yield a cause.[77]

Candida and *Aspergillus* are responsible for most of the FIs during neutropenia.[75] For empirical antifungal therapy, lipid formulations of amphotericin B, echinocandins, and voriconazole can be considered.[77,85]

Preemptive antifungal therapy
The preemptive antifungal therapy employs a combination of clinical, serologic, and CT evidence to initiate antifungal therapy. The aim of preemptive management is to restrict the use of antifungal drugs to selected patients unlike the empirical antifungal therapy, thereby decreasing overuse, toxicity, and cost of antifungal drugs without increasing IFI-related mortality.[87]

There is no consensus regarding definition of preemptive antifungal therapy and it is still an experimental practice. Screening tests based on biomarkers such as serum tests for fungal antigens or DNA [e.g., serum galactomannan (GM) and beta-D glucan] and imaging like high-resolution computed tomography (HRCT) chest may be used for early diagnosis and treatment of FIs. This approach is best applicable for patients receiving anti-yeast prophylaxis where the concern is mainly mold infections. In view of decreased sensitivity of blood cultures (21–71%) and difficulty in obtaining infected tissue, nonculture-based tests have been developed to expedite the diagnosis of IFIs and some of them are described as follows.[82,88,89]

Biomarkers:
- 1,3 beta-D glucan (blood) (cutoff >60–80 pg/mL)— (sensitivity 65–100%, specificity 31–79%):[90-92]
    - beta-D glucan is not specific for *Candida* and can detect fungal organisms like *Aspergillus* and *Pneumocystis jirovecii*.
    - It is also prone to several sources of contamination (e.g., hemodialysis with cellulose membranes, albumin or Igs, amoxicillin–clavulanate or piperacillin–tazobactam, severe bacterial infections, severe mucositis, and glucan-containing surgical sponge or gauze).
- GM in serum and BAL:[92]
    - GM is used to detect invasive aspergillosis (IA). The limitations of this test are:
        - False positive results with some antibiotics, e.g., amoxicillin, beta-lactam/beta-lactamase combination (e.g., piperacillin–tazobactam, augmentin, etc.), plasmalyte, foods (pasta and rice), cross-reactivity with *Fusarium, Alternaria, Mucorales,* and *Histoplasma*[93]

- False-negative results with concomitant antimold therapy
- Serum GM (cutoff 0.5): Sensitivity 60–80%; specificity: 80–95%
- BAL GM (cutoff 0.5–1): Sensitivity 85–90%; specificity: 90–95%.

Antigen–antibody tests:[94]
- Mannan antigen and anti-mannan antibody [blood and cerebrospinal fluid (CSF)]:
    - Both antigen and antibody tests are required for maximum sensitivity. Species-dependent sensitivity is seen—80–100% for *Candida albicans, Candida glabrata,* and *Candida tropicalis,* and around 40–50% for *Candida parapsilosis,* and *Candida krusei*
    - These tests are mainly used for CNS candidiasis and blood culture-negative hepatosplenic candidiasis and may be preferred in circumstances where *Candida* is supposed to be the main pathogen involved and risk of false-positive test with beta-D glucan is high.

Polymerase chain reaction-based methods to detect fungal DNA (blood):
- *SeptiFast (sensitivity 48–72%, specificity 99%):*
    - SeptiFast can detect *C. albicans, C. glabrata, C. krusei, C. parapsilosis, C. tropicalis, Candida auris,* and *Aspergillus fumigatus*
    - The PCR-based assay is more specific for *Candida*. There is a risk of false positive result for *Aspergillus*.

For short-duration neutropenia (<10 days), benefit of preemptive and empirical therapies is similar but for protracted neutropenia, empirical antifungal therapy seems to be better in hematological malignancies.[95]

Besides the importance of timely diagnosis and appropriate antifungal drugs for IFI, another essential step in the management of fungemia is removal of central venous catheter (which may either be the source of infection or get secondarily seeded from hematogenous spread) in order to preclude the fungus from residing relatively protected inside central line biofilm.[82,89,96-100]

Q6. How will you assess a case of neutropenia with continuing fever?

In patients with FN having persistent fever despite initial treatment, then following measures should be instituted.[71,73,74]
- *New or worsening sites of infection:*
    - Comprehensive clinical evaluation to search for infection
    - Blood culture sets and cultures of any suspected sites of infection
    - Search for nosocomial infections such as ventilator-associated pneumonia (VAP), CLABSI, catheter-associated urinary tract infection (CAUTI), *C. difficile* infection (CDI), and sinusitis.
    - Drainage with subsequent microscopy and cultures (bacterial, fungal and viral)
    - Analysis of tissue biopsy specimen for infections, e.g., *Trichosporon beigelii* of skin (fatal FI) may be confused for *Candida* infection.
    - Ultrasonography (USG), CT, magnetic resonance imaging (MRI) scans as indicated.
    - In patients with abdominal pain, look for neutropenic enterocolitis (NEC) and CDIs.
    - Endoscopic evaluation (if bleeding risk is not high or after recovery of thrombocytopenia), e.g., *Candida* esophagitis.
    - Review adequacy of ongoing antibiotic coverage (dosing and spectrum).
    - Broaden antibiotic coverage for hemodynamic instability. Add MRSA coverage if indicated.
    - Consider adding empirical antifungal therapy or switch to a different class of antifungals.
    - Optimize antiviral treatment if required.
- Look for noninfectious sources of infection also.

The approach to persistent fever in patients with FN has been shown in **Flowchart 3**.

Q7. What are the possible noninfectious causes of fever in this patient?
The noninfectious causes of fever are given in **Box 2**.

Q8. What is NEC?
Neutropenic enterocolitis or typhlitis (derived from Greek word Typhlon meaning cecum) is a life-threatening complication seen after intensive chemotherapy in patients with hematological malignancies.[101,102]

The NEC was initially described in leukemic patients in pediatric age group. Of late, it has also been reported in adults with leukemia, lymphoma, multiple myeloma, aplastic anemia, and MDS.

Etiology of NEC:
- *Gastrointestinal mucosal injury (mucositis) by chemotherapeutic agents:* Cytarabine, gemcitabine, doxorubicin, vincristine, cyclophosphamide, 5-fluorouracil, daunorubicin, and leucovorin
- Neutropenia (immunosuppression)
- Intestinal leukemic infiltration.

Pathogenesis of NEC: NEC is believed to be caused by injury to gastrointestinal mucosa in immunosuppressed patients, which results in following changes in intestinal mucosa:
- Intestinal edema
- Vascular engorgement

Flowchart 3: Approach to new-onset fever after 48 hours or persistent fever in febrile neutropenia.

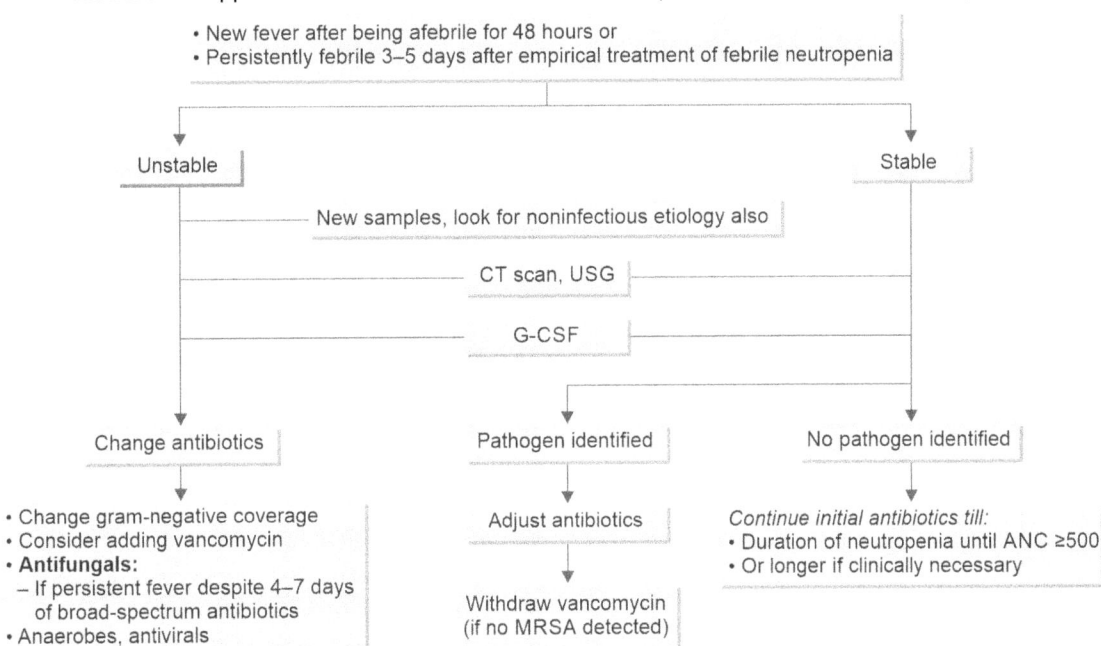

(ANC: absolute neutrophil count; CT: computed tomography; G-CSF: granulocyte colony-stimulating factor; USG: ultrasonography; MRSA: methicillin-resistant *Staphylococcus aureus*)

BOX 2: Noninfectious causes of fever.
- Malignancy (solid organ or hematolymphoid)
- Blood or blood product transfusion
- Gastrointestinal bleed
- Pancreatitis
- Venous or arterial thrombosis
- Intracerebral hematoma or infarct or intraventricular hemorrhage
- Bowel ischemia or infarction
- Pulmonary embolism
- Drug-related, e.g., phenytoin
- Adrenal insufficiency
- Myocardial infarction
- Postoperative fever (within 48 hours postsurgery)

- Disruption of mucosal surface, segmental ulceration, and inflammation with necrosis
- Intramural bacterial invasion
- Bacterial translocation (leading to bacteremia)

The cecum is always affected by the disease and it frequently extends to ileum. Ascending and transverse colon may also be involved. The preference for cecum may be due to its distensibility and limited blood supply.

Microorganisms such as gram-negative rods, gram-positive cocci including enterococci, fungi, and viruses have been implicated in pathogenesis of NEC. Although *Clostridium septicum* has been considered to be associated with generalized peritonitis, peritoneal signs, hemodynamic instability, and other signs of rapid clinical worsening may be suggestive of necrosis and bowel perforation requiring immediate surgical intervention.

Laboratory investigations: Full blood count may show neutropenia and thrombocytopenia. Blood cultures have been found to be positive in 28–84% cases.

Imaging:
- X-ray abdomen may show dilated atonic cecum, ascending colon filled with liquid or gas, small bowel dilatation, and signs of bowel wall thickening (thumb printing) or intramural gas (pneumatosis intestinalis); with NEC, it has not always been implicated among the involved pathogens in many studies.

Q9. How do you diagnose and manage NEC?[103,104]

Clinical presentation: Patients with ANC <500/mm^3 are at increased risk for NEC. The most common symptoms of NEC are abdominal pain, diarrhea, and fever. Nausea, vomiting, and abdominal distension are also commonly seen. Later, localized peritonitis may occur presenting as right iliac fossa tenderness and mass, which may progress to pneumoperitoneum in patients with perforation, but it has limited sensitivity and specificity as compared to USG or CT abdomen.
- Findings in both USG and CT abdomen right lower quadrant mass, pericecal fluid or fat stranding, gross thickening of ileal and cecal walls with intraluminal narrowing

- The CT has higher accuracy than both plain radiography and USG abdomen.
- Endoscopic evaluation of colitis is avoided for fear of hemorrhage and perforation.

Following diagnostic criteria for NEC have been proposed by Gorschlüter et al.[105]
- Fever (axillary temperature 38°C or rectal temperature >38.5°C)
- Abdominal pain
- Bowel wall thickening >4 mm over >30 mm in any segment by USG or CT.

Q10. What are the differential diagnoses of NEC?
The NEC has a nonspecific presentation and can present like following abdominal ailments:
- Inflammatory bowel disease (IBD)
- Intestinal obstruction
- Pseudomembranous colitis
- Appendicitis
- Ischemic colitis
- Infectious colitis
- Other gastrointestinal complications related to chemotherapy

Management of NEC
- *Conservative management:*
  - Bowel rest is commonly used but some authors advise continuing nutrition to prevent villous atrophy and further breach of mucosal integrity.
  - Total parenteral nutrition (TPN) can be used in patients who are malnourished.
  - Prompt administration of broad-spectrum antibiotics against gram-negative, gram-positive, and anaerobic pathogens. In patients with high suspicion for CDI also, metronidazole or vancomycin should be added. Empiric antifungals may be added, if good response to antibiotics is not seen even after 72 hours.

  Resolution of disease will depend upon leukocyte count recovery. Failure of leukocyte normalization may be due to increasing size of bowel lesion, persistent bacterial invasion of bowel mucosa, and bowel wall perforation. Conservative management is the recommended initial step with close monitoring, in case surgical intervention is later warranted.
- *Surgical intervention:*[101,106]
  - Intraperitoneal bowel perforation
  - Persistent gastrointestinal bleeding despite correction of cytopenias and coagulation defects; angiography with embolization may also be done in severe hemorrhage with hemodynamic instability.
  - Appendicitis
  - Intra-abdominal abscess

Necrotic or perforated bowel should be resected. Primary anastomosis is not recommended in these patients because an immunosuppressed state and poor healing predispose them to anastomotic leaks.

Outcome of NEC: Mortality rates are high for NEC despite appropriate therapy. High index of clinical suspicion and aggressive and timely management are essential to decrease the mortality in NEC.

Q11. What is CDI? Describe its clinical features and management.
Clostridium difficile is an anaerobic gram-positive, spore-forming, and toxin-producing bacillus that is transmitted among humans through feco–oral route. It is mainly a hospital-acquired pathogen and can be cultured from stool of 3% healthy adults and as many as 35% of hospitalized patients.[107]

Pathogenesis of CDI[108,109]
The steps crucial in the pathogenesis of CDI are:
- Alteration of normal fecal flora
- Colonization of colon by *C. difficile*
- Production of exotoxins (cytotoxins A and B) locally, which inactivate members of Rho family of guanosine triphosphatases (Rho GTPases) and produce proinflammatory interleukins and tumor necrosis factor-alpha (TNF-α) resulting in:
  - Loss of intestinal barrier function, colonocyte apoptosis
  - Increased vascular permeability
  - Connective tissue degradation leading to pseudomembranous colitis (exudative, inflammatory plaques in colon composed of neutrophils, fibrin, mucin, and cellular debris); occasionally the small bowel may be involved.

Risk factors for CDI:
- Weakening of barrier properties of normal fecal microbiota by antibiotics is the major risk factor: Ampicillin, amoxicillin, cephalosporins, clindamycin and fluoroquinolones are commonly implicated (although any antibiotic may be involved).
- Advanced age, severe underlying disease, and antineoplastic chemotherapy also contribute to susceptibility.
- Infection is transmitted by spores that are resistant to heat, acid, and antibiotics.

Diagnosis of CDI: Patients with unexplained and new-onset more than or equal to three unformed stools in 24 hours with history of antibiotic exposure need to be tested for CDI.[110]

C. difficile infection is diagnosed by:
- *Stool toxin test:*
  - Enzyme immunoassay (EIA) for toxins in stool (toxin A, toxins A and B)

- Stool latex agglutination test for glutamate dehydrogenase (GDH) antigen
- *The PCR-based tests that identify microbial toxin genes in stool:*
  - Nucleic acid amplification test (NAAT) for toxin A (TcdA), toxin B (TcdB) and 16S ribosomal ribonucleic acid
  - Detection of BI/NAP1/027 strain may influence choice of therapy, e.g., fidaxomicin is associated with reduction in recurrence of non-BI/NAP1/027 strains only.[107]

Depending upon institutional criteria, either NAAT alone or stool toxin test as part of multiple step algorithm is used to diagnose CDI.

- *NAAT or multiple step algorithm:* GDH testing is initial screening step in the algorithm that is combined with toxin test and/or molecular test for rapid and better results.
  - GDH + Toxin
  - GDH + Toxin followed by NAAT
  - GDH + NAAT

Stool culture (anaerobic) for *C. difficile* is labor-intensive and not widely used. Biomarkers like fecal lactoferrin are limited by insufficient data.

Types of CDI (with management strategies discussed mainly for adult population)[110-112] Depending upon the clinical presentation and laboratory abnormalities, CDI may be classified into:
- Nonsevere CDI
- Severe CDI
- Fulminant CDI
- Recurrent CDI

Nonsevere CDI: This is characterized by:
- Three to five unformed bowel movements per day
- Afebrile status
- Mild abdominal discomfort or tenderness
- Nonbloody diarrhea
- Nausea, occasional vomiting
- Total leukocyte count (TLC) $\leq 15,000/mm^3$, and Cr <1.5 mg/dL

Mainstays of treatment are:
- Cessation of predisposing antibiotics, hydration, electrolyte replacement, and close monitoring
- Oral vancomycin 125 mg four times a day for 10 days
- Oral fidaxomicin 200 mg twice a day for 10 days
- Alternately, if above agents are unavailable, oral metronidazole 500 mg three times a day for 10 days
- Multidisciplinary approach is required with close collaboration between ICU, microbiology, infectious disease (ID), gastroenterology, and surgery teams.
- Recent data suggest overall superiority of vancomycin over metronidazole in cases of nonsevere infection also.
- Probiotics have uncertain effect on prevention and treatment of CDI and their routine use is not recommended.
- Insufficient data regarding discontinuation of proton-pump inhibitors (PPIs) is present.

Severe CDI:
- Severe abdominal pain, vomiting, and ileus
- Severe or bloody diarrhea
- Temperature >38.9°C, TLC >15,000/mm^3, serum albumin <2.5 mg/dL, serum Cr ≥1.5
- Pseudomembranous colitis

Risk factors include advanced age, severe initial episode of CDI, and concomitant use of antibiotics not directed at *C. difficile*.

Management options comprise following measures:
- Cessation of predisposing antibiotics, hydration, electrolyte replacement, and close monitoring
- Oral or nasogastric vancomycin 125 mg four times per day for 10 days
- Oral fidaxomicin 200 mg twice a day for 10 days

Severe CDI is an independent predictor of urgent colectomy and death.[107]

Fulminant CDI: Fulminant CDI is defined by presence of toxic megacolon (colonic dilation >5 cm), peritonitis, ileus, respiratory distress, and hemodynamic instability in patients with CDI. Management options comprise:
- Vancomycin, 500 mg four times per day orally or by nasogastric tube
- IV metronidazole (500 mg every 8 hours) administered with oral or rectal vancomycin, if ileus is present
- Surgical consultation for subtotal colectomy or diverting ileostomy with vancomycin colonic lavage
- Avoid endoscopic examinations for fear of perforation.
- In patients not responding to vancomycin and metronidazole, IV tigecycline (loading dose of 100 mg followed by 50 mg twice daily) and intravenous immunoglobulins (150–400 mg/kg) have been used but no controlled trials are available.
- Rising WBC count (≥25,000) or rising lactates (≥5 mmol/L) are associated with high mortality and early surgery may be helpful.

Recurrent CDI: Risk of recurrence is from 20% (after initial episode) to 60% (if several prior recurrences).

Treatment of first recurrence:
- Oral vancomycin 125 mg four times per day for 10 days, if metronidazole was used for initial episode
- Oral fidaxomicin 200 mg twice daily for 10 days

Treatment of second or further recurrence:
- Oral vancomycin in a tapered and pulsed regimen:
    - 125 mg four times a day for 1 week
    - 125 mg three times a day for 1 week
    - 125 mg twice a day for 1 week
    - 125 mg daily for 1 week
    - 125 mg once every other day for 1 week
    - 125 mg every 3 days for 1 week
- Oral fidaxomicin 200 mg twice daily for 10 days
- Fecal microbial transplantation (FMT)
- In addition to the above treatment regimens, immunotherapy with human monoclonal antibodies against *C. difficile* toxins A (CDA1) and B (CDB1) as a single IV infusion can also be tried although larger studies are needed for substantiating its role in decreasing the incidence of CDI.

FMT:[113] To allow spontaneous recovery of fecal microbiota and eliminate *C. difficile* from colon, stopping all antibiotics is the best way possible. However, recovery may take 12 weeks or longer, during which patients may have a relapse. Thus, FMT has recently emerged as a safe and effective treatment for recurrent CDI.
- Oral or rectal transplantation of fresh feces (up to 6 hours) from healthy, pretested donor, and the simultaneous cessation of all antibiotic use in the recipient is successful in treating >90% of patients with recurrent CDI.
- In 2013, van Nood and coworkers showed in RCT that administration of vancomycin followed by infusion of donor feces by nasoduodenal tube was safe and superior to vancomycin alone for recurrent CDI.[114]
- Bacteroidetes and firmicutes are thought to comprise critical components that need to be transplanted.
- Future uses may include:
    - FMT for primary CDI
    - Frozen (−80°C), capsulized FMT
    - Cultured fecal bacteria may be used as substitute for stool in FMT

Prevention of CDI spread:[115]
Essential steps to curtail spread of CDI include:
- Hand wash with soap and water by both healthcare personnel and patients
- Use of gloves and gowns
- Use of single use, disposable thermometers; avoid rectal thermometers
- Isolation—private room with dedicated toilet
- Disinfection or terminal cleaning of patient rooms, environmental surfaces, and equipment by hypochlorite (1,000 ppm available chlorine) or other sporicidal agents
- Antibiotic stewardship programs

Contact precautions are continued for at least 48 hours after diarrhea has resolved.

2021 focused update guidelines by Infectious Diseases Society of America (IDSA) and Society for Healthcare Epidemiology of America (SHEA): Three new recommendations are as under:[116]
1. *Initial nonsevere CDI episode (new):*
    a. Oral fidaxomicin is now being recommended over the standard vancomycin regimen for treatment of initial CDI infection. Advantages of fidaxomicin include minimal systemic absorption with high efficacy against *C. difficile*, narrow spectrum with minimal effect on other enteral commensals and fewer recurrences.
2. *Recurrent CDI episode(s) (new):*
    a. Even for recurrent CDI infections, oral fidaxomicin is preferred to standard vancomycin course, although evidence is more robust for initial CDI episodes.
    b. Bezlotoxumab, humanized monoclonal antibody against *C. difficile*, should be used as adjunct to other standard interventions in patients with multiple risk factors for recurrence and a CDI episode in last 6 months, with caution in patients with congestive heart failure (CHF).
3. *Fulminant CDI (similar to IDSA 2017 recommendation):*
    a. Vancomycin, 500 mg four times per day orally or by nasogastric tube
    b. IV metronidazole (500 mg every 8 hours) administered with oral or rectal vancomycin, if ileus is present
    c. Surgical consultation

Q12. Describe in brief about superior vena cava (SVC) syndrome?
Superior vena cava syndrome

Introduction:[117] Superior vena cava is the major vein draining blood from head, neck, and upper limbs to the heart. SVC syndrome results from conditions occluding the drainage of blood through SVC.

Anatomy: SVC is formed by joining of two brachiocephalic veins. Azygos vein is the major tributary of SVC that courses over the anterior borders of thoracic vertebrae and drains posteriorly into SVC at the level of tracheal carina.

Etiology:[118]
- *Malignant causes*: (70%)
    - Non-small cell lung cancer (50%)
    - Small cell lung cancer (25%)
    - Lymphoma (10%)
    - *Others:* Thymoma, mesotheliomas, solid tumors with mediastinal lymph node metastasis, primary germ cell neoplasms

- *Nonmalignant causes:* (30%)
  - Benign causes of SVC syndrome are also increasing nowadays in critically ill population secondary to indwelling catheters, pacemakers
  - Benign tumors, radiation fibrosis, infection, sarcoidosis, idiopathic mediastinal fibrosis, retrosternal thyroid, aortic aneurysm, mediastinal hematoma

Clinical features:[119] Severity of symptoms is inversely related to development of collateral venous pathways for diverting blood to right atrium. Generally, SVC obstruction does not result in hemodynamic instability unless there is significant cardiac compression from underlying malignancy.

Rise in venous pressure proximal to obstruction may be as high as 20–40 mm Hg impeding venous drainage from head, neck, and face. The clinical presentation in descending order of incidence includes facial swelling, distended nonpulsatile neck and chest veins, breathlessness and cough, arm edema, hoarseness of voice and/or stridor, syncope and/or headache, and obtundation.

Grading:[120]

0—Asymptomatic

1—Mild: Head and/or neck edema

2—Moderate: Head and/or neck edema with functional impairment

3—Severe: Cerebral edema, laryngeal edema

4—Life-threatening: Significant cerebral, laryngeal edema, hemodynamic instability

5—Fatal: Death

Stanford Classification based on pattern of obstruction and collateral pathways:[117]
- *Type I:* Both brachiocephalic veins are occluded. Blood returns to SVC through internal thoracic and azygos veins.
- *Type II:* Supra-azygos part of SVC is occluded. Blood returns to SVC through right superior intercostal vein.
- *Type III:* Azygos part of SVC is occluded. Blood returns to SVC through internal mammary and inferior epigastric veins.
- *Type IV:* Infra-azygos part of SVC is occluded. Blood returns to SVC retrogradely via azygos and lumbar veins.

Each of the above types is further classified into three grades based on the degree of occlusion:

1. *Grade A (moderate-to-severe):* 50–90% occlusion
2. *Grade B (preocclusive):* >90% occlusion
3. *Grade C (occlusive):* 100% occlusion

Figure 1 shows Stanford classification of SVC syndrome.

Imaging:[117] Imaging modalities for SVC syndrome include:
- *Chest X-ray:* Chest X-ray may show mediastinal widening (indirect evidence) or even a mediastinal mass compressing SVC.
- *Duplex ultrasound of upper extremities:* Duplex ultrasound helps in evaluating thrombus in jugular, axillary, and subclavian veins. But, direct visualization of SVC and brachiocephalic veins is limited by presence of overlying ribs and lung shadows.
- *Contrast-enhanced computed tomography (CECT) chest:* CECT chest helps in optimally visualizing SVC and also helps in identifying thrombosis versus extrinsic compression of SVC, localizing extent of blockage, and identifying collateral venous pathways.
- *Digital subtraction venography:* Digital subtraction venography is the gold standard modality for identifying thrombus. It also helps in tracing collateral pathways, severity of obstruction, congenital SVC abnormality, and designing an endovascular intervention strategy. However, it fails to detect any extrinsic compression on SVC.
- *Magnetic resonance venography (MRV):* MRV is as sensitive as conventional venography and is especially useful in patients with contrast allergy.

Treatment:[117]

Initial management of SVC syndrome includes head elevation and stabilization of airway, breathing, and circulation, parenteral steroids, and loop diuretics. Histologic diagnosis of tumor is also essential for a comprehensive tumor management plan. Specific management modalities include:
- *Endovascular treatment:* Endovascular treatment is gaining importance in management of SVC syndrome and it includes catheter-directed thrombolysis (CDT), angioplasty, and stenting.
- Open surgical intervention (bypass grafting and SVC reconstruction) is reserved for cases with extensive venous thrombosis not amenable to endovascular intervention.
- *Radiation therapy:* Radiation therapy for tumor is less frequently used due to delayed relief in symptoms, high risk of recurrence, and hindrance in histologic tumor analysis postradiation.

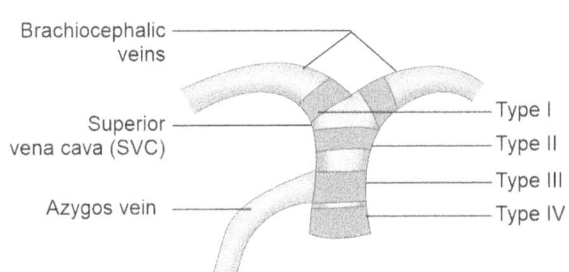

Fig. 1: Classification of superior vena cava (SVC) syndrome.

Flowchart 4 depicts an algorithmic approach for managing SVC syndrome.

Q13. Describe in brief about acute spinal cord compression syndrome?

Acute spinal cord compression[121]

Introduction: Acute spinal cord compression is an emergent condition resulting from conditions disrupting the stability of spinal column and thus leading to compression of spinal cord. It is a devastating but treatable condition if diagnosed and managed timely.

Clinical presentation: Meticulous neurological examination is quintessential in the diagnosis of acute spinal cord compression. Cardinal features comprise sensory level, urinary retention/incontinence, and relatively symmetric limb paralysis. Hyperreflexia and Babinski sign are present in most of the cases, except in cases of traumatic spinal shock where flaccid paralysis and areflexia may be seen in the acute phase of spinal cord injury. Localized neck or back pain may be seen. Depending upon the level and extent of injury, certain spinal cord syndromes have been described:

- *Spinal shock:* Hypotension, cervical and upper thoracic, hypotonia, areflexia, paralysis of limbs, sphincter loss, no Babinski sign
- *Central cord syndrome:* Gray matter damage, weakness and areflexia arms > legs
- *Brown-Séquard (hemicord) syndrome:*
  - Ipsilateral side: paralysis, increased tone, hyperreflexia, reduced vibration
  - Contralateral side: Pain and temperature loss
- *Conus medullaris syndrome:* (L1–L2) Weakness feet and legs, sensation loss lower lumbar and sacral, sphincter loss
- *Cauda equina syndrome:* (L2–S1) Sciatic/radicular pain, sensation loss saddle region and legs to groin, sphincter dysfunction

Figures 2 and 3 describe various spinal cord syndromes.

Etiology: Spinal cord compression results from conditions that arise in spinal column and narrow down the spinal canal, inclusive of trauma, neoplasm, epidural abscess, and epidural hematoma as described in **Table 8**.

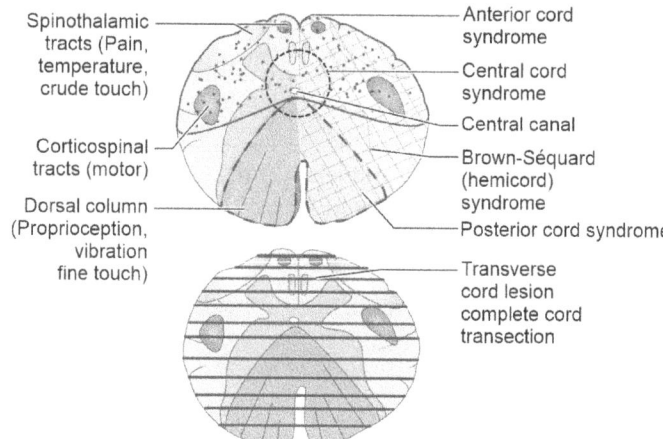

Fig. 2: Spinal cord syndromes.

Flowchart 4: Algorithmic approach to management of superior vena cava (SVC) syndrome.

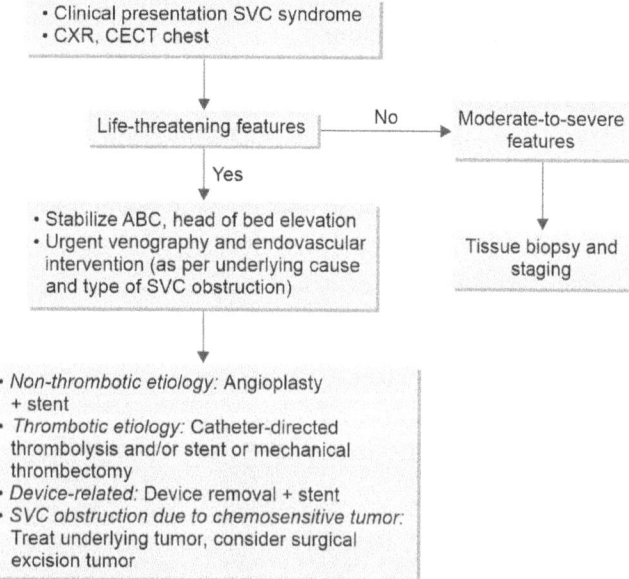

(ABC: airway, breathing, and circulation; CECT: contrast-enhanced computed tomography; CXR: chest X-ray; SVC: superior vena cava)

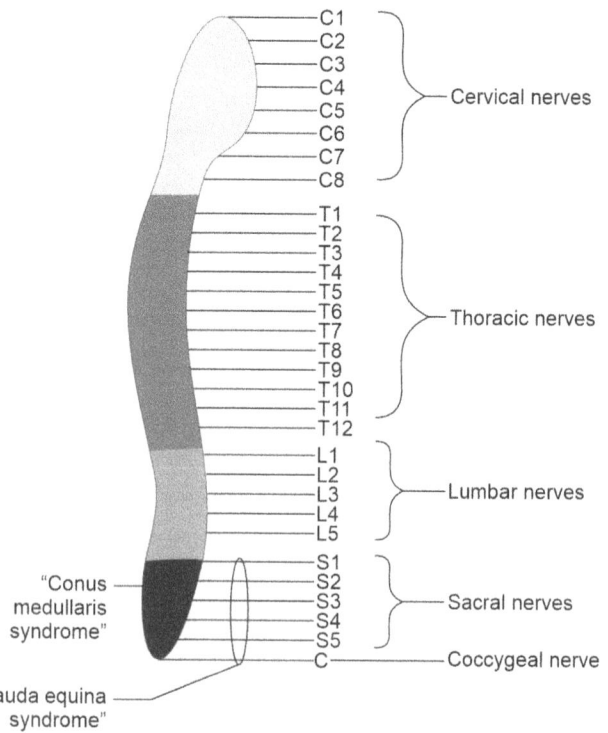

Fig. 3: Conus medullaris and cauda equina syndromes.

TABLE 8: Etiologies of spinal cord syndromes.

	Traumatic	*Neoplastic*	*Spinal epidural abscess*	*Spinal epidural hematoma*
Onset	Sudden	Days/longer	Hours—days/longer	Sudden
Risk factors	High-velocity trauma	Bony metastasis, myeloma, lymphoma	Diabetes, neoplasm, bacteremia, IV drug users, recent spine surgery	Anticoagulants, antiplatelets
Clinical features	Focal spinal pain, Paraplegia/quadriplegia, sensory level, central cord syndrome	Local back/neck pain, radicular pain, sensory level, paraplegia, sphincter dysfunction	Fever, paraparesis, severe midline back pain	Local back pain, paraparesis
Laboratory findings	As per trauma to organs	Depending upon metastasis and bony infiltration	Leukocytosis, increased ESR/hsCRP, positive blood cultures	Coagulopathy, thrombocytopenia
CT scan	Fracture spinal column elements, subluxation	Bony infiltration, pathological fracture, metastasis	Osteomyelitis, diskitis, paraspinal soft tissue fluid collection	Hematoma, spine fracture if trauma
MRI scan	High STIR in ligaments, cord edema/hemorrhage, subluxation	Enhancing tumor extending from spinal column into spinal canal, spared disk space, homogeneous signal changes vertebral body	T1: Reduced signal and T2: Increased signal	T1: Isointense; hyperintense after 24–36 hours T2: Hyperintense

(CT: computed tomography; ESR: erythrocyte sedimentation rate; hsCRP: high-sensitivity C-reactive protein; IV: intravenous; MRI: magnetic resonance imaging; STIR: short tau inversion recovery)

Management: The management approach depends upon the underlying etiology as described below:
- *Traumatic:*
  - Surgical decompression, restoration of alignment, internal fixation and fusion
  - Maintain mean arterial pressure 85–90 mm Hg in acute phase
- *Neoplastic:*
  - Circumferential tumor removal, decompression, internal fixation and fusion
  - High dose glucocorticoids, radiotherapy
- *Spinal epidural abscess:*
  - Surgery with irrigation, biopsy, culture
  - Antibiotics covering *S. aureus*
- *Spinal epidural hematoma:*
  - Surgical evacuation of hematoma
  - Correct coagulopathy and thrombocytopenia.

REFERENCES

1. Azoulay E, Soares M, Darmon M, Benoit D, Pastores S, Afessa B. Intensive care of the cancer patient: recent achievements and remaining challenges. Ann Intensive Care. 2011;1:5.
2. Azoulay É, Schlemmer B. Diagnostic strategy in cancer patients with acute respiratory failure. Intensive Care Med. 2006;32:808-22.
3. Letourneau AR, Issa NC, Baden LR. Pneumonia in the immunocompromised host. Curr Opin Pulm Med. 2014;20:272-9.
4. Azoulay E, Pickkers P, Soares M, Perner A, Rello J, Bauer PR, et al. Acute hypoxemic respiratory failure in immunocompromised patients: the Efraim multinational prospective cohort study. Intensive Care Med. 2017;43:1808-19.
5. Gristina GR, Antonelli M, Conti G, Ciarlone A, Rogante S, Rossi C, et al. Noninvasive versus invasive ventilation for acute respiratory failure in patients with hematologic malignancies: a 5-year multicenter observational survey. Crit Care Med 2011;39:2232-9.
6. Azoulay E, Mokart D, Pene F, Lambert J, Kouatchet A, Mayaux J, et al. Outcomes of critically ill patients with hematologic malignancies: prospective multicenter data from France and Belgium—a groupe de recherche respiratoire en reanimation onco-hématologique study. J Clinb Oncol. 2013;31:2810-8.
7. Azoulay E, Lemiale V, Mokart D, Pène F, Kouatchet A, Perez P, et al. Acute respiratory distress syndrome in patients with malignancies. Intensive Care Med. 2014;40:1106-14.
8. Adda M, Coquet I, Darmon M, Thiery G, Schlemmer B, Azoulay E. Predictors of noninvasive ventilation failure in patients with hematologic malignancy and acute respiratory failure. Crit Care Med. 2008;36:2766-72.
9. Bello G, De Pascale G, Antonelli M. Noninvasive ventilation for the immunocompromised patient: always appropriate? Curr Opin Crit Care. 2012;18:54-60.
10. Azevedo LCP, Caruso P, Silva UVA, Torelly AP, Silva E, Rezende E, et al. Outcomes for patients with cancer admitted to the ICU requiring ventilatory support: results from a prospective multicenter study. Chest. 2014;146:257-66.

11. Antonelli M, Conti G, Rocco M, Bufi M, De Blasi RA, Vivino G, et al. A comparison of noninvasive positive-pressure ventilation and conventional mechanical ventilation in patients with acute respiratory failure. N Engl J Med. 1998;339: 429-35.
12. Hilbert G, Gruson D, Vargas F, Bufi M, De Blasi RA, Vivino G, et al. Noninvasive ventilation in immunosuppressed patients with pulmonary infiltrates, fever, and acute respiratory failure. N Engl J Med. 2001;344:481-7.
13. Wermke M, Schiemanck S, Höffken G, Ehninger G, Bornhäuser M, Illmer T. Respiratory failure in patients undergoing allogeneic hematopoietic SCT—a randomized trial on early non-invasive ventilation based on standard care hematology wards. Bone Marrow Transplant. 2012;47:574-80.
14. Lemiale V, Mokart D, Resche-Rigon M, Pène F, Mayaux J, Faucher E, et al. Effect of noninvasive ventilation vs oxygen therapy on mortality among immunocompromised patients with acute respiratory failure: a randomized clinical trial. JAMA. 2015:314:1711-9.
15. Huang HB, Xu B, Liu GY, Lin JD, Du B. Use of noninvasive ventilation in immunocompromised patients with acute respiratory failure: a systematic review and meta-analysis. Crit Care. 2017;21:4.
16. Soares M, Caruso P, Silva E, Teles JM, Lobo SM, Friedman G, et al. Characteristics and outcomes of patients with cancer requiring admission to intensive care units: a prospective multicenter study. Crit Care Med. 2010;38:9-15.
17. Peñuelas Ó, Esteban A. Noninvasive ventilation for acute respiratory failure: the next step is to know when to stop. Eur Respir J. 2018;52:1801185.
18. Frat JP, Thille AW, Mercat A, Girault C, Ragot S, Perbet S, et al. High-flow oxygen through nasal cannula in acute hypoxemic respiratory failure. N Engl J Med. 2015;372:85-96.
19. Sehgal IS, Dhooria S, Agarwal R. High-flow nasal cannula oxygen in respiratory failure. N Engl J Med. 2015;373:1374.
20. Wawrzeniak IC, Moraes RB, Fendt LC. High-flow nasal cannula oxygen in respiratory failure. N Engl J Med. 2015;373:1373.
21. Ou X, Hua Y, Liu J, Gong C, Zhao W. Effect of high-flow nasal cannula oxygen therapy in adults with acute hypoxemic respiratory failure: a meta-analysis of randomized controlled trials. CMAJ. 2017;189:E260-7.
22. Ni YN, Luo J, Yu H, Liu D, Ni Z, Cheng J, et al. Can high-flow nasal cannula reduce the rate of endotracheal intubation in adult patients with acute respiratory failure compared with conventional oxygen therapy and noninvasive positive pressure ventilation?: a systematic review and meta-analysis. Chest. 2017;151:764-75.
23. Helviz Y, Einav S. A Systematic Review of the High-flow Nasal Cannula for Adult Patients. Crit Care. 2018;22:71.
24. Horr S, Roberson R, Hollingsworth JW. Pseudohypoxemia in a patient with chronic lymphocytic leukemia. Respiratory care. 2013;58:e31-3.
25. Lichtenstein DA. BLUE-protocol and FALLS-protocol: two applications of lung ultrasound in the critically ill. Chest. 2015;147:1659-70.
26. Rosner MH, Perazella MA. Acute Kidney Injury in Patients with Cancer. N Engl J Med. 2017;376:1770-81.
27. Darmon M, Ciroldi M, Thiery G, Schlemmer B, Azoulay E. Clinical review: specific aspects of acute renal failure in cancer patients. Critical Care. 2006;10(2):211.
28. Cavallaro F, Sandroni C, Antonelli M. Functional hemodynamic monitoring and dynamic indices of fluid responsiveness. Minerva Anestesiol. 2008;74:123-35.
29. Guidet B, Soni N, Rocca GD, Kozek S, Vallet B, Annane D, et al. A balanced view of balanced solutions. Crit Care. 2010;14:325.
30. Schulman S, Kearon C. Subcommittee on Control of Anticoagulation of the Scientific and Standardization Committee of the International Society on Thrombosis and Haemostasis. Definition of major bleeding in clinical investigations of antihemostatic medicinal products in non-surgical patients. J Thromb Haemost. 2005;3:692-4.
31. Falanga A, Marchetti M. Venous thromboembolism in the hematologic malignancies. J Clin Oncol. 2009;27:4848-57.
32. Myatra SN, Salins N, Iyer S, Macaden SC, Divatia JV, Muckaden M, et al. End-of-life care policy: An integrated care plan for the dying: A Joint Position Statement of the Indian Society of Critical Care Medicine (ISCCM) and the Indian Association of Palliative Care (IAPC). Indian J Crit Care Med. 2014;18:615-35.
33. Fox MJ, Brody JS, Weintraub LR. Leukocyte larceny: a cause of spurious hypoxemia. Am J Med. 1979;67:742-6.
34. Lele AV, Mirski MA, Stevens RD. Spurious hypoxemia. Crit Care Med. 2005;33:1854-6.
35. Kapoor S, Thakkar J. A Case of Spurious Hypoxemia in an ICU Patient with Leukemic Blast Crisis. J Med Cases. 2015;6:491-2.
36. Charoenratanakul S, Loasuthi K. Pseudohypoxaemia in a patient with acute leukaemia. Thorax. 1997;52:394-5.
37. Schmaier AH. Pseudohypoxemia due to leukemia and thrombocytosis. N Engl J Med. 1980;302:584.
38. Abu-Alfa AK, Younes A. Tumor lysis syndrome and acute kidney injury: evaluation, prevention, and management. Am J Kidney Dis. 2010;55(5 Suppl 3):S1-13.
39. Cairo MS, Coiffier B, Reiter A, Younes A. Recommendations for the evaluation of risk and prophylaxis of tumour lysis syndrome (TLS) in adults and children with malignant diseases: an expert TLS panel consensus. Br J Haematol. 2010;149:578-86.
40. Gertz MA. Managing tumor lysis syndrome in 2010. Leuk Lymphoma. 2010;51:179-80.
41. Cairo MS, Bishop M. Tumour lysis syndrome: new therapeutic strategies and classification. Br J Haematol. 2004;127:3-11.
42. Howard SC, Jones DP, Pui C. The tumor lysis syndrome. N Engl J Med. 2011;364:1844-54.
43. Lieber C, Jones D, Losowsky M, Davidson CS. Interrelation of uric acid and ethanol metabolism in man. J Clin Invest. 1962;41:1863-70.
44. Coiffier B, Altman A, Pui C, Younes A, Cairo MS. Guidelines for the management of Pediatric and Adult Tumor Lysis Syndrome: An evidence-based review. J Clin Oncol. 2008;26:2767-78.

45. Krakoff IH, Meyer RL. Prevention of hyperuricemia in leukemia and lymphoma: Use of allopurinol, a xanthine oxidase inhibitor. JAMA. 1965;193:1-6.
46. Arellano F, Sacristan JA. Allopurinol hypersensitivity syndrome: A review. Ann Pharmacother. 1993;27:337-43.
47. Wilson FP, Berns JS. Tumor lysis syndrome: New challenges and recent advances. Adv Chronic Kidney Dis. 2014;21:18-26.
48. Brogard JM, Coumaros D, Franckhauser J, Stahl A, Stahl J. Enzymatic uricolysis: A study of the effect of a fungal urate-oxydase. Rev Eur Etudes Clin Biol. 1972;17:890-5.
49. Sonbol MS, Yadav H, Vaidya R, Rana V, Witzig TE. Methemoglobinemia and hemolysis in a patient with G6PD deficiency treated with rasburicase. Am J Hematol. 2013;88:152-4.
50. Sherwood GB, Paschal RD, Adamski J. Rasburicase-induced methemoglobinemia: case report, literature review, and proposed treatment algorithm. Clin Case Rep. 2016;4: 315-9.
51. Darmon M, Guichard I, Vincent F, Schlemmer B, Azoulay E. Prognostic significance of acute renal injury in acute tumor lysis syndrome. Leuk Lymphoma. 2010;51:221-7.
52. Montesinos P, Lorenzo I, Martin G, Sanz J, Perez-Sirvent ML, Martinez D, et al. Tumor lysis syndrome in patients with acute myeloid leukemia: identification of risk factors and development of a predictive model. Haematologica. 2008;93:67-74.
53. Sury K. Update on the prevention and treatment of tumor lysis syndrome. J Onco-Nephrol. 2019;3(1):19-30.
54. Kesmarky G, Kenyeres P, Rabai M, Tóth K. Plasma viscosity: a forgotten variable. Clin Hemorheol Microcirc. 2008;39:243-6.
55. Rosencranz R, Bogen SA. Clinical laboratory measurement of serum, plasma, and blood viscosity. Am J Clin Pathol. 2006;125:S78-86.
56. Stone MJ, Bogen SA. Evidence-based focused review of management of hyperviscosity syndrome. Blood. 2012;119:2205-8.
57. Mullen EC, Wang M. Recognizing hyperviscosity syndrome in patients with Waldenstrom macroglobulinemia. Clin J Oncol Nurs. 2007;11:87-95.
58. Buxbaum J. Hyperviscosity syndrome in dysproteinemias. Am J Med Sci. 1972;264:123-6.
59. Behl D, Hendrickson AW, Moynihan TJ. Oncologic emergencies. Crit Care Clin. 2010;26:181-205.
60. Stone MJ. Waldenstrom's macroglobulinemia: hyperviscosity syndrome and cryoglobulinemia. Clin Lymphoma Myeloma. 2009;9:97-9.
61. Fahey JL, Barth WF, Solomon A. Serum hyperviscosity syndrome. JAMA. 1965;192:464-7.
62. Bloch KJ, Maki DG. Hyperviscosity syndromes associated with immunoglobulin abnormalities. Semin Hematol. 1973;10:113-24.
63. MacKenzie MR, Lee TK. Blood viscosity in Waldenstrom's macroglobulinemia. Blood. 1977;49:507-10.
64. MacKenzie MR, Brown E, Fudenberg HH, Goodenday LS. Waldenstrom's macroglobulinemia: correlation between expanded plasma volume and increased serum viscosity. Blood. 1970;35:394-408.
65. Vijay A, Gertz MA. Waldenstrom's macroglobulinemia. Blood. 2007;109: 5096-103.
66. Majhail NS, Lichtin AE. Acute leukemia with a very high leukocyte count: confronting a medical emergency. Cleve Clin J Med. 2004;71:633-7.
67. Marbello L, Ricci F, Nosari AM, Turrini M, Nador G, Nichelatti M, et al. Outcome of hyperleukocytic adult acute myeloid leukaemia: a single-center retrospective study and review of literature. Leuk Res. 2008;32:1221-7.
68. Szczepiorkowski ZM, Bandarenko N, Kim HC, Linenberger ML, Marques MB, Sarode R, et al. Guidelines on the use of therapeutic apheresis in clinical practice: evidence-based approach from the Apheresis Applications Committee of the American Society for Apheresis. J Clin Apheresis. 2007;22:106-75.
69. Adams BD, Baker R, Lopez JA, Spencer S. Myeloproliferative disorders and the hyperviscosity syndrome. Hematol Oncol Clin North Am. 2010;24:585-602.
70. Rajkumar VS, Dispenzieri AS, Kyle RA. Monoclonal gammopathy of undetermined significance, Waldenstrom macroglobulinemia, AL amyloidosis, and related plasma cell disorders: diagnosis and treatment. Mayo Clin Proc. 2006;81:693-703.
71. Kim H, Lee JH, Choi SJ, Kim WK, Lee JS, Lee KH. Analysis of fatal intracranial hemorrhage in 792 acute leukemia patients. Haematologica. 2004;89:622-4.
72. Tsai CC, Huang CB, Sheen JM, Wei HH, Hsiao CC. Sudden hearing loss as the initial manifestation of chronic myeloid leukemia in a child. Chang Gung Med J. 2004;27:629-33.
73. Hsu WH, Chu SJ, Tsai WC, Tsao YT. Acute myeloid leukemia presenting as one-and a-half syndrome. Am J Emerg Med. 2008;26:513,e1-2.
74. Porcu P, Farag S, Marcucci G, Cataland SR, Kennedy MS, Bissell M. Leukocytoreduction for acute leukemia. Ther Apher. 2002;6:15-23.
75. Villafuerte-Gutierrez P, Villalon L, Losa JE, Henriquez-Camacho C. Treatment of febrile neutropenia and prophylaxis in hematologic malignancies: a critical review and update. Adv Hematol. 2014;2014:986938.
76. Keng MK, Sekeres MA. Febrile neutropenia in hematologic malignancies. Curr Hematol Malig Rep. 2013;8:370-8.
77. Freifeld AG, Bow EJ, Sepkowitz KA, Boeckh MJ, Ito JI, Mullen CA, et al. Clinical practice guideline for the use of antimicrobial agents in neutropenic patients with cancer: 2010 update by the Infectious Diseases Society of America. Clin Infect Dis. 2011;52:e56-93.
78. Klastersky J, De Naurois J, Rolston K, Rapoport B, Maschmeyer G, Aapro M, et al. Management of febrile neutropaenia: ESMO clinical practice guidelines. Ann Oncol. 2016;27:v111-8.
79. Klastersky J, Awada A, Paesmans M, Aoun M. Febrile neutropenia: a critical review of the initial management. Crit Rev Oncol Hematol. 2011;78:185-94.
80. Klastersky J, Paesmans M, Rubenstein EB, Boyer M, Elting L, Feld R, et al. The Multinational Association for Supportive Care in Cancer risk index: A multinational scoring system for identifying low-risk febrile neutropenic cancer patients. J Clin Oncol. 2000;18:3038-51.

81. Link H, Böhme A, Cornely OA, Höffken K, Kellner O, Kern WV, et al. Antimicrobial therapy of unexplained fever in neutropenic patients—guidelines of the Infectious Diseases Working Party (AGIHO) of the German Society of Hematology and Oncology (DGHO), Study Group Interventional Therapy of Unexplained Fever, Arbeitsgemeinschaft Supportivmassnahmen in der Onkologie (ASO) of the Deutsche Krebsgesellschaft (DKG-German Cancer Society). Ann Hematol. 2003;82:S105-17.

82. Paul M, Yahav D, Bivas A, Fraser A, Leibovici L. Antipseudomonal beta-lactams for the initial, empirical, treatment of febrile neutropenia: comparison of beta-lactams. Cochrane Database Syst Rev. 2010;11:CD005197.

83. Person AK, Kontoyiannis DP, Alexander BD. Fungal infections in transplant and oncology patients. Hematol Oncol Clin North Am. 2011;25:193-213.

84. Pappas PG, Alexander BD, Andes DR, Hadley S, Kauffman CA, Freifeld A, et al. Invasive fungal infections among organ transplant recipients: results of the Transplant-Associated Infection Surveillance Network (TRANSNET). Clin Infect Dis. 2010;50:1101-11.

85. Bodey G, Bueltmann B, Duguid W, Gibbs D, Hanak H, Hotchi M, et al. Fungal infections in cancer patients: an international autopsy survey. Eur J Clin Microbiol Infect Dis. 1992;11:99-109.

86. Segal BH, Almyroudis NG, Battiwalla M, Herbrecht R, Perfect JR, Walsh TJ, et al. Prevention and early treatment of invasive fungal infection in patients with cancer and neutropenia and in stem cell transplant recipients in the era of newer broad-spectrum antifungal agents and diagnostic adjuncts. Clin Infect Dis. 2007;44:402-9.

87. Kullberg BJ, Arendrup MC. Invasive candidiasis. N Engl J Med. 2015;373:1445-56.

88. Pappas PG, Rex JH, Sobel JD, Filler SG, Dismukes WE, Walsh TJ, et al. Guidelines for treatment of candidiasis. Clin Infect Dis. 2004;38:161-89.

89. Pappas PG, Kauffman CA, Andes DR, Clancy CJ, Marr KA, Ostrosky-Zeichner L, et al. Clinical practice guideline for the management of candidiasis: 2016 update by the Infectious Diseases Society of America. Clin Infect Dis. 2015;62:e1-50.

90. Ostrosky-Zeichner L, Alexander BD, Kett DH, Vazquez J, Pappas PG, Saeki F, et al. Multicenter clinical evaluation of the (1-->3) beta-D-glucan assay as an aid to diagnosis of fungal infections in humans. Clin Infect Dis. 2005;41:654-9.

91. Karageorgopoulos DE, Vouloumanou EK, Ntziora F, Michalopoulos A, Rafailidis PI, Falagas ME. β-D-glucan assay for the diagnosis of invasive fungal infections: a meta-analysis. Clin Infect Dis. 2011;52:750-70.

92. Lamoth F. Galactomannan and 1,3-β-D-glucan testing for the diagnosis of invasive aspergillosis. J Fungi. 2016;2:1-8.

93. Ansorg R, van den Boom R, Rath PM. Detection of Aspergillus galactomannan antigen in foods and antibiotics. Mycoses. 1997;40:353-7.

94. Mikulska M, Calandra T, Sanguinetti M, Poulain D, Viscoli C; Third European Conference on Infections in Leukemia Group. The use of mannan antigen and anti-mannan antibodies in the diagnosis of invasive candidiasis: recommendations from the Third European Conference on Infections in Leukemia. Crit Care. 2010;14:R222.

95. Cordonnier C, Pautas C, Maury S, Vekhoff A, Farhat H, Suarez F, et al. Empirical versus preemptive antifungal therapy for high-risk, febrile, neutropenic patients: a randomized, controlled trial. Clin Infect Dis. 2009;48:1042-51.

96. Labelle AJ, Micek ST, Roubinian N, Kollef MH. Treatment-related risk factors for hospital mortality in Candida bloodstream infections. Crit Care Med. 2008;36:2967-72.

97. Raad I, Hanna H, Boktour M, Girgawy E, Danawi H, Mardani M, et al. Management of central venous catheters in patients with cancer and candidemia. Clin Infect Dis. 2004;38:1119-27.

98. Wade DS, Nava HR, Douglass HO Jr. Neutropenic enterocolitis. Clinical diagnosis and treatment. Cancer. 1992;69:17-23.

99. Rodrigues FG, Dasilva G, Wexner SD. Neutropenic enterocolitis. World J Gastroenterol. 2017;23:42-7.

100. Nesher L, Rolston KV. Neutropenic enterocolitis, a growing concern in the era of widespread use of aggressive chemotherapy. Clin Infect Dis. 2012;56:711-7.

101. Machado NO. Neutropenic enterocolitis: a continuing medical and surgical challenge. N Am J Med Sci. 2010;2:293-300.

102. Cunningham SC, Fakery K, Bass BL, Napolitano LM. Neutropenic enterocolitis in adults: case series and review of literature. Dig Dis Sci. 2005;50:215-20.

103. Dietrich CF, Hermann S, Klein S, Braden B. Sonographic signs of neutropenic enterocolitis. World J Gastroenterol. 2006;12:1397-1402.

104. Cartoni C, Dragoni F, Micozzi A, Pescarmona E, Mecarocci S, Chirletti P, et al. Neutropenic enterocolitis in patients with acute leukemia: prognostic significance of bowel wall thickening detected by ultrasonography. J Clin Oncol. 2001;19:756-61.

105. Gorschlüter M, Mey U, Strehl J, Ziske C, Schepke M, Schmidt-Wolf IG, et al. Neutropenic enterocolitis in adults: systematic analysis of evidence quality. Eur J Haematol. 2005;75:1-13.

106. Alt B, Glass NR, Sollinger H. Neutropenic enterocolitis in adults: Review of the literature and assessment of surgical intervention. Am J Surg. 1985;149:405-8.

107. Leffler DA, Lamont JT. Clostridium difficile infection. N Engl J Med. 2015;372:1539-48.

108. Eaton SR, Mazuski JE. Overview of severe Clostridium difficile infection. Crit Care Clin. 2013;29:827-39.

109. Kelly CP, LaMont JT. Clostridium difficile—more difficult than ever. N Engl J Med. 2008;359:1932-40.

110. McDonald LC, Gerding DN, Johnson S, Bakken JS, Carroll KC, Coffin SE, et al. Clinical practice guidelines for Clostridium difficile infection in adults and children: 2017 update by the Infectious Diseases Society of America (IDSA) and Society for Healthcare Epidemiology of America (SHEA). Clin Infect Dis. 2018;66:e1-48.

111. Nelson RL, Suda KJ, Evans CT. Antibiotic treatment for Clostridium difficile-associated diarrhoea in adults. Cochrane Database Syst Rev. 2017;3:CD004610.

112. Cornely OA, Crook DW, Esposito R, Poirier A, Somero MS, Weiss K, et al. Fidaxomicin versus vancomycin for infection with Clostridium difficile in Europe, Canada, and the USA: a double-blind, non-inferiority, randomised controlled trial. Lancet Infect Dis. 2012;12:281-9.
113. Kelly BJ, Tebas P. Clinical Practice and Infrastructure Review of Fecal Microbiota Transplantation for Clostridium difficile Infection. Chest. 2018;153:266-77.
114. Van Nood E, Vrieze A, Nieuwdorp M, Fuentes S, Zoetendal EG, de Vos WM, et al. Duodenal infusion of donor feces for recurrent Clostridium difficile. N Engl J Med. 2013;368:407-15.
115. Vonberg RP, Kuijper EJ, Wilcox MH, Barbut F, Tüll P, Gastmeier P, et al. Infection control measures to limit the spread of Clostridium difficile. Clin Microbiol Infect. 2008;14:2-20.
116. Johnson S, Lavergne V, Skinner AM, Gonzales-Luna AJ, Garey KW, Kelly CP, et al. Clinical practice guideline by the Infectious Diseases Society of America (IDSA) and Society for Healthcare Epidemiology of America (SHEA): 2021 focused update guidelines on management of Clostridioides difficile infection in adults. Clin Infect Dis. 2021;73(5):e1029-44.
117. Azizi AH, Shafi I, Shah N, Rosenfield K, Schainfeld R, Sista A, et al. Superior vena cava syndrome. JACC Cardiovasc Interv. 2020;13(24):2896-910.
118. Rice TW, Rodriguez RM, Light RW. The superior vena cava syndrome: clinical characteristics and evolving etiology. Medicine (Baltimore) 2006;85:37-42.
119. Wilson LD, Detterbeck FC, Yahalom J. Clinical practice. Superior vena cava syndrome with malignant causes. N Engl J Med. 2007;356:1862-9.
120. Yu JB, Wilson LD, Detterbeck FC. Superior vena cava syndrome–a proposed classification system and algorithm for management. J Thorac Oncol. 2008;3:811-4.
121. Ropper AE, Ropper AH. Acute spinal cord compression. N Engl J Med. 2017;376(14):1358-69.

CHAPTER 28

Acute Heart Failure and Cardiogenic Shock

Kushal Rajeev Kalvit, Atul Prabhakar Kulkarni

CASE STUDY

A 40-year-old female was admitted with shortness of breath and chest pain that began in the morning and progressed over the day. She had a history of fever and cough for 3 days for which she had taken paracetamol. She was conscious with a heart rate (HR) of 140/min, blood pressure (BP) of 80/60 mm Hg, respiratory rate (RR) of 30/min, and oxygen saturation (SpO_2) of 88% on room air. Bilateral crepitations were heard on auscultation with equal air entry on both the sides. Electrocardiography (ECG) showed nonspecific ST-T changes in anterior and lateral leads. 2D echocardiography (Echo) showed left ventricular (LV) systolic dysfunction with a left ventricular ejection fraction (LVEF) of 25% without any pericardial effusion, intracardiac thrombi, or vegetation. She had no known comorbidities and was not on any regular medications. She drank alcohol occasionally but denied the use of tobacco or recreational drugs.

Q1. What is acute heart failure (AHF) and what are its types?

Acute heart failure is the sudden onset of symptoms/signs of heart failure (HF) that warrant medical attention leading to either a hospital admission or a visit to the emergency department. Based on its temporal course, AHF may be de novo acute heart failure (DNHF) or acutely decompensated heart failure (ADCHF). DNHF is a new-onset HF without any previous cardiac dysfunction, while ADCHF is the acute worsening in a known case of chronic HF. ADCHF is more common than DNHF. Overall, AHF carries a high risk of readmission and mortality. Specifically, ADCHF has a worse postdischarge mortality risk as compared to DNHF, while the in-hospital mortality risk may be higher in the case of DNHF.[1]

Q2. What are the causes of DNHF?

- The most common cause is acute coronary syndrome (ACS) leading to dysfunction of a large area of LV and/or right ventricular (RV) myocardium.
- ACS leading to mechanical complications such as papillary muscle or chordae tendinae dysfunction, LV free wall rupture, or interventricular septal rupture.
- Acute valvular dysfunction [prosthetic valve dysfunction, acute aortic regurgitation (AR) caused by leaflet perforation in infective endocarditis (IE), ascending aortic dissection].
- Inflammatory diseases, such as Lyme disease, Chagas disease, giant cell myocarditis, eosinophilic myocarditis, viral myocarditis due to adenovirus, coxsackie virus, COVID-19, parvovirus B19.
- Postpartum cardiomyopathy
- Drugs or toxins (cocaine, amphetamines, alcohol, cancer chemotherapy)
- Takotsubo cardiomyopathy
- Traumatic cardiac contusion
- Cardiac tamponade

Q3. What are the precipitating factors for ADCHF?

- Noncompliance to ongoing medical and/or dietary therapy for HF
- ACS
- Uncontrolled hypertension
- Brady-/tachyarrhythmias
- Anemia
- Hypo- or hyperthyroidism
- Pulmonary infections or any new-onset systemic infection
- Medications with negative inotropy (e.g., verapamil)
- New-onset or worsening renal failure leading to fluid retention
- Pulmonary embolism (PE)

Q4. How will you investigate this patient with likely DNHF?

- 12-lead ECG to diagnose brady- or tachyarrhythmias, ST-elevated myocardial infarction (STEMI), or non-ST-elevated myocardial infarction (NSTEMI).
- Initial blood investigations [complete blood count, troponin, creatinine, blood urea nitrogen (BUN),

electrolytes, thyroid-stimulating hormone (TSH), liver function test (LFT), D-dimer, lactate, brain natriuretic peptide (BNP), or N-terminal pro-brain natriuretic peptide (NT-proBNP)].
- Echo
- Chest X-ray and/or lung ultrasound to look for bilateral pulmonary edema and/or pneumonia.
- If needed, specific investigations such as coronary angiography for suspected ACS, computed tomography pulmonary angiography (CTPA) for suspected PE, and cultures for suspected systemic infection.

Q5. What is the role of cardiac biomarkers in this case?
The biomarkers useful in the assessment of AHF are troponins, BNP, NT-proBNP, and midregional pro-atrial natriuretic peptide (MR-proANP). Troponins represent myocardial injury and are useful to exclude ACS if normal values are obtained. Natriuretic peptides (NP), if normal, can reliably exclude the diagnosis of AHF. The cutoff values for NP to consider AHF are >100 pg/mL for BNP, >300 pg/mL for NT-proBNP, and >120 pg/mL for MR-proANP. Owing to the nonspecific elevation of NT-proBNP in critically ill patients, the rule-in cutoff has been raised to >450 pg/mL for age <55 years, >900 pg/mL for 55–75 years, and >1,800 pg/mL for >75 years.[2]

Elevated troponins and NP may be present in multiple cardiac and noncardiac conditions.

Cardiac conditions: ACS, myocarditis, HF, PE, hypertrophic obstructive cardiomyopathy (HOCM), restrictive cardiomyopathy (RCM), cardioversion, implantable cardioverter defibrillator (ICD) shock, cardiac surgery, cardiac contusion.

Noncardiac condition: Ischemic stroke, subarachnoid hemorrhage (SAH), acute kidney injury (AKI), liver cirrhosis with ascites, sepsis, burns, thyrotoxicosis, advanced age.

Q6. What is the role of pulmonary artery catheterization (PAC) in this case?
The routine insertion of PAC is not recommended in the management of AHF. The ESCAPE trial in HF patients showed that PAC-guided management led to increased adverse effects without any survival benefit or improvement in other outcomes. PAC insertion carries a risk of pneumothorax, line infection, arrhythmias, right bundle-branch block (RBBB), and pulmonary artery (PA) perforation. Moreover, there are no concrete end goals of various parameters to guide hemodynamic management after PA catheter insertion. The only situations where PA catheter insertion may be considered are:
- Mixed origin of shock such as AHF with septic shock or the coexistence of complex congenital heart disease or RV dysfunction.
- Documentation of hemodynamic parameters to assess candidacy for ventricular assist device (VAD) insertion or cardiac transplantation.

Q7. What is the Forrester classification of HF? What are the phenotypes of AHF?
Based on the pulmonary artery occlusion pressure (PAOP) and cardiac index (CI), four classes of HF have been described. An increased PAOP indicates pulmonary edema and hence "wet lungs," while a low CI indicates cardiogenic shock and hence "cold extremities." These classes are not exclusive and may change as the patient's condition worsens.
- *Class I:* Warm and dry (normal PAOP and CI; lowest mortality risk).
- *Class II:* Warm and wet (normal CI and increased PAOP).
- *Class III:* Cold and dry (low CI and normal PAOP).
- *Class IV:* Cold and wet (low CI and increased PAOP).

Similar to these classes, the four clinical presentations/phenotypes of AHF are as follows:
1. ADCHF (wet and warm OR dry and cold)
2. Acute pulmonary edema (wet and warm)
3. Isolated RV failure (dry and cold OR wet and cold)
4. Cardiogenic shock (wet and cold)

Q8. What are the suggested criteria to diagnose cardiogenic shock?
Clinical criteria (both required):
- Systolic blood pressure (SBP) <90 mm Hg for >30 minutes OR mean BP <60 mm Hg for >30 minutes OR requirement of vasopressors to maintain SBP >90 mm Hg or mean arterial pressure (MAP) >60 mm Hg.
- Hypoperfusion defined by decreased mentation, cold extremities, urine output, lactate >2 mmol/L.

Hemodynamic criteria (requires one criterion in addition to SBP and CI):[3]
- SBP <90 mm Hg or MAP <60 mm Hg
- CI <2.2 L/min/m^2
- PAOP >15 mm Hg
- Cardiac power output [CPO = cardiac output (CO) × MAP/451] <0.6 W
- Shock index >1.0
- RV shock [central venous pressure (CVP) >15 mm Hg, CVP-PAOP >0.6, pulmonary artery pulse index <1.0].

Q9. What are the principles of therapy based on phenotypes of AHF?
Acutely decompensated heart failure is the most common presentation and occurs in patients with preexisting HF. The progression of symptoms is gradual over a few days and is mainly related to fluid retention and venous congestion. The usual phenotype is wet and warm and requires diuretic

therapy. Some cases present with the dry and cold phenotype with shock as the predominant feature secondary to systolic failure. The mainstay of therapy then shifts to vasopressors/inotropes.

Acute pulmonary edema is a distinct class and is characterized by a wet and warm phenotype. The symptoms develop rapidly due to lung congestion and are often associated with uncontrolled hypertension. The three important treatment modalities in this scenario are positive pressure ventilation (most commonly noninvasive, with oxygen) therapy and diuretics, and vasodilators for LV afterload reduction. However, vasodilators will need continuous arterial pressure monitoring [preferably invasive, if intravenous (IV) vasodilators are used] and frequent titration.

Isolated RV failure usually presents as dry and cold phenotype. RV failure leads to increased atrial pressure and systemic congestion. At the same time, it leads to reduced CO due to ventricular interdependence necessitating vasopressor support. Fluid loading should be strictly avoided unless a gross hypovolemic state is present.

Cardiogenic shock carries the poorest prognosis and usually presents with the wet and cold phenotype. The mainstay of therapy includes vasopressors/inotropes, mechanical ventilation, and mechanical circulatory support (MCS).

Q10. Discuss the initial stabilization of a patient with AHF.
Airway and breathing: Oxygen therapy is not routinely recommended in nonhypoxemic patients. It should be commenced only when the SpO_2 <90% or partial pressure of oxygen (PaO_2) <60 mm Hg. If oxygen therapy is needed, positive pressure noninvasive ventilation is preferred over traditional oxygen therapy as it has been shown to reduce the need for intubation and mortality. In addition to improving oxygenation, nasal intermittent positive pressure ventilation (NIPPV) helps by reducing the preload and pulmonary congestion via raised intrathoracic pressure. It also reduces LV afterload by Laplace's law and decreases the LV stroke work. Endotracheal intubation is indicated in the event of progressive respiratory failure despite noninvasive ventilation (NIV) or in the presence of cardiogenic shock. Caution needs to be exercised during the application of positive pressure ventilation in isolated RV failure as it may worsen the RV afterload.

Hemodynamics: The hemodynamic management depends on the presentation phenotype. ADHF, isolated RV failure, and cardiogenic shock phenotypes commonly present with hypotension and/or frank shock leading to systemic hypoperfusion. The mainstay of therapy is vasopressors, norepinephrine being the drug of choice. The target is to maintain an MAP sufficient to provide adequate end-organ perfusion. Dopamine has been shown to increase the risk of arrhythmias and may increase mortality in cardiogenic shock and is best avoided. Epinephrine acts as a good inopressor but has been shown in a meta-analysis of more than 2,500 patients that it increases the risk of death in cardiogenic shock threefold as compared to norepinephrine. Vasopressin may be a preferred choice in isolated RV failure or combined biventricular failure, at least theoretically, as it does not increase pulmonary vascular resistance significantly. Inotropes such as dobutamine are not routinely recommended in patients with AHF. Inotropes are associated with tachycardia, peripheral vasodilation, and worsening of hypotension, arrhythmias, and myocardial ischemia. They may be used in cases where hypoperfusion persists with a low CO despite achieving the target MAP with vasopressors. Dobutamine is the commonly used inotrope; however, levosimendan may be preferred in patients on chronic β-blocker therapy. Irrespective of the inotrope chosen, they need to be started at the lowest dose with gradual titration to the target effect. Digoxin may be used in cases of ADHF with atrial fibrillation and HR > 110/min. An initial rapid digitalization ensures quick achievement of therapeutic levels, but needs therapeutic drug monitoring as the pharmacokinetics will be altered in shock states.[4,5]

Acute pulmonary edema phenotype and some cases of ADHF commonly present with hypertensive emergency. These patients require a rapid lowering of BP with vasodilators to reduce the LV afterload. Nitrates such as nitroglycerine or nitroprusside are the most commonly used vasodilators due to the ability to rapidly titrate the doses. They can be started if the SBP is >110 mm Hg but need invasive monitoring of BP to prevent an excessive drop.

Diuretic therapy: Diuretics are the mainstay of treatment in patients with pulmonary edema or isolated RV failure leading to systemic congestion. Diuresis leads to relief of congestion and improvement in oxygenation. However, they should not be used in patients with cardiogenic shock. Loop diuretics are chosen due to their rapid onset of action and effectiveness. The initial dose can be either 20–40 mg IV furosemide or one to two times the dose of oral diuretics if it was already ongoing. The diuretic response should be assessed at 2 or 6 hours with a spot urine Na and hourly urine output. If the urine Na after 2 hours is >50–70 mEq/L and/or the urine output is >100–150 mL/h, the same dose of diuretic needs to be repeated after 6–12 hours. If not, doubling the dose of diuretics with repeated assessment of response is warranted. If there is still not an adequate response, the addition of a second diuretic such as thiazide may be considered. Although the DOSE trial did not demonstrate a better global patient symptom assessment with higher dose diuretics, higher doses led to better relief of dyspnea and net fluid loss. Daily monitoring of creatinine and electrolytes is mandatory. Transition to oral diuretics should be done, only if the patient has stabilized. It is important to achieve adequate decongestion before discharge to prevent rehospitalization.[6]

Q11. What is the role of MCS in AHF?

Cardiogenic shock resulting in end-organ dysfunction has a high risk of mortality and often needs high doses of vasopressors/inotropes. These inopressors have their own adverse effect profile beyond a certain dose. Temporary MCS is indicated in such cases, not responding to optimal medical therapy. It can be initiated as a bridge-to-recovery (BTR), bridge-to-decision (BTD), or bridge-to-bridge (BTB) therapy. The patient may either recover spontaneously after a short duration of MCS or after completion of definitive therapy tailored to the cause (i.e., BTR). Some patients may not recover at all and may require substitution with a permanent/durable MCS device (i.e., BTB). The data regarding the efficacy of MCS as compared to optimal medical therapy is scarce and hence, it has to be employed on a case-by-case basis.

The IABP-SHOCK II trial showed no significant mortality benefit of intra-aortic balloon pump (IABP) over optimal medical therapy in patients undergoing early revascularization in cardiogenic shock post myocardial infarction (MI) at 30 days, 6 months, and 12 months follow-up. Although the trial had some limitations, this led to the recommendation of not using IABP routinely in post-MI cardiogenic shock. However, IABP can still be used in cardiogenic shock due to other causes and also in cases of MI with mechanical complications, till the patient undergoes corrective surgery. The other indication for temporary MCS is when the patient is awaiting either cardiac transplantation or placement of a permanent MCS device.[7,8]

Q12. Which MCS devices can be used in AHF?

The following are the acute percutaneous MCS therapies available:
- IABP
- Axial flow pumps (Impella CP, Impella LP 2.5)
- Left atrial to femoral arterial VADs (TandemHeart)
- Venoarterial extracorporeal membrane oxygenation (VA-ECMO).

Intra-aortic balloon pump is the most commonly used device. It improves coronary perfusion, decreases LV afterload, and modestly improves CO (0.8–1 L/min). It is inserted via an 8Fr sheath in the femoral or axillary artery. The cyclic inflation and deflation of the IABP balloon are dependent on the cardiac cycle and need to be timed properly. The axial flow pumps (Impella) are devices inserted via the femoral artery and pass in a retrograde fashion across the aortic valve into LV. They unload LV by pumping blood from LV to aorta. The Impella CP and Impella 2.5 are used for LV failure and maintain a CO of 2.5–4 L/min. The Impella RP is a right-sided device that pumps blood from the inferior vena cava (IVC) to PA with an output of >4 L/min. These axial flow pumps pump blood continuously independent of the cardiac cycle. The TandemHeart device is inserted via the femoral vein into the right atrium and requires a transseptal puncture to access blood in the left atrium. It then draws blood from LA and pumps it via a returning cannula in the femoral arteries. It requires considerable expertise for insertion and is time consuming as compared to other modalities.[9]

REFERENCES

1. Raffaello WM, Henrina J, Huang I, Lim MA, Suciadi LP, Siswanto BB, et al. Clinical characteristics of de novo heart failure and acute decompensated chronic heart failure: are they distinctive phenotypes that contribute to different outcomes? Card Fail Rev. 2021;7:e02.
2. McDonagh TA, Metra M, Adamo M, Gardner RS, Baumbach A, Böhm M, et al. 2021 ESC Guidelines for the diagnosis and treatment of acute and chronic heart failure. Eur Heart J. 2021;42(36):3599-3726.
3. Heidenreich PA, Bozkurt B, Aguilar D, Allen LA, Byun JJ, Colvin MM, et al. 2022 AHA/ACC/HFSA Guideline for the management of heart failure: a report of the American College of Cardiology/American Heart Association Joint Committee on Clinical Practice Guidelines. Circulation. 2022;145(18):e895-e1032.
4. De Backer D, Biston P, Devriendt J, Madl C, Chochrad D, Aldecoa C, et al. Comparison of dopamine and norepinephrine in the treatment of shock. N Engl J Med. 2010;362(9):779-89.
5. Léopold V, Gayat E, Pirracchio R, Spinar J, Parenica J, Tarvasmäki T, et al. Epinephrine and short-term survival in cardiogenic shock: an individual data meta-analysis of 2583 patients. Intensive Care Med. 2018;44(6):847-56.
6. Felker GM, Lee KL, Bull DA, Redfield MM, Stevenson LW, Goldsmith SR, et al. Diuretic strategies in patients with acute decompensated heart failure. N Engl J Med. 2011;364(9):797-805.
7. Thiele H, Zeymer U, Neumann FJ, Ferenc M, Olbrich HG, Hausleiter J, et al. Intraaortic balloon support for myocardial infarction with cardiogenic shock. N Engl J Med. 2012;367(14):1287-96.
8. Thiele H, Zeymer U, Thelemann N, Neumann FJ, Hausleiter J, Abdel-Wahab M, et al. Intraaortic balloon pump in cardiogenic shock complicating acute myocardial infarction: long-term 6-year outcome of the randomized IABP-SHOCK II trial. Circulation. 2019;139(3):395-403.
9. Vahdatpour C, Collins D, Goldberg S. Cardiogenic shock. J Am Heart Assoc. 2019;8(8):e011991.

Severe Acute Pancreatitis

Subhal Bhalchandra Dixit, Khalid Ismail Khatib

CASE STUDY

A 32-year-old male was brought to casualty with complaints of severe abdominal pain since 3 hours duration. Pain started after a party, where alcohol was served. On examination, patient was conscious, anxious, and in pain. His heart rate was 113 beats/min, blood pressure was 150/100 mm Hg, respiratory rate 25 breaths/min, and saturation was 100% on room air. Arterial blood gas (ABG) was normal and laboratory reports showed elevated serum amylase and lipase (more than five times baseline).

A diagnosis of acute pancreatitis was made, and the patient was admitted for management.

Q1. What are the common causes of pancreatitis?

The common etiologies of pancreatitis are classified as follows:

- *Mechanical:* Cholelithiasis, biliary sludge, pancreatic or periampullary malignancy, stenosis of the ampulla of Vater, and duodenal obstruction or stricture
- *Toxic:* Alcohol, scorpion bite, and organophosphorus poisoning
- *Drugs:*
  - Antibiotics—metronidazole and tetracycline
  - Diuretics (furosemide and thiazides)
  - Sulfa drugs—sulfasalazine, 5-aminosalicylic acid (5-ASA), and salicylates
  - Chemotherapy drugs—L-asparaginase
  - Immunosuppressants—azathioprine
  - Anticonvulsants—valproic acid
  - Others—calcium, estrogen, etc.
- *Metabolic:* Hyperlipidemia and hypercalcemia
- *Infection:*
  - *Viruses:* Mumps, Coxsackie, hepatitis B, *Cytomegalovirus*, varicella-zoster virus, herpes simplex virus, and human immunodeficiency virus (HIV)
  - *Bacteria: Mycoplasma, Legionella, Leptospira,* and *Salmonella*
  - *Fungi: Aspergillus*
  - *Parasites: Toxoplasma, Cryptosporidium,* and *Ascaris*
- *Trauma:* Abdominal injury (blunt/penetrating), post-laparotomy, or post-endoscopic retrograde cholangiopancreatography (ERCP).
- *Congenital malformations of pancreas:* Pancreas divisum and choledochocele
- *Vascular insufficiency:* Pancreatic ischemia, atheroembolism, and vasculitis (polyarteritis nodosa and systemic lupus erythematosus)
- *Genetic:* Pancreatitis due to genetic mutations (CFTR, PRSS1, SPINK1, etc.)
- *Others:* Pregnancy, kidney transplantation, alpha-1-antitrypsin deficiency
- Idiopathic.

Q2. How do you score the severity of pancreatitis?

There are many predictive models which intend to predict the severity of acute pancreatitis. These can be used on admission or are available for use after 2–3 days of hospitalization. However, all these models suffer from low specificity. Also, they are useful for groups of patients, but do not have high accuracy in a given patient's bedside, for predicting results.

The various scoring systems are:

- *Ranson's criteria:* It was developed in 1974 and was the earliest scoring system to be used in patients with acute pancreatitis. It uses 11 parameters [5 on admission (age >55 years, white blood cell (WBC) count >16,000/mm^3, blood glucose level >200 mg/dL or 11.1 mmol/L, lactate dehydrogenase (LDH) >350 U/L, aspartate aminotransferase/serum glutamic pyruvic transaminase (AST/SGPT) >250 U/L) and 6 during next 48 hours (hematocrit reduces by ≥10%, blood urea nitrogen (BUN) raised by ≥5 mg/dL or 1.8 mmol/L despite intravenous (IV) fluids, serum calcium levels <8 mg/dL or 2 mmol/L, PO$_2$ <60 mm Hg, base deficit >4 mEq/L, fluid sequestration, or positive fluid balance >6 L)]. A score of 1 to 3 represents mild pancreatitis (mortality <3%) while as the score increases to >4, mortality increases significantly (>40% when score is >6).[1,2] However, a large meta-analysis found that Ranson's score poorly predicted severity.[3]

- *Acute physiology and chronic health evaluation (APACHE II) score:* It was developed to predict the mortality of critically ill patients in intensive care units (ICUs). It is widely used in these patients and has been applied in patients with acute pancreatitis. Mortality from acute pancreatitis is <4% with a score <8 and is 11-18% with a score >8.[2,4]

  Advantages: (1) Good negative predictive value but modest positive predictive value for predicting mortality in severe acute pancreatitis and (2) Can be performed daily.

  Disadvantages: (1) Complex and cumbersome to use, (2) Does not differentiate between types of pancreatitis (interstitial or necrotizing), (3) Does not differentiate between sterile and infected necrosis, and (4) Poor predictive value at 24 hours.

- *Systemic inflammatory response syndrome (SIRS) score:* The presence of SIRS with pancreatitis is associated with increased mortality as compared to acute pancreatitis without SIRS (25% in patients with persistent SIRS from admission vs. 0% in those with no SIRS).[5]

- *Bedside index of severity in acute pancreatitis (BISAP) score:* It was developed and validated in a large number of patients (approximately 18,000) from 2000 to 2005. It consists of: (1) BUN >25 mg/dL, (2) impaired mental status, (3) SIRS (using the same criteria as the SIRS score mentioned earlier), (4) age >60 years, and (5) presence of pleural effusion. 1 point is awarded to each of these, if present in the first 24 hours.[6] A BISAP score of 0 has mortality <1% while score of 5 has a mortality of 22%.[7]

- *Harmless acute pancreatitis score:* It takes into account the absence of rebound tenderness or guarding, and the presence of normal hematocrit, and normal serum creatinine to predict the harmless course of acute pancreatitis. It can be calculated on admission and has an accuracy of 98%.[8]

- *Organ failure-based scores:* Early (within 72 hours of admission) and persistent organ failure (>48 hours) is associated with prolonged hospital stay and increased mortality (approximately 20-50%).[9,10] The various organ failure scoring systems are: (1) Goris multiple organ failure score, (2) Marshall (or multiple) organ dysfunction score, (3) Bernard score, (4) Sequential organ failure assessment (SOFA), and (5) Logistic organ dysfunction system score (LODSS).

- *CT severity index (Balthazar score):* Described later in this chapter.

International societies [International Association of Pancreatology (IAP)/American Pancreatic Association (APA), and American College of Gastroenterology (ACG)] recommend the use of these severity/predictive scoring systems in patients with acute pancreatitis.

Q3. How will you resuscitate the patient? Describe management of fluids, pain, and nutrition. Discuss the role of antibiotics.

Fluid Resuscitation

Isotonic crystalloid solution (0.9% saline or lactated Ringer's solution) at a rate of 5-10 mL/kg/h were advocated in previous guidelines. Recent randomized controlled trials (RCTs) and guidelines however caution against the use of aggressive fluid resuscitation in milder forms of acute pancreatitis due to deleterious effects of fluid overload. A more judicious rate of fluid administration (1.5 mL/kg/h and if required 10 mL/kg bolus only for those patients who appear hypovolemic) has been advocated.[11,12]

Nonaggressive fluid resuscitation is especially important in patients with cardiovascular, renal, or other related comorbid factors. In patients with severe hypercalcemia, lactated Ringer's solution is contraindicated as it contains calcium (3 mEq/L). Hydroxyethyl starch should not be used for resuscitation. The rate of fluid administration is readjusted frequently as required in the first 6 hours and up to the next 24-48 hours. The goals of resuscitation are: (1) Heart rate <120 beats/minute, (2) Mean arterial pressure (MAP) between 65 and 85 mm Hg, (3) Urine output >0.5 mL/kg/h, (4) Hematocrit of 35-45%, and (5) Reduction of BUN over 24 hours, especially if it was high on admission.

Fluid resuscitation should be done for first 24-48 hours only and over vigorous fluid resuscitation is to be avoided.

Pain Management

Opioid analgesics may be used safely (fentanyl, 20-50 µg bolus followed by infusion, if required). Patient-controlled analgesia (PCA) is preferred, if available.

Nutrition

Mild pancreatitis: IV hydration alone followed by oral diet as tolerated, to be started within 24 hours. If oral diet is not tolerated, enteral nutrition should be tried.

Moderately severe pancreatitis to severe pancreatitis: These patients will usually require nutritional support. Enteral feeding (usually nasojejunal or nasogastric) is preferred over total parenteral nutrition. Patients may be initiated on clear liquids orally within the first 24 hours, in the absence of ileus, nausea, or vomiting. This is then advanced to low residue, low fat, and soft diet, as tolerated. In patients who do not tolerate oral feeds, nasogastric or nasojejunal feeds with high protein, low fat, and semi-elemental feeding formulas are started (20–25 mL/h initially and advanced to meet 30% of daily caloric requirement). Nasogastric route is as good as nasojejunal route. Partial parenteral nutrition may be integrated along with enteral nutrition if patients do not tolerate oral or nasojejunal feeds or if target caloric requirements are not reached even after 72 hours.[13-15]

Antibiotics
Prophylactic antibiotics should not be used. If there is suspicion of infection (usually extrapancreatic), antibiotics may be used. But, if cultures are negative and a source of infection cannot be determined, they should be stopped.

Q4. What is the role of imaging in this patient?
A contrast-enhanced computed tomography (CECT) is performed only in patients with the following indications: (1) Moderately severe or severe acute pancreatitis, (2) signs of sepsis, or (3) clinical deterioration 72 hours after initial presentation. Evaluation is done to assess the presence of acute pancreatic or extrapancreatic fluid collection/necrosis and local complications.

After 48 hours, the patient still complains of pain and is on a fentanyl PCA currently. However, his demand for analgesia is increasing. He has started to have fever spikes also. A CT imaging of abdomen is performed and reveals edematous pancreas and a collection near the tail of pancreas. The patient is also restless and demands to be started on oral feeds.

Q5. Discuss the CT severity scoring in pancreatitis.[16]
Pancreatitis is graded depending on findings on an unenhanced CT
- Grade A—normal pancreas and given a score of 0
- Grade B—focal/diffuse enlargement of the pancreas, no peripancreatic inflammation and given score of 1
- Grade C—peripancreatic inflammation with abnormalities within the pancreas and given a score of 2
- Grade D—fluid collections within/outside the pancreas and given a score of 3
- Grade E—more than and equal to two large collections of gas within the pancreas or in the retroperitoneal area and given a score of 4.

Findings on enhanced CT give a score for presence of necrosis
- Necrosis absent score 0
- Necrosis <33% score 2
- Necrosis 33–50% score 4
- Necrosis >50% score 6

The CT severity index is calculated by adding the two scores for a maximum of 10. A CT severity index of ≥6 indicates severe disease.

Q6. What is the approach for treatment of local collections? What is the role of antibiotics? When and how will you start antibiotic's and how is the treatment guided?
There are two types of acute local collections:
1. *Acute peripancreatic fluid collection (APFC)* usually develops early, does not have well-defined wall, is asymptomatic, and resolves spontaneously within 7–10 days.
2. *Acute necrotic collection* with infection is managed by antibiotics (carbapenem alone or a quinolone, ceftazidime, or cefepime combined with metronidazole) and necrosectomy. Infections usually occur after 10 days and patients will present with signs of infection and presence of gas in the necrosis on abdominal imaging. Necrosectomy may be performed with minimally invasive (endoscopic or percutaneous radiologic) approach or surgical approach.

Q7. What are the indications for early/emergent ERCP? What are the indications for early surgical interventions?
Endoscopic retrograde cholangiopancreatography: Patients with suspected or proven acute gallstone pancreatitis may be candidates for ERCP. However, it is not indicated routinely for all patients with acute gallstone pancreatitis. Only those patients with associated cholangitis or common bile duct obstruction should be subjected to early or emergent ERCP.[15]

Surgical interventions: Surgical interventions may need to be done in the following situations:
- As a follow-up to endoscopic or percutaneous radiologic approach for infected necrosectomy as described earlier
- Abdominal compartment syndrome (ACS) (as described in detail later)
- For treatment of gastrointestinal (GI) bleeding, if other less invasive approaches unsuccessful
- Other complications like ischemic/gangrenous bowel or necrotizing cholecystitis associated with pancreatitis
- Small intestinal or colonic fistula extending into peripancreatic collections.[15]

After starting feeds, he complained of abdominal bloating and abdominal distension. Hence, he is kept further nil by mouth (NBM) and fluids continued. However, his abdominal distension increased. Next day it is noted that he was tachypneic also. Chest X-ray revealed moderate pleural effusion on the left. His abdominal girth had increased by 8 inches and abdomen appeared to be tense and distended. For the past 3 hours his urine output was also gradually trailing.

Q8. What is characteristic of pleural fluid in pancreatitis?
Pleural effusion in acute pancreatitis shows the following characteristics:
- *Size:* Usually small, may be mild to moderate
- *Side:* Left sided (70%), right sided (10%), and bilateral (20%)

- *Appearance:* Clear or hemorrhagic
- *Protein:* >3 g/dL
- *Amylase:* Normal to high (>1,000 U/L)[17]

The two causes of pleural effusion in pancreatitis are:
1. Blockage of lymphatics traversing the diaphragm, and
2. Pancreaticopleural fistula due to leak from pancreatic duct or pseudocyst of pancreas.

Q9. What is the grading of acute GI injury?

Acute gastrointestinal injury (AGI) was defined by the Working Group on Abdominal Problems (WGAP) of the European Society of Intensive Care Medicine (ESICM) in 2012 as malfunction of the GI tract due to acute illness in ICU patients. It is graded as follows:

- *AGI grade I:* Increased risk of developing GI dysfunction/failure
- *AGI grade II:* GI dysfunction (requires interventions to restore GI function)
- *AGI grade III:* GI failure (GI function cannot be restored even with interventions)
- *AGI grade IV:* Life-threatening GI failure.[18]

Q10. What is intra-abdominal hypertension (IAH)? How will you measure it?

Intra-abdominal pressure (IAP) is defined as the steady state pressure present within the abdomen and it is approximately 5-7 mm Hg in adult ICU patients.[17]

Intra-abdominal hypertension is defined as sustained and persistent pathological increase in IAP >12 mm Hg.

Intra-abdominal hypertension is graded as follows:
- *Grade I:* IAP 12-15 mm Hg
- *Grade II:* IAP 16-20 mm Hg
- *Grade III:* IAP 21-25 mm Hg
- *Grade IV:* IAP > 25 mm Hg, termed ACS

Primary IAH is defined as IAH which develops due to injury or disease in the abdominopelvic area, frequently requiring intervention (either surgical, percutaneous, or radiological).

Secondary IAH is defined as IAH due to conditions which are not present in the abdominopelvic region.

Abdominal perfusion pressure (APP) is defined as MAP minus the IAP.

Risk factors for the development of IAH/ACS areas are as follows:
- *Decreased compliance of the abdominal wall:* Due to laparotomy, major burns or trauma, and prone positioning.
- *Increased abdominal contents:* Acute pancreatitis, hemo-/pneumoperitoneum or intraperitoneal fluid collections (ascites, infection, peritonitis, and abscess), laparoscopy with excessive insufflation pressures, intra-abdominal, or retroperitoneal tumors, peritoneal dialysis.
- *Increased contents in the GI lumen:* Gastric distention, paresis of the stomach or intestines (ileus), and volvulus
- *Capillary leak/fluid resuscitation:* Massive fluid resuscitation or positive fluid balance or massive transfusion, acidosis, damage control laparotomy, hypothermia, increased APACHE-II, or SOFA score.
- *Others/miscellaneous:* Age, mechanical ventilation, positive end-expiratory pressure (PEEP), obesity or increased body mass index, bacteremia, sepsis, shock or hypotension, coagulopathy, increased head of bed angle, and massive incisional hernia repair.

Intra-abdominal hypertension is measured by the trans-bladder technique as it is simple to use and also low-cost.

Q11. What is ACS? How will you manage ACS?

Abdominal compartment syndrome is defined as a sustained and persistent IAP >20 mm Hg (with/without an APP <60 mm Hg) associated with new organ dysfunction/failure.[19]

Management of ACS

- *Medical:* Adequate sedation and analgesia, neuromuscular blockade (brief duration as a temporary measure), promotility agents (neostigmine), diuretics, fluid resuscitation strategies (avoiding positive cumulative fluid balance), body positioning, nasogastric/colonic decompression, and continuous renal replacement therapies
- *Minimally invasive:* Percutaneous catheter drainage (PCD)
- *Surgical:* Decompressive laparotomy with temporary abdominal closure (TAC) techniques in patients requiring open abdomen[19]

REFERENCES

1. Ranson JH, Rifkind KM, Roses DF, Fink SD, Eng K, Spencer FC. Prognostic signs and the role of operative management in acute pancreatitis. Surg Gynecol Obstet. 1974;139:69-81.
2. Banks PA, Freeman ML; Practice Parameters Committee of the American College of Gastroenterology. Practice guidelines in acute pancreatitis. Am J Gastroenterol. 2006;101:2379-400.
3. De Bernardinis M, Violi V, Roncoroni L, Boselli AS, Giunta A, Peracchia A. Discriminant power and information content of Ranson's prognostic signs in acute pancreatitis: a meta-analytic study. Crit Care Med. 1999;27:2272-83.
4. Larvin M. Assessment of clinical severity and prognosis. In: Beger HG, Warshaw AL, Buchler MW (Eds). The Pancreas. Oxford: Blackwell Science; 1998. pp. 489.
5. Mofidi R, Duff MD, Wigmore SJ, Madhavan KK, Garden OJ, Parks RW. Association between early systemic inflammatory response, severity of multiorgan dysfunction and death in acute pancreatitis. Br J Surg. 2006;93:738-44.

6. Wu BU, Johannes RS, Sun X, Tabak Y, Conwell DL, Banks PA. The early prediction of mortality in acute pancreatitis: a large population-based study. Gut. 2008;57:1698-703.
7. Papachristou GI, Muddana V, Yadav D, O'Connell M, Sanders MK, Slivka A, et al. Comparison of BISAP, Ranson's, APACHE-II, and CTSI scores in predicting organ failure, complications, and mortality in acute pancreatitis. Am J Gastroenterol. 2010;105:435-41.
8. Lankisch PG, Weber-Dany B, Hebel K, Maisonneuve P, Lowenfels AB. The harmless acute pancreatitis score: a clinical algorithm for rapid initial stratification of nonsevere disease. Clin Gastroenterol Hepatol. 2009;7:702-5.
9. Isenmann R, Rau B, Beger HG. Early severe acute pancreatitis: characteristics of a new subgroup. Pancreas. 2001;22:274-8.
10. Buter A, Imrie CW, Carter CR, Evans S, McKay CJ. Dynamic nature of early organ dysfunction determines outcome in acute pancreatitis. Br J Surg. 2002;89:298-302.
11. Crockett SD, Wani S, Gardner TB, Falck-Ytter Y, Barkun AN; American Gastroenterological Association Institute Clinical Guidelines Committee. American Gastroenterological Association Institute Guideline on Initial Management of Acute Pancreatitis. Gastroenterology. 2018;154:1096-101.
12. de-Madaria E, Buxbaum JL, Maisonneuve P, García García de Paredes A, Zapater P, Guilabert L, et al. Aggressive or moderate fluid resuscitation in acute pancreatitis. N Engl J Med. 2022;387:989-1000.
13. Casaer MP, Mesotten D, Hermans G, Wouters PJ, Schetz M, Meyfroidt G, et al. Early versus late parenteral nutrition in critically ill adults. N Engl J Med. 2011;365:506-17.
14. Kutsogiannis J, Alberda C, Gramlich L, Cahill NE, Wang M, Day AG, et al. Early use of supplemental parenteral nutrition in critically ill patients: results of an international multicenter observational study. Crit Care Med. 2011;39:2691-9.
15. Leppäniemi A, Tolonen M, Tarasconi A, Segovia-Lohse H, Gamberini E, Kirkpatrick AW, et al. 2019 WSES guidelines for the management of severe acute pancreatitis. World J Emerg Surg. 2019;14:27.
16. Balthazar EJ, Robinson DL, Megibow AJ, Ranson JH. Acute pancreatitis: value of CT in establishing prognosis. Radiology. 1990;174:331-6.
17. Basran GS, Ramasubramanian R, Verma R. Intrathoracic complications of acute pancreatitis. Br J Dis Chest. 1987;81:326-31.
18. Reintam Blaser A, Malbrain ML, Starkopf J, Fruhwald S, Jakob SM, De Waele J, et al. Gastrointestinal function in intensive care patients: terminology, definitions and management. Recommendations of the ESICM Working Group on Abdominal Problems. Intensive Care Med. 2012;38:384-94.
19. Kirkpatrick A, Roberts D, De Waele J, Jaeschke R, Malbrain M, De Keulenaer B, et al. Intra-abdominal hypertension and the abdominal compartment syndrome: updated consensus definitions and clinical practice guidelines from the World Society of Abdominal Compartment Syndrome. Intensive Care Med. 2013;39:1190-206.

Acute Liver Failure

Dinesh Ekambaram, Raymond Dominic Savio

CASE STUDY

A 22-year-old male with no previous comorbidities was brought to the intensive care unit (ICU) with a history of fever for 7 days. He was on symptomatic treatment until yesterday when his relatives noted that he was becoming restless and irritable. In the ICU, the patient was restless and drowsy, but arousable. His Glasgow Coma Scale (GCS) was 12/15 (E4M5V3) and there were no focal neurological deficits. His pupils were equal and reacting to light. Icteric hue was noticed all over the body and sclera. His vitals were: Heart rate (HR)—68 beats/min, regular, blood pressure (BP)—130/70 mm Hg, respiratory rate (RR)—24 breaths/min, peripheral capillary oxygen saturation (SpO2)—100% on room air, and temperature—100°F. Laboratory investigation showed hemoglobin (Hb)—12.2 g/dL, total count (TC)—4,800 cells/mm³, differential count—polymorphs 56% and lymphocytes 44%, and platelet count—1.23 lakhs/mm³. The liver function tests revealed bilirubin (T)—12 mg/dL, serum glutamic pyruvic transaminase (SGPT)—10,000 IU/L, serum glutamic oxaloacetic transaminase (SGOT)—14,500 IU/L, and alkaline phosphatase (ALP)—2,300 IU/L. The random blood sugar was 70 mg/dL and the international normalized ratio (INR) was 6.0. His viral markers tested positive for hepatitis E. Hepatitis B surface antigen (HBsAg) was negative.

Q1. How will you classify his liver condition currently?

The patient has a history of acute-onset illness (7 days) with fever, altered mental status (encephalopathy), icterus, elevated liver enzymes, raised INR, and positive markers for hepatitis E viral infection. All of these point toward a working diagnosis of liver failure. The O'Grady system classifies liver failure as hyperacute if encephalopathy sets in within 7 days of onset of jaundice. Although the time since the onset of jaundice is not clear from the available history, the presence of icterus with encephalopathy within 7 days of illness will warrant the classification of the condition as hyperacute liver failure.

There are many systems of classification for acute liver failure (ALF), with the O'Grady system being more commonly used.[1,2] This classifies ALF as follows:

- *Hyperacute*—encephalopathy, which occurs within 7 days of onset of jaundice.
- *Acute*—when encephalopathy occurs between an interval of 8 and 28 days from onset of jaundice.
- *Subacute*—when encephalopathy occurs between an interval of 28 days to 12 weeks from onset of jaundice. The Bernuau, Japanese, and American Association for the Study of Liver Diseases (AASLD) systems for classification given in **Table 1** may also be used for liver failure.[1]

TABLE 1: Alternate systems for classification of acute liver failure (ALF).

Author	Classification		Nomenclature
Bernuau et al. (France)	• <2 weeks after jaundice onset • Between 2 and 12 weeks after jaundice onset		• Fulminant liver failure • Subfulminant liver failure
Mochida et al. (Japan)	Without or with encephalopathy within 8 weeks of disease symptoms' onset	• Within 10 days • Between 11 and 56 days	• ALF without and with coma • Subacute liver failure without and with coma
Polson and Lee (AASLD)	Preexisting disease of <26 weeks' duration		ALF

(AASLD: American Association for the Study of Liver Diseases)

Q2. Why is it important to classify liver failure?

The categorization of ALF into various classes is important as it helps to risk stratify and prognosticate patients. The probability of developing cerebral edema is higher in hyperacute liver failure. The best survival chances likewise are with hyperacute liver failure although it has the most severe presentation.

Paradoxically least survival is seen in patients with subacute liver failure (SALF). It carries a grave prognosis in patients who are managed medically without transplantation.[3]

Q3. What is acute-on-chronic liver failure (ACLF)? What are the various definitions of ACLF?

Acute insult (various causes such as hepatitis and drug-induced) over a preexisting chronic liver condition, leading to the involvement of multiple organ systems along with deterioration in liver function is called ACLF. It is different from decompensation with respect to the severity and involvement of other organ systems.

The recent American College of Gastroenterology (ACG) guidelines defined ACLF as "a potentially reversible condition in patients with chronic liver disease with or without cirrhosis that is associated with the potential for multiple organ failure and mortality within 3 months in the absence of treatment of the underlying liver disease, liver support, or liver transplantation." ACLF involves elevation in serum bilirubin and prolongation of the INR.

Various societies have attempted to define criteria for ACLF, of which the Asian Pacific Association for the Study of the Liver (APASL), the European Association for the Study of the Liver-Chronic Liver Failure (EASL-CLIF) consortium, and the North American Consortium for the Study of End-Stage Liver Disease (NACSELD) are commonly followed **(Table 2)**.[4]

The APASL defines ACLF as "an acute hepatic insult manifesting as jaundice [serum bilirubin >5 mg/dL (85 mmol/L)] and coagulopathy (INR >1.5 or prothrombin activity <40%) complicated within 4 weeks by clinical ascites and/or hepatic encephalopathy (HE) in a patient with previously diagnosed or undiagnosed chronic liver disease/cirrhosis and is associated with a high 28-day mortality." Extrahepatic organ failure is not required to make the diagnosis.

The EASL-CLIF consortium defines ACLF as a specific syndrome in patients with cirrhosis that is characterized by acute decompensation (AD), organ failure, and high short-term mortality. The development of ascites, HE, gastrointestinal hemorrhage, and/or bacterial infections defines AD; however, patients may develop ACLF without a history of AD. Organ failures include liver, kidney, brain, respiratory system, circulation, and coagulation, and they are assessed by the CLIF-consortium organ failures score.

The NACSELD defines ACLF by the presence of at least two severe extrahepatic organ failures including shock, grade

TABLE 2: Defining criteria for ACLF.

Organ	APASL–ACLF research consortium	EASL-CLIF-C ACLF	NACSELD
Liver	Total bilirubin ≥5 mg/dL	Bilirubin level of >12 mg/dL	–
Coagulation	INR ≥1.5	INR ≥2.5	–
Kidney	Acute kidney injury network criteria	Creatinine level of ≥2.0 mg/dL or renal replacement	Need for dialysis or other forms of renal replacement therapy
Brain	West Haven hepatic encephalopathy grade 3–4	West Haven hepatic encephalopathy grade 3–4	West Haven hepatic encephalopathy grade 3–4
Circulatory	Lactate levels	Use of vasopressor (terlipressin and/or catecholamines)	Presence of shock defined by mean arterial pressure <60 mm Hg or a reduction of 40 mm Hg in systolic blood pressure from baseline, despite adequate fluid resuscitation and cardiac output
Respiratory	–	PaO_2/FiO_2 of ≤200 or SpO_2/FiO_2 of ≤214 or need for mechanical ventilation	Need for mechanical ventilation
Major organ failure category	Predominantly hepatic failure variables	Combination of hepatic and extrahepatic organ failure variables	Predominantly extrahepatic organ failure variables

(APASL-ACLF: Asian Pacific Association for the Study of the Liver-Acute-on-chronic Liver Failure; EASL-CLIF-C ACLF: European Association for the Study of the Liver-Chronic Liver Failure Consortium Acute-on-chronic Liver Failure; INR: international normalized ratio; NACSELD: North American Consortium for the Study of End-Stage Liver Disease; PaO_2: partial pressure of arterial oxygen; SpO_2: peripheral capillary oxygen saturation)

III/ IV HE, renal replacement therapy (RRT), or mechanical ventilation.

It should be noted that ACLF may occur both in patients with previously compensated or decompensated cirrhosis and in patients with an underlying chronic liver disease without cirrhosis. In this context, the World Gastroenterology Organization (WGO) proposed a further classification of ACLF into three groups, according to the underlying liver disease:[5]
1. Type A ACLF (patients with underlying noncirrhotic chronic liver disease)
2. Type B ACLF (patients with previous compensated cirrhosis)
3. Type C ACLF (patients with previous decompensated cirrhosis)

Q4. What is Chronic Liver Failure-Sequential Organ Failure Assessment Organ Failure (CLIF-SOFA OF) criteria and its role in prognosticating ACLF?

In cases of AD of chronic liver diseases or in ACLF, organ failure sets in as a result of the precipitating insult and ensuing inflammatory cascade. Previously, the SOFA score was used to assess organ failure as it was considered better than the Model for End-stage Liver Disease (MELD) in the assessment and prognostication of organ failure. Since the components of SOFA score (liver, kidney, brain, coagulation, circulation, and lung function) do not take into account specific characteristics of patients with cirrhosis, a modified version of SOFA score called CLIF-SOFA score was introduced for the diagnosis and prognostication of ACLF. This was simplified further to CLIF Consortium Organ Failure score (CLIF-C OFs) **(Table 3)**.

The accuracy of CLIF-C OFs in predicting short-term mortality was similar to that of CLIF-SOFA score and significantly superior to MELD, MELD-Na, and Child–Pugh–Turcotte score.[5,6]

The CANONIC study showed an overall 28-day mortality of 33% in ACLF. The 28-day mortality rates in patients with ACLF grade 1 (single-organ failure), grade 2 (two-organ failure), and grade 3 (more than or equal to three organ failure) were 22%, 32%, and 73%, respectively.[7]

For each organ system, new cut points were chosen to classify the clinical severity categories, which are directly correlated with the risk of dying at 28 days. The new cutoff values maximized the ability of the aggregated score (ranging 6–18) to predict 28-day mortality. All scores in red will be considered as one organ failure. The number of organ failures decides the grade of ACLF and mortality.[6]

Q5. Describe the management based on 2022 American Gastroenterological Association (AGA) ACLF guidelines.

The management of ACLF focuses on preventing and treating organ failures with diligent efforts to treat sepsis. The focus is also on treating precipitating factors and other core principles of critical care such as fluid resuscitation, maintenance of airway, breathing, and circulation (ABC), early sepsis identification and treatment along with supportive therapies such as ventilation and RRT where required, and liver transplant in some scenarios.

The ACG has recommended organ-specific guidelines for the management of ACLF,[4] and these are summarized in **Tables 4 to 6**.

Q6. What are the etiologies of ALF?
The various etiologies of ALF are discussed in **Table 7**.

Q7. What are the immediate measures to be taken for this patient?

All the patients showing features of acute liver dysfunction must be screened for signs of HE. Once initial stabilization is attempted, other etiologies such as cirrhosis or malignancy, which can resemble ALF, should be excluded. Active search for factors, which are contraindications for an emergency liver transplant, should be carried out, and even in the

TABLE 3: Chronic Liver Failure Consortium Organ Failure score (CLIF-C OFs).

Organ system	Variable	Score 1	Organ failure	Score 2	Organ failure	Score 3	Organ failure
Liver	Bilirubin, mg/dL	<6	No	6 to <12	No	>12	Yes
Kidney	Creatinine, mg/dL	<2	No	2 to <3.5	Yes	≥3.5 or RRT	Yes
Brain	HE (West Haven grading)	0	No	1–2	No	3–4	Yes
Coagulation	INR	<2	No	2 to <2.5	No	≥2.5	Yes
Circulatory	MAP (mm Hg)	≥70	No	<70	No	Vasopressors	Yes
Respiratory	PaO_2/FiO_2 or SpO_2/FiO_2	>300 >357	No	≤300 and >200 >214 and ≤357	No	≤200 ≤214	Yes

(HE: hepatic encephalopathy; INR: international normalized ratio; MAP: mean arterial pressure; PaO_2: partial pressure of arterial oxygen; RRT: renal replacement therapy; SpO_2: peripheral capillary oxygen saturation)

TABLE 4: General and organ-specific guidelines for the management of acute-on-chronic liver failure (ACLF).[4]

Category	Recommendation	Other comments
General critical care management	• Multidisciplinary team approach including expertise in critical care and transplant hepatology • The goal of treatment is reversal of the precipitating cause, treatment of sepsis, support of the failing organ(s), and liver transplant (LT) in selected patients	• HE grades 3 and 4—airway protection • Hypoxemia PaO$_2$ <80—chest X-ray/CT evaluation for hepatopulmonary syndrome. To consider therapeutic thoraco/paracentesis. To increase FiO$_2$ on mechanical ventilation • Hypovolemia—volume challenge using echo monitoring • Hb <7—transfusion of packed RBCs to maintain Hb >7 (>9 in cardiac patients) • MAP <60 mm Hg—volume assessment and to rule out GI bleed. Evaluation of sepsis • Sepsis guidelines—blood, urine, ascitic cultures, lactate measurement, and chest imaging • Treatment of infections—vancomycin 15 mg/kg 6 hourly, meropenem 1 g 8 hourly, and antifungals if no response in 48 hours • MAP <60—norepinephrine infusion, stress dose hydrocortisone for refractory shock • General measures—volume challenge, DVT prophylaxis, stress ulcer prophylaxis, etc.
Brain	• Suggest the use of short-acting dexmedetomidine for sedation as compared to other available agents to shorten time to extubation (very low quality, conditional recommendation) • In patients with cirrhosis and ACLF who continue to require mechanical ventilation because of brain conditions or respiratory failure despite optimal therapy, it is suggested against listing for LT to improve mortality (very low quality, conditional recommendation)	• Consideration for causes other than HE as the reason for altered mental status is important, especially in patients who have not improved despite HE therapies • Careful monitoring of pain and delirium. Avoidance of medication that prolong sedation in order to facilitate return of consciousness
Kidney	• In patients with cirrhosis and stages 2 and 3 acute kidney injury (AKI), it is suggested to use intravenous (IV) albumin and vasoconstrictors as compared to albumin alone, to improve creatinine (low quality, conditional recommendation) • In hospitalized patients with cirrhosis and HRS-AKI without high grade of ACLF or disease, use of terlipressin (moderate quality, conditional recommendation) or norepinephrine (low quality, conditional recommendation) is suggested to improve renal function • In patients with cirrhosis and spontaneous bacterial peritonitis (SBP), use of IV albumin in addition to antibiotics is recommended to prevent AKI and subsequent organ failures (high quality, strong recommendation) • In patients with cirrhosis and infections other than SBP, it is recommended not to use albumin as a measure to improve renal function or mortality (high quality, strong recommendation)	• Kidney failure is the most common organ failure in patients with ACLF • One has to be vigilant for potential precipitating factors for AKI development, with bacterial infections being the most common precipitant • Prompt and judicious treatment of potential bacterial infections may avert the development of renal failure • LT is the definitive treatment for HRS-AKI in cirrhosis. RRT is often required, while patients are waiting for LT • The use of RRT in patients with AKI should be individualized. In general, RRT is recommended for patients with HRS-AKI who are on the LT waiting list and who have failed pharmacotherapy

Contd...

Contd...

Category	Recommendation	Other comments
Lung	In ventilated patients with cirrhosis, it is suggested not to use prophylactic antibiotics to reduce mortality or duration of mechanical ventilation (very low quality, conditional recommendation)	• Endotracheal intubation is mandatory in patients with grade 3–4 HE to facilitate airway management, prevent aspiration, and control ventilation • The risk of developing ventilator-associated pneumonia can be reduced by employing a 30–45° head-end elevation and subglottic suction • Routine use of sedatives is discouraged in patients with grade 3–4 encephalopathy as this may be associated with a delay in extubation • It is suggested to use a proton-pump inhibitor (PPI) in patients with cirrhosis on receiving mechanical ventilation
Circulation	• Higher MAP may decrease the risk of ACLF • Norepinephrine is the vasopressor of choice in patients with ACLF	
Coagulation	• In patients with cirrhosis and ACLF, it is suggested against using INR as a means to measure coagulation risk (very low quality, conditional recommendation) • In patients with cirrhosis, an increased risk of venous thromboembolism (VTE) is suggested as compared to noncirrhotic patients (low quality, conditional recommendation) • In patients with ACLF and altered coagulation parameters, it is suggested against routine transfusion therapy in the absence of bleeding or a planned procedure (low quality, conditional recommendation) • In patients with cirrhosis who require invasive procedures, the use of thromboelastography (TEG) or rotational thromboelastography (ROTEM) is recommended instead of INR, to accurately assess transfusion needs (moderate quality, conditional recommendation)	• Hypocoagulation found on TEG/ROTEM in ACLF is an independent marker of poor prognosis and is usually found in patients with systemic inflammatory response syndrome (SIRS) • In the absence of contraindications, such as recent bleeding and significant thrombocytopenia, hospitalized cirrhotic patients should receive pharmacologic VTE prophylaxis • In patients with well-controlled decompensated cirrhosis, low-molecular-weight heparin (LMWH) may decrease the risk of new decompensation; however, there is inadequate data at this time point concerning anticoagulation of these patients in the absence of thrombosis
	Precipitating factors	
Infections	In patients with cirrhosis and suspected infection, early treatment with antibiotics is suggested to improve survival	
Fungal infections	In hospitalized patients with ACLF because of a bacterial infection and who have not responded to antibiotic therapy, it is suggested to consider an MDR organism or fungal infection	
Medication and prophylaxis	• In patients with cirrhosis with a history of SBP, it is suggested to use antibiotics for secondary SBP prophylaxis to prevent recurrent SBP (low quality, conditional recommendation) • In patients with cirrhosis in need of primary SBP prophylaxis, it is suggested to use daily prophylactic antibiotics (although no one specific regimen is superior to another) to prevent SBP (low quality, conditional recommendation) • In patients with cirrhosis, it is suggested to avoid PPI unless there is a clear indication (such as symptomatic gastroesophageal reflux or healing of erosive esophagitis or an ulcer) because PPI use increases the risk of infection (very low quality)	
Noninfectious precipitating factors: Alcohol-associated hepatitis	• In patients with severe alcohol-associated hepatitis [Maddrey discriminant function (MDF) >32; MELD score >20] in the absence of contraindications, the use of prednisolone or prednisone (40 mg/d) orally is recommended to improve 28-day mortality (moderate quality, strong recommendation) • In patients with severe alcohol-associated hepatitis (MDF >32; MELD score >20), it is suggested against the use of pentoxifylline to improve 28-day mortality (very low quality, conditional recommendation)	

Contd...

Contd...

Category	Recommendation	Other comments
Drug-induced liver injury (DILI)	• Onset of ACLF occurs on average 1 month after taking the offending medication but can be delayed for up to 3 months • Patient education about limiting the use of pharmacological agents and avoiding the use of complementary and alternate medicine (CAM) is key to the prevention of DILI-associated ACLF • Patients with underlying liver disease should be monitored when prescribed new medication(s) with hepatotoxic potential	
Viral hepatitis	• Patients with an underlying liver disease can develop ACLF if they contract any of the known viral hepatitis • Hepatitis B flares are a common cause of ACLF in Asian countries and may present like acute liver failure • Other viral infections that cause ACLF are hepatitis A and E infections superimposed on chronic liver disease or hepatitis D superimposed on hepatitis B viral (HBV) infection. These should be looked for and treated • Bacterial infections are a common trigger of ACLF in patients with viral hepatitis, which should be monitored for and treated promptly • Patients with chronic liver disease should be vaccinated against hepatitis A and hepatitis B if they are not already immune	

(CT: computed tomography; DVT: deep vein thrombosis; echo: echocardiography; GI: gastrointestinal; Hb: hemoglobin; HE: hepatic encephalopathy; HRS-AKI: hepatorenal syndrome-acute kidney injury; INR: international normalized ratio; MAP: mean arterial pressure; MDR: multidrug-resistant; MELD: Model for End-stage Liver Disease; PaO_2: partial pressure of arterial oxygen; RBC: red blood cell; RRT: renal replacement therapy)

TABLE 5: Recommendations governing the use of intravenous (IV) albumin.[4]

Use of albumin	• IV albumin is recommended to prevent AKI and subsequent organ failures in patients diagnosed with spontaneous bacterial peritonitis (SBP) • IV albumin is not recommended to prevent organ failures in patients with cirrhosis who have infections other than SBP • 5% albumin is often used for rapid volume resuscitation, whereas for more sustained volume expansion, 25% albumin is recommended • In hospitalized patients with cirrhosis, daily infusion of albumin to maintain the serum albumin >3 g/dL is not recommended to improve mortality, prevention of renal dysfunction, or infection (moderate quality, strong recommendation)

TABLE 6: Miscellaneous therapies.[4]

Liver assist devices	• Benefit of artificial liver support systems, with or without a biological component, is still unclear • Plasma exchange has been shown to improve survival in patients with acute liver failure; however, its effect in ACLF is not known
Granulocyte colony-stimulating factor (G-CSF)	• In patients with cirrhosis and ACLF, the use of G-CSF to improve mortality is not recommended (very low evidence, conditional recommendation)
Stem cell therapy	• Stem cell therapy is a promising therapeutic strategy to bridge patients with ACLF to more definitive therapy (e.g., control of acute infection, LT), but evidence to support its use in routine clinical practice is currently insufficient
Transplant versus futility for ACLF	• In patients with cirrhosis and ACLF who continue to require mechanical ventilation because of adult respiratory distress syndrome or brain-related conditions despite optimal therapy, it is suggested against listing for LT to improve mortality (very low evidence, conditional recommendation) • In patients with end-stage liver disease admitted to the hospital, it is suggested to discuss early goals of care and where appropriate, refer to a palliative care center to optimize resource utilization (very low evidence, conditional recommendation)

(ACLF: acute-on-chronic liver failure; LT: liver transplant)

presence of such contraindications, the patient must be referred to an experienced tertiary center, especially in the presence of poor prognostic factors such as elevated INR or higher grades of HE. Every attempt to find the cause for the acute deterioration of liver status should be made as it has both prognostic and management implications.[8]

Q8. What are the common clinical features in a case of ALF?

Acute liver failure involves the loss of synthetic and detoxifying function of the liver, resulting in the accumulation of toxins and cytokines that result in severe inflammation. ALF presents with nonspecific symptoms such as

TABLE 7: Etiology of acute liver failure (ALF).	
Viral hepatitis	• Hepatitis B, A, and E • HSV, CMV, VZV (in immunocompromised)
Drug-related	• Acetaminophen • Antituberculosis drugs • Recreational drugs (ecstasy, cocaine) • Idiosyncratic reactions—anticonvulsants, antibiotics, nonsteroidal anti-inflammatory drugs • Aspirin in children may lead to Reye's syndrome
Toxins	• Carbon tetrachloride, phosphorus, *Amanita phalloides*, alcohol • Kava kava
Vascular events	• Ischemia, veno-occlusive disease • Budd-Chiari syndrome (hepatic vein thrombosis)
Pregnancy	• Acute fatty liver of pregnancy • HELLP syndrome • Liver rupture
Miscellaneous	• Wilson disease, autoimmune, carcinoma, hemophagocytic syndrome, malignant infiltration (e.g., lymphoma), heat shock, and seizures • Trauma • Indeterminate (15%)

(CMV: cytomegalovirus; HELLP: hemolysis, elevated liver enzymes, and low platelets; HSV: herpes simplex virus; VZV: varicella-zoster virus)

malaise, fatigue, nausea, and vomiting, along with clinical signs of hypotension, sepsis, and multiple organ failure.

Patients with fulminant hepatic failure usually have circulatory dysfunction in the form of hypotension and tachycardia as a result of reduced systemic vascular resistance, which may be secondary to poor oral intake and third space losses. The presentation is very similar to that of septic shock. Most of these patients are susceptible to serious infections and thorough assessment and investigations should be carried out in all patients with hepatic failure to rule out sepsis. Spontaneous bacterial peritonitis is one such infection, which commonly occurs in this setting, which has to be ruled out.

Altered mental function and coagulopathy are integral parts of ALF, the severity of which has widespread ramifications.

Central nervous system (CNS) dysfunction in ALF manifests as encephalopathy and is mandatory to make a diagnosis of ALF. Systemic and local inflammation in the brain occurs due to the release of cytokines and neurotoxins such as ammonia and results in astrocyte swelling, cerebral edema, and encephalopathy.

The CNS dysfunction can further be aggravated by systemic hypotension, which reduces cerebral perfusion. Cerebral edema and intracranial hypertension (ICH) can be catastrophic and are associated with a mortality of 20–25% in ALF. The prognosis of ALF is related to the severity of encephalopathy and higher grades of encephalopathy are associated with a poor prognosis.

Coagulopathy is common in ALF as the production of almost all clotting factors (except von Willebrand factor and factor VIII) is reduced. The reduced synthesis of clotting factors II, V, VII, IX, and X leads to an elevation of prothrombin time, activated prothrombin time, and INR; however, such elevation need not imply the risk of bleeding. The risk of hemorrhage correlates with the severity of thrombocytopenia rather than the severity of coagulopathy. Common sites of internal bleed in ALF include the gastrointestinal tract, nasopharynx, lungs, and retroperitoneum. Intracranial hemorrhage is rare.

Disseminated intravascular coagulation occurs frequently and leads to a state of consumption. Metabolic acidosis (lactic acidosis), hypothermia, and thrombocytopenia also contribute to coagulopathy.

Acute renal failure occurs commonly in ALF. The causes can be prerenal or renal and are mainly due to hypovolemia, hypotension, or direct effects of toxins resulting in acute tubular necrosis. Acute kidney injury [a serum creatinine (Cr) >300 μmol/L] is one of the transplant criteria among patients with paracetamol-induced ALF. It is vital to anticipate renal failure and prevent it by maintaining adequate circulating volume.

Acute liver failure is associated with metabolic abnormalities such as hypoglycemia, hyponatremia, hypokalemia, hypophosphatemia, and respiratory acidosis. Hypoglycemia occurs due to both impaired gluconeogenesis and increased circulating insulin levels. Hyponatremia is usually hypervolemic hyponatremia, while hypokalemia and hypophosphatemia are secondary to respiratory alkalosis from central hyperventilation.[8]

Q9. What is the pathophysiology of HE and ICH in ALF?

Most of the clinical features seen in ALF arise from the loss of synthetic/detoxification/metabolic and immunologic functions of the liver. The consequent accumulation of various metabolites has been implicated in the development of HE. One such toxin often implicated in a bulk of literature as responsible for HE and ICH is ammonia.[7] It should be stressed upon that the pathogenesis of encephalopathy in ALF is only partially understood. Local and systemic inflammation along with accumulated neurotoxins are implicated.

One popular molecular pathogenetic mechanism, the "Trojan Horse" hypothesis, suggests that glutamine contributes to the pathogenesis of HE. It is postulated that glutamine gets transported into mitochondria where it undergoes hydrolysis to yield high levels of ammonia. This results in deleterious effects such as induction of mitochondrial permeability, transition, and oxidative/nitrative stress.[9] Targeting astrocytic glutamine transport and/or its hydrolysis within the mitochondria, therefore, remains an attractive strategy for the treatment of HE and other hyperammonemic disorders in the future.[9]

The schematic representation of the pathogenesis of HE is shown in **Flowchart 1**.

Q10. Is there any role for ammonia monitoring in ALF?

Although increased circulating levels of ammonia are implicated in the pathogenesis of HE, neither the grade of encephalopathy nor the severity of neurologic dysfunction correlates with arterial ammonia levels. However, there is evidence to suggest that patients who present with high ammonia levels have a higher incidence of HE and ICH. The cutoff levels, at which the increased incidence of HE is noted, have varied between different studies and there is no consensus yet. Plasma ammonia >150–200 µmol/L has generally been considered a risk factor for ICH in ALF.[10,11]

Clemmesen et al. had suggested that cerebral herniation is correlated with arterial ammonia concentration in patients with ALF.[12] However, it is important to note that the presence of inflammation/sepsis and multiple organ dysfunction syndrome (MODS) can themselves foster HE/ICH even with significantly lower levels of ammonia.[13]

There is growing evidence to suggest that ammonia clearance using early continuous renal replacement therapy (CRRT) could improve the outcome, thereby indicating that establishing lower levels of ammonia may reduce the occurrence/severity of HE/ICH. There is, however, no universally accepted threshold. Kandiah et al.[10] suggested that targeting a plasma ammonia level of <100 µmol/L using CRRT is beneficial in treating advanced HE and ICH.

Therefore, measurement of the arterial ammonia level is considered useful in assessing the risk for the development of HE and ICH. The risk of ICH is perhaps greatest with a sustained increase in the arterial ammonia level >150 µmol/L.

Q11. Do metabolic factors contribute to increased circulating ammonia levels?

Hypoxemia, hypokalemia, and metabolic acidosis increase renal ammonia production.[14] In the setting of metabolic acidosis or hypokalemia, the production of renal glutaminase is increased and glutamine is used to facilitate the disposal of acid into or recovery of potassium from the glomerular filtrate. Each glutamine molecule used for either purpose generates two ammonium ions, some of which become ammonia, which then diffuses into circulation.[10,14] Patients with HE and normokalemia that are on the higher side of normal, potassium level, 5.4–5.5 mEq/L, show a quicker improvement in mental status and contribute to longer,

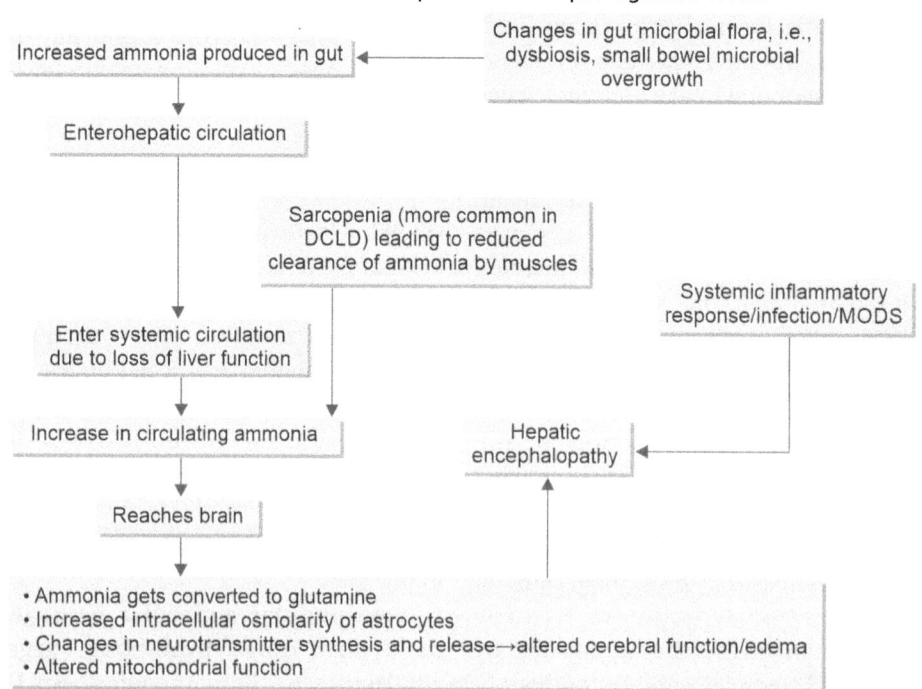

Flowchart 1: Schematic representation of pathogenesis of HE.

(DCLD: decompensated liver disease; HE: hepatic encephalopathy; MODS: multiple organ dysfunction syndrome)

event-free survival than those with normokalemia on the lower side of normal, potassium level, 3.5–3.6 mEq/L.[15] Metabolic alkalosis promotes the conversion of ammonium ion to ammonia, thus increasing its level and its entry across the blood–brain barrier. Needless to say, it must be ensured that hypokalemia and acid–base abnormalities must be avoided in ALF at all times.

Q12. How will you optimize the hemodynamics in a patient with ALF?

Hypotension in ALF is predominantly due to reduced effective circulatory volume, which can be secondary to multiple causes such as due to reduced oral intake, vomiting, and systemic vasodilation.

Initially, they may present with hyperlactatemia although the lactate levels might not entirely be suggestive of reduced perfusion or volume status; rather they may be reflective of the inability of the liver to metabolize the increased lactate production. Clinical examination will reveal signs of hypoperfusion such as cold peripheries, prolonged capillary refill time, peripheral hypoperfusion, acidosis, oliguria, or renal failure. Fluid management in such patients requires care and frequent assessment as both hypovolemia and hypervolemia secondary to aggressive resuscitation can be harmful. Thus, fluid therapy must be guided by bedside basic and advanced hemodynamic monitoring. Continuous noninvasive cardiac output monitoring and fluid responsiveness might be beneficial. These patients should receive fluid boluses guided by biochemical parameters, clinical status, and real-time cardiac output monitoring, keeping in mind the chloride load and the reduced ability of the liver to metabolize buffers such as acetate and lactate. The central venous oxygen saturation ($ScvO_2$) cannot be used as it will be elevated even in ALF, even in the presence of hypovolemia.

As elucidated earlier, overzealous fluid therapy increases the venous pressure and right-sided cardiac pressures that lead to tissue edema and may be detrimental to liver, gut, and kidney function and integrity. Persistent hypotension after adequate fluid resuscitation requires treatment with vasopressors, and norepinephrine is the preferred agent. Low-dose vasopressin (1–2 units/h) may be considered if the requirements of norepinephrine are increasing, although it may be detrimental to cerebral circulation. Ensuring adequate mean arterial pressure (MAP) with vasopressors is paramount to ensuring organ perfusion.

Although a stress dose of steroid has been found to be beneficial in vasopressor-resistant shock in sepsis, its benefit in the setting of ALF is unclear. When the use of steroids is considered, the risk/benefit should be weighed carefully as the benefits obtained by their use could be insignificant in case of worsening sepsis or reactivation of latent viral infections [e.g., cytomegalovirus (CMV) and herpes simplex virus].[8]

Q13. What is the role of neuromonitoring in ALF?

Neuromonitoring can be noninvasive or invasive. Noninvasive methods such as serial head computed tomography (CT) scans, transcranial Doppler, jugular bulb oximetry, and pupillometry have all been studied, but none has been validated.[10]

Invasive intracranial pressure (ICP) monitoring can also be used to detect and treat ICH in ALF; however, the risk of bleeding and further neurologic compromise prevents its routine use. Recent studies, looking at complications arising out of invasive ICP monitoring, have reported lower rates of bleeding though.[16,17] Many studies advocate the use of recombinant factor VII to rapidly correct coagulopathy before attempting invasive monitoring devices without raising concerns of volume overload. Till date, no randomized controlled trial (RCT) has elucidated the role of ICP monitoring and its benefits in ALF, making it difficult to define specific indications. Routine use of ICP monitoring is therefore not recommended. There could be a role for ICP monitoring in patients with ALF with grade 3/4 encephalopathy, pupillary abnormalities, and very high ammonia levels (>150 μmol/L), which could lead to herniation,[12] and possibly as an adjunct to patients scheduled for transplantation.[18,19]

Rajajee et al.[20] suggested that the use of a protocol-based ICP monitoring in patients with grade 4 encephalopathy was able to detect instances of raised ICP, which needed aggressive measures to reduce ICP, thus influencing clinical decisions significantly. Further, this was not accompanied by increased complications. Whether a protocol-based ICP monitoring influences outcomes in patients with ALF needs to be rigorously tested.

Neurological monitoring therefore may benefit a select few patients with severe ICH, requiring aggressive ICP control measures. Outcome and survival benefits are yet to be validated and until then, an individual case-based approach with close clinical monitoring of GCS, pupils, imaging, and laboratories is recommended.

Q14. What is the role of liver-protective measures such as N-acetylcysteine (NAC), branched-chain amino acids (BCAA), and lactulose?

- *N-acetylcysteine:* NAC, when administered early, can reduce liver damage and hasten recovery in patients with acetaminophen-induced ALF. It is the treatment of choice for acetaminophen-induced liver failure.[21] An intravenous loading dose of NAC 150 mg/kg, followed by maintenance infusion at 100 mg/kg until the INR improves to <2.0, is advocated. There is growing evidence to suggest that NAC administration may be clinically beneficial in nonparacetamol-induced ALF as well, though the mechanism of action of NAC in this situation is unclear. The usual loading and maintenance dose recommended for paracetamol overdose is advised in these instances.[19] The use of NAC has been shown to be safe as well as beneficial in terms of reducing nonacetaminophen-induced ALF mortality.[22]

Kortsalioudaki et al. evaluated the safety and efficacy of NAC in children with nonacetaminophen-induced ALF.[23] Survival with native liver occurred in 22% with supportive care versus 43% with NAC, and its use was associated with a higher incidence of native liver recovery without transplantation. Its use was also found to be associated with a shorter length of hospital stay.

Lee et al.[24] showed that intravenous NAC improves transplant-free survival in patients with early stage nonacetaminophen-related ALF. Patients with advanced coma grades did not benefit from NAC and typically required emergency liver transplantation. There was clear survival benefit and evidence to advocate early use of NAC in both acetaminophen- and nonacetaminophen-induced ALF.

- *L-ornithine–L-aspartate (LOLA):* The drug LOLA is believed to aid muscle cells in the detoxification of ammonia to glutamine. However, studies have been unable to establish a clear benefit in terms of reduced ammonia levels, incidence of encephalopathy, and mortality in patients suffering from ALF.[25] There was also no difference in complications such as seizures and acute kidney injury.[25]
- *Branched-chain amino acids:* Gluud et al.[26] identified 16 randomized clinical trials (827 participants) where BCAA was compared with placebo. The analyses found no effect on mortality but that BCAA had a beneficial effect on symptoms and signs of HE. BCAA did not increase the risk of serious adverse events but was associated with nausea and diarrhea. When excluding trials on lactulose or neomycin, BCAA appeared to have a beneficial effect on HE.
- *Lactulose—nonabsorbable disaccharides:*[27,28] Their mechanism of action is multifactorial. First, they decrease colonic transit time, reducing the opportunity for absorption of gut-derived ammonia (purgatory effect). Second, nonabsorbable disaccharides lower colonic pH. This effect converts ammonia to a nonabsorbable ammonium ion, thereby preventing the production of ammonia by gut urea lysis and inhibiting ammonia absorption.

Despite the above plausible explanation, there is no evidence for the role of lactulose in ALF.

Furthermore, prescribing lactulose as overdosage can result in ileus, severe diarrhea, electrolyte disturbances, and hypovolemia. Hypovolemia may be sufficiently severe as to actually induce a flare of encephalopathy symptoms. Despite the benefits, nonabsorbable disaccharides have been associated with poor patient tolerance and the inconvenience of their purgatory effects.

Many authors have suggested that the use of lactulose should be avoided as it can be harmful in ALF and due to the lack of proven survival benefit from trials. There is also a potential risk of worsening ileus in such patients.[28] The recent EASL guidelines do not recommend the use of lactulose or rifaximin as ammonia-lowering agents in the setting of ALF.[8]

Human albumin solution, glycerol phenylbutyrate, ornithine phenylacetate L-ornithine, and zinc are some other compounds being evaluated as measures to reduce ammonia in HE without significant survival benefit.[7]

Q15. What are the characteristics of patients with ALF, which warrant liver transplant?

In ALF, the transplant criteria differ based on whether the ALF is secondary to acetaminophen intake or not (nonacetaminophen).[19]

Till date, the King's College criteria **(Table 8)** are the most commonly used and best validated.[29]

These criteria are not advocated for use in patients with pregnancy-related complications leading to liver failure, acute Budd–Chiari syndrome, and Wilson disease. They are also not applicable in liver failure secondary to trauma or in pediatric liver failure.

TABLE 8: King's College criteria for liver transplantation.	
Acetaminophen-related ALF	**Nonacetaminophen-related ALF**
Single criterion: Arterial pH <7.30 or lactate >3 mmol/L after adequate fluid resuscitation	Single criterion: INR >6.5
Three criteria: 1. Grade III–IV (West Haven) HE 2. INR >6.5 3. Serum creatinine >3.4 mg/dL	Three of five criteria: 1. Age <10 or >40 years 2. Time from jaundice to come >7 days 3. INR >3.5 4. Bilirubin >17 mg/dL 5. *Unfavorable etiology:* Drug-induced, Wilson disease, seronegative hepatitis

Note: Sensitivity—72%, specificity—98%, and PPV—89% for identifying patients needing transplantation. Mortality rate of 90% without OLTx. (ALF: acute liver failure; HE: hepatic encephalopathy; INR: international normalized ratio; OLTx: orthotopic liver transplantation; PPV: positive predictive value)

The EASL advocates transplant for patients with ALF from Budd–Chiari syndrome and Wilson disease associated with any grade of encephalopathy.[30]

The criteria for liver transplantation in nonacetaminophen etiologies have also been developed by the Clichy group from France after an exhaustive study from databases of patients with ALF due to hepatitis B (Clichy-Villejuif criteria). They recommend liver transplantation if there is encephalopathy and low factor V level.[29]

Blood lactate levels remaining high, despite adequate fluid resuscitation, although not included in any criteria, signify poor prognosis and warrant consideration for transplantation.[31] Additionally, the MELD score/MELD-Na score has also been extensively studied for risk prioritization and can be used as a tool to identify patients at high risk for mortality **(Table 9)**. A more important consideration in such patients with high-risk characteristics should be a prompt referral to a transplant center even before the criteria for transplant are met in order to improve survival.[32,33]

For acetaminophen-induced ALF, discussion with a specialist unit should take place, if:

- The INR is >3.0 or the prothrombin time in seconds is greater than the number of hours since overdose or INR of 2.0 at 24 hours, 4.0 at 48 hours, and 6.0 at 72 hours.
- There is an elevated Cr >2.26 mg/dL and INR >2.5.
- There is any evidence of encephalopathy.
- MAP <60 mm Hg following resuscitation
- Metabolic acidosis with pH <7.30/bicarbonate (HCO_3) <20 mmol/L
- Lactate >2.0 mmol/L

In nonacetaminophen-induced acute liver failure (NAI-ALF), the presence of encephalopathy, coagulopathy (INR >1.8), jaundice (bilirubin >8.76 mg/dL), renal failure, hyponatremia, hypoglycemia, ascites, metabolic acidosis, or blood lactate >2 mmol/L following initial resuscitation should prompt urgent discussion with a transplant center. The discovery of a shrinking liver on clinical examination is also a poor prognostic indicator and could be compelling enough a reason for transfer.

Q16. What was the MELD criteria originally meant for?

The MELD score was originally developed at the Mayo Clinic (also referred to as the Mayo End-Stage Liver Disease score) from a series of post-transjugular intrahepatic portosystemic shunt (TIPS) patients to predict their 3-month mortality **(Table 10)**. This was later identified to be useful in risk stratification of patients with liver failure and therefore prioritizing them for a liver transplant. The United Network for Organ Sharing (UNOS) and Eurotransplant currently use the MELD score for transplant allocation. The MELD-Na, which is a mere extension of MELD score, incorporates serum sodium and has been shown to better predict pretransplant mortality (refer to **Table 9** for formulae).

Q17. Does this patient need blood products to correct his coagulopathy—INR 6.0?

No, the patient does not need blood products to correct his coagulopathy since he is not actively bleeding. There is no indication to correct coagulopathy in the absence of clinical bleed since it normalizes INR, which is an important prognostication tool. There is also the concept of rebalanced coagulation wherein the loss of synthetic function of liver leads to decreased production of both the procoagulant and the anticoagulant (proteins C and S) factors, thereby balancing out the net effect on coagulation. In fact, there could be an increased tendency toward coagulation as the extrahepatically produced factor VIII and von Willebrand factor (VWF) increase in the absence of hepatically produced anticoagulant factors.

Thus, INR is not an accurate measure of coagulation homeostasis and there is no indication to treat elevated INR in the absence of clinical bleed or scheduled invasive procedures.[35] Thrombin generation assays, which incorporate the addition of thrombomodulin, may better reflect functional coagulation status in vivo.

Traumatic liver injury and HELLP syndrome are probably two scenarios where a lower threshold for correcting coagulopathy is indicated as they are at a high risk for bleeding.

TABLE 9: Alternate criteria for risk prognostication in acute liver failure (ALF).

Clichy–Villejuif criteria	• Encephalopathy (coma or confusion) and • Factor V level <20% if age <30 years, or • Factor V level <30% if age >30 years
MELD score (predicts mortality at 3 months)	$9.6 \times \log_e$ (creatinine mg/dL) + $3.8 \times \log_e$ (bilirubin mg/dL) + $11.2 \times \log_e$ (INR) + 6.4
MELD-Na	MELD + $1.59 \times (135 - $ Na mEq/L)

(INR: international normalized ratio; MELD: Model for End-stage Liver Disease)

TABLE 10: Model for End-stage Liver Disease (MELD) score and prediction of 3-month mortality.

Score	Mortality (%)
<9	1.9
10–19	6
20–29	19.6
30–39	52.6
>40	71.3

Q18. This patient is negative for HBsAg. Does this exclude hepatitis B infection?

Hepatitis B virus (HBV) infection cannot be excluded. Patients presenting with ALF due to hepatitis B infection usually have a supraphysiological immune response to the infective agent in an attempt to completely eliminate the virus, which can result in hepatocyte necrosis. Such a response would usually clear the surface antigen, and thus HBsAg at presentation could be negative. However, the diagnosis should be sought and confirmed by testing for immunoglobulin M (IgM) anticore antibodies.[33,34]

Q19. What causes renal failure in ALF? What modality would you choose for renal replacement?

Renal failure in ALF is most commonly due to acute tubular necrosis secondary to drug-induced tubular damage or prerenal causes such as hemodynamic instability.

Due to the concomitant presence of raised ICP and hemodynamic instability, CRRT is often the preferred mode of RRT in ALF.[35] CRRT voids rapid fluid shifts and osmolarity changes, thereby providing better fluid management with tight metabolic and acid–base control without a significant alteration in hemodynamics and thereby reducing the risk of cerebral edema exacerbation.

Q20. What is the role of steroids in ALF?

Karkhanis et al.[36] suggested that corticosteroids did not improve overall survival in drug-induced, indeterminate, or autoimmune ALF and were associated with lower survival in patients with the higher MELD scores. Zao et al.[37] suggested that treatment with steroids improved the survival rate in patients with acute and SALF and in patients with liver failure due to viral and nonviral etiology. Corticosteroid use was identified to be an independent predictor of an improved survival rate. These findings indicated that intervention with corticosteroids was effective in preventing the disease progression and improving the prognosis of ALF and SALF. This was inconsistent with the results reported by Karkhanis et al. The discrepancy in the results in these two studies may be due to the different criteria used to define survival. The outcome analyzed in the latter trial was survival without transplantation until 24 weeks versus survival without transplantation for only 21 days in the former. It is important to note that many patients surviving the first 3 weeks may succumb to liver failure after 4–24 weeks.

The study results demonstrated that irrespective of steroid use, the survival rate was extremely low for patients with MELD scores ≥35 and HE grade 4. Moreover, the benefit from steroid use was only observed in patients with MELD scores of 25–35 and without HE or with HE grades 1–3. This implies that corticosteroid treatment may be effective in improving the prognosis for patients with less severe liver failure and ineffective in those with progression to end-stage liver failure. However, further trials are needed to validate this.

Extracorporeal liver support in ALF: During liver failure, endogenous toxins accumulate resulting in an increased capillary permeability, immune dysregulation, HE, and cerebral edema. These toxins are either water-soluble or albumin-bound. Conventional dialysis can remove only the water-soluble toxins and additional techniques such as albumin dialysis will be needed to remove the albumin-bound toxins. Liver-assist devices are developed with an aim to replicate the function of the liver such as removal of putative toxins and improvement of the pathophysiologic features of liver failure, thereby preventing aggravation of liver failure while stimulating a milieu of liver regeneration. Liver support therapies are broadly classified into bioartificial or artificial liver support systems. Bioartificial systems incorporate viable cells into an extracorporeal circuit and support detoxification and synthetic functions. Artificial liver support therapies are devoid of any biological component and depend upon albumin as a binding and scavenging molecule. These artificial liver support systems are intended for detoxification only, i.e., to remove the toxins only (both water-soluble and protein-bound) **(Table 11)**.

Bioartificial extracorporeal liver support provides support to a declining synthetic liver function along with maintaining the detoxification functions of the liver in patients with ALF. This requires incorporation of a cell source to be incorporated into the system. Human hepatocytes are obviously the choice but are limited by availability and poor regeneration capacity within in vitro cultures. C3A human hepatoblastoma cell lines and porcine hepatocytes have

TABLE 11: Bioartificial versus artificial support devices.

	Bioartificial	Artificial
Cellular component	Yes	No
Hepatic function derived	All liver functions	Only detoxification
Efficiency	Promising results	Limited
Ease of use	Difficulty of maintaining cellular components	Relatively easier
Cost	High	Relatively less
Examples	Extracorporeal liver assist device (ELAD), HepatAssist	• Molecular adsorbent recirculating system (MARS) • Single-pass albumin dialysis (SPAD) • Prometheus

been tried as potential alternatives, although they have their drawbacks. The C3A hepatoblastoma cell lines are inferior with respect to their metabolic activity and lack normal metabolic profiles such as ureagenesis. They also have the additional risk of malignancy. Porcine cell lines carry the risk of xenotransmission. These bioartificial systems are costlier and more difficult to maintain.

There are many bioartificial liver systems available **(Table 12)**, but the ones most studied are the HepatAssist, modular extracorporeal liver support (MELS), and extracorporeal liver assist device (ELAD). The HepatAssist (Cedars-Sinai Medical Center, Los Angeles, California, USA) has been evaluated in small case series,[38] a phase I study,[39] and in a large multicenter RCT conducted in the USA and Europe.[40] The multicenter study could demonstrate the safety of the system; however, a survival benefit was seen only in the subgroup of patients with fulminant/subfulminant liver failure. The MELS system (Charité, Berlin, Germany) has been studied in eight patients with ALF (phase I) and appeared to be safe. All patients were successfully transplanted and were alive at a follow-up of 3 years.[41] The ELAD (Vital Therapies Inc., San Diego, California, USA) proved to have a positive effect on ammonia, bilirubin, and HE in an early RCT in 24 patients with ALF.[38] A clear survival advantage has not been proven with any of the above modalities and larger randomized and multicenter trials are warranted.[42,43]

Artificial liver support devices (nonbiological):
- *Molecular adsorbent recirculating system (MARS)*: The MARS was developed by Stange and Mitzner in 1993. In this, the blood is dialyzed across an albumin impermeable membrane that has a molecular weight cutoff of 50 kDa. 20% human albumin is used as the dialysate and the used albumin is continuously stripped by subsequent passage through columns of charcoal and an anion exchange resin. This removes the albumin-bound toxins such as bilirubin, bile acids, and cytokines while the water-soluble waste products (urea, Cr, gamma-aminobutyric acid, ammonia, etc.) are removed by a low-flux dialyzer connected to the secondary circuit. This system removes all toxins with a molecular weight <50 kDa.
- *Single-pass albumin dialysis (SPAD)*: The SPAD uses a normal dialysis system (continuous replacement therapy system) with the blood dialyzed against a dialysate mixture of standard dialysis solution and 4.4% albumin.
- *Prometheus—fractionated plasma separation and adsorption (FPAD)*: The FPAD (Prometheus, Germany) was introduced in 1999 based on the principle of an initial plasmapheresis (where the patient's own albumin and other plasma proteins are separated by a membrane with a molecular weight cutoff of approximately 250 kDa) followed by adsorption, wherein the albumin fraction is passed over two columns containing different adsorbents for purification. Water-soluble substances are cleared by a high-flux dialyzer and directly inserted into the blood circuit.[43]

The use of extracorporeal liver support therapies has provided symptomatic improvement in patients but has failed to translate into a survival benefit.[44] Further studies and experience with these systems are needed before validating their regular use.[43,44]

High-volume plasmapheresis (HVP) is the only therapy that has demonstrated a statistically significant benefit in transplant-free survival in patients with ALF.[44] Larsen et al.,[45] after evaluation of a series of cases, suggested that HVP is defined as an exchange of 8–12 L or 15% of ideal body weight with fresh frozen plasma improved systemic, cerebral, and splanchnic parameters. They noted improved outcomes in the form of transplant-free survival, and this was attributed to possible attenuation of immune responses. These results have to be interpreted with caution as most patients in the trial had ALF secondary to paracetamol toxicity. The benefits of HVP in other etiologies therefore need further validation. Additionally, the trial results did not show improvement in patients who had less severe forms of ALF, thereby questioning its routine use in all patients. There are ongoing trials in the pipeline, which shall hopefully add more clarity.[46] Until then, its use should be judiciously considered in patients awaiting transplant. **Table 13** lists the available artificial liver support devices that have been tested in practice.

Q21. What are the general measures to manage this patient?

The overall management of a patient with ALF has already been discussed and can be summarized as follows:
- Neurological monitoring with a low threshold for neuroimaging in case of unexplained sudden neurological deterioration

TABLE 12: Bioartificial liver support devices (cell-based).	
MELS	Modular extracorporeal liver support system uses primary porcine/human hepatocytes plus albumin dialysis
ELAD	Extracorporeal liver assist device uses hollow fiber cartridges hosting C3A cells
BLSS	Bioartificial liver support system uses hollow fibers with primary porcine hepatocytes
AMC-BAL	Amsterdam Medical Center bioartificial liver primary porcine hepatocytes on polyester fabric
HepatAssist	It uses hollow fiber cartridges lined by primary porcine hepatocytes

TABLE 13: Artificial liver support devices (noncell-based).	
MARS	Molecular adsorbent recirculating system uses dialysis against 20% albumin (membrane cutoff 50 kDa)
FPAD	Fractional plasma separation adsorption and dialysis detoxify by passing through absorbers (membrane cutoff 250 kDa)
SPAD	Single-pass albumin dialysis against 4% albumin across albumin impermeable membrane
SEPET	Selective plasma filtration therapy (membrane cutoff 100 kDa)
High-volume plasmapheresis	Removal of patient plasma and replacement with fresh frozen plasma (FFP)

- Minimizing agitation and using only short-acting benzodiazepines where necessary
- Monitoring hemodynamic status, with judicious use of fluids, albumin, and vasopressors to maintain MAP
- Monitoring for metabolic abnormalities and correction of the same
- Early initiation of discussions for liver transplantation
- Intubation under rapid-sequence intubation (RSI) in case of inadequate ventilatory requirements or compromised airway protection
- Aggressive management of fever and infections with a low threshold for antifungals in a critically ill patient
- Prefer CRRT in case of acute kidney injury
- Stress ulcer prophylaxis
- Providing adequate nutrition (enteral route).

REFERENCES

1. Sugawara K, Nakayama N, Mochida S. Acute liver failure in Japan: definition, classification, and prediction of the outcome. J Gastroenterol. 2012;47:849-61.
2. Willars C. Update in intensive care medicine: acute liver failure. Initial management, supportive treatment and who to transplant. Curr Opin Crit Care. 2014;20:202-9.
3. Singanayagam A, Bernal W. Update on acute liver failure. Curr Opin Crit Care. 2015;21:134-41.
4. Bajaj S, Oleary G, Lai C, Wong F, Long MD, Wong RJ, et al. Acute-on-chronic liver failure clinical guidelines. Am J Gastroenterol. 2022;117:225-52.
5. Hernaez R, Solà E, Moreau R, Ginès P. Acute-on-chronic liver failure: an update. Gut. 2017;66:541-53.
6. Jalan R, Saliba F, Pavesi M, Amoros A, Moreau R, Ginès P, et al. Development and validation of a prognostic score to predict mortality in patients with acute-on-chronic liver failure. J Hepatol. 2014;61(5):1038-47.
7. Ellul MA, Gholkar SA, Cross TJ. Hepatic encephalopathy due to liver cirrhosis. BMJ. 2015;351:h4187.
8. European Association for the Study of the Liver. EASL clinical practice guidelines on the management of acute (fulminant) liver failure. J Hepatol. 2017;66:1047-81.
9. Rao KVR, Norenberg MD. Glutamine in the pathogenesis of hepatic encephalopathy: the Trojan horse hypothesis revisited. Neurochem Res. 2014;39:593-8.
10. Kandiah PA, Olson JC, Subramanian RM. Emerging strategies for the treatment of patients with acute hepatic failure. Curr Opin Crit Care. 2016;22:142-51.
11. Bernal W, Hall C, Karvellas CJ, Auzinger G, Sizer E, Wendon J. Arterial ammonia and clinical risk factors for encephalopathy and intracranial hypertension in acute liver failure. Hepatology. 2007;46:1844-52.
12. Clemmesen JO, Larsen FS, Kondrup J, Hansen BA, Ott P. Cerebral herniation in patients with acute liver failure is correlated with arterial ammonia concentration. Hepatology. 1999;29:648-53.
13. Kitzberger R, Funk GC, Holzinger U, Miehsler W, Kramer L, Kaider A, et al. Severity of organ failure is an independent predictor of intracranial hypertension in acute liver failure. Clin Gastroenterol Hepatol. 2009;7:1000-6.
14. Tapper EB, Jiang ZG, Patwardhan VR. Refining the ammonia hypothesis: a physiology-driven approach to the treatment of hepatic encephalopathy. Mayo Clinic Proc. 2015;90:646-58.
15. Zavagli G, Ricci G, Bader G, Mapelli G, Tomasi F, Maraschin B. The importance of the highest normokalemia in the treatment of early hepatic encephalopathy. Minor Electrolyte Metab. 1993;19:362-7.
16. Vaquero J, Fontana RJ, Larson AM, Bass NM, Davern TJ, Shakil AO, et al. Complications and use of intracranial pressure monitoring in patients with acute liver failure and severe encephalopathy. Liver Transpl. 2005;11:1581-9.
17. Karvellas CJ, Fix OK, Battenhouse H, Durkalski V, Sanders C, Lee WM, et al. Outcomes and complications of intracranial pressure monitoring in acute liver failure: a retrospective cohort study. Crit Care Med. 2014;42:1157-67.
18. Rosen DR, Magee GA, Frankel HL. Who should undergo intracranial pressure monitoring in acute liver failure? A concise clinical review. PulmCCM J. 2015;1:1-11.
19. Kwan Lai W, Murphy N. Management of acute liver failure. Contin Educ Anaesth Crit Care Pain. 2004;4:40-3.
20. Rajajee V, Fontana RJ, Courey AJ, Patil PG. Protocol based invasive intracranial pressure monitoring in acute liver failure: feasibility, safety and impact on management. Crit Care. 2017;21:178.
21. Smilkstein MJ, Knapp GL, Kulig KW, Rumack BH. Efficacy of oral N-acetylcysteine in the treatment of acetaminophen overdose. Analysis of the national multicenter study (1976 to 1985). N Engl J Med. 1988;319:1557-62.
22. Mumtaz K, Azam Z, Hamid S, Abid S, Memon S, Ali Shah H, et al. Role of N-acetylcysteine in adults with non-acetaminophen-induced acute liver failure in a center without the facility of liver transplantation. Hepatol Int. 2009;3:563-70.
23. Kortsalioudaki C, Taylor RM, Cheeseman P, Bansal S, Mieli-Vergani G, Dhawan A. Safety and efficacy of N-acetylcysteine in children with non-acetaminophen-induced acute liver failure. Liver Transpl. 2008;14:25-30.

24. Lee WM, Hynan LS, Rossaro L, Fontana RJ, Stravitz RT, Larson AM, et al. Intravenous N-acetylcysteine improves transplant-free survival in early stage non-acetaminophen acute liver failure. Gastroenterology. 2009;137:856-64.e1.
25. Acharya SK, Bhatia V, Sreenivas V, Khanal S, Panda SK. Efficacy of L-ornithine L-aspartate in acute liver failure: a double-blind, randomized, placebo-controlled study. Gastroenterology. 2009;136:2159-68.
26. Gluud L, Dam G, Les I, Marchesini G, Borre M, Aagaard N, et al. Branched-chain amino acids for people with hepatic encephalopathy. Cochrane Database Syst Rev. 2017;(5): CD001939.
27. Shaker M, Carey WD. (2014). Hepatic Encephalopathy. Clevel and Clinics. Centre for Continuing Education Publication. [online] Available from: http://www.clevelandclinicmeded.com/medicalpubs/diseasemanagement/hepatology/hepatic-encephalopathy/. [Last accessed August, 2023].
28. Olde Damink SW, Jalan R, Dejong CH. Interorgan ammonia trafficking in liver disease. Metab Brain Dis. 2009;24:169-81.
29. Renner EL. How to decide when to list a patient with acute liver failure for liver transplantation? Clichy or King's College criteria, or something else? J Hepatol. 2007;46:553-82.
30. O'Grady J. Timing and benefit of liver transplantation in acute liver failure. J Hepatol. 2014;60:663-70.
31. Bernal W, Donaldson N, Wyncoll D, Wendon J. Blood lactate as an early predictor of outcome in paracetamol-induced acute liver failure: a cohort study. Lancet. 2002;359:558-63.
32. Auzinger G, Wendon J. Intensive care management of acute liver failure. Curr Opin Crit Care. 2008;14:179-88.
33. Willars C, Wendon J. Acute hepatic failure, organ specific problems. PACT—an ESICM multidisciplinary distance learning programme for intensive care training, Update 2012. [online] Available from: http://academy.esicm.org/enrol/index.php?id=175#
34. Tillmann HL, Hadem J, Leifeld L, Zachou K, Canbay A, Eisenbach C, et al. Safety and efficacy of lamivudine in patients with severe acute or fulminant hepatitis B, a multicenter experience. J Viral Hepat. 2006;13:256-63.
35. Bernal W, Wendon J. Acute liver failure. N Engl J Med. 2013; 369:2525-34.
36. Karkhanis J, Verna EC, Chang MS, Stravitz RT, Schilsky M, Lee WM, et al. Steroid use in acute liver failure. Hepatology. 2014;59:612-21.
37. Zao B, Zang HY, Xie GJ, Lui HM, Chen Q, Li RF, et al. Evaluation of the efficacy of steroid therapy on acute liver failure. Exp Ther Med. 2016;12:3121-9.
38. Chen SC, Hewitt WR, Watanabe FD, Eguchi S, Kahaku E, Middleton Y, et al. Clinical experience with a porcine hepatocyte-based liver support system. Int J Artif Organs. 1996;19:664-9.
39. Watanabe FD, Mullon CJ, Hewitt WR, Arkadopoulos N, Kahaku E, Eguchi S, et al. Clinical experience with a bioartificial liver in the treatment of severe liver failure. A phase I clinical trial. Ann Surg. 1997;225:484-91.
40. Demetriou AA, Brown Jr RS, Busuttil RW, Fair J, McGuire BM, Rosenthal P, et al. Prospective, randomized, multicenter, controlled trial of a bioartificial liver in treating acute liver failure. Ann Surg. 2004;239(5):660-7.
41. Sauer IM, Kardassis D, Zeillinger K, Pascher A, Gruenwald A, Pless G, et al. Clinical extracorporeal hybrid liver support—phase I study with primary porcine liver cells. Xenotransplantation. 2003;10:460-9.
42. Ellis AJ, Hughes RD, Nicholl D, Langley PG, Wendon JA, O'Grady JG, et al. Temporary extracorporeal liver support for severe acute alcoholic hepatitis using the BioLogic-DT. Int J Artif Organs. 1999;22:27-34.
43. Stadlbauer V, Jalan R. Acute liver failure: liver support therapies. Curr Opin Crit Care. 2007;13:215-21.
44. Karvellas CJ, Subramanian RM. Current evidence for extracorporeal liver support systems in acute liver failure and acute-on-chronic liver failure. Crit Care Clin. 2016;32:439-51.
45. Larsen FS, Schmidt LE, Bernsmeier C, Rasmussen A, Isoniemi H, Patel VC, et al. High-volume plasma exchange in patients with acute liver failure: an open randomised controlled trial. J Hepatol. 2016;64:69-78.
46. Bernuau J. High volume plasma exchange in patients with acute liver failure. J Hepatol. 2016;65:646-7.

Diabetic Ketoacidosis

Natesh Prabu R, Carol Shayne D Silva, Atul Prabhakar Kulkarni

CASE STUDY

A 52-year-old male, presented to the emergency room (ER) with tachypnea and tachycardia, which has worsened over 1 day. He consumes alcohol once weekly and is an occasional smoker. He is a known case of type 2 diabetes mellitus (DM) for 10 years and he is currently on injection isophane insulin 10 U subcutaneous bid, human regular insulin 6 U tid before meals, and injection glargine 20 U bedtime. His last glycosylated hemoglobin (HbA1c) was 7.2%. He is recently diagnosed as hypertensive, which is controlled with ramipril 5 mg.

He was on an official tour for the past 1 week and had increased daily consumption of alcohol for the past few days and had irregular food intake. He had a fever for 4 days and a cough for 2 days. He also had multiple vomiting episodes, poor food intake, and excessive thirst for 1 day. He himself decreased his insulin dose and missed a few medicines for 2 days. He was having altered sensorium in the ER, with slow response to commands. Heart rate (HR) 126 beats/min, regular, blood pressure (BP) 90/72 mm Hg, and respiratory rate (RR) 40 breaths/min. His saturation was 97% on 4 L/min O_2. There were crepitations and bronchial breathing in the right infra-axillary region on auscultation of the chest. His abdomen was soft and nontender. An arterial blood gas (ABG) showed pH 7.29, partial pressure of arterial carbon dioxide ($PaCO_2$) 24 mm Hg, partial pressure of arterial oxygen (PaO_2) 69 mm Hg, bicarbonate (HCO_3) 16 mmol/L, and lactate 6 mmol/L.

The other laboratory investigations showed serum sodium (Na) 129 mmol/L, serum chloride (Cl) 86 mmol/L, serum potassium (K) 3.2 mmol/L, serum phosphate (PO_4) 2.2 mmol/L, blood glucose (BG) 480 mg/dL, serum urea 82 mg/dL, and serum creatinine 1.4 mg/dL. ECG showed sinus tachycardia. The urinary ketones were 2+.

Q1. How will you approach this patient and what are the possible differential diagnoses in this patient?

The patient is having possible community-acquired pneumonia and complex acid-base disturbance. Resuscitation should proceed with an assessment of airway, breathing, and circulation. After resuscitation, the cause of acid-base electrolyte disturbances, infection, and its complications should be addressed. The ABG shows high anion gap metabolic acidosis with metabolic alkalosis with respiratory alkalosis. Possible causes in him could be sepsis, ketoacidosis (diabetes, alcohol, and starvation), acute kidney injury and hyperlactatemia. Background diabetes with intercurrent infection and missed diabetic medications engender a strong suspicion of diabetic ketoacidosis (DKA) or hyperosmolar hyperglycemic state (HHS), also previously called hyperglycemic hyperosmolar nonketotic coma.[1] Since the patient has blood sugars <600 mg/dL and low bicarbonate with acute history, it does not favor HHS. HHS usually presents with osmolality >320 mOsm/L, severe dehydration and mild or no acidosis. The patient had increased alcohol consumption and poor food intake which increases the possibility of alcoholic ketosis or starvation ketosis (less likely though for just 1 day of poor food intake and both usually do not present with severe acidosis and severe hyperglycemia). Another differential diagnosis is uremia, but usually, patients will have high urea without hyperglycemia and ketosis.

Q2. How are DKA and HHS diagnosed? How do they differ from each other?

Metabolic acidosis, ketosis, and uncontrolled hyperglycemia form the triad of DKA. HHS, on the other hand, is characterized by profound hyperglycemia, hyperosmolality, and dehydration, usually in the absence of significant ketoacidosis.

Diagnostic criteria as per the American Diabetes Association (ADA) guidelines (2009) include:[1]
- Plasma glucose >250 mg/dL
- Arterial pH <7.30
- Serum bicarbonate of <18 mmol/dL
- Anion gap >12
- Positive serum or urine ketones.

The presence of ketosis is the key diagnostic feature in DKA. It is recommended to measure serum ketones to diagnose DKA as the detection of serum ketones is far more sensitive and specific than urine ketones.[2,3] Serum ketones rise early during DKA and if the samples show ketone levels >3 mmol/L, it clinches the diagnosis of DKA.

Diabetic ketoacidosis can be classified based on severity as mild, moderate, and severe with BG levels >250 mg/dL, serum ketone >3.0 mmol/L, and positive urine ketone common for all classes of severity.[1]

- *Mild DKA:* Patients will be alert with arterial pH between 7.25 and 7.30, serum bicarbonate between 15 and 18 mEq/L, and anion gap of >10.
- *Moderate DKA:* Patients will be drowsy with arterial pH 7.00–7.24, serum bicarbonate between 10 and 15 mEq/L, and anion gap of >12.
- *Severe DKA:* Patients will be comatose/stuporous with arterial pH of <7.0, serum bicarbonate <10 mEq/L, and anion gap of >12.

The Joint British Diabetes Societies (JBDS) suggested a few criteria to differentiate patients with severe DKA.[4] The DKA is considered severe if the patient has any one of the following. This helps us to choose the level of care, the urgent need for treatment initiation, and closer follow-up.

- *Acidosis:* Blood ketones >6.0 mmol/L or serum bicarbonate <5.0 mmol/L, anion gap >16 (including potassium in calculation), pH below 7.0
- Hypokalemia on admission (<3.5 mmol/L)
- *Poor sensorium:* Glasgow Coma Scale (GCS) <12 or abnormal AVPU (Alert, Voice, Pain, Unresponsive) scale
- *Hypoxia:* Oxygen saturation below 92% on room air (assuming normal baseline respiratory function)
- *Cardiovascular dysfunction:* Hypotension (systolic BP below 90 mm Hg) and tachycardia (HR >100 or below 60 beats/min).

Diagnosis of Hyperosmolar Hyperglycemic State

The classical features of HHS are BG >600 mg/dL, arterial pH >7.30, serum bicarbonate >18 mmol/L with variable anion gap, serum ketone levels <3.0 mmol/L, negligible urine ketone, and effective serum osmolality >320 mOsm/kg. These patients will be stuporous or comatose. Compared to DKA, the onset is slow, and the patients present with altered mental status and severe dehydration.

Difference between DKA, HHS, and DKA/HHS Overlap

The key features of HHS are: It is relatively less common, the primary physiological abnormality is hyperosmolarity, the key parameter to monitor is osmolality, it takes days to weeks to develop the condition, the key treatment is controlled rehydration, and it has a higher mortality rate compared to DKA. In contrast in the patient with DKA, the primary physiological abnormality is ketoacidosis, insulin infusion is the key treatment and it develops over hours to days. The key parameter to monitor in DKA is the anion gap.

Often patients present with features of both DKA and HHS, and it is a challenge to differentiate at the bedside. Though overlapping presentations of DKA and HHS are recently reported, there is no standard definition.[5,6] Combined DKA/HHS or DKA/HHS overlap patients may have severe hyperglycemia (not common in DKA), severe dehydration, and acidosis. A recent study showed greater mortality (8%) with combined DKA/HHS in comparison to HHS (5%) and DKA (3%) in isolation.[5] The management principles remain the same with key interventions focused on rehydration, electrolyte balance, insulin infusion, and organ support with more vigilant monitoring.

Q3. Describe the pathogenesis and pathophysiology of DKA and HHS.

The development of DKA occurs secondary to two main factors:[1,7-9]
1. Relative or absolute insulin deficiency
2. Unopposed action of counterregulatory hormones, such as glucagon, cortisol, and catecholamines.

In normal individuals, BG levels are kept in tight check by insulin. Insulin promotes the uptake of glucose into skeletal muscle and adipose tissue, and promotes anabolism and glycogen synthesis. Hepatic production of glucose by gluconeogenesis and glycogenolysis is suppressed by insulin. Insulin also inhibits lipolysis, the key factor initiating ketogenesis.

Q4. What happens in DKA?

Hyperglycemia: Hyperglycemia occurs primarily due to unrestrained gluconeogenesis and glycogenolysis, aided by impaired peripheral uptake of glucose into peripheral tissues. High cortisol and catecholamines facilitate proteolysis and lipolysis providing amino acids and glycerol which serve as substrates for gluconeogenesis in the liver and kidney. Impaired tissue perfusion due to volume contraction and the adrenergic response often due to severe underlying precipitating illness result in lactate production, yet another substrate for gluconeogenesis.

The predominant mechanism by which glucose is added to blood is gluconeogenesis due to insulin deficiency. Counterregulatory hormones and other mechanisms play a minor part. The hyperglycemic state promotes osmotic diuresis, leading to volume contraction, hypovolemia, and decreased glomerular filtration rate (GFR) which further worsens the hyperglycemia and causes loss of electrolytes in urine as well **(Fig. 1)**.

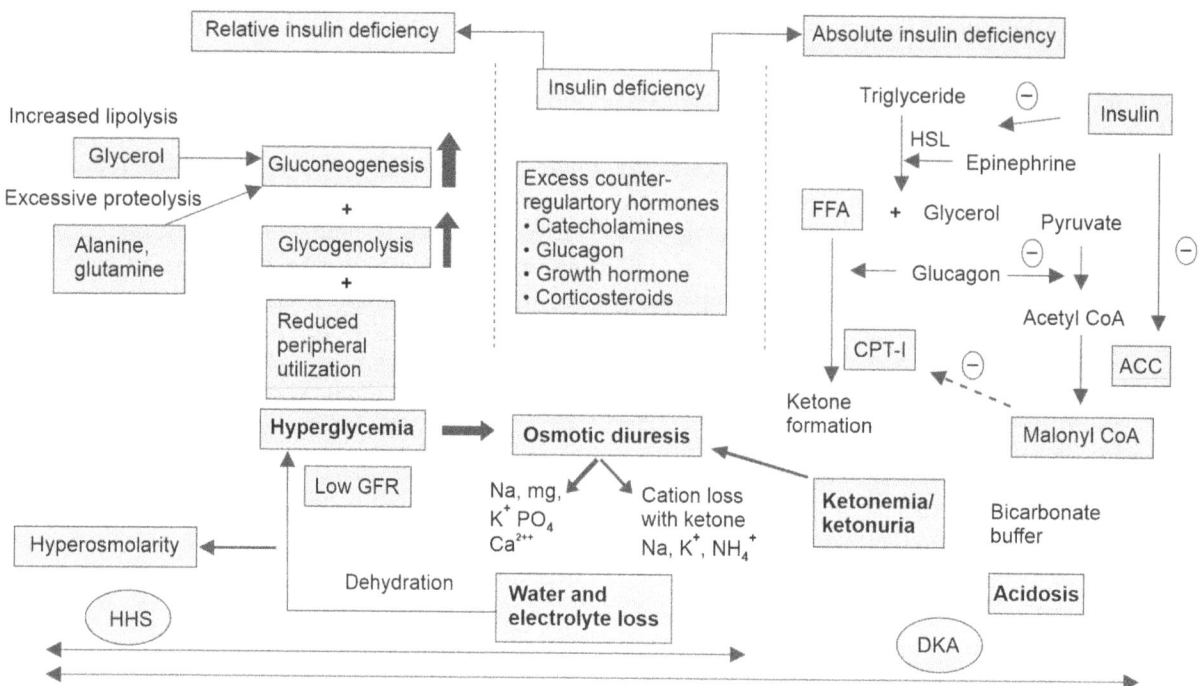

Fig. 1: Pathogenesis and pathophysiology of DKA and HHS.
The width of arrows represents the magnitude of effect and its contribution to pathogenesis.
(ACC: acetyl-CoA carboxylase; Ca^{2+}: calcium; CPT-I: carnitine palmitoyltransferase-I; DKA: diabetic ketoacidosis; FFA: free fatty acid; GFR: glomerular filtration rate; HHS: hyperosmolar hyperglycemic state; HSL: hormone-sensitive lipase; K: potassium; Mg: magnesium; Na: sodium; NH_4^+: ammonium; PO_4: phosphate; –: inhibition)

Ketogenesis and Acidosis

Insulin deficiency and counterregulatory hormones, particularly epinephrine, facilitate lipolysis by activation of hormone-sensitive lipase which breaks down triglycerides (TGs) into free fatty acids (FFAs) and glycerol. The FFA (fatty acyl-CoA) is transported across mitochondria by carnitine palmitoyltransferase-I (CPT-I) where it is oxidized to ketone. Counterregulatory hormones especially glucagon (high glucagon: insulin ratio) blocks the conversion of pyruvate to acetyl-CoA (inhibition of acetyl-CoA carboxylase, rate-limiting step in de novo FFA synthesis) leading to reduced levels of malonyl-CoA. This results in loss of inhibition over CPT-I (malonyl-CoA inhibits CPT-I) which favors more FFA to enter mitochondria leading to the generation of ketoanions by β-oxidation. High glucagon levels alone do not lead to ketone formation,[10] it is the low insulin level that is necessary for ketogenesis (i.e., high glucagon: insulin ratio). The predominant ketones produced are 3-β-hydroxybutyrate (3BHB), acetoacetate (AcAc), and acetone to a lesser extent. AcAc is reduced to β-hydroxybutyrate and during this step. NADH is oxidized to NAD^+. Therefore, the ultimate ratio of 3BHB to AcAc in the blood is dependent on the redox potential (i.e., the $NADH/NAD^+$ ratio) within hepatic mitochondria. The increase in the availability of both CPT-I and fatty acyl-CoA in patients with DKA promotes ketone formation. The ratio of β-hydroxybutyrate to AcAc varies from 0.6:1 to 4.8:1.[11] The variation in ketone levels in untreated DKA is related to the amount of plasma FFA levels.

Not only is the production of ketoanions more in DKA, the excretion of ketoacids are also impaired due to hypovolemia and low GFR. The patients with DKA have acidosis due to the utilization of bicarbonate in buffering ketoacids. Patients with HHS have very less ketone formation. The reason for no or minimal ketone production is not fully known, but it could be because of lower levels of counterregulatory hormones and the presence of some circulating insulin which could be adequate to inhibit lipolysis and subsequent ketogenesis[12] **(Fig. 1)**.

Hyperglycemia and ketosis—a proinflammatory sate: The development of hyperglycemia and ketoacidosis together also results in an inflammatory state characterized by an elevation of proinflammatory cytokines and increased oxidative stress markers, such as tumor necrosis factor-alpha (TNF-α), interleukin-6 (IL-6), IL-1, and IL-8. TNF-α has been implicated in mediating insulin resistance in DKA.[13,14] Increased oxidative stress and generation of free oxygen radicals potentiates the cellular damage. The inflammatory marker levels are reduced after correction of hyperglycemia and ketosis.

Q5. Do normal glucose levels and negative urine ketones rule out DKA? What are the Challenges in diagnosing DKA?

Diabetic ketoacidosis is not always a straightforward diagnosis and the presentation may vary with regards to normal to high blood sugar levels and varying bicarbonate levels. Munro et al.[15] in 1973 observed that out of 211 DKA patients, 37 patients had blood sugar <300 mg/dL and bicarbonate ≤10 mEq/L. He labeled this condition as euglycemic DKA, wherein the blood sugar levels may be normal or even low with ketoacidosis. Other authors have also described DKA with normal blood sugars, hence using blood sugar levels >250 mg/dL as the main feature for diagnosis could be misleading.[1,16,17] The euglycemic DKA is frequently observed in pregnant women with diabetes, alcohol abuse, anorexia, or gastroparesis and more recently, in patients treated with sodium-glucose cotransporter-2 (SGLT2) inhibitors (dapagliflozin and empagliflozin).[1,18] SGLT2 inhibitors that are commonly prescribed for type 2 diabetes and heart failure acts by promoting renal glucose excretion. It is more frequently associated with euglycemic DKA. It is better to stop this drug during DKA episodes or any major surgery and avoid it in future.

Diagnosis of DKA could be even more challenging when there is mixed acid-base disorder (e.g., associated vomiting, which may lead to concomitant alkalosis, so may present with less fall in bicarbonate) or when the anion gap is normal, that occurs due to the loss of ketoanions in osmotic diuresis along with sodium or potassium. Also, if there has been a shift in the redox potential favoring the presence of β-hydroxybutyrate, serum ketones may be negative, especially if the test measuring ketones measures only AcAc.[3]

It is, therefore, important to measure ketones in both the serum and urine. Negative urine ketones should not be used to rule out DKA.[19]

> **Learning Point**
>
> *Normal blood glucose levels and normal urine ketone does not rule out DKA. Diabetic patients with acidosis should be evaluated for presence of elevated serum ketones.*

Q6. Describe the clinical presentation of DKA. What initial laboratory investigations will you send?

Diabetic ketoacidosis usually evolves much faster than HHS, i.e., over 24-48 hours. The clinical presentation[1] is a combined effect of hyperglycemia, ketoacidosis, and the underlying illness. The classical clinical picture is that of polyuria and polydipsia, signs of dehydration occurring due to hyperglycemia. The patient may have symptoms due to ketoacidosis, such as nausea, vomiting, abdominal pain, acetone odor in breath, Kussmaul's respiration, and altered sensorium. The examination may reveal signs of dehydration, such as tachycardia, hypotension, dry mucous membranes, poor skin turgor, decreased tissue perfusion in the form of increased capillary refill time, and hypothermia. Patient can present as acute abdomen in 40-75% of cases, which is associated with the degree of ketoacidosis rather than hyperglycemia itself.[20] Apart from these presentations there could be signs and symptoms of underlying illness that precipitated the DKA.

The following laboratory investigations should be obtained

At presentation and before starting treatment, the following laboratory tests should be sent for plasma glucose, blood urea nitrogen, serum creatinine, serum ketones, electrolytes (with calculated anion gap), serum osmolality, urinalysis for urine ketones: by dipstick, ABGs, and complete blood count with differential count. In addition to the above, appropriate culture (blood, urine, or sputum) and specific necessary tests to evaluate primary or precipitating illness should be sent.

Q7. What are the common precipitating factors for the hyperglycemic crisis?

- Omission of insulin—a common cause
- Infections—a common cause
- Trauma
- Surgery
- Concomitant medical illnesses, such as myocardial infarction (MI), cerebrovascular accident (CVA), and acute pancreatitis
- Drugs that have been implicated in causing DKA are SGLT2 inhibitors, diuretics, glucocorticoids, lithium, and atypical antipsychotics
- Unprovoked ketoacidosis with no precipitating factor has been observed in Afro-Americans and Hispanics.[21]
- New onset type 2 DM can also present as DKA as an initial presentation.[21,22]

Q8. Where should you treat the patient: intensive care unit (ICU)/high-dependency unit (HDU), or ward or emergency department (ED)? How do you triage patients with DKA?

Patients with DKA are often admitted to ICU due to the presence of severe acidosis, the need for strict insulin titration and vigilant monitoring which may be costly and resource intensive. Many recent studies have shown that it is safe and effective to manage mild to moderate DKA in out-of-the-ICU settings with subcutaneous rapid-acting insulin.[23-26] A prospective randomized study from India that compared intravenous insulin versus subcutaneous insulin in DKA patients, intravenous insulin group patients got admitted to ICU and patients on the subcutaneous arm were managed in the emergency department itself. This study showed no difference in mortality, recurrence of acidosis, length of stay, or complications.

Evidence showed that in patients admitted to ICUs,[24,27] a higher number of investigations were sent and hospitalization costs were higher. ICU admission is not always mandatory, treatment in the ED or in a HDU with adequate personnel and monitoring should suffice in uncomplicated mild to moderate DKA. However, patients with severe DKA as suggested by JBDS or with serious precipitating critical illnesses/infections (MI, sepsis, etc.) as cause should be treated in the ICU.[1,4,28]

> The patient had mixed acid-base disorder. Presence of metabolic alkalosis could confound the assessment of severity of acidosis. In the patient, intravenous fluids could have unmasked severe metabolic acidosis. As our patient had pneumonia, sepsis, and severe DKA, he was shifted to ICU and further treatment continued. 0.9% saline continued at 500 mL/h with 30 mEq/L potassium chloride.

Q9. What are the treatment goals for this patient?
- Correcting fluid depletion and restoration of normal circulating volume and adequate tissue perfusion
- Correction of hyperglycemia at an appropriate rate
- Suppression of ketone production and elimination of ketone bodies
- Correction of electrolyte imbalance
- Treat precipitating illnesses.
- Prevention of recurrence.

The management of patients with DKA focus on reversing the fluid, electrolyte, glucose, and metabolic imbalances to normalcy **(Fig. 2)**. The timeline to achieve these vary over time and it is suggested to involve a special diabetic care team if available to improve overall care.[4]

Q10. Describe the fluid management in patients with DKA and the effect of volume expansion.

Intravenous fluid administration is the first-line treatment for patients with DKA and HHS. Patients with DKA and HHS have estimated water loss of approximately 100 mL/kg and 100–200 mL/kg, respectively, leading to both extracellular and intracellular dehydration.[1] Isotonic saline, 0.9% sodium chloride [normal saline (NS)], is the preferred fluid, rushed as boluses when the patients present with hypotension. Typically 500 mL to 1 L over 15–30 minutes or at the rate of 1–1.5 to 2 L/h (15–20 mL/kg) in the first hour in the absence of cardiac compromise.[1,29] Fluid resuscitation restores intravascular volume and renal perfusion leading to a reduction in BG levels by dilution, promoting urinary loss and improving insulin sensitivity by reducing counterregulatory hormones.

Aggressive rehydration is the key to quick correction of hyperosmolar state which itself can enhance the response to insulin therapy. Though 0.9% saline is used worldwide for initial fluid resuscitation, it often leads to hyperchloremic acidosis. Resuscitation using different crystalloids was done in the recent past with varied effect. A study that compared Ringer's lactate (RL) with 0.9% NS showed no difference in the length of stay or other outcomes but the time to correct hyperglycemia was significantly longer in the

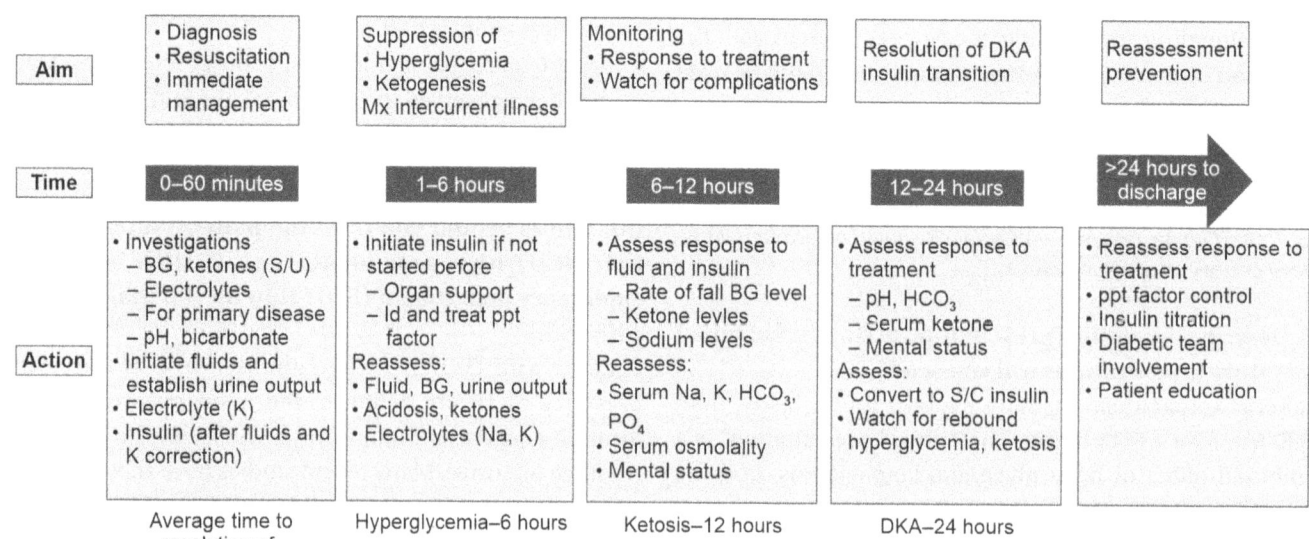

Fig. 2: Summary of DKA management: Simplified and short overview. (BG: blood glucose; DKA: diabetic ketoacidosis; HCO₃: bicarbonate; Id: identification; K: potassium; Mx: management; Na: sodium; PO₄: phosphate; ppt: precipitating; S/C: subcutaneous; S/U: serum/urine)

lactated Ringers' group. A retrospective study that compared Plasma-Lyte with 0.9% NS showed a faster resolution of acidosis.[16,17,30,31] Another study that compared Plasma-Lyte A (PL) with 0.9% NS (with the aim to prevent hyperchloremic acidosis) showed reduced chloride levels and higher bicarbonate levels in Plasma-Lyte A group.[32] Even though there is a lack of evidence many guidelines still prefer 0.9% saline as fluid of choice.[1-3]

A recent clinical trial that compared PL with NS in severe DKA patients admitted to ICU showed faster resolution of DKA (defined as the change in base excess to more than or equal to minus 3 mEq/L at 48 hours) and lesser length of hospital stay with the use of balanced salt solution (BSS) compared to 0.9% NS.[33] Also, a subgroup analysis of DKA patients in SMART[34] and SALT-ED[35] studies showed faster resolution of DKA with a median of 9.8 versus 13.4 hours with balanced solution compared (RL and PL) to NS.[36] A recent meta-analysis including these two trials (both had bias with blinding) though showed faster resolution of DKA with BSS, the results are from small, randomized trials. It is logical that the resolution of DKA may not be fully dependent on the choice of fluid but also on the rate and volume of infusion. BSS may be a preferred solution, but RL or NS can be an alternative pending large good quality studies and this may be beneficial in resource-limited settings.

Once initial fluid resuscitation is completed, subsequent fluid administration should be guided by patient's hemodynamics, urine output, electrolyte levels, and cardiorenal status.[29] The estimated fluid deficit should be repleted in the first 24 hours. The choice of fluid, either 0.9% saline or 0.45% saline depending on serum sodium levels, is given at the rate of 250–500 mL/h. The rate of fluid administration should be reassessed frequently and could be altered based on serum sodium, osmolality, fall in blood sugar levels, and urine output. Patients with DKA require more free water due to increased water losses. These losses are far greater in patients with HHS.

Once the blood sugar levels reach <200–250 mg/dL, it is prudent to start 5% dextrose (or 10% dextrose, dextrose concentration adjusted for blood sugar level) with the maintenance fluids to allow for continued insulin infusion for control of ketonemia, and more importantly, to avoid hypoglycemia.[1,29]

Q11. How will you initiate insulin in a patient with DKA?
Insulin is the mainstay treatment in patients with hyperglycemic crisis. Insulin helps control blood sugar levels, preventing lipolysis and ketone body formation. Intravenous insulin regimens are the initial choice to control blood sugar levels, halt lipolysis, and ketone body formation. After a low-dose insulin regimen was found to have equal efficacy and lesser complications compared to a conventional high-dose regimen,[37,38] it has become common practice to use only low-dose insulin in managing patients with hyperglycemic crisis.[1] Start insulin infusion in all patients with moderate to severe DKA having serum potassium above 3.3 mEq/L. The insulin is either started with a priming bolus 0.1 units/kg followed by continuous infusion of 0.1 U/kg/h or continuous infusion without priming bolus at the rate of 0.14 U/kg/h. Insulin infusion is titrated to achieve a steady decline in glucose level by 50–75 mg/h as well as to achieve a reduction in blood ketones levels (0.5 mmol/h) and an increase in bicarbonate levels (3 mmol/L).[2,39] As BG falls with hydration due to dilution and urinary glucose excretion, insulin infusion should be started only after achieving good urine output and hydration should be checked when there is no expected fall in BG levels before increasing insulin dosage. When BG levels fall below 200–250 mg/dL, insulin infusion is reduced to half and dextrose infusion is added to prevent rapid fall in osmolality and blood sugar. Insulin and dextrose infusion are titrated to achieve glucose concentration between 140 and 200 mg/dL until resolution of ketoacidosis. Though intravenous regular insulin is widely recommended[1,29] several other studies showed good control with subcutaneous shorter-acting insulin (aspart and lispro), particularly in patients with mild to moderate DKA.[1,32,40,41] Subcutaneous insulin is commonly given in doses of 0.2–0.3 U/kg followed by 0.1–0.2 U/kg every 1–2 hours subcutaneously till blood sugar falls to 250 mg/dL, then continued with a reduced dose of 0.05 Us/kg every 1–2 hours till DKA resolves. Managing patients on continuous intravenous insulin is more resource intense and recommended in sick patients with hypoperfusion, hypotension, and critically ill. Subcutaneous regimens allow easy and effective treatment particularly in out-of-the-ICU settings.[29] Recently fixed rate intravenous insulin infusion (FRIII) is recommended by Joint British Societies since the patient profile is changing with more obese patients, and patients with more insulin resistance. FRIII has good ketone clearance and is easy to administer.[2] It is recommended to start with 0.1 U/kg/h when the blood sugar is >250 mg/dL and to reduce the rate to 0.05 U/kg/h when the blood sugar falls below 250 mg/dL.[4]

Q12. Compare the different insulin regimens used for the treatment of hyperglycemic emergencies.
Comparison of the different insulin regimens used for the treatment of hyperglycemic emergencies is given in **Table 1**.

TABLE 1: Comparison of various insulin regimens used in the management of diabetic ketoacidosis (DKA).

Regimens	Dose	Advantages	Comments
Intravenous continuous infusion with loading	0.1 U/kg f/b infusion	• Time tested • Quickly achieves target blood insulin levels • Good glucose control	• Precipitous fall in blood glucose can happen • Labor intensive
Intravenous continuous without loading	0.14 U/kg/h	Equally effective, good blood glucose control and less hypoglycemia (vs. with loading)	• Less precipitous fall of blood sugar and better sugar titration • Labor intensive
Fixed rate intravenous insulin infusion (FRIII)	0.1 U/kg/h (0.05 U/kg/h when blood sugar <250 mg/dL)	No need to alter the dose as it is fixed dose*	Good ketone clearance and less hypoglycemia
Subcutaneous insulin	0.2–0.3 U/kg, f/b 0.1–0.2 U/kg every 1–2 hour	• Equally effective in reducing blood sugars • Compared to the intravenous route, it requires less resource and is cost-effective	• Only for mild to moderate DKA • Can be used in out-of-the-ICU settings • Avoided in patients with shock and severely ill • Not patient friendly and absorption may be a problem
Intravenous + Subcutaneous glargine	Early glargine coadministration	• Reduced rebound hyperglycemia • Shorter hospital stay	Need more studies
Intramuscular	7 U/kg	Bolus can be given and slow release	• Risk of hematoma • Not commonly practiced

*The dose of insulin is kept constant, the dose depend on the starting blood sugar levels (more or less than 250 mg/dL).
(DKA: diabetic ketoacidosis; f/b: followed by; U/kg: units per kilogram; h: hour; ICU: intensive care unit)

Q13. How will you approach electrolyte disturbances in DKA?

Potassium correction: Total potassium deficit in DKA patients is around 3–5 mEq/kg body weight. Even if the serum values are normal, the total body stores are often depleted by renal losses and intracellular shifts. With poor insulin sensitivity and hyperosmolarity, uptake of potassium into the skeletal muscle is also impaired and potassium efflux from the cells ensues. This can cause depletion of body stores of potassium and phosphate. The potassium level is influenced by amount and rate of volume expansion, insulin therapy, and correction of acidosis.

- If serum K⁺ is <3.3 mmol/L, insulin therapy is withheld. Give potassium chloride 20–40 mmol/h intravenously until K⁺ >3.3 mmol/L.
- If >3.3 mmol/L and <5.3 mmol/L give potassium chloride 20–30 mmol in every liter of intravenous fluid.
- If K⁺ >5.3 mmol/L, no supplementation is required, check potassium every 2 hours.

The goal is to maintain serum potassium around 4–5 mEq/L and administration of 20–30 mmol/L of potassium into fluids is sufficient in most patients.[1]

Phosphate therapy: Hypophosphatemia is commonly seen in patients with DKA. Serum phosphate is either low or normal despite a loss of 1 mmol/kg. Studies have not shown any beneficial effect with phosphate replacement[18-20,42] and routine replacement is not recommended.[29] Correction, however, is indicated if the patients have cardiac dysfunction, respiratory depression and levels less than 1.0–1.5 mg/dL.[1] Hypocalcemia is a deadly complication with phosphate supplementation. When there is a need, 20–30 mmol/L of potassium phosphate can be added to fluids.

Sodium balance: Serum sodium deficits occur in the range of 7–10 mmoL/kg in patients with DKA. Patients with DKA/HHS will have reduced serum sodium concentration due to shift of water out of cells due to hyperosmolar state. There will be a drop of 1.6 mmol/L sodium for every 100 mg/dL increase in serum glucose concentration >100 mg/dL. There will also loss of sodium due to osmotic diuresis. DKA is frequent cause of hypertonic hyponatremia and the corrected sodium values should be calculated basis on the glucose levels at the time of presentation. The serum sodium trend during treatment should be closely monitored. If patient has normal or high corrected serum sodium it indicates severe dehydration.

Bicarbonate therapy: Whether to give bicarbonate in patient with DKA having severe acidosis is subject of a long-standing debate. Severe acidosis causes impaired cardiac contractility, vasodilation, and coma. A study that evaluated role of bicarbonate in patients with pH between 6.9 and 7.1 did not show any benefit[43] but there are no randomized studies done with pH <6.9.[44] Considering possible adverse cardiovascular effects, it is suggested to administer bicarbonate to such patients. The recent Canadian guidelines suggest bicarbonate therapy for severe DKA cases with pH ≤7.0.[3] Sodium bicarbonate infusion is not without adverse effects, it can cause hypokalemia, hypercarbia, and cerebral edema, especially in pediatric population.[3,45] Bicarbonate therapy in DKA patients with pH <7.0 did not result in either faster resolution of acidosis or time to discharge from hospital.[46] Still many guidelines and different societies[1,3,29] suggest administering sodium bicarbonate in patients with severe acidosis with pH <6.9. Common practice is to give 50–100 mmol of sodium bicarbonate as an isotonic solution with 200 ml 5% dextrose in water and repeated every 2 hours until the pH recovers to >7.0.

> Patient was continued with 0.9% saline with 30 mEq/L potassium chloride at rate of 250 mL/h for 2 hours. Potassium correction was given to maintain K^+ >3.3 mEq/L before starting insulin. After 3 hours at ICU, HR—102 bpm, BP—110/74 mm Hg, urine output—40 mL/h past hour, ABG: pH—7.23, partial pressure of arterial oxygen (PaO_2)—6 mm Hg with 5 L/min O_2, partial pressure of arterial carbon dioxide ($PaCO_2$)—28 mm Hg, bicarbonate—12 mEq/L, lactate—2.5 mmol/L, serum sodium—140 mEq/dL, K^+—3.6 mEq/L, Cl⁻—99 mEq/L, blood sugar—402 mg/dL. Insulin was started at 10 U/h infusion. After 1 hour, blood sugar—388 mg/dL, urine ketone—2+, blood ketones—6.2 mmol/L, serum osmolality—301 mOsm/L.

Q14. What are the problems encountered?
The decrease in blood sugar is less than expected 50 mg/dL and increase in serum sodium and not much change in acidosis. When there is less than expected drop in BG levels with increasing serum sodium—check the fluid status, type of fluid rather than increasing insulin dose. This condition indicates severe dehydration.

Learning Point

Intravenous fluid therapy is the first-line treatment for hyperglycemic crisis. Good hydration reduces blood sugar levels by dilution, glycosuria, and reducing counterregulatory hormones. Whenever there is less than expected response with insulin, recheck hydration status. Aggressive hydration and correction of hyperosmolar state enhances response to low-dose insulin therapy. So, good hydration and establishment of good urine output are necessary before initiating and titrating insulin therapy.

Learning Point

When serum sodium becomes normal or high, it reflects severe dehydration and such patients require more free water. When serum osmolality drops despite addition of dextrose (either with or without drop in serum sodium) then more saline infusion is given to increase sodium concentration.

Q15. How will you monitor this patient?
The patient with hyperglycemic crisis should be monitored for effectiveness of treatment, resolution of DKA, and onset of complications. During treatment, the following should be closely monitored: vital signs, volume status, urine output, rate of fluid administration, insulin infusion, and blood sugar levels. While measuring blood sugar levels, it should be ideally measured every 1–2 hours. Capillary BG levels may not be reliable in patients with severe acidosis and shock.[3]

In addition, laboratory measurements of electrolytes (sodium and potassium), bicarbonate, and anion gap should be repeated every 2-4 hours. Venous blood gas is recommended rather arterial and blood ketone should be measured and monitored for rate of fall with treatment.[2] A recent meta-analysis showed superior outcomes when blood ketones are measured and monitored rather urine ketones.[47]

Q16. How will you assess the response to therapy?
The response could be assessed by achieving the desired targets.

- Reduction of BG levels by 50–75 mg/dL/h
- 0.5 mmol/L/h reduction in blood ketone concentration
- Increase in venous bicarbonate by 3.0 mmol/L/h.

Other targets are maintaining good urine output, potassium concentration between 4 and 5 mEq/L, and reduction in plasma anion gap.

Q17. How will you detect resolution of DKA/HHS?
The resolution of DKA happens when hyperglycemia is controlled and most importantly when there is suppression of ketogenesis.

The resolution criteria of DKA as per ADA 2009 are:[1]
Blood glucose levels <200 mg/dL and two of the following:
1. Serum bicarbonate level ≥15 mmol/L
2. Venous pH >7.3
3. Calculated anion gap ≤12

Resolution of DKA as per JBDS:[2]
1. Serum bicarbonate level >15 mmol/L
2. pH >7.3
3. Blood ketone levels <0.6 mmol/L.

Resolution of HHS:[1]
1. Serum osmolality <310 mOsm/kg
2. Improvement in altered sensorium with glucose levels, 250 mg/dL.

> Insulin and hydration continued with 0.45% normal saline at 250 mL/h. Dextrose containing fluid was added when blood sugar was <250 mg/dL and insulin infusion reduced to 5.0 U/h targeting blood sugar around 140–200 mg/dL. At 12 hours postadmission, HR—90 bpm, BP—120/68 mm Hg, urine output—80–100 mL/h, blood sugar—152 mg/dL, pH—7.35, PaO_2—90 mm Hg, O_2—5 L/min, $PaCO_2$—38 mm Hg, bicarbonate—20 mEq/L, serum sodium—138 mEq/L, chloride—98 mEq/L, serum potassium—2.9 mEq/L, urine ketones—3+, serum lactate—0.9, blood ketones—2.8 mmol/L, serum osmolality—288 mOsm/L.

Q18. What are the problems encountered during treatment of DKA and what are the possible reasons?

The problems are occurrence of hypokalemia with therapy and increase in urine ketones from 2+ to 3+.

During therapy, β-hydroxybutyric acid will be converted to AcAc and acetone and there will be increased detection of ketones in urine since nitroprusside test done on urine samples detects only AcAc while β-hydroxybutyrate is the predominant ketone body formed which is directly measured in serum samples. Hence, ketones are detected much longer in urine samples even though DKA is resolving or resolved and this can be misleading. So, direct measurement of β-hydroxybutyrate levels in serum samples is far more accurate to detect the resolution of ketosis[9,16] and is currently recommended to measure serum ketones to guide insulin infusion and to assess response to therapy.[2,10]

Q19. What will you do when blood sugar drops below 200 mg/dL?

When there is a drop of blood sugar below 200–250 mg/dL, dextrose-containing fluid should be initiated to avoid a fall in serum osmolality and prevent hypoglycemia. 5–10% dextrose infusion should be added, and dextrose concentration can be titrated to achieve blood sugar 140–200 mg/dL. Insulin should not be stopped as it will cause rebound ketosis. Insulin infusion should be continued at half the dose, i.e., 0.05 U/kg/h.

Q20. What will you do when there is no expected response?

When you did not get the expected response after initiating the treatment, i.e., lesser change in the blood sugar or serum ketone or bicarbonate, then it may be due to technical problems or patients precipitating illness is not addressed. First check for cannula blockage, quality of insulin (temperature sensitive), infusion lines were primed with insulin, and the measurement is correct. Insulin resistance is not common but to keep in mind correctly. Some patients may need surgical intervention for source control, especially who have intra-abdominal sepsis with peritonitis, soft tissue infection, obstructive uropathy, etc. Patients with mixed etiologies for acidosis such as coexisting renal failure or bicarbonate loss after diarrhea may not show bicarbonate improvement as expected with DKA management protocol.

Q21. What are the common complications that occur during the treatment of DKA?

Hypoglycemia: Hypoglycemia is the most common complication and it can occur during treatment because of wrong titration of insulin infusion, not starting dextrose-containing fluids once blood sugar levels fall below 250 mg/dL, and failure to monitor it at frequent intervals. The classical signs of hypoglycemia, such as sweating, tachycardia, hunger, and fatigue, may not be evident, so the recognition may be difficult, and these signs may be clouded by the precipitating conditions. So, identification requires vigilant and frequent (1–2 hourly) monitoring of blood sugars.[48]

Hypokalemia: Hypokalemia is another common complication of DKA treatment and it frequently occurs due to the intracellular shifts of potassium following insulin administration. It can rarely occur as a side effect to bicarbonate therapy for severe acidosis. For every liter of fluid, 20–30 mmol of KCL should be routinely added to avoid hypokalemia. Serum potassium levels should be checked every 4–6 hours and if found to be <3.3 mmol/dL, insulin infusion is stopped until potassium levels are >3.3 mmol/dL with supplementation.

Cerebral edema: It is commonly seen in children with DKA/HHS and uncommon in adults. The exact mechanisms have not been understood. Proposed mechanisms include the role of cerebral ischemia and hypoxia, the generation of various inflammatory mediators, an increased cerebral blood flow, the disruption of cell membrane ion transport, and a rapid shift in extracellular and intracellular fluids that results in changes in osmolality. It occurs due to rapid changes in osmolality. The serum osmolality is quite variable in patients with DKA of all severity.[1] Patients with higher osmolality have a higher risk of mental status changes, risk of cerebral edema, and higher mortality.[49] So, serum osmolality should not have been allowed to reduce quickly during initial hours of DKA/HHS management (rate of fall not >3 mmol/kg/h). It is important to follow measured osmolality, especially in patients with HHS. Criteria for the severity of DKA/HHS could be revised by including serum osmolality since a recent estimate suggests that 20–30% of patients present with combined ketoacidosis and hyperosmolality(may be in combination with increased lactates).[48] High-risk period is 4–12 hours after initiation of treatment but may occur within 48 hours. Initial treatment is with either 20% mannitol or hypertonic saline and tight control over the rate of fall of blood sugar and sodium levels. To rule out other causes, neuroimaging should be done.

Other rare complications are acute respiratory distress syndrome (ARDS) and pulmonary edema.[50,51]

Acute respiratory distress syndrome or pulmonary edema can occur due to change in osmolality during treatment of DKA and fluid overload particularly in patients with renal and cardiac compromise.

Q22. When will you stop intravenous insulin?

Once there is the resolution of DKA, suppression of ketogenesis and patient resumes oral diet, intravenous insulin can be stopped but simultaneously initiate subcutaneous insulin regimen.

> **Learning Point**
> The time of resolution of hyperglycemia and ketosis is on average 6 hours and 12 hours. Ketosis resolution lags blood sugar. Stopping insulin before suppression of ketogenesis will cause rebound ketoacidosis. So, intravenous insulin should be continued until resolution of DKA.

Q23. How will you make a transition from treatment infusion to maintenance insulin regimen?

Maintenance insulin is always started along with initial insulin infusion to avoid rebound ketosis and hyperglycemia as intravenous insulin has a very short half-life (around 10 minutes). Resolution of DKA and the ability of the patients to take adequate oral intake are important prerequisites to initiate maintenance insulin regimens. Current practice and ADA recommendation is to initiate a combination of subcutaneous NPH (isophane/neutral protamine Hagedorn) and regular insulin twice a day.[1] Subcutaneous regimens are usually started 2–4 hours before the stoppage of intravenous insulin depending on chosen insulin, i.e., intermediate versus long-acting. Patients with known diabetes on insulin therapy (on regimen with controlled sugars) can be started with their own regimen. In insulin-naïve patients multidose insulin regimen should be started with the dose of 0.5–0.8 U/kg/day or the previous 24 hours insulin requirement can be taken as a guide to starting insulin. Newer trials that compared NPH+ regular insulin versus basal bolus (glargine) + shorter-acting insulin (glulisine) before meals have shown similar glycemic control but with less hypoglycemic episodes with basal-bolus insulin regimen.[52] The practice to use basal-bolus insulin has increased in the recent past due to its nonpeak blood levels, better blood sugar control with less hypoglycemic episodes. It also behaves as physiological basal insulin secretion. Because of its advantages and equal efficacy with less adverse effects, it is preferred along with preprandial insulin, especially after the resolution of DKA.[48]

Q24. Comment on protocols in managing DKA.

Recently DKA management protocols and computerized protocol management have been tried with varied success.[53-55] The possible advantages could be following protocols may increase adherence to key principles of management of DKA that may translate into better outcomes. Studies have shown poor adherence to protocols and guidelines[56] even as low as around 30%.[53] Moreover, there is only limited evidence to support that following protocols or guidelines will improve adherence and outcome.[54,56] Many interventions of DKA management are currently based on poor quality evidence and expert opinion/consensus statement and it requires randomized control trials (RCTs) to affirm treatment and to formulate guidelines based on it.[55]

Q25. What is the blood sugar target for critically ill patients? Discuss the major blood sugar trials.

The subject of glucose control in the critically ill has always sparked debate. Van den Berghe et al.[57] brought to the fore the concept of tight glucose control in 2001 through their landmark single-center prospective RCT in surgical intensive care patients (primarily cardiac surgical), which showed reduced mortality, reduced renal impairment, and decreased bloodstream infection but higher rate of hypoglycemia in intensive insulin therapy (blood sugar target 80–110 mg/dL) compared to conventional group (blood sugar 180–200 mg/dL). However, when repeated in medical intensive care patients, intensive insulin therapy did not improve mortality but was associated with significantly higher rates of hypoglycemia (BG <40 mg/dL) 18.7 versus 3.1%.[58] NICE-SUGAR trial performed in critically ill patients showed increased mortality and hypoglycemia with the intensive insulin group and favored a target BG <180 mg/dL.[59] Many other studies done in different critically ill populations, such as septic shock, MI, neurocritical care, and surgical patients did not show any benefit in tight control of blood sugar and the patients in this group had more episodes of hypoglycemia.[60-64] Though there is no mortality benefit, controlling blood sugar has shown to decrease ICU length of stay, infections, mechanical ventilator days, and improved neurological outcome (especially after traumatic brain injury).[59,65] Different societies recommend insulin starting threshold if BG >180 mg/dL and to target BG between 140 and 180 mg/dL.[66,67] However, they do mention stringent goals of 110–140 mg/dL to be achieved in select populations of critically ill when it can be achieved without causing hypoglycemia.

> The patient improved and started on oral diet. Intravenous insulin continued. Patient was started on his previous insulin regimen with inj. Glargine 20 U at night and started on inj. NPH 10 U bid. Patient urine output, electrolytes, blood sugar and ketone urine/blood monitored. Insulin dose were titrated further, and patient was discharged to high-dependency unit next day.

Q26. How will you modify the DKA management in special populations?

Patients with chronic kidney disease and pregnancy are common populations we come across in ICU. Patients with CKD may have less insulin clearance, so DKA is not very common but if it occurs it poses a significant diagnostic and therapeutic challenge to the treatment team. Advanced CKD patients may have metabolic acidosis that may pose diagnostic challenges. They may not have osmotic diuresis due to hyperglycemia since they are oliguric or anuric. So, they may not be dehydrated but still may have ketosis and hyperglycemia. It will be difficult to titrate fluids in patients on dialysis and they will be at risk of hypoglycemia (long half-life of insulin, removal of glucose during dialysis). So, such patients may not need much hydration and if required should be infused in small-volume aliquots (250 mL). Considering these it is suggested to start with a lower rate of insulin (0.05 U/kg/h) and watch for glucose reduction.[4] Also, the electrolyte should be monitored closely since dialysis may alter the electrolyte dynamics.

The patients with pregnancy are usually young and many have type 1 diabetes. DKA in pregnancy is a medical emergency where the risk of fetal mortality and complications is very high.[68] The common presentation may be abdominal pain, nausea, vomiting, and tiredness that may be mistaken as labor pain or pregnancy-related diseases, e.g., pregnancy-induced hypertension. It is important to keep sugars under control and reverse acidosis to prevent complications to the fetus as well. The common precipitating factors identified are infection, vomiting, steroid treatment, or medication errors.[68] Severe dehydration may further increase the risk of venous thrombosis and organ dysfunction.

The majority of the time the patients will have euglycemic DKA with moderate elevation of blood sugars. The principles of DKA management remain the same with due diligence on both mother and fetus monitoring and the involvement of a multidisciplinary team.

SUMMARY

Diabetic ketoacidosis and HHS are severe metabolic complications of diabetes. Absolute or relative insulin deficiency coupled with increased counterregulatory hormones plays major role in pathogenesis. The common derangements are severe dehydration, hyperosmolality, hyperglycemia, ketosis, and electrolyte imbalance of varying severity. DKA can present with varied blood sugars and negative urine ketones, so measuring blood ketones and high index of suspicion in acidotic diabetic patients with normal blood sugar is important. Intravenous fluids and insulin are keys to the treatment of DKA. Blood sugar, sodium, potassium, and ketone levels should be closely monitored, and intravenous insulin infusion should be continued till resolution of DKA/HHS (bicarbonate >15 mmol/L, pH >7.3/ serum osmolality <320, improved sensorium) and patients takes oral diet. Intravenous insulin should be bridged with subcutaneous regimen preferable basal insulin with short-acting insulin or intermediate-acting with regular insulin or if patient was already on insulin, it is better to continue same regimen.

REFERENCES

1. Kitabchi AE, Umpierrez GE, Miles JM, Fisher JN. Hyperglycemic crises in adult patients with diabetes. Diabetes Care. 2009;32(7):1335-43.
2. Dhatariya K, Savage M. (2013). The Management of Diabetic ketoacidosis in adults. Joint British Diabetes Societies Inpatient Care Group, Second edition. [online] Available from: http://www.diabetologists-abcd.org.uk/jbds/jbds_ip_dka_adults_revised.pdf [Last accessed September, 2023].
3. Goguen J, Gilbert J. Hyperglycemic Emergencies in Adults. Can J Diabetes. 2018;42:S109-14.
4. Dhatariya KK; Joint British Diabetes Societies for Inpatient Care. The management of diabetic ketoacidosis in adults-An updated guideline from the Joint British Diabetes Society for Inpatient Care. Diabet Med. 2022;39(6):e14788.
5. Pasquel FJ, Tsegka K, Wang H, Cardona S, Galindo RJ, Fayfman M, et al. Clinical Outcomes in Patients With Isolated or Combined Diabetic Ketoacidosis and Hyperosmolar Hyperglycemic State: A Retrospective, Hospital-Based Cohort Study. Diabetes Care. 2019;43(2):349-57.
6. Singh B, Kaur P, Majachani N, Patel P, Reid RR, Maroules M. COVID-19 and Combined Diabetic Ketoacidosis and Hyperglycemic Hyperosmolar Nonketotic Coma: Report of 11 Cases. J Investig Med High Impact Case Rep. 2021;9: 23247096211021231.
7. Chiasson JL, Aris-Jilwan N, Bélanger R, Bertrand S, Beauregard H, Ékoé JM, et al. Diagnosis and treatment of diabetic ketoacidosis and the hyperglycemic hyperosmolar state. CMAJ. 2003;168(7):859-66.
8. Kitabchi AE, Umpierrez GE, Murphy MB, Barrett EJ, Kreisberg RA, Malone JI, et al. Management of hyperglycemic crises in patients with diabetes. Diabetes Care. 2001;24(1):131-53.
9. Laffel L. Ketone bodies: a review of physiology, pathophysiology and application of monitoring to diabetes. Diabetes Metab Res Rev. 1999;15(6):412-26.
10. Stojanovic V, Ihle S. Role of beta-hydroxybutyric acid in diabetic ketoacidosis: a review. Can Vet J. 2011;52(4):426-30.
11. Stephens JM, Sulway MJ, Watkins PJ. Relationship of blood acetoacetate and 3-hydroxybutyrate in diabetes. Diabetes. 1971;20(7):485-9.
12. Kitabchi AE, Fisher JN, Murphy MB, Rumbak MJ. Diabetic ketoacidosis and the hyperglycemic hyperosmolar nonketotic state. In: Kahn CR, Weir GC, (Eds). Joslin's Diabetes Mellitus 13th edition. Philadelphia: Lea & Febige; 1994. pp. 738-70.
13. Hotamisligil GS, Murray DL, Choy LN, Spiegelman BM. Tumor necrosis factor alpha inhibits signaling from the insulin receptor. Proc Natl Acad Sci U S A. 1994;91(11):4854-8.
14. Feinstein R, Kanety H, Papa MZ, Lunenfeld B, Karasik A. Tumor necrosis factor-alpha suppresses insulin-induced tyrosine phosphorylation of insulin receptor and its substrates. J Biol Chem. 1993;268(35):26055-8.
15. Munro JF, Campbell IW, McCuish AC, Duncan LJ. Euglycaemic diabetic ketoacidosis. Br Med J. 1973;2:578-80.
16. Dhatariya KK, Umpierrez GE. Guidelines for management of diabetic ketoacidosis: time to revise? Lancet Diabetes Endocrinol. 2017;5(5):321-3.

17. Rawla P, Vellipuram AR, Bandaru SS, Pradeep Raj J. Euglycemic diabetic ketoacidosis: a diagnostic and therapeutic dilemma. Endocrinol Diabetes Metab Case Rep. 2017;(2017):17-0081.
18. Rosenstock J, Ferrannini E. Euglycemic diabetic ketoacidosis: a predictable, detectable, and preventable safety concern with SGLT2 inhibitors. Diabetes Care. 2015;38(9):1638-42.
19. Kuru B, Sever M, Aksay E, Dogan T, Yalcin N, Seker Eren E, et al. Comparing finger-stick β-hydroxybutyrate with dipstick urine tests in the detection of ketone bodies. Turkiye Acil Tip Dergisi. 2014;14(2):47-52.
20. Umpierrez G, Freire AX. Abdominal pain in patients with hyperglycemic crises. J Crit Care. 2002;17(1):63-7.
21. Umpierrez GE, Smiley D, Kitabchi AE. Ketosis-prone type 2 diabetes mellitus. Ann Intern Med. 2007;144:350-8.
22. Balasubramanyam A, Nalini R, Hampe CS, Maldonado M. Syndromes of ketosis-prone diabetes mellitus. Endocr Rev. 2008;29(3):292-302.
23. Mendez Y, Surani S, Varon J. Diabetic ketoacidosis: Treatment in the intensive care unit or general medical/surgical ward? World J Diabetes. 2017;8(2):40-4.
24. Umpierrez GE, Cuervo R, Karabell A, Latif K, Freire AX, Kitabchi AE. Treatment of diabetic ketoacidosis with subcutaneous insulin aspart. Diabetes Care. 2004;27(8):1873-8.
25. Karoli R, Salman T, Shankar R, Fatima J, Sandhu S. Managing diabetic ketoacidosis in non-intensive care unit setting: Role of insulin analogs. Indian J Pharmacol. 2011;43(4):398-401.
26. Cohn BG, Keim SM, Watkins JW, Camargo CA. Does Management of Diabetic Ketoacidosis with Subcutaneous Rapid-acting Insulin Reduce the Need for Intensive Care Unit Admission? J Emerg Med. 2015;49(4):530-8.
27. Javor KA, Kotsanos JG, McDonald RC, Baron AD, Kesterson JG Tierney WM. Diabetic ketoacidosis charges relative to medical charges of adult patients with type I diabetes. Diabetes Care. 1997;20(3):349-54.
28. May ME, Young C, King J. Resource utilization in treatment of diabetic ketoacidosis in adults. Am J Med Sci. 1993;306(5):287-94.
29. Nyenwe EA, Kitabchi AE. Evidence-based management of hyperglycemic emergencies in diabetes mellitus. Diabetes Res Clin Pract. 2011;94(3):340-51.
30. Van Zyl DG, Rheeder P, Delport E. Fluid management in diabetic-acidosis—Ringer's lactate versus normal saline: a randomized controlled trial. QJM. 2012;105(4):337-43.
31. Chua HR, Venkatesh B, Stachowski E, Schneider AG, Perkins K, Ladanyi S, et al. Plasma-Lyte 148 vs 0.9% saline for fluid resuscitation in diabetic ketoacidosis. J Crit Care. 2012;27(2):138-45.
32. Mahler SA, Conrad SA, Wang H, Arnold TC. Resuscitation with balanced electrolyte solution prevents hyperchloremic metabolic acidosis in patients with. Am J Emerg Med. 2011;29(6):670-4.
33. Ramanan M, Attokaran A, Murray L, Bhadange N, Stewart D, Rajendran G, et al. Sodium chloride or Plasmalyte-148 evaluation in severe diabetic ketoacidosis (SCOPE-DKA): a cluster, crossover, randomized, controlled trial. Intensive Care Med. 2021;47(11):1248-57.
34. Wang L, Byrne DW, Stollings JL, Pharm D, Kumar AB, Hughes CG, et al. Balanced crystalloid versus saline in critically ill adults. J Intensive Care Soc. 2019;20(2):171-3.
35. Self WH, Semler MW, Wanderer JP, Wang L, Byrne DW, Collins SP, et al. Balanced crystalloid versus saline in Noncritically ill adults. N Engl J Med. 2018;378:891-28.
36. Self WH, Evans CS, Jenkins CA, Brown RM, Casey JD, Collins SP, et al. Clinical effects of balanced crystalloids vs saline in adults with diabetic ketoacidosis: a subgroup analysis of cluster randomized clinical trials. JAMA Netw Open. 2020;3(11):e2024596.
37. Kitabchi AE, Ayyagari V, Guerra SM. The efficacy of low-dose versus conventional therapy of insulin for treatment of diabetic ketoacidosis. Ann Intern Med. 1976;84(6):633-8.
38. Kitabchi AE, Young R, Sacks H, Morris L. Diabetic ketoacidosis: reappraisal of therapeutic approach. Annu Rev Med. 1979;30:339-57.
39. Dhatariya KK, Vellanki P. Treatment of diabetic ketoacidosis (DKA)/hyperglycemic hyperosmolar state (HHS): novel advances in the management of hyperglycemic crises (UK Versus USA). Curr Diab Rep. 2017;17(5):33.
40. Ersöz HÖ, Ukinc K, Köse M, Erem C, Gunduz A, Hacihasanoglu AB, et al. Subcutaneous lispro and intravenous regular insulin treatments are equally effective and safe for the treatment of mild and moderate diabetic ketoacidosis in adult patients. Int J Clin Pract. 2006;60(4):429-33.
41. Kitabchi AE, Umpierrez GE, Fisher JN, Murphy MB, Stentz FB. Thirty years of personal experience in hyperglycemic crises: diabetic ketoacidosis and hyperglycemic hyperosmolar state. J Clin Endocrinol Metab. 2008;93(5):1541-52.
42. Fisher JN, Kitabchi AE. A randomized study of phosphate therapy in the treatment of diabetic ketoacidosis. J Clin Endocrinol Metab. 1983;57(1):177-80.
43. Morris LR, Murphy MB, Kitabchi AE. Bicarbonate therapy in severe diabetic ketoacidosis. Ann Intern Med. 1986;105(6):836-40.
44. Latif KA, Freire AX, Kitabchi AE, Umpierrez GE, Qureshi N. The use of alkali therapy in severe diabetic ketoacidosis. Diabetes Care. 2002;25(11):2113-4.
45. Chua H, Schneider A, Bellomo R. Bicarbonate in diabetic ketoacidosis—a systematic review. Ann Intensive Care. 2011;1(1):23.
46. Duhon B, Attridge RL, Franco-Martinez AC, Maxwell PR, Hughes DW. Intravenous Sodium bicarbonate therapy in severely acidotic diabetic ketoacidosis. Ann Pharmacother. 2013;47(7-8):970-5.
47. Klocker AA, Phelan H, Twigg SM, Craig ME. Blood β-hydroxybutyrate vs. urine acetoacetate testing for the prevention and management of ketoacidosis in Type 1 diabetes: a systematic review. Diabet Med. 2013;30(7):818-24.
48. Umpierrez G, Korytkowski M. Diabetic emergencies-ketoacidosis, hyperglycaemic hyperosmolar state and hypoglycaemia. Nat Rev Endocrinol. 2016;12(4):222-32.
49. Kamel KS, Halperin ML. Acid-base problems in diabetic ketoacidosis. N Engl J Med. 2015;372:546-54.
50. Konstantinov NK, Rohrscheib M, Agaba EI, Dorin RI, Murata GH, Tzamaloukas AH. Respiratory failure in diabetic ketoacidosis. World J Diabetes. 2015;6(8):1009-23.

51. Catalano C, Fabbian F, Di Landro D. Acute pulmonary oedema occurring in association with diabetic ketoacidosis in a diabetic patient with chronic renal failure. Nephrol Dial Transplant. 1998;13(2):491-2.
52. Umpierrez GE, Jones S, Smiley D, Mulligan P, Keyler T, Temponi A, et al. Insulin analogs versus human insulin in the treatment of patients with diabetic ketoacidosis: a randomized controlled trial. Diabetes Care. 2009;32(7):1164-9.
53. Hassan IS, Al-Otaibi AD, Al-Bugami MM, Salih S Bin, Saleh Y Al, Abdulaziz S. The impact of a structured clinical pathway on the application of management standards in patients with diabetic ketoacidosis and its acceptability by medical residents. J Diabetes Mellitus. 2014;4:264-72.
54. Ilag LL, Kronick S, Ernst RD, Grondin L, Alaniz C, Liu L, et al. Impact of a critical pathway on inpatient management of diabetic ketoacidosis. Diabetes Res Clin Pract. 2003;62(1):23-32.
55. Tran TTT, Pease A, Wood AJ, Zajac JD, Mårtensson J, Bellomo R, et al. Review of evidence for adult diabetic ketoacidosis management protocols. Front Endocrinol (Lausanne). 2017;8:106.
56. Jervis A, Champion S, Figg G, Langley J, Adams GG. Prevalence of diabetes ketoacidosis rises and still no strict treatment adherence. Curr Diabetes Rev. 2013;9(1):54-61.
57. Van den Berghe G, Wouters P, Weekers F, Verwaest C, Bruyninckx F, Schetz M, et al. Intensive insulin therapy in critically ill patients. N Engl J Med. 2001;345(19):1359-67.
58. Van den Berghe G, Wilmer A, Hermans G, Meersseman W, Wouters PJ, Milants I, et al. Intensive insulin therapy in the medical ICU. N Engl J Med. 2006;354(5):449-61.
59. NICE-SUGAR Study Investigators; Finfer S, Chittock DR, Su SY, Blair D, Foster D, et al. Intensive versus conventional glucose control in critically ill patients. N Engl J Med. 2009;360(13):1283-97.
60. Annane D, Cariou A, Maxime V, Azoulay E, D'honneur G, Timsit JF, et al. Corticosteroid treatment and intensive insulin therapy for septic shock in adults: a randomized controlled trial. JAMA. 2010;303(4):341-8.
61. Kramer AH, Roberts DJ, Zygun DA. Optimal glycemic control in neurocritical care patients: a systematic review and meta-analysis. Crit Care. 2012;16(5):R203.
62. Chatterjee S, Sharma A, Lichstein E, Mukherjee D. Intensive glucose control in diabetics with an acute myocardial infarction does not improve mortality and increases risk of hypoglycemia-a meta-regression analysis. Curr Vasc Pharmacol. 2013;11(1):100-4.
63. Silva-Perez LJ, Benitez-Lopez MA, Varon J, Surani S. Management of critically ill patients with diabetes. World J Diabetes. 2017;8(3):89-96.
64. Yamada T, Shojima N, Noma H, Yamauchi T, Kadowaki T. Glycemic control, mortality, and hypoglycemia in critically ill patients: a systematic review and network meta-analysis of randomized controlled trials. Intensive Care Med. 2017;43(1):1-15.
65. Zhu C, Chen J, Pan J, Qiu Z, Xu T. Therapeutic effect of intensive glycemic control therapy in patients with traumatic brain injury: a systematic review and meta-analysis of randomized controlled trials. Medicine (Baltimore). 2018;97(30):e11671.
66. Professional Practice Committee for the Standards of Medical Care in Diabetes—2016. Diabetes Care. 2016;39(Suppl 1):S107-8.
67. Jacobi J, Bircher N, Krinsley J, Agus M, Braithwaite SS, Deutschman C, et al. Guidelines for the use of an insulin infusion for the management of hyperglycemia in critically ill patients. Crit Care Med. 2012;40(12):3251-76.
68. Diguisto C, Strachan MWJ, Churchill D, Ayman G, Knight M. A study of diabetic ketoacidosis in the pregnant population in the United Kingdom: Investigating the incidence, aetiology, management and outcomes. Diabet Med. 2022;39(4):e14743.

Out-of-Hospital Cardiac Arrest, Brain Death, and Organ Donation

Anand M Tiwari, Kapil Gangadhar Zirpe

CASE STUDY

A 44-year-old man was brought to the casualty following a witnessed cardiac arrest in the street. A bystander had immediately started cardiopulmonary resuscitation (CPR) and called for help. Paramedics arrived after 15 minutes and return of spontaneous circulation (ROSC) was attained after 18 minutes. The patient was shifted to intensive care unit (ICU) for further management. In the ICU, he was brought unconscious, [Glasgow Coma Scale (GCS) 4T (E1M3VT)], pupils were equal and reactive. His heart rate (HR) was 98 beats/min and the blood pressure (BP) was 90/60 mm Hg with 8 μg/h adrenaline. He was being ventilated with an Ambu bag by emergency department team and was maintaining oxygen saturation (SpO$_2$) 98% with 8 L/min O$_2$.

Q1. How will you elicit the cause of cardiac arrest?

This patient has been brought as case of out-of-hospital cardiac arrest (OHCA). As this patient had witnessed cardiac arrest, history from care giver and relatives will give important clues. However, eliciting cause for OHCA is at times difficult and presumed mostly to be of cardiac origin. Among the cardiac causes acute myocardial infarction, lethal arrhythmia without ischemic heart disease (IHD), myocardiopathy, myocarditis, acute heart failure due to valvular disease, pulmonary embolism, and acute aortic dissection are common. A recent study from Japan looked at etiology of OHCA diagnosed via detailed examination including perimortem computed tomography (CT).[1] Sudden cardiac arrest due to noncardiac causes account for 15–25% of these patients.[2] These causes included respiratory causes such as hypoxia due to pneumonia, asthma, and worsening of chronic obstructive pulmonary disease (COPD), neurological emergencies inclusive of cerebral hemorrhage, cerebral infarction, subarachnoid hemorrhage (SAH), and epilepsy. Other causes were organ failures such as liver failure, gastrointestinal bleeding, intra-abdominal bleeding (ectopy), renal failure, septic shock, dehydration and malnutrition, and airway obstruction. Other important conditions included hypoglycemia, hypothermia, ingestion of toxic substances, trauma to neck from hanging, and submersion.

Q2. What are the important points in history and investigations for OHCA patient?

History: Sudden cardiac arrest is often linked to coronary artery disease (CAD) and non-CAD cardiac problems. Therefore, enquiry regarding risk factors such as detailed history of CAD, high BP, cardiac arrest, and/or any other relevant cardiac-related medical history (e.g., congenital heart defects, conduction disorders, cardiac failure, and cardiomyopathy); preexisting in the family members should be delved into. History related to addiction such as smoking and alcohol intake should be probed. Modern lifestyle disorders such as obesity, diabetes, and hypertension should be enquired. The importance of noting down age and sex in the complete history is that higher incidence of sudden cardiac arrest is observed in males and also with increasing age. Use of illegal drugs, such as cocaine or amphetamines should be enquired into. Nutritional imbalance, such as low potassium or magnesium levels can precipitate OHCA.[3]

Investigations: Diagnostic tests are performed depending on the history and the availability of required test in the center treating the patient.[4] Resuscitation and stability during the test are of prime importance. Basic investigations and imaging, such as complete blood count (CBC), arterial blood gas (ABG), serum electrolytes, chest X-ray, 12-lead electrocardiogram (ECG) recording, and two-dimensional (2D) echocardiography should be carried out. Coronary angiography should be performed emergently for OHCA.[5] Ultrasonography of thoracic cavity, abdominal cavity, and neck-chest-abdominal great vessels should be considered.

Q3. How will you prognosticate the case? What are the factors favoring better outcome in patients with sudden cardiac arrest?

Postcardiac arrest prognostication requires integrated approach from data obtained clinically, biochemical investigations, and imaging details.[6] All patients who continue to be comatose state with absent or extensor response to pain after 72 hours of ROSC are likely to have poor prognosis. In all such patients, it is mandatory to exclude confounders such as residual sedation and body temperature. Clinical test bedside which suggest guarded prognosis includes absence of bilateral pupillary light reflex, bilateral absence of the corneal reflex, and witnessed myoclonic jerks. Although bilateral absent pupillary light reflex ≥72 hours from ROSC has high specificity for predicting poor neurological outcome, yet it has limitations of having low sensitivity as it relies on subjective assessment.[7] On the contrary, automated infrared pupillometer provides quantitative pupillary size measurement which is an objective parameter. Bilaterally absent corneal reflex has sensitivity and specificity lower than pupillary light reflex testing. It is also prone to interference from residual effects of sedatives or muscle relaxants. Myoclonus is sudden brief involuntary jerks caused by muscle contraction or inhibition.[7] Presence of myoclonic jerks early (<48 hours); following postanoxic state lasting >30 minutes; indicates poor outcome. It can be used in combination with other predictors. Electroencephalography (EEG) is recommended in patients with myoclonic jerks to rule out Lance–Adams syndrome (which is benign form of postanoxic syndrome). EEG can assess severity of hypoxic–ischemic brain injury (HIBI). However European Resuscitation Council-European Society of Intensive Care Medicine (ERC-ESICM) 2021 guidelines emphasize on multimodal approach for neuroprognostication **(Flowchart 1)**. The updated algorithm can be used bedside for both counseling the patient's relative and guiding the clinician to base therapy on patient's chances of making a neurologically significant recovery.

Take in consideration other associated predictors along with malignant EEG patterns for prognostication of poor neurological outcome; this is due to lack of consistent differentiation of EEG patterns.[8] Amplitude-integrated EEG provides a simplified and suitable method for monitoring EEG. Bispectral index (BIS) is an automated analysis of EEG signal at the bedside. It can be an adjuvant prognostic tool during targeted temperature management (TTM). Generally BIS scores range from 100 (awake patient) to 0 (flat EEG). BIS signal ≤6 predicted a poor neurological outcome in few studies.[9,10] Somatosensory evoked potential (SSEP) is an additional tool to record as it is less affected by sedation. Bilateral absent N20 SSEP is a predictor of poor outcome; however, it is prone to electrical interference. Brain imaging and biochemical enzymes (neuron specific) analysis can be considered in centers where facilities are available. On CT scan of the brain, the main finding of HIBI is cerebral edema and attenuation of gray matter to white matter interface. For attenuation of gray matter and white matter this gray white ratio (GWR) is radiologically sampled at three levels, viz., basal ganglia, central semiovale, and high convexity.[11] There is no consensus on optimal technique and timing of performing GWR and CT scan. However, for predicting poor outcome; GWR measured 24 hours to 7 days after ROSC; had sensitivity of 47.3–65.3%, and specificity was close to 87.9–100%.[12] Current prognostication guidelines suggest performing MRI brain 2–5 days after ROSC. HIBI, which is generally quantified with the help of apparent diffusion coefficient (ADC), appears as hyperintense area

Flowchart 1: Prognostication algorithm ERC/ESICM 2021 guidelines.

Unconscious patient, M ≤3 at ≥72 hours without confounders (1)	
Yes (go to next step)	No → Includes (1)–Major confounders–sedation, neuromuscular blockade, hypothermia, severe hypotension, hypoglycemia, sepsis, metabolic/respiratory derangements

At least 2 of:					
No pupillary and corneal reflexes at ≥72 hours	Status myoclonus ≤72 hours	Highly malignant EEG at ≥24 hours	Diffuse and extensive anoxic injury on brain CT/MRI	NSE 60 µg/L at 48 hours and/or ≤72 hours	Bilateral absent N20 SSEP wave

Yes	No
Poor outcome likely	Observe and reevaluate

(EEG: Electroencephalography; ESICM: European Society of Intensive Care Medicine; ERC: European Resuscitation Council; SSEP: Somatosensory evoked potential)

on diffusion-weighted image (DWI). Occipital cortex, deep gray nuclei, hippocampus, and cerebellum are commonly affected ADC area of brain. Performing these imaging studies however is not always feasible in most of the unstable patients. Imaging studies should be used in conjunction with other predictors and not alone. Biomarkers such as neuron-specific enolase (NSE), S100B, and tau protein are released after neuronal injury. Tau protein is a marker of axonal injury; a threshold of 11.2 ng/L at 72 hours had predictive value of poor outcome with 98% specificity and 66% sensitivity (cerebral performance category—3-4) at 6 months.[13] Biomarker levels are presumed to correlate with extent of HIBI and are unlikely to be affected by sedatives and easy to assess.[14] Recent studies on micro-ribonucleic acid (miRNA) and noninvasive near-infrared spectroscopy (NIRS) are experimental. miRNA is released after global brain ischemia and miRNA crosses the disrupted blood–brain barrier and can be measured in plasma. It looks promising in preliminary studies not only for severity of damage but also neuronal cell function. NIRS which monitors regional oxygen saturation noninvasively; however, further studies are needed to confirm their clinical utility.

Q4. What are the factors favoring better outcome in patients with sudden cardiac arrest?

Early recognition and CPR: ROSC within 8 minutes was associated with up to two times higher survival as compared with no CPR before emergency medical service (EMS) arrival.[6] A recent study from Taiwan looked at factors leading to improved survival in OHCA patients.[15] In this study, initial cardiac rhythm, time to CPR, and defibrillation were important variables apart from patient variables such as age, gender, and comorbidities and hospital variables such as postcardiac arrest care.

Q5. How will you manage this patient in the ICU?

Goals of management in postcardiac arrest patients are to determine and treat cause of cardiac arrest and minimize brain injury.[5] Emergency Cardiovascular Care (ECC) guidelines (2015) recommend emergency coronary angiography in ST-elevation myocardial infarction (STEMI) patients and also in non-STEMI (NSTEMI) ones, but where there is a high clinical suspicion of cardiovascular lesion. Hemodynamic goals for postcardiac arrest patient are to avoid hypotension and target a mean arterial pressure (MAP) >65 mm Hg and systolic blood pressure (SBP) above 90 mm Hg. Normocarbia [end-tidal carbon dioxide ($ETCO_2$) 30-40 mm Hg] or partial pressure of arterial carbon dioxide ($PaCO_2$) 35-45 mm Hg should be targeted unless patient factors prompt individualized treatment. Avoid hyperventilation-induced cerebral vasoconstriction. Hypoxia should be avoided after ROSC, with highest fraction of inspired oxygen (FiO_2) until arterial oxyhemoglobin saturation or partial pressure of arterial oxygen (PaO_2) can be measured. When resources are available try to titrate FiO_2 to achieve SpO_2 >94%. As far as use of titrated and controlled sedation or use of any analgesic in critically ill patients is concerned, the ECC guidelines agree to their use in a setting of hypothermia to suppress shivering or if the patient requires mechanical ventilation. Tight glycemic control may have adverse patient outcomes that may be attributed to hypoglycemic episodes. Role of steroids in postcardiac arrest patients is debatable.

Q6. What is the role of TTM in patients with OHCA?

Targeted temperature management should be considered in all postcardiac arrest patients with ROSC who continue to remain comatose. Earlier it was suggested that target temperature should be around 33°C at least 24 hours. TTM consists of lowering the body temperature with goal of reducing ischemia-mediated and reperfusion-mediated neurological injury. The American Heart Association (AHA) 2020 guidelines recommend TTM for all unresponsive adults post- ROSC: OHCA with any initial rhythm, IHCA with non-shockable or shockable rhythms (class 1 recommendation). To achieve and maintain TTM generally a combination of methods is used like those of surface cooling or core cooling. Simple use of ice packs on the body is used for surface cooling whereas cold saline administered intravenously is one of the methods for core cooling. A recent trial, however, found that there is no additional benefit of lowering the temperature to 33°C as compared to 36°C.[16] In light of current evidence, updated ERC-ESICM guidelines 2021 recommend TTM for all adults who remain unresponsive after ROSC in OHCA or IHCA (with any initial rhythm), duration of TTM (between 32 and 36°C) for at least 24 hours, and avoidance of fever (>37°C) for at least 72 hours after ROSC in patient who remain unconscious.[17] Sedatives and paralytic agents may be required for ensuring comfort and prevent shivering. Rewarm the patient at the rate of 0.25-5°C/hour to avoid hyperthermia. Once normothermia is achieved, sedation and paralytic agents are discontinued to monitor recovery. Still some questions remain unanswered such as what is the best time to initiate TTM in OHCP patients? ERC-ESICM recommends not using intravenous cold fluids prehospital to initiate hypothermia.[17]

Q7. How will you manage hypoxic seizures?

Hypoxic seizures or posthypoxic myoclonus (PHM) is abrupt and irregular contractions of muscles that may be focal or generalized. Hypoxic seizures which start within 24 hours of cardiac arrest have poor prognosis, however, myoclonic jerks in isolation should not be considered for prognostication.[18] This has important clinical implications because an inaccurate prognosis of a poor outcome can result in premature withdrawal of care, whereas an excessively optimistic prediction can lead to futile prolongation of medical treatment.

Multiple large controlled treatment trials are not available for guiding treatment. Following principles should be followed:[19]
- Early identification of patients with nonconvulsive seizures using EEG monitoring
- Supportive care to facilitate adequate perfusion and nutrients to brain.

Hypothermia to reduce cerebral metabolic rate of oxygen ($CMRO_2$):
- Prevent hyperthermia and hypoglycemia
- Antiepileptic agents are usually used and *valproic acid* is the preferred drug [likely mechanism of action of valproic acid is elevation of brain gamma aminobutyric acid (GABA) in synaptic region].

Q8. What is the role of brain imaging and EEG in these patients?

Brain imaging: The commonly performed imaging techniques done are CT scan and MRI.[7]

CT scan: Main finding of HIBI is cerebral edema, attenuation of gray matter to white matter.

MRI brain: It is used for assessing the cause of encephalopathy, severity, and timing. MRI brain with DWIs and spectroscopy is technique of choice. Timing of imaging should be at least 24 hours post-ROSC, full extent of hypoxic–ischemic encephalopathy is rarely evident early. Conventional T1 and T2 typically show abnormality in 2–3 days in T1 and 6–7 days in T2. DWIs show changes 4 days after injury. Pattern of injury seen on MRI correlates with outcome, central pattern involving deep gray nuclei seen are associated with worst outcome. HIBI occurs as hyperintense area on DWI, the changes can be quantified using ADC. Occipital cortex, deep gray nuclei, hippocampus, and cerebellum are commonly affected ADC areas of brain. Limitation of imaging studies is limited feasibility in most unstable patients.

Electroencephalography: It can be used to assess severity of HIBI.

Amplitude-integrated EEG (aEEG-augmented) is obtained from small number of channels, has several advantages such as ease of application and interpretation by bedside nursing staff and physician.

However, the limitation of EEG is lack of consistent classification of different EEG patterns associated with poor neurological outcome. It should not be considered in isolation and the intensivist should consider malignant EEG pattern as adjuvant test with other predictors.

After 5 days there has been no significant improvement in patient condition. His GCS has worsened and remained at E1VTM1 even after stopping sedation for >2 days. His other laboratory parameters are normal.

Q9. How will you diagnose brain death in this case?

The American Academy of Neurology (AAN)[20] defined brain death with three cardinal signs, cessation of function of brain including brainstem, coma or unresponsiveness, and apnea. The diagnosis of brain death is clinical and can be confirmed by apnea testing. Ancillary tests can be considered when the apnea test cannot be completed or is inconclusive.

Four steps for diagnosis of brain death at the bedside by clinician are as follows:[20]

1. *Coma:* Absence of response to noxious stimulus (supraorbital pressure or pressure on the nailbed) with the exception of spinally mediated reflexes.
2. *Brainstem reflexes absent:*

Bilateral pupillary light reflex	Absent
Bilateral corneal reflex	Absent
Oculocephalic reflex/doll's eye movement	Absent
Oculovestibular reflex	Absent
Pharyngeal (gag reflex)	Absent
Laryngeal (cough reflex)	Absent

3. *Apnea test*:
   Prerequisites:
   - Patient should be normothermic (core temperature ≥36.5°C).
   - Patient should be hemodynamically stable (systolic pressure ≥100 mm Hg).
   - Patient should not be under the effects of sedative and paralytic drugs.
   - The ABG shows normal oxygenation (PaO_2 ≥200 mm Hg on FiO_2 1.0) and near normal $PaCO_2$ (35–45 mm Hg).
   - The apnea test should be *conducted twice at interval of 6 hours (as per Indian law)*. The certified team of doctors should document both tests with neurologist and intensivist registered with the state.

   Procedure for conducting the apnea test:
   - Adjust vasopressors to achieve SBP ≥100 mm Hg.
   - Preoxygenate for at least 10 minutes with 100% oxygen, to obtain a PaO_2 >200 mm Hg.
   - Reduce ventilation frequency to 10 breaths per minute to get eucapnia.
   - Reduce positive end-expiratory pressure (PEEP) to 5 cmH_2O (oxygen desaturation with decreasing PEEP suggests difficulty with apnea testing).

- If the SpO_2 remains >95%, obtain a baseline blood gas (PaO_2, $PaCO_2$, pH, bicarbonate, and base excess).
- Disconnect the patient from the ventilator and put him on a T-piece.

Observation and interpretation:
- Preserve oxygenation (e.g., place an insufflation catheter through the endotracheal tube and close to the level of the carina and deliver 100% O_2 at 6 L/min).
- Look closely for respiratory movements for 8-10 minutes. Respiration is defined as abdominal or chest excursions and may include a brief gasp.
- Abort if SBP decreases to <90 mm Hg.
- Abort if the SpO_2 is <85% for >30 seconds. Retry procedure with piece, continuous positive airway pressure (CPAP) 10 cmH_2O, and 100% O_2 12 L/min.
- If no respiratory drive is observed, repeat blood gas (PaO_2, $PaCO_2$, pH, bicarbonate, and base excess) after approximately 8 minutes. If respiratory movements are absent and arterial $PaCO_2$ is ≥60 mm Hg (or 20 mm Hg increase in arterial $PaCO_2$ over the baseline $PaCO_2$), the apnea test result is positive (i.e., supports the clinical diagnosis of brain death). Patient can be declared and documented to be brain dead after second apnea test.
- If the test is inconclusive but the patient is hemodynamically stable during the procedure, it may be repeated for a longer period of time (10-15 minutes) after the patient is again adequately preoxygenated.

4. *Ancillary tests:*[20] These are carried out when there is uncertainty about whether the patient is brain dead on apnea testing or apnea test could not be performed or had to be aborted (for reasons mentioned earlier).

Types of ancillary tests:
- Tests that document cerebral blood flow (CBF):[21]
  - *Digital subtraction angiography (DSA):* Brain death is confirmed by demonstrating the absence of intracerebral filling at the level of the carotid bifurcation or vertebral arteries.
  - *CT angiography:* It is a safer alternative that can accurately document CBF.
  - *Transcranial Doppler:* The presence of diastolic reverberation flow and little or no forward flow is diagnostic.
  - *Tests that evaluate electrical activity of brain:* An isoelectric recording of EEG from 18 channels to 20 channels for 30 minutes is suggestive of brain death (prior to interpretation of the same, hypothermia, or use of sedatives should be excluded).[21]

Limitations: Operator variability and inconsistent availability.

Final word: Interpretation of each test requires expertise. In adults, ancillary tests are not needed for the clinical diagnosis of brain death and cannot replace neurological examination. Rather than ordering ancillary tests, physician may decide not to proceed with declaration of brain death, if clinical findings are uncertain.

The relatives have understood the futility of further treatment and have consented for organ donation.

Q10. How will you manage a potential organ donor?

In management of potential organ donor, focus should switch to maintaining physiological stability and understanding pathophysiology of brain death with reference to organ perfusion and critical care management to retain quality of grafts. Management of potential organ donor can be remembered by the mnemonic *GIFT A LIFE*.

G: General critical care
The potential organ donor is managed in the ICU. Apart from basic facilities of good medical and nursing support, the backbone of managing the potential organ donor requires invasive hemodynamic monitoring. The general critical care management bundle includes the insertion central line, arterial line cannulation with monitoring, nasogastric tube insertion, Foley catheter insertion, maintaining head of bed at 30–40° elevation, side-to-side body positioning, warming blankets to maintain body temperature around 36.5°C, pneumatic compression device to prevent deep vein thrombosis, eye protection, ulcer prophylaxis, and broad-spectrum antibiotics. Additionally, one cannot deny the important aspect of counseling of relatives and support.

I: Investigations
Routine blood investigations to be done includes, complete blood count, blood group typing, serum electrolytes panel with (sodium, potassium, calcium, magnesium, and phosphate), blood glucose, blood urea nitrogen, serum creatinine, liver function test panel (total bilirubin, direct bilirubin, aspartate aminotransferase, alanine transferase, alkaline phosphatase, gamma-glutamyl transferase, serum protein, and albumin), serum amylase, lipase, total cholesterol, triglycerides, uric acid, C-reactive protein, erythrocyte sedimentation rate, procalcitonin, creatinine phosphokinase, CK-MB, and N-terminal prohormone of brain natriuretic peptide (NT-proBNP), troponin I, carcinoembryonic antigen, prostate-specific antigen, CA125, alpha-fetoprotein activated partial thromboplastin time (aPTT), prothrombin time, hemoglobin A1C (HbA1C), urine analysis, and ABG studies. Barring overwhelming sepsis, bacteremia, or fungemia in the donor, there are no absolute contraindications to organ donation. Infections with human immunodeficiency virus (HIV), herpetic

meningoencephalitis, and T-cell leukemia-lymphoma virus also preclude organ donation. CBC, HIV, hepatitis B surface antigen (HBsAg), venereal disease research laboratory (VDRL), cytomegalovirus (CMV), hepatitis C virus (HCV), ECG, and echocardiography are performed. Coronary angiogram may be indicated. Bronchoscopy and bronchoalveolar lavage are carried out, followed by lung recruitment maneuvers. Chest X-ray should be performed after lung recruitment.

F: Fluids/electrolytes/nutrition

Optimum hemodynamic management should target maintaining euvolemia with isotonic crystalloid solution. A balanced crystalloid should be considered when initial sodium level is <150 mEq/L. In cases of hypernatremia with initial sodium level >150 mEq/L, the fluid of choice differs as combination of 5% dextrose along with 0.45% normal saline as to aim normal sodium level. Colloids, such as hydroxyethyl starches, with adverse effect on renal epithelial cell, needs to be avoided. Albumin solutions (4% and 20%) can be used with intention to reduce the amount of volume administrated; however, high content of sodium in albumin-based solution should not be overlooked. Administer maintenance fluids (you can use enteral route to administer plain water in cases of hypernatremia), but avoid positive balance and hypernatremia. Monitor urine output and maintain at 0.5–2.5 mL/kg/h. If urine output is >4 mL/kg/h, consider diagnosis of diabetes insipidus and treat with vasopressin infusion or add desmopressin (DDAVP). Continuing enteral feeding in the potential donors may help in providing beneficial effects for organ function. Maintain feeding or glucose source and insulin infusion (1 unit/h minimum) may be needed to achieve the blood glucose target concentrations between 4 and 8 mmol/L.[22] Correct electrolyte abnormalities, if any.

T: Temperature management

Patient loses temperature control and becomes poikilothermic after brain death. The aim is to keep the core temperature >35°C prior to organ donation. Circulating hot air blankets, warmed intravenous fluids, and adjustments of ambient temperature may be needed to achieve this goal.

A: Anticipate autonomic storm

Brain death is also proposed to induce organ dysfunction via ischemia reperfusion injury, due to vasoconstriction and low flow associated with autonomic storm, followed by vasodilatation and reflow. Recent studies suggest that there is upregulation of inflammatory cytokines, increased expression of cell adhesion molecule/antigen, and widespread microvascular and endothelial changes.[23] Therefore, use of methylprednisolone 15 mg/kg bolus immediately after confirmation of brain death may help.[22]

L: Lung protection

Use "lung protective" ventilation, i.e., use tidal volume 6–8 mL/kg predicted body weight, with optimal PEEP. Maintain tracheal cuff pressure at 25 cmH$_2$O and nurse the organ donor with the head of the bed elevated to reduce the risk of aspiration. Avoid the administration of excessive intravenous fluids. Consider diuretics if there is a marked fluid overload.

I: Inotropes, vasopressors, and cardiovascular system

Optimize fluid balance with the help of dynamic tests for fluid responsiveness. Invasive hemodynamic monitoring to target MAP >65 mm Hg, urine output >1 mL/kg/h, serial lactate measurement along with echocardiographic measurements will help titrate fluid and vasopressor requirement. Norepinephrine is indicated as primary vasopressor of choice for vasodilatory component after judicious correction of hypovolemia. Alternative inotropic agents such as dopamine, dobutamine, or epinephrine can be considered, if primary cardiac dysfunction is evident on assessment with echocardiography. High dose of catecholamines should be avoided to achieve target MAP. Vasopressin 2–4 units/h may be used to decrease the catecholamine requirements in refractory cases. Hormone replacement therapy should be considered as if hemodynamic targets as described earlier are not met and left ventricular ejection fraction remains <45%. Triple therapy with methylprednisolone, vasopressin, and thyroxine is considered in patients particularly when optimal fluid therapy and maximum vasoactive medication fails to correct hemodynamic instability.[23] Recommended dosage of triple hormonal replacement as shown in **Table 1**.

F: Follow rule of 100[24]

Maintain SBP ≥100 mm Hg, urine output ≥100 mL/h, hemoglobin of ≥100 g/L, PaO$_2$ ≥100 mm Hg, and blood sugar targeted at 100% normal.

TABLE 1: Recommended dosage of triple hormonal therapy.

Hormonal therapy	Recommended dosage	Comments
Methylprednisolone	• 15 mg/kg bolus • Alternatively 250 mg bolus and 100 mg/h infusion	• Immediate after diagnosis of brain death and every 24 hour there after • Infusion till organ retrieval
Vasopressin	1 unit bolus followed by 0.5–4 U/h	
• Thyroxine (T4) • T3	• 20 µg bolus followed by 10 µg/h • 4 µg bolus with 3 µg/h	If intravenous not available, alternatively 300 µg (oral tablet thyroxine) through Ryles tubes

E: Endocrine

Diabetes insipidus (DI): The posterior pituitary function is lost early in brain death with occurrence of diabetes insipidus with polyuria and hypernatremia. Arginine vasopressin and DDAVP can be given as replacements. The anterior pituitary functions are preserved for a slightly longer period. Thyroid hormone levels decrease and a state similar to the sick euthyroid state in critical illness can occur.

Hyperglycemia management

Aim to keep euglycemia, i.e., blood sugar level between 120 and 140 mg%. Hyperglycemia worsens with stress, alteration in carbohydrate metabolism, and use of glucose solutions. Hyperglycemia-induced pancreatic cell damage may affect the pancreatic graft and measures aimed at strict euglycemia may minimize this risk. Hyperglycemia can also affect the outcomes after renal transplantation.

REFERENCES

1. Moriwaki Y, Tahara Y, Kosuge T, Suzuki N. Etiology of out-of-hospital cardiac arrest diagnosed via detailed examination including perimortem computed tomography. J Emerg Trauma Shock. 2013;6(2):87-94.
2. Drory Y, Turetz Y, Hiss Y, Lev B, Fisman EZ, Pines A, et al. Sudden unexpected death in person less than 40 year of age. Am J Cardiol. 1991;68(13):1388-92.
3. Mayo Clinic. (2023). Sudden cardiac arrest. [online] Available from: http://www.mayoclinic.org/diseases-conditions/sudden-cardiac arrest/symptoms-causes/syc-20350634?p=1. [Last accessed August, 2023].
4. BMJ Best Practice. (2022). Cardiac Arrest. [online] Available from: https://bestpractice.bmj.com/topics/en-gb/283. [Last accessed August, 2023].
5. Callaway CW, Donnino MW, Fink EL, Geocadin RG, Golan E, Kern KB, et al. Part 8: post–cardiac arrest care: 2015 American Heart Association Guidelines Update for Cardiopulmonary Resuscitation and Emergency Cardiovascular Care. Circulation. 2015;132(18 Suppl 2):S465-82.
6. Hasselqvist I, Riva G, Herlitz J, Rosenqvist M, Hollenberg J, Nordberg P, et al. Early cardiopulmonary resuscitation in out of hospital cardiac arrest. N Engl J Med. 2015;372:2307-15.
7. Sandroni C, D'Arrigo S, Nolan JP. Prognostication after cardiac arrest. Crit Care. 2018;22(1):150.
8. Sandroni C, Cavallaro F, Callaway CW, Sanna T, D'Arrigo S, Kuiper MA, et al. Predictors of poor neurological outcome in adult comatose survivors of cardiac arrest: a systematic review and meta-analysis. Part 1: patients not treated with therapeutic hypothermia. Resuscitation. 2013;84(10):1310-23.
9. Seder DB, Fraser GL, Robbins T, Libby L, Riker RR. The bispectral index and suppression ratio are very early predictors of neurological outcome during therapeutic hypothermia after cardiac arrest. Intensive Care Med. 2010;36(2):281-8.
10. Stammet P, Werer C, Mertens L, Lorang C, Hemmer M. Bispectral index (BIS) helps predicting bad neurological outcome in comatose survivors after cardiac arrest and induced therapeutic hypothermia. Resuscitation. 2009;80(4):437-42.
11. Lee BK, Kim WY, Shin J, Oh JS, Wee JH, Cha KC, et al. Prognostic value of gray matter to white matter ratio in hypoxic and non-hypoxic cardiac arrest with non-cardiac etiology. Am J Emerg Med. 2016;34(8):1583-8.
12. Moseby-Knappe M, Pellis T, Dragancea I, Friberg H, Nielsen N, Horn J, et al. Head computed tomography for prognostication of poor outcome in comatose patients after cardiac arrest and targeted temperature management. Resuscitation. 2017;119:89-94.
13. Mattsson N, Zetterberg H, Nielsen N, Blennow K, Dankiewicz J, Friberg H, et al. Serum tau and neurological outcome in cardiac arrest. Ann Neurol. 2017;82(5):665-75.
14. Stammet P, Dankiewicz J, Nielsen N, Fays F, Collignon O, Hassager C, et al. Protein S100 as outcome predictor after out-of-hospital cardiac arrest and targeted temperature management at 33°C and 36°C. Crit Care. 2017;21(1):153.
15. Lai CY, Lin FH, Chu H, Ku CH, Tsai SH, Chung CH, et al. Survival factors of hospitalized out-of-hospital cardiac arrest patients in Taiwan: A retrospective study. PLoS One. 2018;13(2):e0191954.
16. Nielsen N, Wetterslev J, Cronberg T, Erlinge D, Gasche Y, Hassager C, et al. Targeted temperature management at 33°C versus 36°C after cardiac arrest. N Engl J Med. 2013;369(23):2197-206.
17. Nolan JP, Sandroni C, Böttiger BW, Cariou A, Cronberg T, Friberg H, et al. European resuscitation council and European society of intensive care medicine guidelines 2021: post-resuscitation care. Resuscitation. 2021;161:220-69.
18. Morris HR, Howard RS, Brown P. Early myoclonus status and outcome after cardiorespiratory arrest. J Neurol Neurosurg Psychiatry. 1998;64:267-8.
19. Gupta HV, Caviness JN. Post-hypoxic myoclonus: current concepts, neurophysiology, and treatment. Tremor Other Hyperkinet Mov (NY). 2016;6:409.
20. Wijdicks EF, Varelas PN, Gronseth GS, Greer DM, American Academy of Neurology. Evidence-based guideline update: determining brain death in adults: report of the Quality Standards Subcommittee of the American Academy of Neurology. Neurology. 2010;74(23):1911-8.
21. Kumar L. Brain death and care of organ donor. J Anaesthesiol Clin Pharmacol. 2016;32(2):146-52.
22. Oxford University Press. Summary of the principles of donor management. [online] Available from: https://academic.oup.com/view-large/91172199. [Last accessed August, 2023].
23. Anwar AT, Lee JM. Medical management of brain-dead organ donors. Acute Crit Care. 2019;34(1):14-29.
24. Gelb AW, Robertson KM. Anaesthetic management of the brain dead for organ donation. Can J Anaesth. 1990;37(7):806-12.

CHAPTER 33

End-of-life Care in Intensive Care Unit

Sheila Nainan Myatra, Suhail Sarwar Siddiqui, Naveen Salins

"Dying can be a peaceful event or a great agony when it is inappropriately sustained by life support."

—Roger Bone

CASE STUDY

A 73-year-old male, a known case of chronic obstructive pulmonary disease (COPD), hypertension, obstructive sleep apnea (OSA), coronary artery disease (CAD), and atrial fibrillation on warfarin, is brought to the casualty with complaints of acute loss of consciousness while reading the newspaper at home. On examination, the patient was unconscious, gasping for breath, and the Glasgow Coma Scale (GCS) is E1V1M2. The heart rate (HR) was 50 beats/min, the blood pressure (BP) was 170/100 mm Hg, and the respiratory rate (RR) was 12 breaths/min and irregular. The pupils were bilaterally fixed and dilated. Given the low GCS, the patient was immediately intubated and shifted for computerized tomography (CT) scan of the brain. The CT scan revealed an intracerebral, intraventricular bleed with a midline shift of 8 mm, diffuse cerebral edema, and signs of imminent herniation. The neurosurgeon evaluated the patient and suggested conservative management because of a poor prognosis.

Q1. How will you discuss the prognosis with the relatives?
At this stage, our objective is to thoroughly assess the patient, reach an agreement among the medical team regarding the prognosis and treatment, furnish the family with precise details about the disease, prognosis, and future care plan, and address any questions or worries raised by the family.

Evaluating the case
In the given vignette, the patient has multiple comorbidities and has now presented with intracerebral bleed (possibly secondary to warfarin therapy) with a significant midline shift. His presenting GCS is low, and he has bilateral fixed dilated pupils. Given his clinical findings (bradycardia, hypertension, and bilateral fixed dilated pupils), the patient has raised intracranial pressure with imminent brain herniation. The CT scan of the brain confirms these findings and that the patient is likely to have a poor prognosis. The neurosurgeon has thus ruled out performing surgery as operating on this patient is unlikely to improve his condition or change his outcome. Performing a surgical intervention at this point will constitute a *"potentially inappropriate treatment"* (interventions aimed at a cure that carries far greater possibilities of harm than reasonable possibilities of benefit).[1] A conservative treatment was opted. If the medical management fails, the patient will likely suffer brain herniation.

Consensus
Based on the clinical and imaging results, it appears likely that this patient's prognosis is poor. However, it is important to note that this is not always the case. If there is any doubt about the prognosis, seeking additional opinions from a neurosurgeon or a specialist like a neurologist is recommended. Additional imaging or tests may also be necessary. Before discussing the patient's condition with their family, the intensivist, neurosurgeon, and primary attending physician must agree on the patient's prognosis, management goals, and future care plan.

Process
Remember that you are only disclosing the patient's prognosis to the family at this point and not *making* an end-of-life care (EOLC) decision. The discussion should be made with a family member who is responsible for the patient and to whom all patient-related matters have been communicated since admission. At the time of admission itself, or soon after, the clinicians must ascertain who the decision-maker is. Other family members may join the discussion if desired.

The intensivist, the primary attending physician, and the neurosurgeon should jointly discuss the patient's prognosis with the family, including further management options. If available, any other doctor involved in prognosticating the patient may also be part of the discussion. An honest, accurate, and early disclosure of the patient's prognosis should be made to the family. The family must be aware of the patient's poor prognosis early rather than at the time of making an EOLC discussion. It gives the family time to be better prepared for such a discussion.

The discussion should include providing information about the patient's present condition, prognosis, and further management plan. Concerns and queries of the family should be elicited and addressed at this time. Any conflict related to the prognosis and further management should be addressed and resolved at this point.

Q2. How will you initiate EOLC?
End-of-life care is an approach to a terminally or critically ill patient that shifts care focus to symptom control, comfort, dignity, quality of life, and dying rather than treatments aimed at cure or prolonging life.[1] During EOLC, the physician does not abandon the patient; only the goal shifts from *"cure"* to *"care."* EOLC is a fundamental human right. Everyone has a right to a good, peaceful, and dignified death.[2,3]

To initiate EOLC, two things are essential: First, the acknowledgment of medical futility and second, the recognition that death is approaching. Recognizing "medical futility" is the first step in planning effective EOLC. It should be based on the physician's objective and subjective assessment of the patient's medical condition.[4] The official policy statement of the American Thoracic Society, the American Association for Critical Care Nurses, the American College of Chest Physicians, the European Society for Intensive Care Medicine, and the Society of Critical Care Medicine,[5] regarding responding to requests for potentially inappropriate treatments in an intensive care unit (ICU), encourage the use of the term *"potentially inappropriate"* rather than *"futile"* (to avoid a negative overtone and it is difficult to define) to be used, to describe nonbeneficial or unnecessary treatment, that have greater possibilities of harm than benefit.

Once any member of the treating team has identified medical inappropriateness, it should be reviewed by the other members to achieve consensus about the poor prognosis and initiate an EOLC plan. The intensivist usually helps to coordinate this process. The treating physician should take the lead in addressing the plan to initiate an EOLC discussion. If there is a difference of opinion regarding the patient's prognosis, the EOLC decision should be deferred, and the clinical condition should be reviewed later as the clinical state unfolds. Opinions from experts should be taken as required. Once consensus is achieved among the treating team about the patient's poor prognosis and to initiate an EOLC decision, the family should be communicated. The clinician should communicate the most appropriate treatment plan to the family. The patient's family should be counseled in a compassionate way, that the death is imminent and that any treatment modality, even if available, will not be beneficial at this juncture. If there are family requests for inappropriate treatment that are intractable, further communication is required, which should be managed through conflict resolution. A stepwise approach to the EOLC process is detailed below. In our case, the patient has been intubated and receives mechanical ventilation given a low GCS. The patient has fixed and dilated pupils and has an intracerebral and intraventricular bleed with a significant midline shift and diffuse cerebral edema with impending brain herniation. The neurosurgeon thinks surgery will not benefit the patient, and conservative treatment has been advised. In this setting, the patient will develop complications of raised intracranial pressure and imminent herniation of the brain, leading to the patient's death. The treating team has a consensus regarding the prognosis and further management plan. The poor prognosis has already been explained to the family. The patient has been on a mechanical ventilator, receiving conservative treatment in the ICU for some time with no improvement. Hence, this may be the right time to initiate an EOLC discussion with the family.

In our patient, one might argue why intubation was performed, considering the patient on the presentation showed clinical signs of a poor prognosis, and an EOLC decision was likely. However, these decisions are never to be made in haste. When the patient got admitted, he had a low GCS and an inability to protect his airway, and thus there was a medical indication for intubation. However, on complete objective and subjective assessment of the patient's condition, the chance of reversibility of the illness was found to be practically nil. Further, subjecting such a patient to surgery would only give a false sense of hope to the family and it would not benefit the patient nor is ethically justified. Thus, in this case, though the initial management was done aggressively, considering the poor prognosis, a consensus among the treating team should be achieved to initiate EOLC.

Though presently in India, legal guidelines and provisions regarding issues around EOLC are evolving, we are well within the ethical framework while acting in the best interest of the patients. The four basic fundamental ethical principles of *"autonomy"* (it is the right of an individual to make a free and informed decision), *"beneficence"* (a principle that makes it obligatory on the part of physicians to act in the best interests of patients), *"nonmalfeasance"* (physicians should first do no harm), and *"social justice"* (all people should be treated without prejudice and healthcare resources should be used equitably)[1] should be respected and followed while making an EOLC decision.

Q3. What are the components of EOLC including bereavement care?

The Indian Society of Critical Care Medicine (ISCCM) and the Indian Association of Palliative Care (IAPC) jointly published guidelines for EOLC with an integrated care plan for the dying.[4] They proposed the stepwise EOLC process pathway **(Flowchart 1)**. The steps of this pathway are detailed below.

Step 1

Physician's objective and subjective assessment of medical futility and the dying process: Identifying that the patient has an irreversible condition, despite ongoing optimal treatment, and that the dying process has set in is the first step toward EOLC in ICU. Any doctor may identify it from the treating team. When there is no treatment benefit, continuing therapy only prolongs the suffering and pain and increases the economic burden.[3,4] A reasonably good mortality prediction is required to identify the patients for whom an EOLC discussion can be initiated. However, this is not always easy to identify and often needs experience. In addition, the clinician's judgments may sometimes be influenced by his biases and attitudes toward death. Thus, this needs to be discussed with other team members to reach a consensus on the patient's prognosis.

Step 2

Consensus among all healthcare providers: Once medical futility has been identified, this should be communicated to the treating team members, and discussion should follow to obtain a consensus among all the treating physicians about the poor prognosis of the patient and the need to initiate an EOLC plan. The primary responsibility for initiating an EOLC discussion lies with the patient's attending physician. Suppose there is a difference of opinion among the treating team members regarding the prognosis of the patient, in that case, the decision to initiate an EOLC should be deferred, and the patients should be reviewed again later as the clinical condition unfolds. If required, inputs from various experts should be sought. Achieving consensus is essential as this will prevent conflicting messages communicated to the family regarding the patient's prognosis. A known cause of family dissatisfaction is inconsistency in the information given by the caregivers.[6]

Step 3

Honest, accurate, and early disclosure of the prognosis to the family: The physician has a moral and legal obligation to disclose to the family, with honesty and clarity, the poor prognosis of the patient, the imminence of death, and that further treatment may not be beneficial and the appropriateness of allowing natural death. A surrogate decision-maker should be identified for the patient for regular communication by any member of the treating team, who will, in turn, communicate the discussion with the rest of the family. This could be the spouse, parents, children, siblings, the next of kin who is available, or even a trusted friend. Hierarchy of surrogates as described in the organ transplant act is considered.

Clear, candid communication is a determinant of family satisfaction during EOLC.[7] While "hope" should be respected during such communication, a realistic view should be maintained.[8] Family members' concerns should be addressed practically without making unrealistic promises. The physician should be able to distinguish between the intellectual and emotional components of conversation with

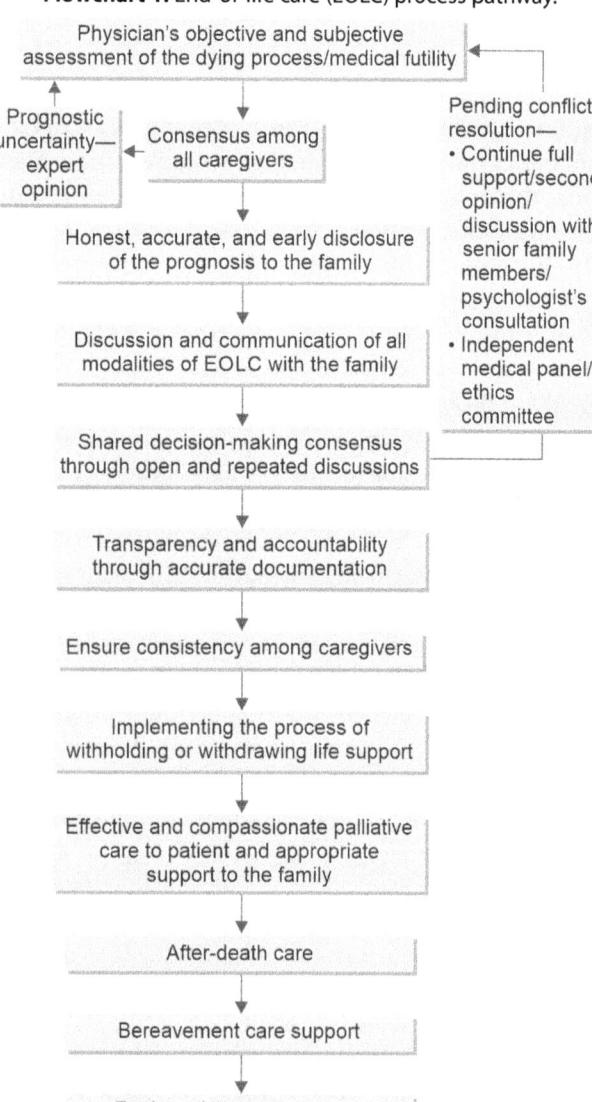

Flowchart 1: End-of-life care (EOLC) process pathway.[4]

the family and respond to them with empathy. The physician should be able to clarify doubts and queries, address concerns. They should spend over 75% of the discussion time listening empathically.[9] Most family members are concerned about common distressing symptoms such as pain, agitation, thirst, and other physical symptoms. The physician should ease their anxiety and reassure them that the patient will always be made comfortable.

Good communication skills include being attentive, following verbal and nonverbal cues, and demonstrating interest using appropriate speech and body language. The physician should be careful not to impose personal biases to influence the family. Effective communication should empower the family to implement what they perceive to be the patient's wishes and lead them to an EOLC plan. Proper communication between the healthcare staff and formulation of care goals help avoid conflicts between the family and healthcare staff. Several approaches have been developed to help clinicians with effective and empathetic communication. These include the "SOLER" model for nonverbal communication, which is a way to physically demonstrate interest and engagement in what a person is saying and "SPIKES," which is a six-step protocol for breaking bad news to cancer patients[10,11] **(Tables 1 and 2)**.

Step 4
Discussion and communication of all modalities of EOLC with the family: Once the family accepts to shift the overall treatment goal to "comfort care only," discussion and communication of the following three standard available options for limiting support should be discussed with the family:[12]

1. *Do not attempt resuscitation:* A decision not to initiate or perform cardiopulmonary resuscitation (CPR) on the background of a terminal illness[1]
2. *Withholding of life-sustaining treatment:* A decision made not to initiate or escalate a life-sustaining treatment in a terminal illness[1]
3. *Withdrawal of life-sustaining treatment:* A decision to cease or remove a life-sustaining intervention in a terminal illness.[1]

Step 5
Shared decision-making—consensus through open and repeated discussions: The physician must respect the choices of the patient expressed directly or through his family and work toward shared decision-making. In the shared decision-making model, the discussions should include discussing the present condition of the patient, the prognosis, a discussion of the patient's values and choices, physician recommendations, and family opinion to work toward joint decision-making for limiting or withdrawing therapy for the patient. This model helps the physician respect the patient's autonomy while acting in the patient's best interest. There are various decision-making models.[13-15] One extreme is the paternalistic approach, where the physician informs the surrogate about the patient's condition but takes responsibility for making the decision. The other extreme is that the patient/family makes the decision together, and the physician only has an facilitatory role. Moreover, worldwide there is a shift toward a shared decision model.

The surrogate should be made free from anxiety and be well informed if they have to function well as a decision-maker for the patient. The surrogate may sometimes lack confidence as a decision-maker, especially if they have not had a prior discussion with the patient about his treatment preferences or has no previous experience as a surrogate.[16] Ample time should be provided, and multiple meetings arranged, if required. Till consensus is achieved, all existing life-supporting interventions should be continued. If the family requests a second opinion, it should be respected.

Pending consensus or if there is a conflict with the family/patient, all existing life-supporting interventions should

TABLE 1: SOLER: The active listening model.[10]

Model initials	Expanded form
S (square)	*Face squarely:* By doing this, it shows you are involved
O (open)	*Keep an open posture:* Keeping an open posture means not crossing arms and legs. Open postures make people feel engaged and welcome
L (lean)	*By leaning forward* when a person is talking to you, it shows that you are involved and listening to what they have to say
E (eye contact)	*Use good eye contact:* Good eye contact shows you are listening and not distracted
R (relax)	It is essential to stay calm and avoid fidgeting when a person is talking to you to show you are focused

TABLE 2: SPIKES: A six-step protocol for delivering bad news to cancer patients.[11]

Step initials	Expanded form
S	*Setting up* the interview
P	Assessing the *patient's perception*
I	Obtaining the patient's *invitation*
K	Giving *knowledge* and information to the patient
E	Addressing the patient's *emotions* with empathic responses
S	*Strategy* and *summary*

continue. The physician is not morally or legally obliged to institute any new therapies that the family demands if it goes against his professional judgment of not being in the best interest of the patients. Conflicts may be resolved through repeated meetings, better communications, taking a second opinion, involving a psychologist in communication, or seeking help from senior colleagues, in or outside the hospital. If required, a medical panel or ethics committee guidance may be sought to mitigate conflict.

Step 6
Transparency and accountability through accurate documentation: There should be honest documentation of the discussion with the family and the accepted care plan. Documentation implies transparency, clarity, and proof of an evolving decision-making process, suggesting that the physician has taken appropriate care. Such documentation could be helpful to the physician to demonstrate his bona fide intent in case of any litigation. It also avoids any confusion among the caregivers about the care plan, thus avoiding unnecessary drug administration or therapy. The bedside nurse should be aware of the documented care plan.

Step 7
Ensure consistency among caregivers regarding care goals: Once an EOLC plan has been made for the patient, all the disease-directed treatment is stopped, and comfort care is instituted. Every member of the treating team and the healthcare personnel caring for the patient should be aware of the goals of care. They should ensure that any visiting physician or therapist attending to the patient or family member is made aware of the goals of therapy. It can avoid unnecessary consults, investigations, or medications being administered to the patients, thus avoiding trauma to the family.

Step 8
Implementing the process of withholding or withdrawing life support: Once a shared decision has been made for EOLC with the family and documented, withholding or withdrawing of life support can be initiated according to the plan. The goal now shifts from "cure" to "comfort." The objective is to give the patient a right to have a life free from the pain, distress, and agony of a prolonged dying process.

Before implementing EOLC, it is essential to prepare the healthcare providers, the family members, and the patient's environment. The standard life-prolonging therapies and artificial organ supports such as mechanical ventilation, vasopressors or renal replacement therapy, and other disease-directed therapies and investigations should be withdrawn or limited according to the EOLC plan. If the patient/family desires, the patient may be shifted to the ward or home if feasible, where the palliative care team can pay home visits and teach the family to take care of the patient's common symptoms if required. In the wards or the ICU, if possible, an isolated area, which will be more comfortable for patients and families for free visitation and privacy, may be provided. The patient should be kept comfortable, and unnecessary monitoring devices and tests should be stopped. It is essential to ensure that the patient is calm and pain-free before implementing a withholding or withdrawing therapy care plan.

Step 9
Effective and compassionate palliative care to the patient and appropriate support to the family: The provision of compassionate care at EOL is not only about merely controlling pain and physical symptom but also respecting the patient's and family's choices and providing emotional, psychological, and spiritual support. Any request for a preferred place of care should be respected and facilitated, if possible. Adequate sedation and analgesia should be provided to patients to ensure that they are pain-free and always comfortable. Therapies should focus on symptom control, such as dyspnea, delirium, and respiratory secretions. Care protocols and medication charts should be reviewed, and unnecessary medications should be stopped. The family should be counseled regarding the comfort care for their loved one.

Family requests for religious and cultural rituals should be honored whenever feasible. There should be a relaxation in the visitation policy for the family members. The family should feel satisfied, involved, supported, and empowered during the entire period. They should be counseled and prepared to accept that their loved one is dying and be willing to provide EOLC.[17,18] There should be continued communication throughout the process.

Step 10
After-death care: As emphasized in American Thoracic Society guidelines,[19] palliative care does not end with the patient's life but continues beyond it to support the family in grief. It seems prudent to be aware of the major religion's rituals. However, in today's multicultural society, it seems complicated, and family members should be sought where applicable.[9]

After death, the body should be laid in a culturally appropriate manner, and logistic support should be provided to avoid delays in the transfer of the deceased person in a dignified manner. Death certificates and other relevant documents should be provided to the family on a priority basis to avoid delay.[20] Any assistance in transporting the deceased person's body and funeral rituals may be arranged if needed.

Step 11

Bereavement care support: Bereavement care and family support should be initiated even before the patient's death. A family member at high risk of grief should be identified and prepared to cope with the loss, utilizing multiprofessional care provided by a team of medical social workers, a psychiatrist, and a clinical psychologist. Bereavement care support system should play an essential role in counseling-based and/or pharmacological management of those bereaved relatives.[21]

Step 12

Review of care process: A review of the care process is essential and akin to a quality assurance audit. The feedback from the family and healthcare providers is reviewed for improvement in all aspects of the EOLC process.

REFERENCES

1. Salins N, Gursahani R, Mathur R, Iyer S, Macaden S, Simha N, et al. Definition of terms used in limitation of treatment and providing palliative care at the end of life: the Indian Council of Medical Research Commission Report. Indian J Crit Care Med. 2018;22:249-62.
2. Welie JVM, Have HAT. The ethics of forgoing life-sustaining treatment: theoretical considerations and clinical decision making. Multidiscip Respir Med. 2014;9(1):14.
3. Cook D, Rocker G. Dying with dignity in the intensive care unit. N Engl J Med. 2014;370:2506-14.
4. Myatra SN, Salins N, Iyer S, Macaden SC, Divatia JV, Muckaden M, et al. End-of-life care policy: an integrated care plan for the dying: a joint position statement of the Indian Society of Critical Care Medicine (ISCCM) and the Indian Association of Palliative Care (IAPC). Ind J Crit Care Med. 2014;18(9):615-35.
5. Bosslet GT, Pope TM, Rubenfeld GD, Lo B, Truog RD, Rushton CH, et al. An official ATS/AACN/ACCP/ESICM/SCCM policy statement: responding to requests for potentially inappropriate treatments in intensive care units. Am J Respir Crit Care Med. 2015;191:1318-30.
6. Azoulay E, Pochard F, Kentish-Barnes N, Chevret S, Aboab J, Adrie C, et al. Risk of post-traumatic stress symptoms in family members of intensive care unit patients. Am J Respir Crit Care Med. 2005;171:987-94.
7. Heyland DK, Rocker GM, Dodek PM, Kutsogiannis DJ, Konopad E, Cook DJ, et al. Family satisfaction with care in the intensive care unit: results of a multiple center study. Crit Care Med. 2002;30:1413-8.
8. Simpson C. When hope makes us vulnerable: a discussion of patient-healthcare provider interactions in the context of hope. Bioethics. 2004;18(5):428-47.
9. Halpern J. Empathy and patient-physician conflicts. J Gen Intern Med. 2007;22:696-700.
10. Back A, Arnold R, Tulsky J. Mastering Communication with Seriously Ill Patients: Balancing Honesty with Empathy and Hope. Cambridge: Cambridge University Press; 2009.
11. Baile WF, Buckman R, Lenzi R, Glober G, Beale EA, Kudelka AP. SPIKES-A six-step protocol for delivering bad news: application to the patient with cancer. Oncologist. 2000;5(4):302-11.
12. Prendergast TJ, Claessens MT, Luce JM. A national survey of end-of-life care for critically ill patients. Am J Respir Crit Care Med. 1998;158:1163-7.
13. Carlet J, Thijs LG, Antonelli M, Cassell J, Cox P, Hill N, et al. Challenges in end-of-life care in the ICU. Statement of the 5th International Consensus Conference in Critical Care: Brussels, Belgium, April 2003. Intensive Care Med. 2004;30:770-84.
14. Crippen DW, Kilcullen JK, Kelly DF (Eds). Three Patients: International Perspective on Intensive Care at the End of Life. USA: Kluwer Academic Publishers; 2002.
15. Levy MM. Shared decision-making in the ICU: entering a new era. Crit Care Med. 2004;32:1966-8.
16. Majesko A, Hong SY, Weissfeld L, White DB. Identifying family members who may struggle in the role of surrogate decision maker. Crit Care Med. 2012;40:2281-6.
17. Sawkins N, Bawn R. The gold standards framework competency document. End Life Care. 2010;4:58-9.
18. Chan R, Webster J. End-of-life care pathways for improving outcomes in caring for the dying. Cochrane Database Syst Rev. 2010;(1):CD008006.
19. Lanken PN, Terry PB, Delisser HM, Fahy BF, Hansen-Flaschen J, Heffner JE, et al. An official American Thoracic Society clinical policy statement: palliative care for patients with respiratory diseases and critical illnesses. Am J Respir Crit Care Med. 2008;177(8):912-27.
20. Olausson J, Ferrell BR. Care of the body after death. Clin J Oncol Nurs. 2013;17(6):647-51.
21. Forte AL, Hill M, Pazder R, Feudtner C. Bereavement care interventions: a systematic review. BMC Palliat Care. 2004;3(1):3.

CHAPTER 34

Tips and Tricks for the Table Viva Voce

Khalid Ismail Khatib, Subhal Bhalchandra Dixit, Rahul Anil Pandit, Atul Prabhakar Kulkarni

INTRODUCTION

Please remember at the outset, there are no shortcuts to success, only hard work can get you through the examination.

There is a trick to make it easier for yourself during the examination, but it may boomerang! You can try to lead the examination in a very subtle manner, in the direction of your choice. But this is an art, since the examiners are not fools and may see through your subterfuge. Like I say all the time (My hairs have not grayed because of sunlight).

DURING THE TRAINING PERIOD

- Study regularly and diligently all through the training period. Keep aside some time (1 hour or half an hour) every day when you can read about the cases seen/clinical problems faced on that day.
- Take a look at the syllabus and the competency skills required. Try to achieve all the skills which are required. If it is not possible to achieve them at your institute, discuss with your teacher and find a way to learn those skills (attending workshops/simulation courses, etc.).
- Have a positive attitude toward learning. Do not think of it as a chore or something of a burden. Try to enjoy your time during the training period in learning new things (this pertains to only critical care medicine; other things you try to do at your own risk).

FEW DAYS PRIOR TO THE EXAMINATION

- Know the location of the examination (in which hospital or in which hall). If required, confirm it from your colleagues/seniors/administrators. If the examination is in another city, arrange for confirmed transportation/place to stay, and reach there at least a day in advance.
- Keep all the required documents for the examination together in one bag (hall ticket, ID card, etc.). Also keep ready a clean and professional dress and an apron (if required). One must not search for these items on the morning of the day of examination, as it may lead to anxiety and panic.
- Practice your speaking skills. It may be done either in front of your friends/colleagues or in front of the mirror.
- Stay calm and control your anxiety. This may be done either by meditation/breathing exercises, talking to friends, reading newspapers, watching television, or anything that works for you. The examination is in a few days and no amount of anxiety will bring the examination quicker or earlier.
- Revise the common topics and the common questions which may be asked. The examiner may ask you anything, but generally it is the common things which are asked first. Once you answer the common things, the examiner will ask you in depth about the topic.
- Know the pattern of the examination [how many cases/which tables are there for objective structured clinical examinations (OSCEs), etc.]. Prepare accordingly.

ON THE MORNING OF THE EXAMINATION

- Get up nice and early so as to reach the venue of the examination well in time. Keep some margin of time for unforeseen circumstances.
- Be properly dressed and groomed. Take along the bag, which was prepared in advance.
- Do not get worked up and nervous.
- You have prepared for this day for a long time and you have the knowledge required to pass the examination. It is just a matter of presenting it properly.

- Keep a positive and confident attitude. The examiners sympathize and empathize with you and your situation. They are not your enemies.
- Do not be in a hurry to answer the questions posed to you. Even if you know the answer, think about it for a second and then answer in a calm and composed manner. Do not get excited and be overconfident.
- If the examiner criticizes you or you do not know the answer to some questions, do not get anxious/angry/flustered. Stay calm and move on to the next question.
- If given a choice to talk about your favorite topic, always take it and discuss the topic which you have prepared well. The examiners are interested in knowing what you know and what you do not know.
- *About last minute revision*: Some people like to read till it is the time to enter the examination hall, while others like to stop well before that. Do what works best for you. There is no right or wrong choice or preference in this.

Finally, all the best to you and we hope you enjoy yourselves.

Index

Page numbers followed by *b* refer to box, *f* refer to figure, *fc* refer to flowchart, and *t* refer to table.

A

Abbreviated injury scale 218
Abruptio placenta 238
Abscess
    annular 244
    perivalvular 248
    splenic 249
Absolute neutrophil count 317, 319
Acetaminophen 278
Acetylcholine 130*f*
Acetylcholinesterase 284
Acetyl-CoA carboxylase 356
Acid-base abnormalities 30
Acidemia 43
Acidosis 110, 225, 299, 347, 355, 356, 360
Acinetobacter 33
Acquired immunodeficiency
        syndrome 266, 308
Actinomyces 19
Activated charcoal 280, 280*b*
    role of 283
Activated partial thromboplastin time 78, 146, 234,
        236, 239, 371
Active cells, metabolically 310
Acute coronary syndrome 141, 330
    clinical features of 141
Acute ischemic stroke 174, 180, 182
    management of 181
Acute kidney injury 111, 127*t*, 235, 289, 307, 344, 345
    causes of 310*t*
    classification of 289
    network 289
        score 125
    sepsis-associated 125, 126*fc*
Acute liver failure 339, 345, 348, 349*t*
    classification of 339*t*
    etiology of 345*t*
Acute respiratory distress syndrome 30, 33, 35, 41,
        42, 54, 70, 86, 87, 87*t*, 90*t*, 91*t*, 98*t*, 103,
        110, 122, 221, 230, 309, 362
    Berlin definition of 89*t*
    management of 93*b*
Acute spinal cord compression syndrome 324
Acyclovir 198, 201
Adaptive support ventilation 26
Adenosine
    deaminase activity 14
    triphosphate depletion 224
Adenovirus 197, 330
Adrenal diseases 262
Adrenal insufficiency 255, 262, 270
    acute 30
    secondary 262
Adrenaline 62
Adrenocorticotropic hormone 130*f*
    secretion 126
Adult T-cell lymphoma 314
Advanced cardiac life support 65, 216*b*, 227, 277
Advanced glycosylation end-product 87
Advanced trauma life support protocols 216

Aerosol delivery devices 52
Aerosol therapy 52
Aggressive bronchodilator therapy 67
Air bronchogram 91*f*
Airway 1, 2, 4, 197, 216, 217*t*, 324, 332
    bifurcation of 101
    management of 34, 147
    obstruction 282*t*
    pressure release ventilation 102
Akin criteria 289*t*
Alanine aminotransferase 112, 150
Albumin
    bound toxins 350, 351
    dialysis, single-pass 351
    use of 344
Alcohol 278, 354
    abuse, excessive 189
Alkalinization 285, 286
Allergy 198
Allopurinol 312
Alpha1 antitrypsin deficiency 44
Alteplase 180
Alternaria 317
Alveolar interstitial syndrome 91*f*
Alzheimer's disease 37
Amaurosis fugax 179
American Academy of Neurology 370
American Association for Study of Liver Diseases 339
American College of Obstetricians and Gynecologists
    Classification of Hypertensive Disorders
        of Pregnancy 146
American European Consensus Conference 88, 89, 89*t*
American Gastroenterological
    Association 341
American Heart Association 181, 193*fc*, 194*fc*, 369
American Stroke Association 165, 193*fc*, 194*fc*
    Guidelines 181
American Thoracic Society 10, 15
Aminoglycoside 133, 247
Aminopenicillins 133
Ammonia monitoring 346
Ammonium 356
    ions 346
Amnesia, post-traumatic 212
Amoxicillin 198, 317, 320
Amphetamines 278
Ampicillin 198, 247, 320
    sodium 247
Amplitude, maximum 304
Analgesia 5
Anaphylaxis 60
Ancillary support 281
Ancillary tests 371
    types of 371
Anemia
    hemolytic 30, 149
    severe 110
Aneurysm
    cerebral 163
    rupture of 152
Angiodysplasia 295, 298

Angioedema 184
Angiopoietin 122
Angiotensin receptor blockers 48
Anion gap 279*t*
Ankle dorsiflexors 36
Anterior cerebral artery territory, infarcts of 179
Anterior hemisphere 177*f*
Anti-B-cell therapy 275
Antibiotic 16, 17, 31, 245, 336
    administration 41
    choice of 18, 246
    exposure 31
    intraventricular 200
    resistance, risk of 56
    role of 335, 336
    selection of 32*fc*
    therapy 14, 246
        minimum duration of 199
    treatment 16
Antibody 112, 201
Anticholinergic agent 283
Anticipate autonomic storm 372
Anticoagulant therapy, principles of 145
Anticoagulation 189
Anticomplement therapy 275
Anticonvulsant 280
Antidepressants, tricyclic 279, 280
Antidote 284
Antiepileptics 148
Antifibrinolytic therapy 165
    administration of 165
Antifungal prophylaxis 316
Antifungal therapy 246, 316
    preemptive 317
Antiganglioside antibodies 272
Antigen-antibody tests 318
Antihypertensive therapy 179
Antimalarial drugs 111
Anti-Mannan antibody 318
Antimicrobial peptides 114
Antimicrobial susceptibility test 136
Antimicrobial therapy 247*t*
Antimuscarinic agent, short-acting 61
Anti-neutrophilic drugs 45
Antinuclear antibody 7
Antiphospholipid antibody syndrome 149
Antiplatelet agents 300
    role of 181
Antiplatelet therapy 181
    principles of 144
Antipseudomonal penicillin 33
Anti-pseudomonas aeruginosa 316
Antipsychotic drugs 71
Antiseizure treatment 191
Antisnake venom 235
Anti-tumor necrosis factor 45
Anxiety 47
Aortic aneurysm, abdominal 252
Aortic dissection 143, 252, 252*t*
    classification of 253*t*
    clinical features of 253*t*

detection of 253
presence of 253
signs of 144
symptoms of 144
treatment for 254
Aortic emergencies, acute 252
Aortic regurgitation 330
Aortic syndrome, acute 252
Aortoenteric fistula 296
Apnea test 370
Apolipoprotein 195
Apoptotic pathways 206
Appendicitis 320
Areflexia 273
Arginine vasopressin 257f, 262
Arm drift 175
Arrhythmias 16, 47, 71, 331
    cardiac 148
    risk of 332
Artemether 110
Artemisinin 110
    derivatives 111
Arterial blood 89, 93, 98, 101
    gas 6, 43t, 46, 49, 51, 64, 73, 101, 198, 221, 278, 283, 309, 367
    sample 89
Arterial carbon dioxide, partial pressure of 43, 51, 61, 64, 163f, 216
Arterial occlusions 152
Arterial oxygen, partial pressure of 33, 216, 231, 310, 341, 344, 369
Arterial pulse 210f
Arterial vasodilatation 55
Arterioarterial embolism 179
Arteriovenous malformation 152, 189
Artery
    intracerebral 162
    thrombosis, large 179
Artesunate 110
Arthralgia 6
Artificial liver support
    devices 351, 352t
    systems 350
Ascaris 334
Ascites 297
    development of 340
Aspartate aminotransferase 146, 150
Aspergillus 316, 334
    fumigatus 318
Aspiration
    pneumonitis 7
    signs of 204
Asthma 44, 71, 86
    acute severe 61-62
    exacerbation, classification of 61
    severe 68
    signs of 60
Atherosclerosis 47
Atherosclerotic disease 252
Atherothrombosis
    extracranial 152
    intracranial 152
Atrial fibrillation 43, 374
Atrial natriuretic peptide 18, 257f
Atropine 282, 284
    infusion 283
    psychoses 283
    requirement 284
Augmentin 317
Auscultation 2, 3, 4
Autoimmune
    disorder 150
    encephalitis 202

Automated weaning systems 26
Automatic tube compensation 25
Autonomic dysfunction 47, 274
    signs of 275
Autonomic nervous system
    dysfunction 237
    function 36
Autonomy 375
Auto-positive end-expiratory pressure 63
Autoregulation 158, 159f, 162
    loss of 166
Avibactam 133
Axolemma 272
Azathioprine 334
Azithromycin 115

B

Babinski sign 324
Back pain 250
Bacteremic seeding causing 249
Bacterial infections, secondary 113
Balanced salt solution, use of 359
Balloon pressure 301
Balloon-occluded retrograde transvenous obliteration 302
Balthazar score 335
Barbiturate 162, 278, 281
    coma 212
Barotrauma 96
Basal ganglia hemorrhage, left 189f
Bean syndrome 296
Behçet's disease 252
Benzodiazepines 96, 148, 278, 280
Bereavement care support 379
Best motor response 157
Beta-adrenergic blockade 165, 277
Beta-agonists, short-acting 47, 61
Beta-amyloid protein, deposition of 190
Beta-blockers 72, 191, 253, 280, 281
    nonselective 301-303
Beta-lactam 14, 20, 33, 114, 198
    classification of 132
Bicarbonate 277, 357, 358f, 361
    level, high 48
    loss 362
    lower 91
    therapy 360
Bickerstaff's brainstem encephalitis 272
Bilevel positive airway pressure 6
Bilirubin 351
    raised 149
Bioartificial liver support devices 350t, 351t
Biochemical theory 231
Biotrauma 96
Blatchford score 294, 294t
Bleeding
    gastrointestinal 298t
    lesions, management of 300
    management 229
    severe 298
    time 235
B-lines-alveolar interstitial syndrome 90
Blood
    brain barrier 122, 129, 148, 161, 205, 267
        disruption of 206
    components, management of loss of 299
    consumption, assessment of 221
    culture 11, 244
    eosinophils 44
    glucose 358f
    loss 299
        estimated 215
    oozing of 235

    pressure 41, 101, 146, 147, 283, 289, 293, 330, 334, 367
        control of 147, 165, 191
        systolic 71, 110, 147, 204, 282, 294
    streaked stool 298
    tests 273
    transfusion of 239
    urea nitrogen 10, 43, 198, 234-236, 241
Bloodstream infection 30
    catheter-related 317
Blue rubber bleb nevus syndrome 296
Botulism 271
Brachiocephalic veins 323
Bradyarrhythmias 143
Bradycardia 204, 275
Brain 340, 342
    abscess 174
    cells, swelling of 256
    computed tomography of 177f, 374
    death 367, 370
        diagnosis of 370
    dysfunction 54
    imaging 370
    injury
        early 166
        moderate risk for 205
        primary 205, 206
        secondary 205
    natriuretic peptide 27, 41, 46, 74, 77
        N-terminal prohormone of 371
    parenchymal strain gauge devices 159
    tissue oxygen 216
        monitoring 210
        tension 209
Brainstem
    acute 271
    reflexes 157, 370
    response 156, 157
Branched-chain amino acids 347, 348
Breast, carcinoma of 176f, 177f
Breathing 1, 2, 4, 97, 160, 216, 217, 217t, 324, 332
    management of 147
    work of 29
Breathlessness 252
Broad-spectrum antibiotics 315
Bronchiectasis 44, 86
    acute exacerbation of 7
Bronchitis 7
Bronchoalveolar lavage 11, 31
Bronchogenic lung reduction 56
Bronchoscopy 12
Bronchospasm, persistent 67
Brownian motion 52
Brown-Séquard syndrome 324
B-type natriuretic peptide 90
Budd-Chiari syndrome, acute 348
Bulbar paralysis 237
Bulk flow 101
Bullectomy 56
Bupivacaine 279
Burkholderia pseudomallei 18
Burns, major 143
Burst suppression pattern 202
Butyrylcholinesterase 285

C

Cachexia 37
Caffeine 278
Calcium 356
    blockers 280
    channel
        antagonists 280
        blocker 253, 281, 285, 286

Index

gluconate 312
sign 252
Cameron lesions 296
Campylobacter 273
    infection 276
    jejuni 272
Candida
    albicans 318
    auris 318
    esophagitis 318
    glabrata 318
    infection 318
    krusei 318
    parapsilosis 318
    tropicalis 318
Carbamazepine 280, 281
Carbapenems 33
Carbohydrate, use of 280
Carbon dioxide 91
    generation of 281
    partial pressure of 41, 93, 101, 117, 123*fc*, 204
Carbon monoxide 56, 279, 280
Carboxyhemoglobin 279
Carcinoma, bronchogenic 7
Carcinomatous meningitis 197
Cardiac arrest 148
    causes of 367
    out-of-hospital 367
    situation 78
Cardiac dysfunction 67, 113, 124*fc*, 289
    high risk for 55
    weaning-induced 55
Cardiac failure
    congestive 41, 261
    signs of 90
Cardiac function 26
Cardiac medications 3
Cardiac overload, transfusion-associated 221
Cardiac troponins, level of 47
Cardiobacterium hominis 245, 247, 249
Cardioembolism 152
Cardiomyopathy, sepsis-induced 124*fc*
Cardiopulmonary bypass 224
Cardiothoracic valvular surgery 224
Cardiovascular disease 47
Cardiovascular dysfunction 54, 355
Cardiovascular instability, management of 275
Cardiovascular system 4, 372
Carnitine palmitoyltransferase 356
Carvedilol 303
Cauda equina syndrome 324, 324*f*
Cavities, abdomen 299
Cefazolin 247
Cefepime 33, 247, 316
Cefiderocol 133
Cefotaxime 132
Ceftazidime 33, 133, 316
Ceftriaxone 198, 203, 247
    sodium 247
Cell cycle, dysregulation of 206
Cellular autoregulation, loss of 206
Cellular component 350
Cellulose membranes 317
Centipoise 313
Central cord syndrome 324
Central nervous system 29, 30, 112, 130*f*, 240, 282, 345
Central venous
    catheters 316
    line, prolonged 243
    oxygen saturation 120, 123*fc*, 347
    pressure 3, 207
Cephalosporins 14, 33, 198, 320
    first generation of 132

Cerebellar ataxia 6
Cerebellar hemispheres 178, 190
Cerebral artery, middle 166, 176*f*, 177*f*
Cerebral autoregulation 162
Cerebral blood
    flow 157, 158, 206
        autoregulation of 159*f*
    volume 205
Cerebral edema 361, 362
    formation 148
    pathophysiology of 154
    risk of 256
Cerebral hemispheres, bilateral 156
Cerebral hemorrhage, acute 191
Cerebral hypoperfusion 225
Cerebral infarction 167, 167*b*, 367
Cerebral ischemia, delayed 167, 167*b*
Cerebral microbleeds 185
Cerebral microdialysis 209, 210
Cerebral perfusion pressure 157, 163*f*, 205-207, 211
Cerebral salt wasting 257*f*, 262, 267*t*
Cerebral trauma 225
Cerebral vasospasm 166
    treatment of 168
Cerebral venous
    outflow 207
    sinus thrombosis 189
    thrombosis 146, 152
        management of 153
Cerebrospinal fluid 36, 192, 198, 207, 209, 318
    analysis 146
    drainage 211
    examination 273
    withdrawal 161
Cerebrovascular accident 50, 357
Cervical arteries, dissection of 179
Cervical collar 218
Cervical spine
    clearance 217
    imaging 219*t*
    injury 204
Cesarean section 148
Chandipura encephalitis 201
Chemotherapeutic agents 318
Chemotherapy 310
    drugs 334
    neoadjuvant 176*f*, 177*f*
Chest
    pain 72
    radiograph 7, 10, 22
    wiggle factor 101
    X-ray 13, 46, 101, 317, 324, 367
Chikungunya 272
    encephalitis 201
Chlamydia
    pneumoniae 20
    psittaci 20
Chlamydophila
    pneumoniae 9
    psittaci 9
Chloramphenicol 115
Chlorine 322
Chlorpromazine 279
Chlorpyrifos 282
Cholecystitis 149
    acalculous 30
Cholelithiasis 334
Cholinergic receptor blockers 278
Chronic liver disease 257*f*, 261, 299, 302*t*, 340, 341*t*
    evidence of 297
Chronic obstructive pulmonary disease 7, 8, 26, 35, 41-43, 47, 70, 71, 86, 307, 367, 374

acute exacerbation of 7, 41, 43, 43*t*, 46*t*, 49*fc*, 50, 51*b*, 60
assessment test 48
classification of 48*fc*
Cilastatin 133, 316
Cincinnati stroke scale 175, 189
Circulation 1, 3, 4, 160, 197, 217*t*, 324, 343
Cirrhosis 262, 309
Citrate
    phosphate dextrose 299
    toxicity 221
Citrobacter freundii 133
Clavulanate 317
Clichy-Villejuif criteria 349
Clindamycin 320
Clinical pulmonary infection score 33, 33*t*
Clomipramine 279
Clonidine 278, 285, 286
Clostridium difficile 136, 316, 320
    infection 192
        diagnosis of 120
        pathogenesis of 320
        prevention of 322
        risk factors for 320
        severe 321
        types of 321
Clostridium septicum 319
Clot firmness, maximum 304
Clotting time 235
Cloxacillin 132
Coagulation 343
    abnormalities 149, 235
    disorder, advancement of 131*fc*
    theory 231
Coagulopathy 225
    development of 299
    scoring systems, sepsis-induced 131*t*
    sepsis-induced 131
Cocaine 278
Coccidioides immitis 9
Cognitive behavior therapies 275
Cold fluids, infusion of 299
Colitis
    infectious 320
    ischemic 320
Coma 50, 283
Combination therapy 303
Community-acquired pneumonia 6-8, 10, 15, 31
    management of 8, 13, 17, 18
    severe 243
    treatment of 14, 16, 20
Compartment syndrome 218, 221, 310
    diagnosis of 230
Complete blood count 113, 114, 198, 222, 367
Compound muscle action potential 36, 285
Compression ultrasonography 73
Computed tomography 46, 167, 304, 316, 319, 325, 367
    angiography 177*f*
    contrast-enhanced 324
    high-resolution 7
    pulmonary angiography 73, 75, 77
    thorax 13
Confusion 50, 313
Conjunctival suffusion 109, 113
Consciousness
    altered 179
    course of loss of 156
    impaired 110
    level of 156, 176
    loss of 205
    moderate-to-severe impairment of 198
Continuous positive airway pressure 25, 89
Continuous renal replacement therapy 120, 312, 346

Controlled positive-pressure ventilation 55
Contusion, cortical 212
Conus medullaris 324f
    syndrome 324
Convective gas exchange 101
Conventional coagulation tests 229
Conventional oxygen therapy 8
Cord sign 153
Corneal reflex, bilateral 370
Coronary artery
    disease 298, 367, 374
    spasm 143
    vasculitis 143
Coronary syndrome, acute 141, 330
Cortical venous thrombosis 201
Corticosteroids 36, 350
    administration of 149
    treatment 17, 350
Corticotrophin-releasing hormone 262
Cortisol deficiency 268
Cough 41
    reflex 370
COVID-19 89, 330
Coxiella burnetii 9, 245
Coxsackie 334
    virus 330
Cranial nerve
    dysfunction 237
    palsies 6, 284
Craniectomy, decompressive 212
Crash prognostic model 214
C-reactive protein 31, 45, 46, 119, 122
    high sensitivity 122, 325
Creatine phosphokinase, raised 109
Critical illness
    chronic 37
    myopathy 35, 36
    neuropathy 35, 271
    polyneuropathy 36
Crush injury 229
Cryptococcal antigen test 120
Cryptococcus neoformans 9
Cryptosporidium 334
Cuff leak test 28
Cyanide 279, 280
Cyanotic congenital heart disease 86
Cyclophosphamide 318
Cystitis, uncomplicated 133, 134
Cytarabine 318
Cytomegalovirus 9, 197, 272, 297, 334, 345, 372
    encephalitis 201
Cytopenia 113

D

Damage associated molecular pattern 122, 126
Damage control
    resuscitation 225, 229
    surgery 229
Dapagliflozin 357
Dapsone 280
Daptomycin 247
De novo acute heart failure 330
De Winter's T waves 142
Deafness 313
Death
    cardiac 142
    lethal triad of 224
    neonatal 149
    primary cause of 41
Deep tendon reflexes
    absence of 148
    loss of 148
Deep venous thrombosis 16, 42, 70, 72, 77, 344

Dehydration 262
    signs of 357
Delirium 54
Demeclocycline 269
Dementia 313
Demyelination 274
Dengue 112, 113, 201
    first attack of 112
    pathophysiology of severe 112
    primary 112
    secondary 112
    severe 109, 112, 113
    syndrome 113
Dense triangle sign 153
Dental infections 30
Deoxyhemoglobin 279
Deoxyribonucleic acid metabolism 312*fc*
Desmopressin 268
Dexamethasone 149
Dextrose concentration 362
Diabetes
    insipidus 269, 373
        diagnosis of 372
    mellitus 185, 354
Diabetic ketoacidosis 354-356, 358f, 360, 364
    management of 360t
    treatment of 364
Diaphoresis 27, 141, 252
Diaphragm 54
Diarrhea 6, 19, 262, 362
Diastolic dysfunction 55
Diazepam 148, 285, 286
Dicrotic waves 159
Dieulafoy's lesion 296
Diffuse axonal injury 206
Diffusion-weighted imaging 178, 369
Digestive tract 34
Digital subtraction
    angiography 165, 371
    venography 323
Digoxin 279, 280
    antibody 277
Dilutional coagulopathy 221
Diphenoxylate 278
Disability, long-term 237
Disseminated intravascular coagulation 122, 129, 131, 131t, 241
    evidence of 114
    management of 235
Diuretic therapy 332
Dobutamine 77, 332
Doll's eye movement 370
Dopamine 332
Doppler mitral annulus 27
Doxorubicin 318
Doxycycline 115
Driving pressure 94
Drowsiness 283
Drowsy 117
Dry mucous membranes 357
Duke's criteria 248
    modified 249t
Duodenopathy 295
Dupuytren's contracture 297
Dysarthria 175
Dyselectrolytemia 28, 54, 307, 309
Dyspepsia 47
Dyspnea 6, 41, 43, 56
    acute-onset 70, 70t
    persistent 308

E

Echocardiogram 244
Echocardiography 46, 344

E-cigarette 87
Eclampsia 146, 147, 152
    treatment of 147
Edema 37, 207
    cardiogenic pulmonary 90, 90t
    peripheral 3
Ehlers-Danlos syndrome 252
Eikenella corrodens 245, 247, 249
Electrocardiogram 7, 77, 141f, 234, 236, 241, 367
Electrocardiography 46, 54
Electrocution 143
Electroencephalogram 163f
Electroencephalography 201, 368, 370
Electrolyte 358, 361, 372
    abnormalities 221
    disturbances 54
    imbalance 67
    panel 198
Electromyography 271
Elevated cardiac troponins 143
Emergency
    cardiovascular care 369
    transfusion score 221
Empagliflozin 357
Empirical antibiotic therapy 198, 316
Empty triangle sign 153
Empyema 16
Encephalitis 6, 201
    acute viral 197
Encephalopathy
    hepatic 303, 340, 341, 344, 346, 348
    hypertensive 174
    sepsis-associated 128, 129fc, 130f
End-expiratory lung volumes 43
Endocrine 54, 373
End-organ dysfunction 147
Endoscopic retrograde cholangiopancreatography 336
Endoscopic variceal ligation therapy 293, 303
Endothelin antagonists, role of 170
Endotracheal aspirate 11, 33
Endotracheal tube 26, 29, 30, 160
    blockage 66
    cuff leak 66
    displacement 65
Endovascular therapy 169
Endovascular trauma 229
    options for 229
End-tidal carbon dioxide 369
Enterobacter cloacae complex 133
Enterobacteriaceae 31, 33
Enterovirus 201
Enzyme-linked immunosorbent assay 74, 114
Enzymes, cardiac 230
Eosinopenia 43
Eosinophils 45
Ephedrine 278
Epidural pressure monitor 159
Epilepsy 367
Epinephrine 278
Epstein-Barr virus 197, 272
Erythrocyte sedimentation rate 31, 45, 231, 325
Escherichia coli 31
Esophageal balloon catheter 95
Esophageal varices 302
Esophagitis 295
Ethylene glycol 280, 281
Etomidate 226
European Cooperative Acute Stroke Study-3 Trial 182
European Resuscitation Council 368
European Society of Intensive Care Medicine 368
Ex vivo metabolism 310
Excitotoxicity 205
External ventricular drainage 163f, 193, 194
    system 159

Extracellular fluid 256f, 257, 259
Extracorporeal carbon dioxide removal 98
Extracorporeal life support 67
Extracorporeal liver
    assist device 351
    support 350
        therapies, use of 351
Extracorporeal membrane oxygenation 68, 101, 280
Extrapontine myelinolysis 267
Extrarenal sodium loss 262
Extravascular coagulation cascade 88
Extravascular fluid collection 293
Extubation failure 56t, 286
    high risk for 55
Eye
    movement, conjugate 179
    opening response 157
    response 157

F

Facial
    injury 216
    palsy 176
Falciparum malaria 111
    pathophysiology of severe 110
    severe 110, 111
Fat embolism 87, 230
    syndrome 86, 218, 231, 231t
        pathogenesis of 231t
Fatal arrhythmias 47
Favipiravir 15
Febrile 197
    infection-related epilepsy syndrome 203
    neutropenia 315, 316, 316b, 317fc, 319fc
Febuxostat 312
Feeding 5
Femoral arteries 333
Fentanyl 226
Fetal lung maturity 149
Fetus, delivery of 147, 148
Fever 197, 201
    high-grade 41
    noninfectious causes of 319b
    persistent 113
Fiberoptic bronchoscopy 309
Fibrin degradation product 131
Fibrinogen
    consumption 219
    functional 304
Fibrinolysis 144
Fidaxomicin 321
First aid 239
Fixed rate intravenous insulin infusion 359
Fluid 1, 372
    balance 3
    management of 96, 335
    resuscitation 239, 277, 283, 335
    therapy 110
Fluoroquinolones 14, 320
Focal neurologic deficit, new-onset 201
Food and Drug Administration 127
Forced vital capacity 3, 48
Forrester classification 331
Francisella tularensis 20
Free fatty acid 356
Free oxygen radical injury 205
Fresh frozen plasma 185, 285, 293, 304
Frusemide 290
    stress test 290
Fundo-variceal varices 302
Furosemide 334
Fusarium 317

G

Gag reflex 370
Galactomannan antigen 119
Gamma-aminobutyric acid 278, 370
Gamma-hydroxybutyrate 278
Ganciclovir 201
Gastric
    antral vascular ectasia 296
    balloon 301
    decontamination 280
    distension 66
    lavage, role of 283
    pH 151
    varices 302, 303
Gastrointestinal
    dysfunction 282
    injury, acute 337
    mucosal injury 318
    symptoms 47
    tract 345
Gastropathy 298
Gastrorenal shunts 302
Gemcitabine 318
Gentamicin 247
Giant cell arteritis 252
Giemsa-stained blood smears 109
Glargine 363
Glasgow Coma Scale 3, 27, 156, 157t, 167, 194, 197, 207, 207t, 215, 218, 282, 285, 367, 374
Glasgow-Blatchford score, modified 294
Glomerular filtration rate 356
Glomerulonephritis 6
Gluconeogenesis 355
Glucose 261, 358
    6-phosphate dehydrogenase 111, 312
    control 5
    management 191
Glulisine 363
Glutamate 205
Glycerol phenylbutyrate 348
Glycoprotein, routine administration of 145
Glycopyrrolate 282
Graft-versus-host disease 221
Gram-negative bacteria, multidrug resistance 133t
Granulocyte colony-stimulating factor 319
Guanosine triphosphatases 320
Guillain-Barré syndrome 35, 271-275
    fulminant 237
    prognosis of 275
Gurd's criteria 231
Gynecomastia 297

H

Haemophilus influenzae 9, 31, 45, 197
Hand hygiene 34
Harmless acute pancreatitis score 335
Head injury 216
    moderate 37
    penetrating 212
Headache 6, 190, 313
    asymptomatic 163
    mild 163
    moderate-to-severe 163
Heart
    disease
        ischemic 185, 367
        structural 243
    failure 16, 255, 298, 330, 331
        acute 330
        congestive 7, 33, 185, 244, 249, 262
        signs of 330
        symptoms of 330
    lung interaction 45, 54
    rate 41, 93, 101, 215, 284, 330
Heliox 62, 67
Hematemesis 298
Hematochezia 298
Hematocrit 258
Hematologic dysfunction 307
Hematoma expansion, development of 190
Hematoma
    epidural 206, 213
    extradural 206
    subdural 206, 213
Hematopoietic stem cell transplant 317
Hemiplegia, acute onset of 177f
Hemoadsorption 127
Hemobilia 297
Hemodialysis, intermittent 290
Hemodynamic 332
    alterations 151
    augmentation 168
    criteria 331
    instability 71, 75, 269
    management 125, 212
    parameters 284
Hemoglobin 109, 234, 236, 294, 307, 344
    optimization 169
Hemoglobinuria 110
Hemolysis 146, 235
    elevated liver enzymes, low platelet count 149, 345
    intravascular 235
Hemolytic transfusion reactions 221
Hemolytic uremic syndrome 146, 149
Hemoperfusion 281, 285
    indication for 281b
Hemophagocytic lymphohistiocytosis, secondary 113
Hemoptysis 19, 109
Hemorrhage 181, 201, 293
    abdominal 228
    alveolar 113
    aneurysmal subarachnoid 164fc
    anticoagulation-related 192, 193fc
    cerebral 367
    diffuse subarachnoid 156
    intracranial 207, 345
    intraventricular 149, 206
    radiographic appearance of 184
    retinal 235
    risk of 302, 345
    score, trauma-associated severe 221
    subdural 206
    symptomatic intracerebral 184
Hemorrhagic infarcts 189
Hemosuccus pancreaticus 297
Hemothorax 230
Hepatic disease 294
Hepatic venous pressure gradient 302t
Hepatitis
    A-E viruses 272
    alcohol-associated 343
    B 334
        infection 350
        surface antigen 372
        virus 350
    C virus 372
Hepatorenal syndrome 344
Herniation
    cerebral 204
    syndrome 157
Heroin 278
Herpes simplex virus 197, 297, 334, 345
    encephalitis 201
High peak airway pressure alarm 65fc

High-flow nasal
　cannula 8, 35, 61, 90, 114, 308, 309
　　oxygenation, role of 49
　oxygen 8
High-frequency
　nasal oxygen 89
　oscillatory ventilation 98, 100, 101t
Histoplasma 317
　capsulatum 9
Home oxygen therapy 48
　indication for 48
Homeostasis 257
Horizontal eye movement 176
Hormone replacement therapy 372
Hormone
　antidiuretic 256
　sensitive lipase 356
Human albumin solution 348
Human immunodeficiency virus 8, 20, 197, 201, 297, 334, 371
Human organophosphorus poisoning 286
Hydralazine 147, 165
Hydrocephalus
　acute 207
　management of 170
Hydrocortisone 17
　group 17
Hydrogen
　potential of 216
　sulfide 279
Hydrolyze cefotaxime 132
Hydromorphone 278
Hyperammonemic disorders 346
Hypercalcemia 334
Hypercapnia 48, 67
Hypercarbia 361
Hyperglycemia 36, 355-357, 363, 364, 373
　management 373
Hyperglycemic crisis 357, 361
Hyperinflation, dynamic 43, 64, 65
Hyperkalemia 221, 224
Hyperlactatemia 110
Hyperleukocytosis 307
Hyperlipidemia 260, 334
Hypernatremia 309
Hyperosmolar hyperglycemic state 354, 356
　diagnosis of 355
Hyperosmolar therapy 191
Hyperparasitemia 110
Hyperphosphatemia, management of 312
Hyperreflexia 324
Hypertension 152, 168, 185, 275, 374
　chronic 147
　control of 195
　gestational 147
　intra-abdominal 113, 337
　intracranial 161, 345
　persistent 147, 148
　portal 300
　preexisting 147
　pregnancy-induced 147
　severe 143, 165
　systemic 159
　treatment of 165
Hyperthermia, malignant 30
Hypertonic saline 226
Hyperuricemia 307, 309
　management of 312
Hyperviscosity syndromes 313
Hypocalcemia 202, 221, 360
Hypochondriac pain, right 109
Hypoglycemia 110, 174, 202, 362, 363, 367
　signs of 362

Hypoglycemic episodes 363
Hypokalemia 221, 346, 355, 361, 362
　periodic paralysis 237
Hypomagnesemia 202, 299
Hyponatremia 202, 255, 256, 257, 257f, 260, 261, 264, 265, 267, 268
　acute 255, 265
　　severe 267
　causes of 258, 261
　chronic 256, 263, 267, 268
　chronicity of 265
　classification of 258, 258t
　diagnosis of 259fc
　differential diagnosis of 259
　etiology of 261fc
　hypervolemic 255
　hypotonic 261-263
　hypovolemic 255
　isotonic 260
　management of 263fc, 265, 268, 269t, 270
　nonhypotonic 260, 260t
　pathophysiology of 257f
　severe chronic 268
　symptomatic 255, 263
　translocational
　　hypertonic 260
　　redistributive 260
　treatment of 263
Hypoperfusion
　peripheral 347
　sepsis-induced 117
　severe 143
Hypotension 19, 204, 215, 226, 235, 357
　causes of 227t
　permissive 226
　principle of permissive 226
　refractory 113
Hypothalamic-pituitary-adrenal axis 130f
Hypothermia 221, 225, 299, 367, 370
Hypothyroidism 262, 270
Hypovolemia 255, 268, 309
　mild-to-moderate 298
Hypoxemia 308
　refractory 88, 98
Hypoxia 48, 355
　management of 8
　postintubation 65
　prevention of 8
　severe 143
Hypoxic-ischemic brain injury 368
Hysteria 175

I

Icterus 113
Imipenem 33, 133, 316
Immobilization 36, 71, 239
Immune
　cells 130f
　complex deposition 235
　injury, pathologies of 272
　thrombocytopenic purpura 150
Immunization, role of 22
Immunoglobulin 272, 275
　E 7
　intravenous 275, 321
　M 350
　　detection of 201
Immunomodulation, transfusion-associated 221
Immunosuppressants 334
Immunosuppression
　reduction of 201
　sepsis-induced 130f

Immunotherapy 275, 310
Indian Association of Palliative Care 376
Indian Society of Critical Care Medicine 376
Infections 37, 343
　bacterial 16, 44
　fungal 343
　previous 179
　screen for 274
　systemic 202
　transmission of 221
　uncontrolled 248
　worsening sites of 318
Infectious Diseases Society of America 10, 15, 133t
Infective endocarditis 30, 243, 243b, 244b, 247t, 249, 249t
Infective focus
　signs of 316
　symptoms of 316
Inflammation, internal milieu of 219
Inflammatory bowel disease 320
Inflation, sustained 98
Influenza 9, 14, 16, 272
　virus 9, 56
Infusion therapy, low-dose 235
Inhalational injury 87
Inhaler, metered-dose 53
Injury
　cancer-related 309
　incidence of 227
　severity score 218
　　modified 218
Inotropes 3, 372
Inspiratory positive airway pressure 50
Inspiratory pressure, maximum 30
Inspired oxygen, fraction of 10, 25, 33, 34, 49, 50, 64, 89, 93, 98, 308, 369
Insulin
　dose of 360
　euglycemia 280
　　high-dose 280
　high-dose 277
　infusion 359
　intravenous 362
　regimen 359, 360t
　shorter-acting 359, 363
　subcutaneous 360
Intensive care unit 10, 15, 26, 35, 53t, 54, 62, 87, 119, 122, 136t, 146, 180, 235, 239, 258, 290, 357, 360, 367, 374
　examination of 1
　protocols 75
Intensive insulin therapy 363
Interleukin 122
Intermittent bolus therapy, high-dose 235
Internal carotid artery
　aneurysms 166
　stenosis 179
International normalized ratio 193, 216, 221, 234, 235, 236, 241, 341, 344, 348, 349
International Society on Thrombosis and Hemostasis 129, 131
Intestinal fatty acid binding protein 122
Intestinal leukemic infiltration 318
Intra-abdominal pressure 337
Intra-aortic balloon pump 3, 333
Intracellular fluid 257
Intracerebral hemorrhage 184, 189, 193, 194, 206
　post-thrombolysis 184
　primary 194
　score 194, 194t
Intracranial bleed 235
Intracranial compliance 158
　pathophysiology of 156
　physiology of 157

Intracranial pressure 157, 158f, 160f, 163f, 205, 207, 209t, 210f, 211, 256
    invasive 347
    measurements 211fc
    signs of raised 190
    symptoms of raised 190
    transient increases in 204
    waveform 210f
Intraparenchymal monitor 209
Intravenous calcium channel blockers 191
Intravenous crystalloid fluid 277
Intravenous drug
    abuse 271
    therapy 243
Intraventricular hemorrhage 149, 206
    management of 193, 194fc
Intubation
    drug-assisted 277
    endotracheal 197, 308
Ipsilateral cranial nerve palsy 179
Iron 279, 280
    poisoning 280
Irregular respiration, Cushing triad of 204
Ischemia 54, 201
    localization of 142t
Isophane insulin 354
Isopropanol 281
Isoxsuprine 239

J

Jarisch–Herxheimer-like reaction 114
Jaundice 109, 297, 340
Jugular venous
    blood 210
    oximetry 209, 210
    pressure 3

K

Ketamine 226
    infusion 67
    intravenous 62
Ketanserin 147
Ketoacidosis 354, 357
Ketogenesis 356
Ketolide 20
Ketone formation 356
Ketosis 356
Kidney 340, 342
    disease 290
        chronic 289, 363
        end-stage 289
    injury
        acute 111, 127t, 235, 289, 307, 344, 345
        molecule 127
Klebsiella aerogenes 133
Kussmaul's respiration 357
Kyphoscoliosis 86, 95

L

Labetalol 147, 165, 182, 191, 253
Lactate dehydrogenase 150, 314, 334
Lactic acidosis 224, 299, 345
Lactulose 347
    nonabsorbable disaccharides 348
Lacunar stroke 179
Lance–Adams syndrome 368
Langfitt curve 158, 158f
Laninamivir 15
Laplace's law 332
Large-vessel occlusion 176
Larson score 221

Laryngeal edema 28, 282
Laryngeal muscle dysfunction 286
L-asparaginase 334
Left ventricle 71
Left ventricular
    ejection fraction 330
    end diastolic area 152
    hypertrophy 143
Legionella 197, 334
    urinary antigen test 12
Legionella pneumonia 20
    infection 6
Legionnaire's disease 8, 20
Leptospira 113, 334
Leptospirosis 109
    pathophysiology of severe 114
    severe 109, 113
Lesion, storage 223
Lethal triad 225t
Lethargy 50, 112
Leukemia 313
    acute 313
        lymphoblastic 314
        myeloid 314
    chronic 313
        lymphoid 314
        myeloid 314
Leukoaraiosis 185
Leukocyte 33
    count 234, 236
    failure of 320
Leukostasis treatment 315
Leukotriene inhibitors, intravenous 62
Levetiracetam 148
Levofloxacin 33
Levosalbutamol 47
Life-threatening cardiac arrhythmias, prevention of 312
Limb
    ataxia 176
    temperature of 3
Lindeque's criteria 231
Linezolid 247
Linton–Nachlas tube 300
Lipid peroxidation 205, 224
Lipocalin 127
Lipo-oligosaccharides 272
Lipopolysaccharide 31, 126
Lipoprotein
    high density 122
    low-density 122
Listeria 197
    monocytogenes 198
Lithium 269, 279, 281
    poisoning 280
    toxicity 174
Liver 340
    assist devices 344, 350
    cirrhosis 255
    enlargement 112
    function of 344
    injury, drug-induced 344
    profile 113
    support therapies 350
    transplantation 340, 348t, 349
Liver disease 346
    chronic 257f, 261, 299, 302t, 340, 341t
    end-stage 341, 344, 349, 349t
Liver enzymes 149
    elevated 146
Liver failure 281, 340, 350
    acute 339, 345, 348, 349t
    acute-on-chronic 340, 342t, 344

    chronic 340
    subacute 340
Liver function 114
    test 149t, 278, 331
Lobar territories 190
Lorazepam 148
L-ornithine–L-aspartate 348
Lower limb
    compression ultrasound 74
    ultrasound, role of 74
Lower lobe pneumonia, right 6
Lower respiratory tract sample 12
Low-molecular weight heparin 78, 281
Lumbar puncture 198, 199
Lung 265, 343, 345
    biopsy, open 12
    cancer, small cell 314
    compliance 88
    consolidation 91f
    contusion 87
    examination, ultrasonographic 91f
    scintigraphy 77
    sliding 42
    small cell carcinoma of 265
Lung disease
    chronic obstructive 48
    granulomatous 86
    interstitial 7, 41, 307
Lung function 45
    tests 274
Lung injury
    acute 221
    pressure-mediated 96
    transfusion-associated 230
    transfusion-related acute 87, 299
    ventilator-induced 90
Lung protection 372
    ventilation 92
Lung transplantation 56
    listing for 57
Lyme disease 197
Lymphocytic predominance 14
Lymphoid tissue, mucosa-associated 314
Lymphoma virus 372
Lymphomatous meningitis 197
Lysine analog 223

M

Macrolide 20
Macrophages later 273
Magnesium 285, 356
    intravenous 286
    regimens 148
    role of 170
    sulfate 147, 148
        anticonvulsant mechanism of action of 148
Magnetic resonance imaging 165, 178, 325
Malaria 110, 197
    rapid diagnostic tests in 109
    severe 109-111
Malignancy 71
    hematologic 310, 313
Mallory-Weiss syndrome 296
Malnutrition 36
Mannan antigen 318
Marfan syndrome 179, 252
Marginal ulcers 296
Marshall computed tomography classification 207, 208t
Massive blood
    loss, management of 299
    transfusion
        complications of 221b, 299
        protocol 299

Massive pleural effusion 230
Massive transfusion 219, 220, 221t, 222, 223, 299
    protocol 220, 222fc
    score 221
Mclaughlin score 221
Mean airway pressure 100, 101, 117, 123, 163f, 211, 341, 344, 369
Mean pulmonary artery pressure 71
Mechanical interventions 183
Mechanical tamponade, role of 301
Mechanical thrombectomy 182
Mechanical ventilation 5, 25-28, 51, 62, 67
    failures 27
    invasive 51, 95, 308
    noninvasive 8
Melena 298
Membrane attack complex 273
Meningitis 6, 30, 175, 199, 200, 203
    acute bacterial 199
    bacterial 157, 203
    causes of 197
    community-acquired bacterial 198
    cryptococcal 197
    etiology of 199
    fungal 197
    healthcare-associated 200
Meningococcus 198, 199
Meningoencephalitis 197, 243, 372
    epidemiology of 197
Mental status, altered 43
Meropenem 33, 133, 316
Metabolic abnormalities 202
Metabolic acidosis 125, 346
    hyperchloremic 225
    severe 125
Metabolic alkalosis 347
Metabolic components 309
Metabolic imbalances 358
Methadone 278
Methamphetamine 189
Methanol 280, 281
Methemoglobin 279
Methemoglobinemia 280
Methicillin-resistant *Staphylococcus aureus* 11, 20, 31, 32, 136, 246, 247, 316, 319
Methicillin-sensitive *Staphylococcus aureus* 198, 247
Methylenedioxymethamphetamine 266, 278
Methylprednisolone 17, 28, 372
    treatment 17
Methylxanthines 67
Metronidazole 321, 322, 334
Microangiopathic hemolytic anemia 149
Microangiopathic stroke 179
Microcirculatory dysfunction 166
Micro-ribonucleic acid 369
Midazolam 226
Migraine 175
Migrating pain 253
Miller-Fisher syndrome 272, 273
Miller-Fisher variant 272
Minimally invasive surgery 192, 193
Minnesota tube 300, 301, 301f
Minute ventilation 26
Mississippi triple-class system 150t
Molecular adsorbent recirculating system 351
Monoamine oxidase inhibitors 266
Monro-Kellie
    doctrine 157, 206, 207, 207f
    theory 158
Moraxella catarrhalis 9
Morphine 278
Motor arm 176
Motor axonal neuropathy, acute 271, 274

Motor deficit 163
Motor leg 176
Motor response 156, 157
Mouth, angle of 2
Moxifloxacin 33
Mucosal bleed 112
Mucositis 318
Mucus membrane 313
Mucus metaplasia 44
Multiorgan dysfunction syndrome 16, 36, 224, 346
Multiorgan failure 16
Multiple convulsions 110
Multiple organ dysfunction syndrome 346
Mumps 334
Muscle
    biopsy 36
    injury, development of 28
    pain 109
        severe 113
    problems 35
    spasms 47
    weakness
        generalized 237
        proximal 284
Muscular pain 273
Myalgia 6
Myasthenia gravis 35, 271
Mycobacterium tuberculosis 9, 203
Mycoplasma 197, 273, 334
    infections 18, 272
    pneumoniae infection 6
Myeloma, multiple 313, 314
Myeloperoxidase 122
Myocardial depression 124fc
Myocardial infarction 16, 333
    acute 141, 142
Myocardial injury, acute 141
Myocardial ischemia, symptoms of 142
Myocardial oxygen supply 142
Myocardial trauma 143
Myocardial tumor 143
Myocarditis 113, 143
Myocyte metabolism 280
Myofascial compartment 230
Myopathy 36t

N

N-acetyl cysteine 285, 286, 347
Nadolol 303
Nafcillin 247
Nafithromycin 20
Nasal intermittent positive pressure ventilation 332
Nasal mucosa 8
Nasogastric feed, type of 1
Nasopharynx 345
National Institutes of Health Stroke Scale 176t
National Institutes of Health Stroke Scale Score, interpretation of 176t
Native valve endocarditis, treating 245
Natriuretic peptides 331
Nausea 6, 269, 357, 364
Nebulizer 52
Necrotic collection, acute 336
Necrotizing pneumonia, severe 19
Neoplasm 174
Nephrotic syndrome 262, 309
Nephrotoxicity
    direct 235
    incidence of 246
Nerve conduction 273
Nervous system 130f
Neurocritical Care Society 166

Neuroinflammation, uncontrolled 128
Neuroinvasive disease 271
Neuroleptic malignant syndrome 30
Neurologic leukostasis 315
Neurologic manifestation 256, 313
Neurological dysfunction, rapid-onset 190
Neurological examination 156
Neurological impairments 237
Neurological manifestations 236
Neurological system 3
Neuromuscular blockade 36, 98
    improves 226
Neuromuscular junction involvement 236
Neuromuscular transmission defects 284
Neuromuscular weakness 67
    acute 271
Neuron-specific enolase 122, 369
Neuropathy
    acute motor demyelinating 271
    inflammatory 272
    peripheral 313
Neurotoxic snake bite 237, 238
    complications of 237
    features of 236
    treatment of 237
Neurotoxic venoms 237
Neutropenia 315, 318
    profound 315
    protracted 315
    severe 315
Neutropenic enterocolitis, pathogenesis of 318
Neutrophil gelatinase 127
Neutrophilic infiltration leading 87
Neutrophilic inflammation 45
Nicardipine 182, 191
Nifedipine 147, 239
Nimodipine 147, 168
Nipah virus encephalitis 201
Nitrofurantoin 133
Nitroglycerin 55
Nitroprusside 362
Nocardia 307
Nodal axolemma 272
Nonadrenergic vasoactive drugs 277
Nonaggressive fluid resuscitation 335
Noncardiac condition 331
Noncardiac manifestations 244
Noncompressible veins 42
Noncontact-argon plasma coagulation 301
Noninfectious precipitating factors 343
Noninvasive near-infrared spectroscopy 369
Noninvasive ventilation 8, 35, 45, 49, 50b, 51b, 61, 90, 307, 308t, 332
    failure 50t
        risk factors for 309t
    therapy 50
Nonmalfeasance 375
Nonmalignant causes 323
Non-neurotropic virus 201
Nonpandemic steroid 17
Non-poisonous snake 234t
Non-ST-elevated myocardial infarction 142, 330
Nonsteroidal anti-inflammatory drug 266, 297, 298
Noradrenaline 277
Norepinephrine 278, 347, 372
Nosocomial infection 18
N-terminal pro-brain natriuretic peptide 54, 122, 230
Nuchal rigidity 163
Nucleic acid 11
    amplification test 12, 321
Nutrition 4, 96, 192, 335, 372

O

Obesity 86
Obstruction, intestinal 320
Obstructive airway disease 41
Obstructive hydrocephalus 192
Obstructive shock 227
Obstructive sleep apnea 374
Oculocephalic reflex 370
Oculovestibular reflex 370
Oliguria 215, 290t, 347
Oliguric requiring dialysis 315
Oncologic emergencies 307
Opiate 278
Opioids 280
Optic nerve sheath diameter 160, 209
Oral antibiotics 18
Oral anticoagulant 189
   direct 193
   newer 222
Oral contraceptive pills 71
Oral fidaxomicin 321, 322
Oral glucocorticoids 45
Oral vancomycin 321
Organ donation 367, 372
Organ dysfunction 114
Organ failure 237
   assessment, high sepsis-related 91
   based scores 335
Organocarbamate 286
   compounds 286, 286t
   poisoning 286
Organophosphate 271
   pesticides 278
   poisoning 237
      acute 285t
Organophosphorus 286
   coma, delayed 285
   compound 282, 283, 285, 286t
   effects of 283
   poisoning 271, 280, 282, 282t, 283-286
      acute 282, 283, 284
Orientia tsutsugamushi 115
Orthotopic liver transplantation 348
Oscillating intracardiac mass 244
Oseltamivir 14, 15
   initiation of 14
Osmolal gap 279t
Osmoreceptive neurons 257
Osmotherapy 161, 191
Osmotic
   demyelination syndrome 255, 256f, 266
   diuresis 261, 360
   therapy 211
Otitis 20
Ottawa Subarachnoid Hemorrhage Rule 164b
Oxacillin 132, 247
Oxazolidinones 22
Oxidative stress 356
Oxime 284
   therapy, role of 284
Oxygen 22
   consumption 26
   gradient, alveolar-arterial partial pressure of 86
   partial pressure of 89, 93, 98
   requirement 34
   saturation of peripheral 86, 93
Oxygen saturation 41, 60, 367
   measurement of 210
   monitoring of 45
   peripheral 308, 309
Oxygen therapy 48, 48b, 49fc
   long-term 49
Oxygenation 2, 30, 92
   normal 370
   status 33
Oxyhemoglobin 279
Oxyimino-cephalosporins 132

P

Pacemaker problems 282
Packed cell volume 257f
Packed red blood cells 224t
Pain 269
   abdominal 6, 112, 253, 357, 364
   control, postoperative 152
   epigastric 297
   flank 253
   management 239, 335
Palmar erythema 297
Pancreatic cell damage, hyperglycemia-induced 373
Pancreatitis 30, 336
   acute 334, 335
   causes of 334
   mild 335
   moderately severe 335
   severe 335
      acute 334
Pandysautonomia 272
Panton-valentine leukocidin gene 19
Paracetamol 280
Paradoxical worsening 114
Parapneumonic effusion 14, 16
Parasitic meningitis 197
Parasympathetic nervous system 240
Parathyroid hormone 299
Parenchymal fibrosis 32
Parenchymal lesions 19
Paresthesia 273
Parvovirus B19 330
Pathogen-specific biomarkers 119
Pathologic Q waves, development of 142
Pelvic injuries, severe 229
Penicillin 132, 198
Penicillin-resistant
   meningococcus 198
   pneumococcus 198
Penicillin-sensitive
   meningococcus 198
   pneumococcus 198
Peptic ulcer disease 298
Peramivir 15
Percussion wave 159
Percutaneous coronary intervention 142
Percutaneous dilatational tracheostomy 274
Perfusion pressure, abdominal 337
Pericarditis, acute 143
Periodic paralysis 271
Peripancreatic fluid collection, acute 336
Peripheral capillary oxygen saturation 204, 341
Peritoneal lavage 228
Phagocytic cells engulf 114
Pharyngitis 20
Phenytoin 148, 279
Phosphate 41, 356, 358f
   therapy 360
Physiologic parameters 215
Pinpoint pupils 285
Piperacillin 33, 34, 133, 316, 317
Plasma
   ammonia 346
   cell dyscrasias 313
   exchange 275
   magnesium 148t
Plasmalyte 309

Plasmapheresis 275
   high-volume 351, 352
Plasma-protein concentration 55
Plasmodium falciparum 109
Plateau waves, abnormal 159
Platelet 109
   count 236
   dysfunction 219, 293
   transfusion, role of 192
Pleural effusion 32, 90, 252, 336
Pleural fluid, characteristic of 336
Pleural line, loss of 42
Pleural pressure 95
Pleuritis 13
   signs of 199
Pneumatosis intestinalis 319
Pneumococcal pneumonia 11
Pneumococcus 198, 199
Pneumoconiosis 86
Pneumocystis 307
   jirovecii 9, 317
   pneumonia 119
Pneumonia 13, 19, 20, 28, 30, 32, 41, 54, 66, 86, 230, 265, 293
   atypical 14, 20
   bacterial 16
   community-acquired 6-8, 10, 15, 31
   fungal 13
   necrotizing 16
   nonresponding 13, 18, 19
   nonsevere 15
   prevention of 22
   severe 14, 15
   severity index 9
   slow resolving 19
   suspect 66
   ventilator-associated 274
Pneumonitis, hypersensitivity 7
Pneumothorax 41, 65, 86, 230
Poison 271, 277
   acute 283, 284
   management 277
   reduces gastric motility 284
Poisonous snake 234t
Poliomyelitis 271
Polycythemia 313
Polydipsia 255
   primary 270
Polymerase chain reaction 113, 318
Polymyxin B 127
Polyneuropathy 36t
   acute inflammatory demyelinating 273
Polyradiculoneuropathy, chronic inflammatory demyelinating 273
Polytrauma 207, 215
   injuries 215
Porphyria neuropathy 271
Portacaval shunt surgery 303
Portal hypertension, complications of 295
Positive end-expiratory pressure 2, 25, 34, 44, 51, 64, 78, 89, 92, 93, 98, 99f, 308, 370
   titration 92
Posterior cerebral arterial territory, infarcts of 179
Posterior fossa 177f
   hemorrhage 192
   lesions 176
Postextubation respiratory failure 55
Postictal paresis 175
Postinfluenza pneumonia 16
Postpolypectomy 296
Postrenal causes 310
Post-thrombolysis reperfusion injury 184
Potassium 41, 356, 358f, 361
   correction 360

Povidone iodine, use of 213
Pralidoxime 284
Precipitate ascites 293
Prednisolone 17
Pre-eclampsia 147, 147t, 152
Preexisting organic cardiovascular disease 179
Pregnancy, acute fatty liver of 149
Prerenal causes 310
Prerequisite 311
Pressure time scalar waveforms 95f
Pressure volume loop 94f
Primaquine, single dose of 111
Proadrenomedullin 18, 31
Procalcitonin 18, 31, 45, 122
    role of 18, 45
    use of 31
Procoagulant–anticoagulant misbalance 130
Proinflammatory factors 103
Prophylactic antibiotics 56, 336
Prophylactic antifungal therapy 316
Prophylactic platelet transfusions, role of 113
Prophylaxis 268, 343
    preprimary 302
    primary 302
    secondary 303
Propofol 226
Proportional assist ventilation 26
Propranolol 303
Prosthetic valve 243
    dehiscence of 244, 248
    dysfunction 330
Proteases leads, activation of 206
Protein 337
Prothrombin complex concentrate 193, 223, 304
Prothrombin time 131, 234-236
Proton-pump inhibitor 299
Pseudoephedrine 278
Pseudohyponatremia 260
Pseudomembranous colitis 320
Pseudomonas 33
    aeruginosa 9
Psychiatric illnesses 175
Pulmonary angiography 77
Pulmonary artery
    catheterization, role of 331
    hypertension 86
    occlusion pressure 331
    vasoconstriction 67
    wedge pressure 90
Pulmonary cachexia phenotype 44
Pulmonary capillary wedge pressure 89
Pulmonary contusion 230
Pulmonary edema 27, 32, 41, 55, 60, 86, 110, 230, 248, 362
    acute 7, 332
    cardiogenic 230
    nonhydrostatic 90
    re-expansion 32
    weaning-induced 55
Pulmonary embolism 32, 41, 50, 70, 72, 72fc-74fc, 77, 80t, 81t, 86, 143, 243
    rule-out criteria 73, 73t
    severity index 75
    score 71
    thrombolysis 79, 80
    treatment of 79t
Pulmonary fibrosis 86
Pulmonary function tests 274
Pulmonary hypertension 27, 49, 88
Pulmonary leukostasis 313
Pulmonary necrosis 13
Pulmonary vascular pressure index 90

Pulse
    oximetry 45
    pressure 215
        variation 152
Pulseless electrical activity 51
Pupillary abnormalities 347
Pupillary light reflex, bilateral 370
Pure inodilators 77
Purpura fulminans 130
Pyelonephritis 133, 134
Pylorus cephalad 151

Q

Quadri-Sialosyl groups 272
Quinine 110, 280
Quinolone 20, 22

R

Rabies encephalitis 201
Radiation
    pneumonitis 7
    therapy 323
Radicular pain 273
Radiotherapy 310
Raised intracranial pressure 156
    causes of 158t
    pathophysiology of 156
Rankin scale, modified 166
Ranson's criteria 334
Rapid antigen test 13
Rapid sequence intubation 226t
Rapid shallow breathing index 30
Rasburicase 312
Recombinant tissue
    plasminogen activator 176
    type plasminogen activator 168
Recruitment maneuver 98, 99
Red blood cell 110, 224, 235, 344
Red-cell storage duration study 224
Refractory bronchospasm, management of 67
Refractory intracranial hypertension 212
Refractory status epilepticus 202
    new-onset 203
Relebactam 133
Renal abnormalities 149
Renal biopsy, indication for 291
Renal causes 310
Renal disease 298
Renal dysfunction 27
Renal failure 143, 236, 262, 281, 347, 350, 362
    management of established 312
Renal function 114
    tests 278
Renal hypoperfusion 309
Renal impairment 110, 185
Renal profile 113
Renal replacement therapy 290, 291t, 309, 341, 344, 350
Renal sodium loss 261
Renal tubular cells, destruction of 235
Renin-angiotensin
    aldosterone system 126, 257f, 261
    system 262
Reperfusion injury 87
Reperfusion therapy, acute 181
Rescue therapies 98
Respiration pattern 157
Respiratory acidemia 308
Respiratory components 309
Respiratory distress 2, 27, 50, 110
    signs of 27
    syndrome, incidence of 149
Respiratory emergencies, acute 42fc

Respiratory failure 41, 48b, 49, 71, 283
    acute 41t, 42t, 43, 307, 308t, 309, 309t
    hypoxemic 86
    severity of 283
Respiratory fluoroquinolone 20, 33
Respiratory muscle
    function 238
    weakness 54, 284
Respiratory paralysis 148, 237
    severe 238
Respiratory rate 6, 30, 41, 64, 293, 308, 374
Respiratory syncytial virus 9
Respiratory system 4, 43, 340
    analysis of 2
Restlessness 112
Resuscitation
    cardiopulmonary 78, 277, 367
    fluid 226
    intensity 222
Resuscitative endovascular balloon occlusion 229
Resuscitative thoracotomy 229
Retained illicit drug packets 280
Retroperitoneum 345
Revised trauma score 218
Rhabdomyolysis 218, 235
Rheumatic heart disease 243
Rheumatoid arthritis 313
Ribonucleic acid 122, 201
Rickettsial infection, severe 109
Rickettsial meningitis 197
Rifampicin 115, 203
RIFLE criteria 289t
Right atrium 333
Right bundle-branch block 77, 331
Right ventricular
    dysfunction 45
    failure 88
Ringer's lactate 309, 358
Rockall score 294t
Rocuronium 226
Rotterdam score 208t

S

Salbutamol 47
Salicylates 279, 281
Salivation 284
Salmonella 334
Salt-wasting nephropathy kidney disease 262
Scars 4
Schistosomiasis 197
Schonfeld criteria 231
Sclerosants agent 303
Sclerosis, multiple 174
Scorpion
    anti-venom 241
        role of 241
    bites 234
    sting 240, 241
        complications of 241fc
Scrub typhus
    pathophysiology of severe 115
    severe 115
Sedation 5, 96
Sedative agents 202
Seizure 6, 148, 201, 212, 313
    hypoxic 369
    management of 170
    post-traumatic 212
    prevention of 147
        recurrence of 147, 148
    prophylaxis 199
        routine 212
    treatment of 147, 148

Selective serotonin reuptake inhibitors 266
Sengstaken-Blakemore tube 300, 300f, 301
Sensorium
　altered 6, 197
　poor 355
Sensory 176
　axonal neuropathy 271
　nerve action potential 36
Sepsis 27, 31, 36, 41, 117, 121f, 126, 131fc, 230
　campaign, surviving 117
　signs of 250
Sepsis-induced cardiomyopathy, mechanisms of 124, 124fc
Septal perforation 248
Septic cardiomyopathy 124
Septic shock 117, 120, 122-127, 363
Sequential organ failure assessment 131
Serum
　albumin 14
　biochemistry 46
　creatinine 289, 345
　electrolytes 367
　fibrinogen 222
　galactomannan 317
　glutamic
　　oxaloacetic transaminase 234, 236, 241
　　pyruvic transaminase 234, 236, 241
　lactate 278
　osmolality 256, 258, 260
Serum sodium 256, 359
　concentration 255, 258
　raise 267
　rise, rate of 268
Severe tropical infection, suspected 114
Shallow breathing 282
Shellfish poisoning 271
Shock
　cardiogenic 227, 247, 277, 330-333
　circulatory 118, 130
　distributive 227
　hemorrhagic 215t
　hypovolemic 227
　index 221, 222
　type of 227
Shunt 88
Simple weaning 28, 53
Single donor platelets 192
Sinus
　tachycardia 41, 289
　venous thrombosis 174
Sinusitis 30
Sjögren's syndrome 313
Skin
　changes 20
　turgor 3
Skull fracture, depressed 212
Smear examination, peripheral 110
Snake bite 234, 235
　management of 238
　neuroparalytic 237
Snake envenomations 236, 238
　cardiac effects of 239
Sodium 356, 358f, 361
　balance 360
　bicarbonate
　　role of 125, 291
　　use of 125
　fractional excretion of 127
　nitroprusside 182
Sodium-glucose cotransporter-2 357
Soluble intercellular adhesion molecule 122
Soluble vascular cell adhesion molecule 122
Speech 176

Spherocytosis 313
Sphincterotomy, endoscopic 296
Spider angiomata 297
Spinal cord syndromes 324f
　etiologies of 325t
Spinal epidural hematoma 325
Spinal shock 324
Spirometry classification 47
Spontaneous bleeding 110
Spontaneous breathing 55, 67
　trial 29, 53, 56
Spontaneous intracerebral hemorrhage 189
Spontaneous thrombotic myocardial infarction 142
Spot urine sample 258
Sputum
　culture 11
　eosinophilia 45
Stanford classification 323
Staphylococcal shock syndrome 19
Staphylococcus aureus 6, 9, 246, 248
　community-acquired methicillin-resistant 15, 19
Statins, role of 170
Status epilepticus 197, 201, 202
ST-elevation myocardial infarction 369
Stem cell therapy 344
Stem intubation, right main 65
Sterofundin 309
Steroid 97
　dose 97
　　timing of 97
　effects of 17
　resistance, peripheral 126
　role of 17, 97, 126, 199, 229, 350, 369
Stevens-Johnson syndrome 20
Stool
　occult blood in 298
　toxin test 320
Strain 95
Streptococcus
　pneumoniae 6, 9, 31, 197
　viridans 247
Stress 95
　cardiomyopathy 143
　index 95, 95f
　ulcer prophylaxis 16, 192
Stretch-sensitive receptors 257
Stridor 70
Stroke 16, 143, 179, 182, 201
　acute 178
　　ischemic 174, 180, 182
　hemorrhagic 174, 175, 207
　ischemic 152, 174, 180
　minor 176
　moderate 176
　moderate-to-severe 176
　severe 176
　volume variation 3, 45, 152
Subarachnoid bolt 159, 209
Subarachnoid hemorrhage 143, 156, 165-167, 170, 174, 206, 265, 367
　causes of 163t
　complications of 170t
　management of 165
Substantial bleeding 222
Succinylcholine 226
　use of 226
Sudden cardiac arrest 367, 369
Sulfhydryl variable 132
Sulfonylureas 280
Superior vena cava 324
　syndrome 322
　　classification of 323f
　　management of 323, 324fc

Supplemental fibrinogen 223
Suppress intracellular glucocorticoid function 126
Supratentorial hemorrhage, surgical management in 192
Surgical therapy, role of 192
Suxamethonium 226
Sweating 2
Sweet-tasting substances 269
Sylvian fissure sign 177f
Symmetric peripheral gangrene 141t
Sympathetic nervous system 240
Symptomatic intracranial hemorrhage, management of 185
Synchronized intermittent mandatory ventilation 27
Syndrome of inappropriate
　antidiuresis hormone 261, 266t, 267b, 267t
　secretion of antidiuretic hormone 257f, 259, 262, 269
Systemic bleeding 184
Systemic embolism 179
Systemic hypoperfusion 332
Systemic inflammatory response 207
　syndrome 36, 122, 299, 335
Systemic lupus erythematosus 149, 150, 313
Systemic phenotype 44
Systemic steroids 28
　role of 45

T

Tachyarrhythmias 143
Tachycardia 2, 19, 27, 47, 275, 297, 332, 357
　resting 298
Tachypnea 6, 19, 27, 215
Takayasu arteritis 252
Tazobactam 33, 34, 133, 316, 317
T-cell leukemia 372
Temoneira 132
Temperature management 191
Tenderness, abdominal 112, 199
Tenecteplase 180, 181
Tennessee classification 149
Tension pneumothorax 230
Terlipressin 301
Testicular atrophy 297
Tetracycline 20, 334
Theophylline 47, 278-281
Therapeutic hypothermia 199, 212
Therapy-related injury 309
Thiazide 334
　diuretics 268
Thiopentone 226
Thoracentesis 12
Thoracic aortic aneurysm 252
Thoracoscopic surgery, video-assisted 309
Thrombin generation 349
Thrombocytopenia 147, 149, 151, 297, 318
　spectrum 310
Thrombocytopenic purpura 146
Thrombocytosis 313
Thromboelastography 304, 305
　role of 304
Thromboelastometry 304, 305
　rotational 220, 221
Thromboembolic illness 281
Thromboembolism 230
Thrombolysis 189, 193
　intraventricular 194
　low-dose 79
Thrombolytic therapy 78, 184
　complications of 184
Thrombophlebitis 30
Thromboprophylaxis 5, 192

Thrombotic microangiopathy 150
Thrombotic thrombocytopenic purpura 149
Thyroid-stimulating hormone 331
Thyrotoxicosis 30
Thyroxine 372
Tick paralysis 271
Tidal volume 308
Tidal wave 159
Tier one 161
Tigecycline 20
  role of 20
Tiredness 364
Tissue
  abnormalities, signs of connective 179
  plasminogen activator, instillation of 193
Todd's paralysis 175
Tongue falling back 282
Toxic substances, ingestion of 367
Toxidrome 278, 286
Toxin 282, 345
Toxoplasma 334
Toxoplasmosis 197
Tracheal secretions 33
Tracheostomy 37, 274
Tramadol 278
Tranexamic acid 165, 192, 223, 304, 305
  military application of 223
Transaminases 109
Transcranial Doppler 160, 209, 371
Transdermal sodium loss 262
Transformation, hemorrhagic 177f
Transfusion
  guidelines 293
  thresholds 301
Transgastric jejunal feeding 213
Transient ischemic attacks 179
Transjugular intrahepatic portosystemic
  shunt 302, 303
Transmural pressure 26
Transpulmonary pressure 95
  measurement of 95
Trauma 223
  abdominal 228, 229
  and injury severity score 218
  emergency resuscitation 223
  index, acute 218
  recent 179
  score 218
  severe 118
  unstable 228
Trauma-induced coagulopathy 219, 220fc
  clinical score 221
Traumatic bleeding severity score 221
Traumatic brain injury 157, 202, 204, 205fc, 206t,
  213, 229
  management of severe 211fc
  pathophysiology of 205
Traumatic intubation 282
Trichosporon beigelii 318
Tropical infection
  differential diagnosis of 109
  severe 114
Tube compensation 25
Tuberculosis 119
Tuberculous meningitis 197
Tubular damage, drug-induced 350
Tubular necrosis, acute 235
Tumor
  bleeding 189
  identification of 152
Tumor lysis syndrome 311t, 313
  Bishop classification of 311t
Tumor necrosis factor 124fc
  alpha 122, 124

TURP syndrome 260
Typhoid, severe 109
Typical atherogenic risk factors 179

U

Ulcer prophylaxis 5
Ulinastatin 128
Ultra-early tranexamic acid 165
Unfractionated heparin 78, 185, 281
  administration of 130
Upper cervical spinal cord disease 271
Upper extremities 157
  duplex ultrasound of 323
Upper gastrointestinal
  bleeding 293
  tumors 297
Upper limb 35
Upper respiratory involvement 20
Urea 261, 294
Uric acid 258
Urinary alkalinization 312
Urinary antigen 12
  testing, limitations of 12
Urinary bladder 289
Urinary tract infections 136
Urine
  alkalinization 280, 281b
  osmolality 258
  output, monitoring of 268
  pregnancy test 278
  sodium concentration 258
  toxin screen 278
Urokinase-streptokinase pulmonary embolism trial 80

V

Vaborbactam 133
Valproic acid 281, 334
Valvular heart disease 152, 243
Vancomycin 246, 247, 321, 322
  resistant enterococci 136
Vandromme score 221
Variceal band ligation 301
Variceal bleeding 303t
  risk of 302
Varicella-zoster virus 197, 201, 334, 345
Vascular injury 218
Vascular insufficiency 334
Vascular lesions 295
Vasculitides 252
Vasculitis 175, 189
Vasculotoxic snake bite 236
  management of 238
  risks of 239
Vasoactive drugs 3
Vasodilators, intra-arterial 169
Vasopressin 332, 372
  activity 258
  levels 123
  renal actions of 257
Vasopressin release
  baroregulation of 257
  osmoregulation of 257
  unregulated 257
Vasopressors 77, 372
  adrenergic 36
Vena cava
  filter, role of 81
  inferior 90, 152
Venereal disease research laboratory 372
Venoarterial extracorporeal membrane
  oxygenation 78
Venomous snakes 235
Venous oxygen saturation, role of 120

Venous thromboembolism 70, 71t, 310
  prophylaxis 275
Venous thrombosis, Virchow's triad of 70
Ventilation 28, 98, 217
  control mode of 67
  low 86
  positive pressure 65
  pressure support 25
Ventilator dyssynchrony 2, 26
Ventilator settings 51, 52
Ventilator-associated
  pneumonia 17, 25, 31, 32fc, 34, 318
    bundle 35t
  tracheobronchitis 17, 33, 52
Ventilatory circuit 52
Ventilatory support 274
  long-term 37
Ventriculitis 199, 200
  healthcare-associated 200
Ventriculostomy 159
Verapamil 279
Vertebrobasilar arterial territory, infarcts of 179
Vincristine 318
Viral encephalitides 201
Viral encephalitis 198, 200
Viral hepatitis 344, 345
Viral organism 16
Viral pneumonia 14, 16, 60
Viremia 112
Viscoelastic hemostatic assays, role of 229
Viscoelastic testing 304
Visual field test 176
Vitamin K antagonists 78, 189
Vivax malaria, severe 111
Volume optimization 77
Volume-assist control 51
Vomiting 6, 19, 357, 364
  persistent 112
von Willebrand factor 349

W

Waldenstrom's macroglobulinemia 313
Water intake
  excessive 263
  regulation of 257
Weakness 37
Weaning
  classification of 29fc, 53t
  difficult 28, 53
  indices 30t
  trial 52
Weaning failure 28, 29, 53, 67
  causes of 29fc, 54t
Weaning-induced pulmonary edema 54
  management of 55
Well's criteria 72
Well's score, modified 72t
West Nile encephalitis 201
West Nile virus 271
Wheeze, bilateral 70
White blood cell 46, 109, 314
Whole blood clotting time 234-236, 241
Whole-bowel irrigation 280
Wide-bore cannulae 289
Wilson disease 348
Windscreen injury 216
Wounds incisions, operative 4

Z

Zika 272
  virus encephalitis 201
Zollinger-Ellison syndrome 297
Zolpidem 278

EU GSPR Authorised Reprsentative
Logos Europe, 9 rue Nicolas Poussin
1700, La Rochelle, France
Phone: +33 (0) 6 67 93 73 78
E-mail: contact@logoseurope.eu

www.ingramcontent.com/pod-product-compliance
Ingram Content Group UK Ltd.
Pitfield, Milton Keynes, MK11 3LW, UK
UKHW050458150426
5217IPUK00025B/1737